AN EXPOSITION ON THE
EIGHT EXTRAORDINARY VESSELS

AN
EXPOSITION
ON THE EIGHT
EXTRAORDINARY VESSELS

*Acupuncture, Alchemy,
and Herbal Medicine*

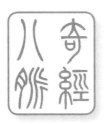

CHARLES CHACE AND MIKI SHIMA

EASTLAND PRESS ▼ SEATTLE

Eastland Press, Inc.
P.O. Box 99749
Seattle, WA 98139, USA
www.eastlandpress.com

Library of Congress Catalog Card Number: 2009938276
ISBN: 978-0-939616-69-5

Printed in the United States of America

4   6   8   10   9   7   5

Plates of the eight extraordinary vessels drawn by Bruce Wang
Cover design by Patricia O'Connor and Lilian Bensky
Cover illustration is a reproduction of the Daoist energetic map
of inner luminosity from the White Cloud Temple in Beijing

Book design by Gary Niemeier

Table of Contents

v

Part IV　　**Legacy of *Exposition on the Eight Extraordinary Vessels* ⋯ 321**

Part V　　**Appendices ⋯ 379**

Acknowledgments

We would first like to thank Dan Bensky, Lilian Lai Bensky, and John O'Connor for their considerable efforts in making our ideas both readable and visually attractive. Professors Matthias and Antje Richter of the University of Colorado provided invaluable assistance in answering endless sinological questions. Professor Terry Kleeman of the University of Colorado, Harrison Moretz, and Daniel Burton-Rose clarified some of the murky waters of the inner cultivation literature. Yan Yu-Shu, Shuang Fu, and Luo Yi-Yi helped in editing the Chinese text. Special thanks to Cindy Wang Yue, our research assistant in Beijing, who spent hours in photocopying articles and manuscripts and mailing them to us. Graham Chamness helped in preparing the bibliography. Merlin Young, Steven Birch, Arnaud Versluys, Craig Mitchell, Sharon Weizenbaum, Jason Blalack, Volker Scheid, Z'ev Rosenberg, and Will Morris read various sections of the book and provided many thoughtful suggestions. Others who helped in the preparation of this book include Eric Stoger and Leo Lok. We thank them all for their contributions. Whatever errors remain are our own.

Foreword

A number of years ago, Chip Chace and I spent a sunny afternoon in an outdoor café in Rothenberg, Germany discussing the eight extraordinary vessels. In the course of a far-reaching conversation, I mentioned that it was a pity Li Shi-Zhen's *Exposition on the Eight Extraordinary Vessels* had never been translated into English as this text held the potential for clarifying many commonly held misconceptions regarding the extraordinary vessels. I recounted to him that although Kiiko Matsumoto and I had translated significant portions of Li Shi-Zhen's book while compiling materials for our book *Extraordinary Vessels*,[1] much of Li's text had remained opaque to us because Ms. Matsumoto and I were not herbal practitioners, nor did we have the resources to investigate its Daoist layers. We discussed the fact that Li Shi-Zhen did not describe the pairing of the eight vessels treatment points most commonly used in acupuncture today. This struck me as especially curious since this methodology was described in 1437 and must have been known to Li in the 1570s. I suggested that perhaps Li did not agree with this treatment model. This conversation apparently made an impression on Chip. The next thing I heard, he and Miki Shima were working on a translation of the *Exposition*.

As this project proceeded, I have awaited its publication with excitement. Not only was Li Shi-Zhen one of the most important historical figures in the field of traditional East Asian medicine (TEAM), making enormous contributions, but the nature of his small text on the extraordinary vessels always fascinated me. What was Li's purpose in bringing together Daoist lore and practices with herbal medicine and acupuncture? I am thus honored that Chip Chace and Miki Shima have asked me to write this foreword to their translation. They are both rare individuals in this field: scholar-practitioners. Historically, the field had many more scholar-practitioners, but today, with specialization, one rarely has time to be both scholar and practitioner; one is usually one or the other. Chace and Shima have produced a translation that reflects this synthesis of interests.

At the time of the *Inner Classic* and *Classic of Difficulties*, the theories of the channels and vessels and the 12 primary channels had solidified and reached a mature enough state to allow a series of therapeutic strategies to be formulated.[2,3] But the *qi jing ba mai* had not yet reached the same level of coherent description in the medical

---

1. Kiiko Matsumoto and Stephen Birch, 1986.

2. Stephen Birch and Robert Felt, *Understanding Acupuncture.* Edinburgh: Churchill Livingstone, 1999.

3. Paul Unschuld, 1986a.

literature. There were gaps and contradictions among the various descriptions one finds in these early acupuncture texts. While the *Classic of Difficulties* gave at least a coherent and systematic description, it was not detailed enough to allow a clear treatment approach. It was not until later that enough descriptions could be found in medical texts, such as Hua Shou's *Comprehensive Elucidation of the Fourteen Channels*, Xu Feng's *Comprehensive Compendium of Acupuncture and Moxibustion*, Gao Wu's *Gathering of the Blossoms of Acupuncture* and Yang Ji-Zhou's *Grand Compendium of Acupuncture and Moxibustion*, to allow the development of systematic treatment approaches.[4] These later texts focused especially on the selection (diagnosis and treatment) of the extraordinary vessels to treat a broad range of different problems. They are more treatment oriented and have less theoretical discussion about the extraordinary vessels. This is in stark contrast to the earlier literature, which evokes a number of interesting (and often different) theoretical descriptions, with less clinically focused details.

We know that the extraordinary vessels have been used in various Daoist practices and these uses appear to be quite old, but precise dating is difficult. It is possible that the traditions that gave birth to the idea of the extraordinary vessels were different than those that gave birth to the channel and vessel, and viscera and bowel, and that the earliest medical texts, such as the *Inner Classic,* attempted to bring these different streams of thought together. However, it is also probable that the Daoist-influenced ideas of the extraordinary vessels remained of a different nature than the channels and vessel model, which became more overtly accessible. Li Shi-Zhen's treatise on the extraordinary vessels appears to be the first medical text that attempts to bring these diverse medical and alchemical influences squarely into focus. Not only will acupuncturists and herbal practitioners find this treatise interesting and useful, it will illuminate ideas of interest to Daoist practitioners as well. To my knowledge, no TEAM medical text that describes the integration of internal cultivation techniques coming from Daoist practices with herbal and acupuncture treatments has been translated into English, thus this will be a unique text much discussed in the field for a long time to come.

Chace has written elsewhere about how early Daoist ideas from meditation traditions seem to have influenced the practice of acupuncture, as found in the *Divine Pivot.*[5] While that description focuses on the state of the practitioner in order to needle correctly, and is thus different than what is described in Li Shi-Zhen's text, his ideas are almost unique in the field for tracing Daoist influences within the medical traditions.

Exactly what Li Shi-Zhen intended to say is often not clear on first reading, and how he intended these ideas to be used will inevitably remain open to different interpretations. Yet it is clear that Li Shi-Zhen refers to practices linked to the disciplines of internal cultivation, meditation, and breath control. It is also evident that

4. Kiiko Matsumoto and Stephen Birch, 1986.

5. Charles Chace, 2006, "On greeting a friend, an approach to needle technique" in *The Lantern,* 3(3):4-7.

he had an understanding of the extraordinary vessels that differed substantially from that documented in the medical literature before him. Although Li's perspectives have influenced some later acupuncturists, they have largely been overshadowed by the powerhouse of the four pairs of the eight extraordinary vessels and their eight treatment points, advanced by Xu Feng. However, with the publication of this excellent translation and commentary by Chace and Shima, this may change. Their translation provides equally novel treatment approaches and perspectives in the field of herbal medicine. There will undoubtedly be much to discuss. A number of sacred cows will go into hiding and more rigid arguments about the nature of the extraordinary vessels or the field of TEAM in general will have to soften.

The text itself is difficult to translate, in contrast to standard TEAM medical texts. Today we have various resources and developing methodologies for translation of TEAM medical literature, but references of a Daoist nature often remain obscure to medical readers. Chace and Shima's incisive explanations of the Daoist references, concepts, and allusions clarify the text considerably, making it much more accessible to medical practitioners. It is likely that this book will foment a revolution in perspectives, models, and practices pertaining to the extraordinary vessels.

—*Stephen Birch*
AMSTERDAM 2009

Plates of the Eight Extraordinary Vessels

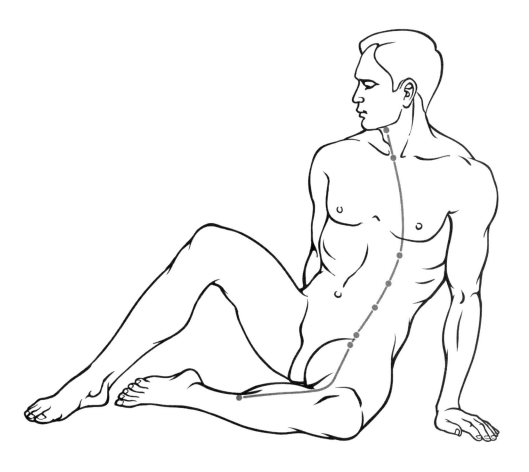

The *Yin Wei* Vessel

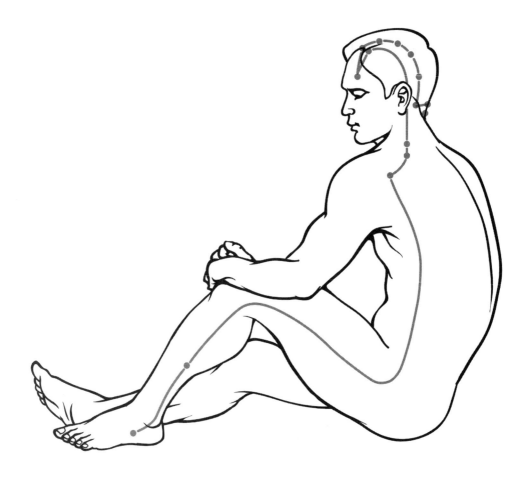

The *Yang Wei* Vessel

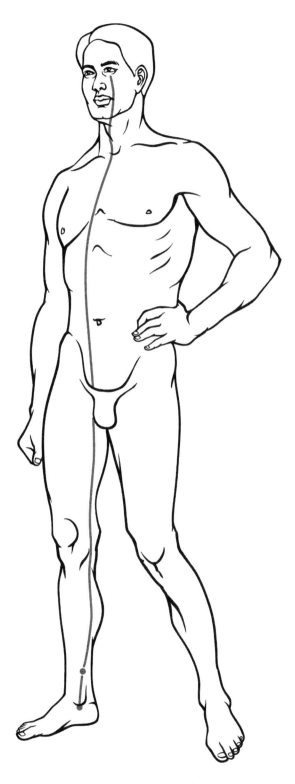

The *Yin Qiao* Vessel

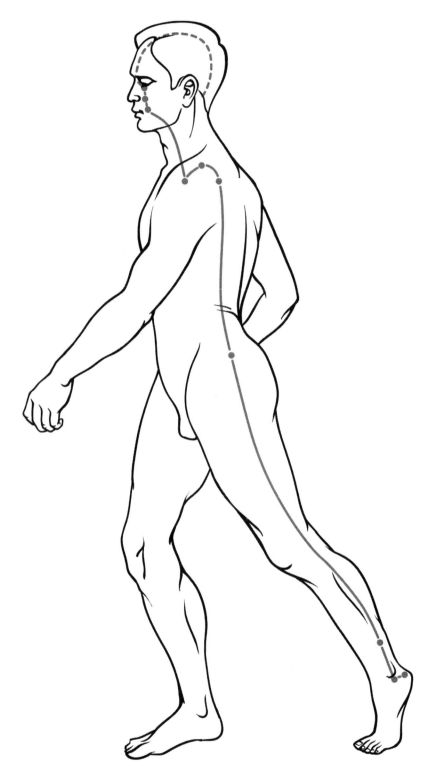

The *Yang Qiao* Vessel

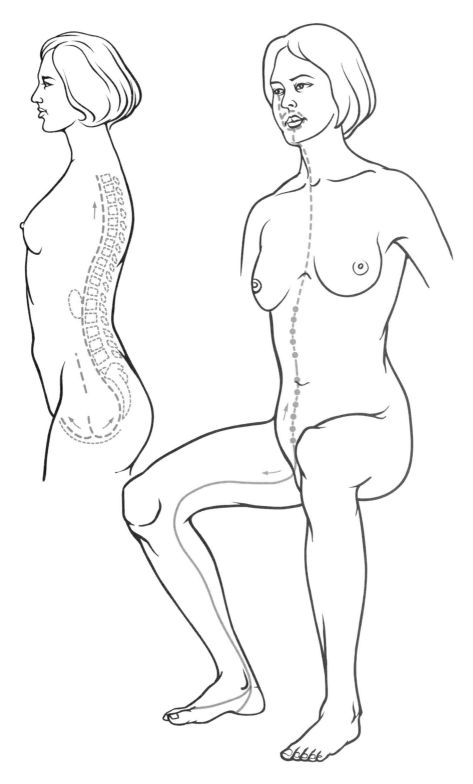

The *Chong* Vessel

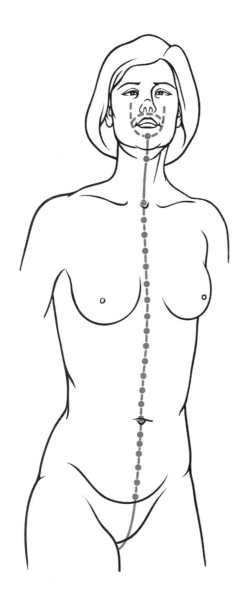
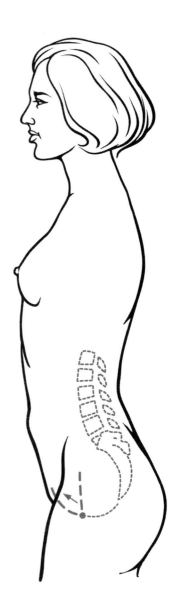

The *Ren* Vessel

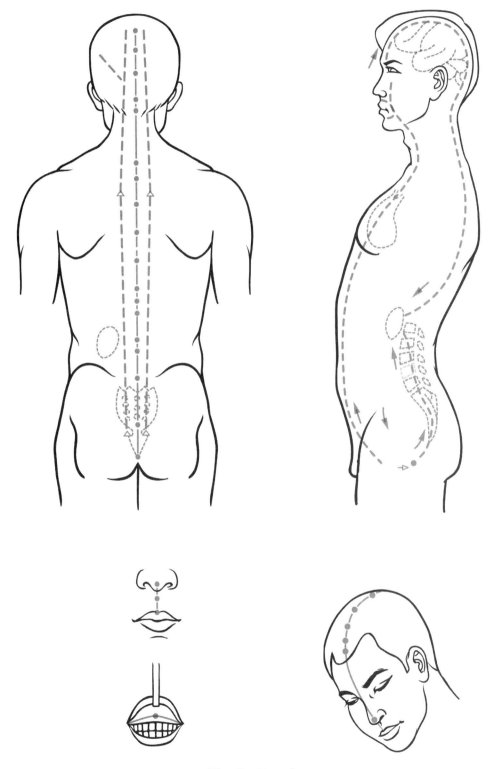

The *Du* Vessel

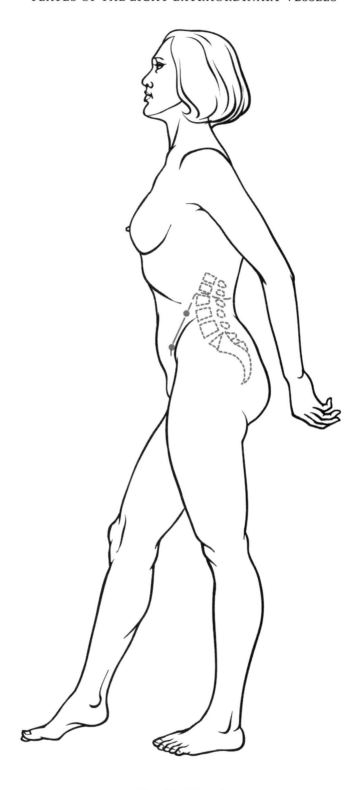

The *Dai* Vessel

Part I

Preliminaries

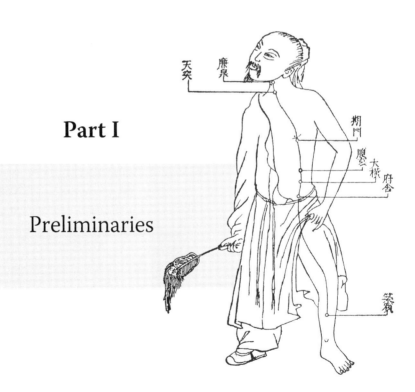

Part I contains six chapters that provide an overview of the main themes running through the text.

CHAPTER A

Introduction

One can be forgiven for regarding Li Shi-Zhen's (李時珍) *Exposition on the Eight Extraordinary Vessels (Qi jing ba mai kao* 奇經八脈考, between 1577 and 1578) as a footnote in a career marked by more monumental achievements. He certainly had other interests. Li's *Comprehensive Outline of the Materia Medica (Ben cao gang mu* 本草綱目, 1590), the product of a lifetime of work, is widely regarded as the culmination of the Chinese literature on pharmaceutics.[1] His *Pulse Studies of the Lakeside [Recluse] (Bin-Hu mai xue* 濱湖脈學, 1564) was equally innovative in its organization and presentation of pulse lore. Both texts definitively shaped how Chinese medicine is conceptualized and practiced today.

The *Exposition on the Eight Extraordinary Vessels* and *Pulse Studies* are the only remaining examples of a series of shorter works written by Li on various topics. His biographers typically portray these efforts as pleasant diversions from his daunting work on the *Comprehensive Outline.* Yet the *Exposition* has been no less pivotal in the development of its topic than the *Comprehensive Outline* and *Pulse Studies* have been to theirs. In bringing together writings from acupuncture, herbal medicine, pulse diagnosis, and internal cultivation, the book is quite literally the cornerstone of the literature on the extraordinary vessels.

Li's *Exposition* straddles the border between the familiar and the unexplored. Interest in the book has focused largely on the well-traveled territory that forms the basis for mainstream thinking on the extraordinary vessels, and the focus of scholarship has thus far been directed toward understanding how Li's work fits into the larger landscape of extraordinary vessel lore. Indeed, much of this material has now been so well-rehearsed that it seems almost pedestrian and is part of the curriculum of first-year acupuncture students. Yet the *Exposition* contains a great deal of material that has been left largely unexamined.

Few texts in the mainstream medical literature draw as deeply and explicitly from the literature of internal cultivation as the *Exposition.* Although tantalizing, these portions of the text are often rather opaque to medical readers. At first reading, such passages appear to shed little light on the medical material, and in some cases, they openly contradict our common assumptions regarding the extraordinary vessels. It is not surprising, then, that the alchemical stratum of the text has been uniformly ignored by medical readers. Yet Li states at the outset that he is writing for both physicians and those involved in internal cultivation, and to truly comprehend the extraordinary vessels, each must become intimately familiar with the territory of the

3

other. The authors of both of the original prefaces to the *Exposition* comment specifically on the importance of the text in creating such a synthesis.

The challenge of *Exposition on the Eight Extraordinary Vessels* is not limited to the layers of the text dealing with internal alchemy. When considered on its own terms, the book presents novel perspectives on even the most unremarkable topics. Modern acupuncturists and herbalists tend to think about the extraordinary vessels primarily in terms of the literature of their respective modalities; however, a more nuanced picture emerges when one is forced to consider the extraordinary vessels in the light of both these disciplines together. The *Exposition* is a very short book, yet the scope of its discourse demands that the extraordinary vessels be approached in new ways.

Even within the bounds of the various disciplines it addresses, the *Exposition* presents a variety of fresh perspectives. What are we to make of an extraordinary vessel acupuncture that ignores the so called 'master-couple' holes that form the basis for nearly all extraordinary vessel therapeutics today? What are the implications of an approach to extraordinary vessel herbal prescriptions based not on individual ingredients entering specific extraordinary vessels but on entire herbal formulas that address generalized extraordinary vessel pathologies?

Li Shi-Zhen juxtaposes all of these ideas, and then leaves the reader to somehow make them all fit together. He explains almost nothing, simply pointing his audience in the right direction. It is a text that must be read with attention and care. On initial examination, the *Exposition* appears to be little more than a laundry list of earlier writings punctuated with an occasional cryptic annotation by Li himself. Yet in classical Chinese, the structure and organization of a discourse often conveys as much information as the words and sentences it frames. This is particularly true in the *Exposition*, where Li's own perspectives on the extraordinary vessels are most evident in how he shapes the writings of others. Typically starting with a scrap of text from the *Classic of Difficulties (Nan jing* 難經, ca. 260), Li builds upon its ideas, interpreting the extraordinary vessels in innovative ways.

Li's message is defined by his editorial decisions, by his inclusion of material that originally only inferred the involvement of the extraordinary vessels, and by the material that is conspicuously omitted. Throughout the course of the book, Li requires that his audience attend to the structure of his argument as well as its substance. The reader's sensitivity to this aspect of his writing significantly influences what she makes of the text.

Then, too, the questions one asks of a text determine the answers one gets. When one asks "How does *Exposition on the Eight Extraordinary Vessels* fit it into the larger corpus of extraordinary vessel lore?" one is rewarded with what is now a fairly predictable picture of the extraordinary vessels, some interesting new tidbits of information, and a great deal of loose ends that do not seem to really fit anywhere. By contrast, if one attempts to suspend one's preconceptions about even the most familiar of the passages in the book in an effort to discern how Li has used them to make his own point, then a substantively different image emerges, one that is genuinely fresh and creative.

This translation and commentary aims to define Li Shi-Zhen's unique understanding of the extraordinary vessels.

Questions without Answers

Practitioners of Chinese medicine typically study the historical literature because we hope to be able to do something with it; at the very least, it inspires us to think about what we do in fresh ways. For us, this literature is, potentially, still very much alive.

For this reason, we tend to approach the literature in very practical terms. For instance, our interests in the social or cultural milieu in which a premodern Chinese medical text developed is circumscribed by how that type of information might inform our application of the material in that text. The modern cold damage (*shang han* 傷寒) specialist Huang Huang (黃煌) has made much of the cultural milieu in which Zhang Zhong-Jing (張仲景 fl. 220 CE) developed and used his herbal formulas.[2] For Huang, the historical context in which those prescriptions were originally formulated and administered sheds fresh light on how we understand and apply those formulas today.

In reading historical literature, one is rewarded with new herbal formulas or needling strategies less often than one gains more generalized insights into diseases and their treatments. Even so, the counsel of many if not most medical texts can be maddeningly ambiguous, even as they seem to present detailed treatment strategies. Early medical texts in particular were written with the assumption that their meaning would be verbally transmitted from teacher to student.[3] As the commentary literature makes clear, a remarkable amount of information is left open to interpretation.

Then too, one need not delve very deeply into the history of the development of the *Inner Classic* (*Nei jing* 內經) to appreciate that the received version is far different from what physicians had to work with in the Han dynasty (206 BCE–220 CE). The text had, even by that time, deteriorated to the point that while compiling his *Systematic Classic of Acupuncture and Moxibustion (Zhen jiu jia yi jing* 針灸甲乙經), Huang-Fu Mi (皇甫謐, 215–282) grumbled about the sad state of the *Inner Classic*.[4] For its part, the *Discussion of Cold Damage* (*Shang han lun* 傷寒論, ca. 220) lay moldering for centuries before it was resurrected and reconstituted in a form that is unquestionably different from the original. By the time Li Shi-Zhen was parsing such texts in the latter half of the 16th century, many of their passages may well have seemed as opaque to him as they do to us today. Thus, in reading a text like *Exposition on the Eight Extraordinary Vessels,* we do well to ask not just what a passage in *Divine Pivot (Ling shu* 靈樞) might have meant to its authors, but what it might have meant to Li Shi-Zhen. How might Li have put a given piece of information to practical use? In this, our present attempt to make sense of the material in *Exposition on the Eight Extraordinary Vessels* is part of an ongoing interpretive tradition spanning millennia.

Many, if not most, of the questions that clinicians ask of a text are unanswerable in any definitive way. In most cases, we can never really know how physicians applied the principles of the *Inner Classic* in the early Han or how Li Shi-Zhen interpreted that book 1500 years later. The purpose of reading a book like *Exposition on the Eight Extraordinary Vessels* is not to try to practice precisely as Li did, but to bring its ideas to life. We do our best to understand the ramifications of those principles as thoroughly as possible and then extrapolate from them using modern tools and techniques.

Like many premodern medical texts, on initial reading, one is left wondering what relevance Li's work has to one's daily practice. It is a book that clearly requires some explanation. However, our translation and commentary on the *Exposition* is not intended to be a clinical manual. Any attempt to posit definitive treatment protocols based on our interpretation of the *Exposition* would be contrary to the spirit of the text itself and would only serve to limit its possible range of meanings. In this book, we have tried to present readers with an intermediate step, providing them with the necessary tools to make independent decisions regarding how the *Exposition* might be applied without dictating what those decisions should be. First, we have produced a reliable translation as a basis for our inquiry. In our commentary on the text, we have then tried to elucidate the fundamental principles that are characteristic of Li Shi-Zhen's approach to the extraordinary vessels. Finally, we have asked the questions that clinicians will inevitably ask of the text, and questions regarding its clinical application arise on every page. For instance, the pulse material in the *Exposition* is particularly opaque, derived as it is from a part of the *Pulse Classic (Mai jing 脈經*, 3rd century) that was unquestionably corrupted by the time Li was working with it.[5] Virtually every line of the text requires the reader to make significant interpretive decisions just to gain the slightest clue about how this material might be used. How strictly must the pulses described in the text be interpreted, and what are the criteria for using them? Must they accompany the symptoms that are presented with them? How one chooses to answer such questions determines how and if the reader will use the extraordinary vessel pulses.

Insightful physicians since Li have nevertheless interpreted the *Exposition* in ways that have yielded clinically effective strategies. From Ye Tian-Shi's (葉天士 1667-1746) extraordinary vessel herbal prescriptions in the 17th century to Kido Katsuyasu's extraordinary vessel pulse strategies in the modern era, clinicians have not only kept Li's ideas alive, but have pushed them in new directions.[6] We have included a few essays of our own detailing how we have approached Li's material. These musings are in no way meant to be definitive. They are presented here to illustrate how we have attempted to engage the *Exposition* in a creative manner to produce a clinically relevant result.

Texts that maintain their currency throughout the ages are those that remain open to ongoing interpretation. Once a book is saddled with a definitive interpretation, it ossifies and dies. In the hope that we have left Li's *Exposition* at least as vital as we found it, we have tried to accommodate the greatest possible range of plausible interpretations. Although we have freely speculated on a range of interpretive possibilities, we have nevertheless done our best to maintain clear boundaries between the facts presented in Li's *Exposition* and our own suppositions about the book. Much as Li Shi-Zhen left his material very open-ended, we have tried to present it in a manner that encourages readers to make the material their own.

Organization

This book is divided into five parts. Part I contains a biography of Li Shi-Zhen and provides an introductory overview of the main themes that run through the text. These include chapters on theory, acupuncture, herbal medicine, internal alchemy, and pulse diagnosis in the *Exposition*. For instance, the rather arcane method of pulse diagnosis described in the *Exposition* is first outlined in an introductory chapter on the pulse, providing the reader with some context for understanding this material prior to encountering it in the text itself. A much more detailed discussion of extraordinary vessel pulse diagnosis appears in Ch. 17 of the *Exposition*, and in our commentary in Ch. 33.

Part II contains the Chinese text and our annotated translation of *Exposition on the Eight Extraordinary Vessels*, and Part III presents our commentary on the text. These commentaries assume a familiarity with the general themes presented in Part I, and explore those ideas in greater detail. As noted above, the structure and organization of the *Exposition* is Li's primary medium for expressing his own perspective. For this reason, our commentaries attend closely to how Li Shi-Zhen builds on a core set of ideas throughout the course of each chapter. The translation is easily read independently of the commentaries for those wishing to form their own impression of the text.

Readers will note that our commentaries to certain portions of the Li's text are considerably longer than others. For instance, we have a great deal to say about the *chong* vessel and relatively little to say about the *ren*. This is because Li himself had much more to say about the *chong* than the *ren*. We have not attempted to provide a more generalized discussion of the extraordinary vessels but have instead focused our remarks on those topics that bear directly on Li's perspective.

In understanding the role of *Exposition on the Eight Extraordinary Vessels* in Chinese medical history, it is helpful to know what later writers did with Li's ideas. Part IV discusses the influence of Li Shi-Zhen's extraordinary vessel writings on three later physicians: Luo Dong-Yi (羅東逸, 1662–1722), Ye Tian-Shi, and Shen Jin-Ao (沈金鰲, 1717–1777). In his commentary on the *Inner Classic*, Luo Dong-Yi presents a perspective on the extraordinary vessels that resonates strongly with the alchemical perspective presented in the *Exposition*. Ye Tian-Shi is himself one of the great figures of Chinese medicine, and is indelibly linked to the use of the extraordinary vessels in herbal medicine. While Li Shi-Zhen left no case records detailing how he used the extraordinary vessels in clinical practice, Ye Tian-Shi's writings, and those attributed to him, consist primarily of case records. Shen Jin-Ao's writings are, by contrast, entirely theoretical in nature, and his thinking on the extraordinary vessels suggests that he adhered closely to Li's methodology.

Part IV also contains a selection of modern case records that reflect acupuncture and herbal approaches to the extraordinary vessels that are consistent with Li's ideas. There are also two essays by Charles Chace. The first illustrates the potential clinical value of critically examining variant readings of early acupuncture texts, and the other examines the roots of extraordinary vessels in China's early philosophical literature.

Acupuncture texts compiled after Li's *Exposition,* most notably Yang Ji-Zhou's (楊繼洲) *Grand Compendium of Acupuncture and Moxibustion (Zhen jiu da cheng* 針灸大成, 1601), contain extensive extraordinary vessel acupuncture formularies making use of the so-called 'master-couple' holes. This information is now well-represented in the Western language literature and moreover constitutes the basis of most modern extraordinary vessel therapeutics. Perhaps more importantly, the present book is concerned specifically with Li Shi-Zhen's approach to the extraordinary vessels, and the master couple holes were clearly of little interest to him. For these reasons, we have left this material for others to develop. Readers are referred to Kiiko Matsumoto and Steven Birch's *Extraordinary Vessels* for translations of this material.[7]

Part V contains appendices presenting historical prefaces to the *Exposition* as well as tables of herbs, prescriptions, acupuncture holes, people, and books mentioned in the *Exposition.*

Various Editions of *Exposition on the Eight Extraordinary Vessels*

Exposition on the Eight Extraordinary Vessels was apparently published between 1576 and 1578 (the precise date is unknown), during Li's lifetime, but it is not known where or by whom. The text was accompanied by two prefaces, dated 1572 and 1577. The earliest extant edition of the book dates to 1606, shortly after Li's death, and was published by Zhang Ding-Si (張鼎思) in a compilation of Li's writings that included his *Pulse Studies of the Lakeside Recluse* and *Exposition and Explication of the Pulse Rhymes (Mai jue zheng kao* 脈訣證考). Zhang contributed his own preface to the work.

Our translation is based on the earliest extant edition of *Exposition on the Eight Extraordinary Vessels* that appears in *Catalog of the Complete Collection of the Four Treasuries (Si ku quan shu mu lu* 四庫全書目錄, 1784). This edition also appears to be the basis for all the other editions we consulted.[8] No commentaries were written on the *Exposition* until modern times. Wang Luo-Zhen (王羅珍) and Li Ding's (李鼎) *An Annotated Exposition on the Eight Extraordinary Vessels (Qi jing ba mai kao jiao zhu* 奇經八脈考校註, 1985) is the first true commentary on the text. Katsuda Masayasu's (勝田正泰) *Modern Language Translation of the Exposition on the Eight Extraordinary Vessels (Gendaigo Yaku Kikei Hachimyaku Kou* 現代語訳(奇經八脈考校注, 1995) is essentially a more thoroughly annotated extrapolation on Wang and Li's work, accompanied by a translation into Japanese. We have made extensive use of both texts. For a listing of the various editions of *Exposition on the Eight Extraordinary Vessels,* see Appendix 5.

Notes on the Translation

The original edition of *Exposition on the Eight Extraordinary Vessels* that appears in *Catalog of the Complete Collection of the Four Treasuries* is unpunctuated, and that is how we have presented the Chinese version of the text here. Much of Li's text consists of passages that are direct quotations or paraphrases of other texts. Sometimes, Li delineates his own comments with a prefatory "Bin-Hu says," but more often than not, he simply inserts his own two-cents worth directly into the flow of the passage he is citing. This can make it difficult for a reader who is not intimately familiar with the full breadth of the Chinese medical literature to know whether one is reading Li or, for instance, the *Inner Classic.* Subsequent editors have attempted to clarify this matter by placing Li's comments in a smaller typeface, in parentheses, or both, and we have adopted this convention in our translation. Moreover, classical Chinese is typically telegraphic in style, and in the interest of readability, it is often necessary to make interpretive additions to an English translation. Such additions in our own translation are placed in brackets [ ].

Our primary source for term selection is the Eastland Press house glossary. However, there are many instances where we have chosen other words that we believe more clearly and transparently convey the meaning of the Chinese.[9] A few words, in particular, bear mentioning.

We refer to the directions that the extraordinary vessels travel as 'trajectories' rather than pathways to remind the reader that these vessels are not lines or even pathways in the same sense as the primary channels, but are instead general directions of flow. Although they may intersect with specific holes on the pathways of the primary channels and are generally depicted as lines in graphic representations, the extraordinary vessels function more like tides than streams.

Similarly, we refer to acupuncture loci as 'holes' rather than points, both because this is a more accurate translation of the term *xué* (穴) and to remind the reader that these loci are three dimensional in nature. We have identified acupuncture holes by their English translations in *Practical Dictionary of Chinese Medicine*[10] and by their World Health Organization alphanumeric designation.

The names of the extraordinary vessels have been translated in a number of ways, none of which is (in our view) optimal, and at present there is no real consensus on how they should be translated. It has been our experience, in discussing the extraordinary vessels with both students and colleagues, that we often find ourselves running through a litany of possible translations—the yin linking vessel, the yin binding vessel, and so on—searching for the term with which our interlocutor is most familiar. Often it is only when we resort to the Chinese—in this case, the *yin wei* vessel—that our interlocutor's eyes light up in recognition. To be sure, the *chong, ren,* and *du* vessels are just as often recognized as the penetrating, conception, and governing vessels, but these translations are problematic as well in that they are by no means entirely accurate. In any event, because the Chinese names of the extraordinary vessels have become part of the common terminology in the West and are the terms most readily identified by the greatest number of readers, we have chosen to use them in our text.

Chinese measure words, too, tend to be either as familiar to most readers as their English translations or they tend to lack meaningful English language equivalents. We have therefore not translated Chinese measure words into English. Thus, the word 寸 remains simply *cun* and not inch, body inch, or cubit.

Li Shi-Zhen cobbles his narrative together from a wide range of sources, and, in keeping with the scholarly style of his time, each of Li's citations lie somewhere on a continuum between a direct quotation and a rough paraphrase. Those passages that are closer to paraphrase often, but not always, begin with 云 *yun* rather than 曰 *yue*. Regardless of the prefatory words that he uses, when Li's references stray closest to paraphrase, we have omitted quotation marks and begun the translation with "xxx says that ... ."

In pre-modern times, Chinese writers were typically known by a number of different names throughout the course of their lives. In his writing, Li Shi-Zhen refers to people in a variety of ways. For instance, he refers to himself by his pen name *(bie hao* 別號), Bin-Hu (濱湖). When referring to people in our own discussion of the text, however, we have used the names that Western readers of Chinese medicine are likely to recognize. This is most often, though not invariably, some form of their literary name *(hao* 號), or their courtesy name *(zi* 字). For instance, we refer to Ye Gui (葉桂) as Ye Tian-Shi (葉天士), and Li Gao (李杲) as Li Dong-Yuan (李東垣).

Chinese proper names appear with Chinese characters when they are first mentioned. Subsequent mentions are in pinyin only. Book titles appear in English followed by the pinyin and Chinese characters when they are first mentioned. Subsequent mentions are in English only. Lists of the significant people and books mentioned in this book are included in Appendix 6.

In the interest of clarity, we have translated premodern anatomical terms using their modern anatomical equivalents. For instance, *jue gu* 絕骨, literally the extreme or terminal bone, is translated as the fibula, and *que pen* 缺盆, literally the empty basin, as the supraclavicular fossa.

Biographical Sketch of Li Shi-Zhen

Because Li Shi-Zhen is among the most eminent figures in Chinese medical history, the essential details of his life are reasonably well documented. He was born in 1518 into a family of medical practitioners in Hu Guang (湖廣) in what is now known as Qi Zhou (蘄洲) county, in the Qi Chun (蘄春) prefecture of modern day Hubei province. His grandfather was an itinerant doctor *(ling yi* 鈴醫)[1] who traveled from town to town in this region, offering his services as a physician. His grandfather's place in Ming society was so low that there is no record of his given name. By contrast, Li Shi-Zhen's father, Li Yue-Chi (李月池), became locally famous for his medical skills and was registered as Medical Secretary of the Imperial Academy of Medicine *(tai yi yuan li mu* 太醫院吏目). He is known to have written a selection of texts, including *Illumination of the Four Diagnostic Methods (Si zhen fa ming* 四診發明), *Commentaries on Medical Studies of the Eight Vessels (Yi xue ba mai zhu* 醫學八脈註), *Diagnosis, Pattern [Discrimination] and Treatment of Pox Diseases (Dou zhen zheng zhi* 痘診證治), and *Lore of Ginseng (Ren shen zhuan* 人參傳), all written at the end of the 15th and the beginning of the 16th centuries. Once Li's father managed to acquire some farmland and his practice of medicine was no longer the basis of their livelihood, he was able to distance himself from his own father's lowly station in life. Li Yue-Chi was also able to pass the central state exams, attaining the rank of cultivated talent *(xiu cai* 秀才), further enhancing his status.

Li Shi-Zhen was a sickly child who was considered dull and slow by his family. Despite this perceived handicap, at six years of age he began learning how to read and write, and he soon developed a love of books. While still a young boy, he completed a subject for the first-level examination for the appointment of local officials. By age 12, Li was studying the *Four Classics (Si shu* 四書) for the second-level examination, which he passed at age 14. Despite his diligent preparation, Li twice failed to pass the subsequent county, provincial, and state level examinations. His progress stalled, and in response to his father's admonitions to study harder, Li worked so intently that he contracted tuberculosis and nearly died. His father is reported to have treated Li Shi-Zhen for this condition exclusively with Scutellaria Decoction *(huang qin tang)*, which cured him. Fully recovered, two years later Li again failed the examinations for the third time.

With this third humiliating failure, Li finally gave up on a bureaucratic career and began studying medicine with his father. At age 25, after only a year of medical study, he joined his father's practice. His lack of aptitude for governmental examinations

11

notwithstanding, Li remained a voracious reader. According to the *Qizhou Gazetteer* (*Qi zhou zhi* 蘄州誌), Li spent his days reading books, and reportedly did not leave his house for ten years. If this was true, then like most doctors of his day, he must have seen patients at his home. His interests were eclectic, and his reading ranged from medicine and the classics to history. According to this gazetteer, he never wasted one moment in his studies. The picture that emerges is that of a young man struggling to compensate for his shortcomings in mainstream scholarship by immersing himself in a less formalized but no less rigorous course of study.

In 1545, when Li was 28, a plague broke out in his hometown of Huchang and spread throughout the populace, killing rich and poor alike. Li and his father treated many of the plague victims, prompting a commendation in the *Qizhou Gazetteer* for their invaluable service to the community. As a consequence, shortly thereafter, Li's father was promoted to the position of Official of the Imperial Academy of Medicine (*tai yi yuan li* 太醫院吏) and became very famous. This made it possible for both Li Yue-Chi and his son to mingle in high society and allowed Li Shi-Zhen to make many important acquaintances, including the Hao (郝) family, whose extensive library contained numerous medical books. Li borrowed many books from the Hao library, comparing various editions, which helped deepen his medical knowledge.

Over the course of his research, Li Shi-Zhen came to believe that the number of medicinals contained in *Divine Husbandman's Classic of the Materia Medica* (*Shen nong ben cao jing* 神農本草經) was insufficient for clinical practice and that its three-level classification was impractical. Li was not quite 30 years old when he began developing his idea of a *Comprehensive Outline of the Materia Medica* (*Ben cao gang mu*) to remedy this situation.

In 1552, 12 years after failing the imperial service exams, Li Shi-Zhen began the Herculean task of completely revising the pharmaceutical knowledge of the time. Where previous efforts of this kind were the product of committees composed of 20 to 50 scholars, Li undertook this project on his own, an endeavor that would stretch over the course of 40 years. Li Shi-Zhen's first step was to review the *Materia Medica Arranged According to Pattern* (*Zheng lei ben cao* 證類本草, 1108). He emulated its principles of herbal classification in his own *Comprehensive Outline of the Materia Medica*.

During this period of Li's life, his fame spread and he maintained a busy clinical practice in addition to his scholarly pursuits. He also began teaching medicine. Li's father was a noted scholar in his own right who had done a significant amount of first-hand research in his own writing projects, and Li Shi-Zhen followed this example. Li Shi-Zhen researched a famous local medicinal called Qi [province] snake (*Qi she* 蘄蛇). His monograph on *The Lore of [White] Pattern Snakes* (*Hua she zhuan* 花蛇傳) has been lost, although at least some of its content appears to have survived in the *Comprehensive Outline of the Materia Medica*.

In 1556, Li was invited to have an audience in the court of Chu (楚) where he cured the ruler's eldest son of epilepsy. As a result, he was appointed to the Sacrificial Office of the Princely Establishment *(Wang fu feng ci zheng* 王府奉祠正*)*, which combined the roles of head of court proceedings and of head physician. Deeply interested in Daoist alchemy and immortality, the King of Chu surrounded himself with Daoist priests who clashed with Li over political matters. It is curious that much of Li's work, particularly his *Exposition on the Eight Extraordinary Vessels*, reflects an affinity for Daoist sensibilities since the only mention of Li's interaction with Daoists in the official histories concerns his conflict with them.

Li's tenure as a court physician lasted just three years, but it allowed him to continue his herbal research in an environment that gave him access to extensive literary resources until he was recommended for employment at the Imperial Academy of Medicine in Beijing *(Bei jing tai yi yuan* 北京太醫院*)*. He spent a year in Beijing where he was again exposed to a large number of medical books and medicinals.

In 1561, a year after returning to his hometown, Li had a new home built in the Safflower Garden *(Hong hua yuan* 紅花園*)* on the northern side of Rain Lake *(Yu hu* 雨湖*)*. It was then that he adopted the nickname of Lakeside Recluse *(Bin hu shan ren* 濱湖山人*)*. During this time, Li completed a series of smaller monographs including *The Case Records of the Lakeside [Recluse] (Bin hu yi an* 濱湖醫案*)*, *Difficulties of the Triple Warmer due to Guest [Qi] (San jiao ke nan* 三焦客難*)*, *An Exposition on the Life Gate (Ming men kao* 命門考*)*, and *An Illustrated Discourse on the Five [Yin] Viscera (Wu zang tu lun* 五臟圖論*)*, none of which survives.

Li remained at his home on the lake where he continued to work on his *Comprehensive Outline of the Materia Medica* in addition to proceeding with research on pulse diagnosis and herbal medicine. In 1564, at the age of 47, Li completed his famous *Pulse Studies of the Lakeside [Recluse]*. Around this time, he also began work on *Exposition on the Eight Extraordinary Vessels*, a topic of some interest to his father as well, and *Textual Research on the Pulse Rhymes (Mai jue kao zheng* 脈訣考證*)*. It was also around this time that Li Shi-Zhen's father died, and his own eldest son took his first imperial examination.

Lacking the resources available to the materia medica commissions of the Tang (618–907) and Song (960–1279) dynasties, which benefited from imperially ordered collection drives, Li was compelled to do his own herb collecting. In the three to four years that followed, Li embarked on a series of research trips to Hunan, Jiangxi, and Anhui provinces, collecting herbs and talking to local herbal producers, herbal merchants, farmers, wood choppers, fishermen, miners, and old women about medicinal plants. He took extensive notes and returned home with a large number of herbal samples, which became the models for the illustrations that would appear in his *Comprehensive Outline of the Materia Medica*.

By 1569, with enough information to begin writing, Li retired to his lakeside home and began work on the first draft of his *magnum opus*. As an apparent diversion from this monumental task, he published *Collected Simple Prescriptions of the Lake-*

side [Recluse] (Bin hu ji jian fang 濱湖集簡方). Taking another break from work on *Comprehensive Outline of the Materia Medica,* Li completed *Exposition on the Eight Extraordinary Vessels* a few years later, in 1572, but then shelved it. In the years that followed, Li completed the first draft of *Comprehensive Outline of the Materia Medica,* producing an 800-page document, only to spend another four years on revisions.

Exposition on the Eight Extraordinary Vessels was finally published between 1576 and 1578 when Li was about 60 years old. *Comprehensive Outline of the Materia Medica* was completed a year later, after being revised three times over 27 years. In the preface to the first edition, Li noted:

> [I] began [this project] in 1552 and finished in 1578, after rewriting the entire manuscript three times over. [I] divided [the contents into] 52 volumes, consisting of 16 parts, each part [broken into] 60 categories in total. Monographs on each medicinal are referred to as 'guiding principles' *(gang* 綱*)* while the technical material within each category are referred to as 'items' *(mu* 目*)*.

The book contains 1,892 medicinals, including 374 substances added by Li himself, with 1,109 illustrations drawn by his second son, Li Jiang-Yuan, and 1,096 formulas. Having finally completed this masterpiece, his life's work, Li must have been devastated to find that no one was interested in publishing it. In 1579, he began traveling around China in the hopes of finding a publisher, a quest that would consume much of the remainder of his life. After first visiting Hangzhou and Wuchang, to no avail, he continued on to Nanjing where he remained for several years in negotiations with a publisher there. These labors were ultimately fruitless. In early September of 1580, Li paid a visit to Wang Shi-Zhen (王世禎), one of the most famous scholars of his time, who was visiting Nanjing. According to Wang, Li appeared at his house "emaciated in face and body," a shadow of his former self, who had once been "an enthusiastic debater and a unique man [born] under the sign of the Great Bear."[2] After spending a few days together, Li asked Wang to write a preface to *Comprehensive Outline of the Materia Medica,* and Wang happily agreed, additionally composing a poem in admiration of Li's work. Unfortunately, even these accolades failed to impress the publishers of his day.

After three fruitless years of travel in search of a publisher, Li returned home, humiliated. From this time until his death in 1593, at the age of 75, he retreated to his lakeside home, practicing medicine, entertaining friends, drinking wine, composing poems, and generally trying to enjoy himself. Yet even then he was unable to set the *Comprehensive Outline of the Materia Medica* aside, undertaking a final revision of the work.

In 1590, the Nanjing publisher Hu Cheng-Long *(胡承龍)* finally agreed to finance and publish *Comprehensive Outline of the Materia Medica.* Li's sons and grandsons had all contributed to the completion of the text. The illustrations were compiled by his son Li Jian-Zhong (李建中) and drawn by his grandson Li Jian-Yuan (李建元). Sadly, however, Li did not live to see his life's work published. The first edition did not appear until 1596, three years after his death.

Where previous materia medica were confined largely to medicinal substances, Li had produced a comprehensive encyclopedia that often went beyond the scope of pharmaceuticals. This was ultimately a source of criticism by subsequent authors who complained that his book was too large and unwieldy, and contained too many digressions into areas of marginal interest to anyone other than scholars. Nevertheless, it represented the climax of the development of the materia medica literature, and quickly superseded the book upon which Li had based his own work, Tang Shen-Wei's (唐慎微, 1056–1136) *Materia Medica Arranged According to Pattern*, the previous contender for the title of most comprehensive materia medica.[3] It remains a benchmark of the literature to the present day.

Li Shi-Zhen's Work on the Pulse

Even if Li had never written *Comprehensive Outline of the Materia Medica,* he would certainly be remembered for his much shorter, but no less influential, contributions to the study of the pulse. Of his two monographs on the pulse, *Textual Research on the Pulse Rhymes* and the *Pulse Studies of the Lakeside [Recluse]*, only the latter survives. Books dealing with pulse diagnosis were quite popular during the Ming dynasty, many of which were commentaries and corrections of *Wang Shu-He's Pulse Rhymes (Wang Shu-He mai jue* 王叔和脈訣), attributed to the eponymous author.[4] Many historians believe that *Pulse Rhymes* was actually written by Gao Yang-Sheng (高陽生) during the Six Dynasties, but in either case, the original work had been lost long before Li's era. Like many critics of his time, Li believed that although physicians would often commit *Pulse Rhymes* to memory, the text failed to truly clarify the principles of pulse examination. Moreover, he believed that both *Pulse Rhymes* and many of its subsequent corrections were narrow-minded and full of mistakes. Using his father's work, *Illumination of the Four Diagnostic Methods,* as his primary reference, Li composed his own interpretation of *Pulse Rhymes* with the stated goal of correcting the errors it contained.

In *Pulse Studies of the Lakeside [Recluse],* Li divided all pulse images into 27 types, which were analyzed in great detail in the first section of the book. Then, in *Essentials [of Pulse Diagnosis] in Quatrain (Si yan ju yao* 四言舉要), he composed quatrains for easy memorization of the three aspects of each pulse—the pulse quality (*ti zhuang* 體狀), its classification among different qualities of pulses (*xiang lei* 相類), and the primary disorders it reflects (*zhu bing* 主病). Lastly, Li included a critical commentary on *Pulse Rhymes* by Cui Xi-yuan (崔希范) entitled *Textual Research on the Pulse Rhymes.*

Li Shi-Zhen as Daoist

Paul Unschuld has observed that the use of the title and arrangement of *Comprehensive Outline of the Materia Medica* into *gang* and *mu* reflects the respect that Li felt for the Neoconfucian scholar Zhu Xi (朱熹, 1130–1200), author of *Comprehensive Outline of the General Mirror (Tong jian gang mu*通鑒網目, 12th century), whose school of thought constituted the official government version of Confucianism during Li Shi-Zhen's lifetime.[5] Li's entire project of collating and reorganizing the herbal lore is consistent with Zhu Xi's maxim of obtaining a clear picture of things on one's own, which consequently led Li to a fresh understanding of the material.[6]

Although the title and structure of *Comprehensive Outline of the Materia Medica* reflect the influence of his early training for a Confucian civil service career, the contents of the work belies other sensibilities as well. Like most scholars of his time, Li was at once a Confucian and a Daoist. One would have expected that Li the Confucian might have rejected demonological concepts on principle, yet it is clear from *Comprehensive Outline of the Materia Medica* that he believed in possession by corpse spirits and demons to the extent that he even composed prescriptions containing peach kernels as a key ingredient to remedy such conditions.[7] At the very least, Li's many references to the literature of internal cultivation in his writing on the extraordinary vessels suggest a substantive familiarity with this branch of Daoist practice.[8] Li's familiarity with Daoist practice is also evident in his many references to internal cultivation in *Exposition on the Eight Extraordinary Vessels*.

Conclusion

The intellectual climate in China during the Ming dynasty was one of inquiry, of testing and questioning the suppositions of previous ages. In this, Li Shi-Zhen was very much a product of his times. Although all of his extant writings clearly rely heavily on the writings of his predecessors, it would be a mistake to view him as a mere collator, exhaustively recapitulating the ideas of others. That he spent almost 40 years traveling around the country to ensure that the information in his *Comprehensive Outline of the Materia Medica* was indeed accurate is evidence of his commitment to an approach to knowledge based on methodical investigation. Li's own innovative contributions to medicine sprang from precisely this mindset. In the course of his own research, he added many medicinals to the repertoire of Chinese medicine and made significant contributions to the classification of medicinals. This capacity to expand the theoretical framework of a field while collating and synthesizing related materials is a hallmark of his genius. It is evident throughout his work on the materia medica, pulse studies, and the extraordinary vessels.

Many of the sources cited by Li in his writings may strike the modern reader as remarkably abstruse and arcane, dealing as they do with the esoterica of Daoist practice. Yet Li was typical of nearly every scholar of his time who were all familiar with such texts and to whom it probably never occurred to distinguish themselves as either Confucian or Daoist. The presence of such explicitly Daoist writings in his *Exposition on the Eight Extraordinary Vessels* is remarkable only in that they are so prominent. In this, too, Li's primary contribution to the medicine is that, in the process of bringing material together, he places it in a new and creative context in which it can be most effectively put to use.

Theoretical Considerations

Broad Trends and Fundamental Principles

The first two chapters of Li Shi-Zhen's *Exposition on the Eight Extraordinary Vessels* present a cogent and succinct synopsis of the basic principles of extraordinary vessel function. Although these chapters draw primarily from the 27th, 28th, and 29th Difficult Issues of the *Classic of Difficulties*, Li's organization of the material reflects his own understanding of extraordinary vessel functions and relationships. By and large, his own comments simply summarize the passages that he has presented. In only a few instances does he directly interject ideas of his own. Yet throughout the text, Li expresses his perspective through his arrangement and editing of other authoritative sources. A presentation strategy such as this allows Li to articulate his opinions without appearing rashly innovative or controversial.

It is not known whether the extraordinary vessels were originally developed as an entirely independent system of channels that were subsequently superimposed upon the primary channels or whether the two channel systems evolved together. Certainly, by the time of *Basic Questions* and *Divine Pivot*, in the early Han (206 BCE-8 CE), the extraordinary vessels and the primary channels had become inextricably intertwined. In these texts, the eight extraordinary vessels are presented as overarching regulators of yin and yang, and, by extension, the modulators of the rest of the channel system. The *Classic of Difficulties* most clearly defines their role as absorbers of the overflow of qi from the primary channels. In the *Classic of Difficulties*, qi may flow into but not out of the extraordinary vessels.

One of the more remarkable examples of subtle editing in the early chapters of the *Exposition* alters one of these passages from the *Classic of Difficulties* to establish a reciprocal flow of qi between the primary channels and the extraordinary vessels, a milestone development in the theoretical understanding of the channel system. By adding a single word, 'reciprocal' *(xiang* 相*)*, to an otherwise verbatim discussion of the *Classic of Difficulties*, Li changes its meaning entirely. He states:

> The overflow of qi [from the channels and networks] enters the extraordinary vessels providing reciprocal irrigation, internally warming the viscera and receptacles, and externally moistening the interstices.

In the *Exposition,* the extraordinary vessels are no longer the passive recipients of the spillover from the primary channels described in the *Classic of Difficulties*; they have become full participants in the ebb and flow of qi within the system as a whole. This is a dynamic only hinted at in *Basic Questions* and *Divine Pivot*. The *Exposition* contains a number of subtle changes such as this, all of which have ramifications for our understanding of extraordinary vessel function.

Despite their close associations with the rest of the channels, the extraordinary vessels nevertheless maintain a degree of autonomy. They are not bound to the primary channels in the same way as the secondary vessels. All of the other secondary vessels are directly linked to an associated primary channel. For instance, the channel sinew of the bladder is in many ways simply a conceptual extension of the foot greater yang bladder channel. The same is true of its network vessels *(luo mai* 絡脈*)* and channel divergences *(jing bie* 經別*)*. With the exception of the *ren* and *du* vessels, none of the extraordinary vessels has holes of its own. Of course, this is also true of all the networks and channel sinews. Yet, because these ancillary vessels are all bound to a single primary channel, it is clear that they must be accessed in relation to that primary channel, even if that means pricking a sore spot in the general proximity of its trajectory.

In the case of the extraordinary vessels, the situation is considerably more complex. To be sure, the holes of the *yang qiao* are situated predominantly on the bladder channel, and those of the *yin qiao* on the kidney channel; however, each extraordinary vessel exerts its own influence on every channel to one extent or another, and no single extraordinary vessel may be conceptualized in relation to any one primary channel. In very practical terms, each of the extraordinary vessels exercises its regulatory effect on the entire body. They are the matrix that provides the gross structure for the rest of the channel system. For this reason, the converse is also true: Disease states of the extraordinary vessels also tend to express systemically.

General Pathodynamics of the Eight Extraordinary Vessels

The *Classic of Difficulties* presents a remarkably concise description of extraordinary vessel pathology. Each vessel is characterized by a core pathological presentation that is summarized in a sentence or less (Table C-1). These statements are the foundation upon which Li builds his own presentation of each of the eight vessels. Methodically expanding upon them with quotations drawn mainly from *Basic Questions* and *Divine Pivot*, Li then moves further afield to include sources ranging from the *Discussion on Cold Damage* to others contemporary to his own time. His sources often do not mention the extraordinary vessels directly. Li infers an extraordinary vessel relationship simply because the pathology described in such passages is consistent with that of the extraordinary vessels.

For instance, from Li's perspective, many if not most pathodynamics characterized by counterflow and abdominal pain or stagnation are expressions of a *chong* vessel disorder. This rationale is the basis for Li's inclusion of material such as the following

Yang wei	Disregulation of the nutritive and protective qi
Yin wei	Heart pain, including epigastric pain
Combined *wei* vessel pathologies	Inability to hold oneself together
Yang qiao	Slack yin and tense yang
Yin qiao	Slack yang and tense yin
Combined *qiao* vessel pathologies	Regulation of yin and yang between the interior and exterior
Chong	Counterflow of qi and abdominal urgency, yang brightness insufficiency
Ren	Internal binding and bulging
Du	Contracture and counterflow in the *du*
Dai	Transverse control of all the channels

Table C-1 General Pathodynamics of the Eight Extraordinary Vessels from *Classic of Difficulties*

passage by Sun Si-Miao, found in Ch. 10 of Li's text:

> When there is a cough that causes one to spit up saliva accompanied by frigidly cold extremities, qi from the lower abdomen surges upward into the chest, mouth, and throat, [and] the face will be flushed and boiling hot as if one were intoxicated. [The patient feels] as if she will experience either urinary or fecal incontinence that will flow down the inner thigh, [and] there will be urinary difficulty [although the patient] remains anxious about the possible return of these symptoms. The distal pulse will be deep, and the proximal pulse will be faint. It is appropriate to use Poria and Schisandra Decoction *(ling wu wei zi tang)* to treat this surging of qi.[1]

Despite this open-ended approach to the interpretation of extraordinary vessel pathology, Li's book contains some notable gaps in the diseases it covers, particularly when compared to the current understanding of extraordinary vessel therapy. The pathology of the *du* vessel is particularly sparse, limited to localized symptoms of the spine and head. Also notable is the absence of gynecological symptoms associated with the *chong*. Although he expands the scope of extraordinary vessel pathology considerably, Li develops the core ideas from the 27th, 28th, and 29th Difficult Issues just so far. He seems to have been content to provide some practical examples of this inferential approach to extraordinary vessel pathology, leaving ample room for a more detailed interpretation.

Chronic Diseases Ultimately Afflict the Extraordinary Vessels

Extraordinary vessel pathology is often characterized by pathodynamics that are long-standing in nature. This is because pathological processes do not, as a general rule, directly afflict the extraordinary vessels. They must, as the 28th Difficult Issue describes, spill over *(yi* 溢*)* from the primary channels. Nowhere in Li's *Exposition* is this important principle of extraordinary vessel pathodynamics directly stated, although the vast majority of the conditions described in the book appear to be chronic. Nevertheless, subsequent writings have explicitly acknowledged the close association between chronic disease and the extraordinary vessels. Most notable among these are the case records of Ye Tian-Shi (also known as Ye Gui 葉桂), which are most responsible for directly linking long-standing illnesses to the blood and network vessels, and for associating this pathodynamic with the extraordinary vessels.[2]

Extraordinary Vessel Patterns are Mixed Presentations

Li's extrapolations on the conditions discussed in the *Classic of Difficulties* are typically characterized by patterns of excess overlaying deeper, often more subtle, deficiencies. Although such a juxtaposition of excess and deficiency is apparent to some degree in the early literature of the extraordinary vessels, Li's work amplifies this trait considerably. The mixed nature of extraordinary vessel pathology is most apparent when it is considered within the context of the herbal material appearing in the *Exposition.* Taken as a whole, these formulas plainly reflect pathodynamics that are characterized by simultaneous excess and deficiency.

   If one were to rely on the early acupuncture and pulse literature quoted in the *Exposition,* one might conclude that eight vessel diseases are predominantly presentations of excess. This is particularly true of the *Classic of Difficulties,* which forms the basis for Li's discussions of pathology. As already mentioned, its description of extraordinary vessel function posits them only as receivers of overflow from the rest of the channel system.

> The main channels are like irrigation ditches, and the extraordinary channels are like lakes and marshes. When the vessels of the main channels are swollen and abundant, they overflow into the extraordinary channels. Thus it was that Qin Yue-Ren compared it to when the "rains pour down from heaven, the irrigation ditches overflow, the rain floods rush wildly, flowing into the lakes and marshes." This is the revelation of the secret meaning not presented in *Divine* [*Pivot*] and *Basic* [*Questions*].

In the *Classic of Difficulties,* qi may flow into the extraordinary vessels but not out, and that is why the qi cannot return to the normal circulation. The only method of treating the extraordinary vessels mentioned in the *Classic of Difficulties* is "piercing with a sharp stone and letting blood out," a modality consistent with a view of pathology centered on excess. Of all the sources cited in the *Exposition,* the *Classic of Difficulties* appears to be the most unambiguously biased toward presentations of excess in the extraordinary vessels.

The basis for Li's discussion of extraordinary vessel pulses is Wang Shu-He's *Pulse Classic.* In this text, extraordinary vessel pulse descriptors such as hard, pill-like, tapping, beating straight up and down, tense, and confined are all generally considered to be pulses of excess. For instance, the *ren* pulse is "tight, fine, excessive, and long from below [in the proximal position] up to the middle position." According to the *Pulse Classic,* its accompanying symptom picture includes "lesser abdominal pain and periumbilical pain. Men will suffer from the seven types of bulging and women will suffer from accumulations and masses."

The pulses associated with the *wei* vessels bend this rule somewhat. Because they are described solely in terms of their oblique orientation on the wrist, they are not linked to any other identifying pulse qualities. Yet even here, their auxiliary pulse qualities and the symptoms associated with them leave little room for doubt that the clinical picture is one of at least localized excess.

> When examination reveals that the *yang wei* pulse is floating, vertigo will occur when standing. This is due to the yang being overabundant and overfull [such that the patient also] suffers from raised-shoulder breathing [3] and shivering, as if cold.
>
> When examination reveals that the *yin wei* pulse is deep, large, and excessive, [the patient] suffers from pain in the chest, propping fullness below the hypochondrium,[4] and heart pain. If the pulse[5] feels like a string of pearls, then in men there will be an excess below both rib-sides and lumbar pain, while in women there will be genital pain, as if sores have formed.

Despite the apparent bias toward excess in the *Classic of Difficulties*, a careful examination of Li's other sources reveals that some element of deficiency is discernable in most patterns. *Basic Questions* is definitely more balanced in its presentation of extraordinary vessel function. Still, most of the descriptions of deficiency in extraordinary vessel patterns tend to express dynamics that are so fundamental to the normal arc of human maturation and decline that therapy is not even mentioned. For instance, the discussion of the waning of the *chong* and *ren* in Ch. 1 of *Basic Questions* is presented as a physiological fact rather than as a disease process requiring treatment.

> It also states that: "Women at the age of two times seven [years] attain their heavenly measure, [during this time] the *ren* vessel flows freely and the great thoroughfare vessel fills, the menses come according to their time, and [a woman] can bear offspring. At the age of seven times seven [years], the *ren* vessel is empty and the supreme *chong* vessel weakens and the heavenly measure is exhausted. The passages of earth are obstructed, the body deteriorates, and [a woman] can no longer bear children.

There is no question that the authors of the *Inner Classic* and *Pulse Classic* recognized that the extraordinary vessels may become pathologically deficient. However, in these texts, such deficiencies do not tend to occur on the level of the day-to-day functioning of correct qi *(zheng qi 正氣)*; rather, they manifest their insufficiencies on the related but fundamentally deeper level of former heaven or prenatal *(xian tian 先天)* essence *(jing 精)* and primal qi *(元氣 yuan qi)*, a topic we will return to below. At the very least, the contents of the *Exposition* suggest that even relatively minor deficiencies of the extraordinary vessels tend to reflect a significant compromise in one's health. This is particularly evident in the pulse qualities associated with the extraordinary vessels. In their most pronounced presentation, two of the defining extraordinary vessel pulses, tapping *(tan 彈)* and pill-like *(wan 丸)*, both signal such a profound debilitation of qi that their associated viscera is on the verge of collapse. Insofar as extraordinary vessel pathologies tend to be more severe than those of the primary channels, the pulse qualities themselves may be understood as reflecting a profound erosion of qi despite their apparent strength. The extraordinary vessel symptoms associated with these pulses may appear to be those of excess, but deficiency lies at the core of these patterns. This theme, too, is discussed in greater depth in Ch. 17 of the *Exposition* on pulse diagnosis, and in our commentary in Ch. 33.

Ch. 10 of *Divine Pivot* contains one of the few passages that clearly delineates excess and deficiency patterns for an extraordinary vessel. Even here, it is a branch of the *du* vessel and not its primary trajectory that may become depleted. "When excessive, it presents with arched back rigidity, and when deficient, it presents with heavy-headedness such that one wobbles one's head in an attempt to hold it up. For problems with the bone such as this, then select this diverging branch."[6]

Distinctions such as these are the exceptions to the rule in the early medical literature. In general, evidence of deficiency is submerged in an overall presentation of surfeit. Even the few appearances in the *Pulse Classic* of symptoms typically associated with extraordinary vessel deficiency tend to occur in contexts that also suggest an etiology of excess. For instance, frequent urination and female infertility are commonly associated with deficiency. They appear in the *Pulse Classic* along with the decidedly excessive symptoms of accumulation, bulging, and a hard and excessive *chong* vessel pulse, suggesting a predominantly excessive presentation.

By the Ming dynasty, this tendency had shifted and patterns more overtly reflecting deficiency began to be more prevalent in the literature of the extraordinary vessels. Even so, the extraordinary vessel treatments recommended in two of the seminal acupuncture anthologies of this time, Gao Wu's *Gathering of the Blossoms of Acupuncture and Moxibustion* and Yang Ji-Zhou's *Grand Compendium of Acupuncture and Moxibustion*, are still heavily weighted toward presentations of excess.

Li Shi-Zhen's discussion of the seas from Ch. 33 of *Divine Pivot* explicitly establishes that the *chong* vessel may present in states of either excess or deficiency:

[In Ch. 33 of *Divine Pivot*], Qi Bo states: Just as there are Northern, Southern, Eastern, and Western Seas, so [too do] humans have four seas that correspond to them. "The stomach is the sea of water and grains. Its transport [holes] include Qi Thoroughfare (ST-30) above and Three Li (ST-36) below. The *chong* vessel is the sea of the 12 channels. Its transport [holes] include Great Shuttle (BL-11) above and below it issues from both Upper and Lower Great Hollow (ST-37 and ST-39). The center of the chest is the sea of qi. Its transport [holes] are above and below the neck bone,[7] and at Man's Prognosis (ST-9) in front. The brain is the sea of marrow. Its transport [holes] are on top of the head above[8] and at Wind Pool (GV-16) below.

When there is a surplus in the sea of qi, there will be qi fullness in the chest, rapid breathing, and a red face. When there is an insufficiency of the sea of qi, the breath is reduced and insufficient for speech. When there is a surplus in the sea of blood, commonly there will be the illusion [that] one's body is enlarged, depression and peevishness, and an inability to tell exactly where one feels sick. When there is an insufficiency in the sea of blood, commonly there will be the illusion that one's body is small and cramped and there will be an inability to tell exactly where one feels sick. When there is a surplus in the sea of water and grains, there will be abdominal fullness. When there is an insufficiency in the sea of water and grains, there will be hunger with an inability to ingest food. When there is a surplus in the sea of marrow, [the body] will be light, agile, possessed of great strength, and one will have the ability to accomplish what is normally beyond oneself. When there is an insufficiency in the sea of marrow, the brain will spin, the ears will ring, there will be aching pain in the lower legs, dizziness, and loss of vision, indolence, and somnolence.

The dynamic between excess and deficiency is more plainly evident in Li's use of herbal formulas, such as Cinnamon Twig Decoction *(gui zhi tang)* and Regulate the Middle to Augment the Qi Decoction *(tiao zhong yi qi tang),* that tonify even as they address pathogenic factors. This is exemplified in Li's discussion of diseases of the *dai* vessel, where he clearly delineates between patterns that are primarily excessive and those that are primarily deficient.

In other instances, [one may experience] fear and fright such that wood overwhelms the seat of earth, and turbid fluids flow downward; or persistent lamentation may produce a withering of the [ancestral] sinew, and this is what is referred to as diseases of the two yang developing in the heart and spleen; or the other channels have damp-heat that concentrates and stagnates in the inferior aspect of the lower abdomen. In other instances, the primal [qi] of the lower [burner] may be deficient and chilled, causing the womb to become excessively damp. The methods for treating [these conditions] include purgation, or emesis, or simultaneously supplementing while discharging, simultaneously promoting [urination] while supplementing the middle, simultaneously raising and discharging while drying, simultaneously warming and nourishing while moistening, or warming and tonifying, or restraining and binding. All cases require different [treatment techniques] as well as their flexible application based on the [particular expression] of the pathodynamic.

In the early acupuncture literature, the day-to-day nutritive qi tends to become excessive and subsequently overflows into the eight extraordinary vessels. Deficiency presentations in the extraordinary vessels tend to present on deeper levels more closely associated with blood and prenatal influences.

The Nature of the Qi Conveyed in the Extraordinary Vessels

In Chinese medicine, the most basic species of qi in the body is source qi (*yuan qi* 原 氣). It is comprised of the essential qi of the kidney, the qi of grain and water through the transformational functions of the spleen, and air drawn in through the lungs. All other forms of qi in the body are considered to be manifestations or derivatives of source qi. Source qi springs from the kidney and is stored in the lower abdomen. It is closely tied to the concept of essence, the qi responsible for growth, maturation, and development. Essence qi has both prenatal aspects that are inherited from the parents and postnatal aspects produced from food. It, too, is stored in the kidney. Primal qi is often conflated with source qi in medical texts, but in the literature of internal alchemy, it typically refers to the primordial, extracorporeal qi of the cosmos. Source, primal, and essence qi are present to one extent or another throughout the channel system, but for most acupuncturists in the West, they have a particularly intimate relationship with the extraordinary vessels. This is also the prevailing opinion among those involved in the modern practice of *qigong*. Any mention of the extraordinary vessels in modern textbooks of *qigong* tends to equate them with source qi.

For many, if not most, practitioners of Chinese medicine in the West, it is axiomatic that the extraordinary vessels carry source/primal qi. The basis for this assumption in the primary Chinese medical literature is ambiguous at best, although it finds some support in the literature of internal alchemy *(nei dan* 內 丹). *Exposition on the Eight Extraordinary Vessels* addresses the question of source/primal qi extensively, if often obliquely, in the contexts of both pathology and internal alchemy. Source qi does indeed play a prominent role in Li's understanding, but for him it is by no means the only kind of qi at work in the extraordinary vessels, nor is it necessarily the most important.

Li presents a description of qi in the extraordinary vessels that is both nuanced and inconsistent. Nevertheless, a careful reading of the *Exposition* reveals a discernable pattern of thinking that is even evident in the arrangement of its chapters. Given his interest in internal alchemy, Li might well have begun with the vessels most important to spiritual cultivation, the *ren*, *du*, or *chong*, yet he arranges his material in a manner that progresses inward from the exterior. Even this is consistent with the sensibilities of internal cultivation. One must control more rudimentary forms of qi before one takes on the most fundamental dynamics of life. Internal cultivation cannot take place in a vacuum. There must be a physical substrate to give form to the primordial qi, and this form must be regulated and maintained on a day-to-day basis. The protective and nutritive qi perform this role, and so this is where Li begins.

Li Shi-Zhen follows the *Classic of Difficulties* in describing the two *wei* vessels as a functional pair that regulates yin and yang in its general relationship to the interior and exterior. "The *yang wei* governs the exterior of the body while the *yin wei* governs the interior." He then develops this idea, quoting a passage from Zhang Yuan-Su (張元素 1151–1234), referred to below by his courtesy name Zhang Jie-Gu (張潔古), asserting that the *wei* vessels specifically regulate the protective and nutritive qi within the body.

> Zhang Jie-Gu says that the protective is yang, and it governs the exterior. When the *yang wei* contracts a pathogen, it produces a disease in the exterior, and therefore [the patient] suffers from chills and fever. The nutritive is yin, and it governs the interior.

On this point, Li's understanding of extraordinary vessel function is unambiguous. He makes no mention of source qi in his discussion of the *wei* vessels; however, his perspective on the role of source qi in the *qiao* vessels is more problematic. According to him, the *qiao* vessels are responsible for the overall mastery of yin and yang, and for the sides of the body. "The *yang qiao* governs the yang [aspect] of the left and right sides of the body while the *yin qiao* governs the yin [aspect] of the left and right sides of the body, so they are referred to as east and west." While the *wei* vessels deal with yin and yang as they pertain to the protective and nutritive levels, the *qiao* vessels address the diurnal regulation of yin and yang and the structural balance of left and right. Again, source qi is not mentioned on this purely medical level of discussion. It appears only in his citation of texts concerned with internal alchemy.

By contrast, Li unambiguously states that the *chong, ren,* and *du* vessels are directly associated with source/primal qi. In his discussion of the *chong*, he cites Wang Hao-Gu (王好古, fl. 1306), who explicitly links this vessel with the functions of the triple burner, heart master, and ministerial fire, and, by extension, with the source/primal qi.

> The hand lesser yang triple burnert is one dwelling place of the minsterial fire, the right kidney life gate is the ministerial fire, and the heart envelope master[9] is also called the ministerial fire. These vessels are all diagnosed in the same manner. The kidney is the gate of qi generation.[10] It emerges from and governs [the area] below the umbilicus, and it is divided into three forks surging upward through the umbilicus via the Celestial Pivot (ST-25), ascending to reach the Chest Center (CV-17) beside both breasts. This is where the primal qi is tied in.

Li continues:

> The *Classic* [*of Difficulties*] states: The source qi is the triple burner's director of separation. The moving qi between the kidneys is the true primal unitary qi that divides into three routes. It is the life force of a person and the root of the 12 channels.

While it could be argued that these passages provide rather circumstantial evidence of the relationship between source qi and the extraordinary vessels, Li's own concluding comments leave little room for doubt. He clearly states that the source/primal qi is communicated via the triple burner to the *chong, ren,* and *du.* "Li Bin-Hu states: The triple burner performs the life gate's function of communicating with the *chong, ren,* and *du.*"

Li concludes his discussion of each individual vessel with a presentation of the *dai,* the vessel that ties all the others together. Citing Zhang Zi-He, he acknowledges the direct communication between this vessel and the *chong, ren,* and *du,* all channels that he has already established as containing source qi. "The three vessels of the *chong, ren,* and *du* all arise [from the same place], but their trajectories differ. They are of a single source but have three branches, and all network with the *dai* vessel."

The *qiao* vessels appear after the *wei* and before the *chong* in the *Exposition's* flow of ideas. Although they have much in common with the *wei* vessels, Li highlights the special role of the *yin qiao* in internal alchemy. In the course of one remarkable discussion on the pivotal role of the *yin qiao* in facilitating the alchemical activation of the rest of the extraordinary vessels, Li asserts, "The eight vessels are the root of the great way of former heaven and the ancestor of all qi." The implication of this pronouncement is that all of the extraordinary vessels are linked to the primal qi of former heaven.

References to source/primal qi occur primarily in the alchemical literature and, to a lesser extent, in medical references to the physiological roles of the *chong* and *ren* in physiological development. This thread runs throughout the *Exposition,* and we will return to it in subsequent chapters.

Channel Pairings of the Extraordinary Vessels

In the opening chapter of *Exposition on the Eight Extraordinary Vessels,* Li establishes a defining characteristic of the eight vessels. He points out that they are "not controlled by the 12 main channels nor are they arranged in exterior-interior combinations." Although the notion of the extraordinary vessels as separate from the 12 primary channels originates in the 27th Difficult Issue of the *Classic of Difficulties,* the observation that the extraordinary vessels are not arranged in interior-exterior combinations appears to have originated with Li himself. Because Li makes no mention of the so-called 'master-couple' holes commonly associated with the extraordinary vessels today, the pairings associated with them are also absent from his writing. For instance, the *yin wei* is not paired with the *chong* by virtue of their sharing the master couple holes Yellow Emperor (SP-4) and Inner Pass (PC-6). This is not to say, however, that Li does not recognize more fundamental extraordinary vessel pairings. Moreover, Li's pairings shed light on how the extraordinary vessels function in health and disease.

What follows is a rough overview of the key functional relationships linked to the extraordinary vessels. Each of these dynamics will be discussed in greater detail in subsequent chapters. For the present, however, we will concern ourselves with their most general characteristics.

The *Exposition* explicitly couples the two *wei* vessels and the two *qiao* vessels as functional pairs, particularly with respect to their pathologies. Moreover, despite Li's statements to the contrary, these pairings have many of the characteristics of exterior-interior relationships attributed to the 12 primary channels. For instance, in most cases it is difficult to talk about the pathology of the *yang wei* outside of its relationship to the *yin wei*. This is even more true for the *qiao* vessels.

Wei Vessels

Li's first statement regarding the pathology of the *wei* vessels is based on the 28th Difficult Issue of the *Classic of Difficulties*. The pathology presented reflects a dual disharmony afflicting both the *yin wei* and *yang wei*.

> [Qin] Yue-Ren says: The *yang wei* and *yin wei* are a binding network in the body. When they overflow from accumulation, [their contents] stagnate and they are unable to circulate and irrigate all the other [primary] channels. Therefore, the *yang wei* arises from the [places it] meets with all the yang, and the *yin wei* arises from [the places it] intersects with intersection of all the yin. The *yang wei* binds to the yang, and the *yin wei* binds to the yin such that when yin and yang are unable to bind with one another, then one experiences such disappointment that one loses one's sense of purpose. One becomes sluggish and unable to support oneself. (Sluggish, as in a lethargic bearing.)

Li elaborates on this point by citing Zhang Jie-Gu's perspective that the *yang wei* and *yin wei* vessels are responsible for the harmonization of the protective and nutritive qi. While the problem may lie predominantly in either the *yang wei* or *yin wei*, the protective or the nutritive, the relationship between them is the central issue.

> The protective is the yang, and it governs the exterior. When the *yang wei* contracts a pathogen, it produces a disease in the exterior, and therefore [the patient] suffers from chills and fever. The nutritive is in the yin, and it governs the interior. When the *yin wei* contracts a pathogen, it produces a disease in the interior, and therefore [the patient] suffers from heart pain.

When the yin and yang are bound together, then the nutritive and protective are all harmonized.

Li takes the protective/nutritive dynamic between the *yang wei* and *yin wei* quite seriously, going so far as to reinterpret Zhang Zhong-Jing's *Discussion on Cold Damage* from the perspective of the extraordinary vessels. In Li's view, because Zhang identifies Cinnamon Twig Decoction *(gui zhi tang)* as addressing a disharmony between the protective and nutritive aspects, this formula therefore treats disorders of the *yang wei*. In summary, as a functional pair, the *wei* vessels are primarily concerned with the regulation of yin and yang on the level of the protective and nutritive levels.

Qiao Vessels

Both the *wei* and *qiao* vessels are intimately connected to the network vessels. In terms of their functional pairings, this relationship with the networks is especially pronounced in the *qiao* vessels. According to Li, the seminal characteristic of the *qiao* is the slackness or tenseness of the yin and yang channels and tissues described in the *Classic of Difficulties.*

> Qin Yue-Ren states in the *Classic of Difficulties*: "The yin networks are the networks of the *yin qiao*. The yang networks are the networks of the *yang qiao*.[11] When the *yin qiao* is diseased, the yang is slack and the yin is tense. When the *yang qiao* is diseased, the yin is slack and the yang is tense."

This slackness or tension typically presents as a range of disorders, from mild structural imbalances to seizures. One vessel may be more fundamentally disordered than the other, but once again, that is ultimately secondary to the functional relationship between the two *qiao* vessels.

The *qiao* vessels also modulate the diurnal transmission of protective qi, and arguably nutritive qi, between the exterior and the interior. Li synthesizes both *qiao* functions in his citation of Zhang Jie-Gu's counsel on treating seizures: "For diurnal seizures, moxa the *yang [qiao]*, and for nocturnal [seizures], moxa the *yin [qiao]*." 癲癇晝發灸陽夜發灸陰

The *wei* and *qiao* vessels are best understood as two functional pairs devoted to regulating the yin and yang in relatively superficial expressions of qi, even as they are grounded in deeper reserves of vitality within the body.

Ren and Du Vessels

The pairing of the *ren* and *du* in the *Exposition on the Eight Extraordinary Vessels* is most clearly expressed in Li's presentation of material pertaining to internal alchemy. The communication of qi between these two vessels is so well established in Daoist practice that they are almost invariably referred to together.

They are paired by virtue of their complementary roles in internal cultivation, as opposed to any fundamental commonality in their pathological expression, and indeed, their respective pathologies are quite different. Nevertheless, Li is careful to illustrate the importance of the essential relationship between the *ren* and *du* in acupuncture practice, pointing out that some diseases associated with the *du* may be treated on the *ren* vessel.

Chong and *Dai* Vessels

With the other six vessels comfortably paired, the *dai* and *chong* appear to be thrown together by default, almost as an afterthought. On initial inspection, it is difficult to think of two less similar vessels, and yet the *dai* and *chong* do indeed perform complementary functions. The role of the *dai* vessel as the transverse or horizontal belt that girds the vertical trajectories of all the other channels is quite clear. Problems arise when the belt is either too tight or too loose, adversely affecting one or more of the primary channels. The *dai* is best understood as the most exterior of all the vessels in its function of regulating and defining the outer perimeter of all the channels and networks.

By contrast, the *chong* is inarguably the deepest vessel in the body, and yet as the 'sea of the channels and vessels,' it performs a similar function in regulating the 12 channels, not from the outside in, as in the case of the *dai*, but from the inside out. The *chong* may be conceptualized as an interior boundary for all the channels and vessels. Because the channels and vessels must all be in some relationship with the *chong* vessel, it acts as a center of gravity. The *chong* exerts its influence outward from the interior, maintaining a longitudinal regulation of the channels, while the *dai* imposes its influence from the exterior inward, imposing horizontal regulation of the channels. In this way, the *chong* and *dai* form a complementary pair.

These broad concepts provide the foundation upon which Li develops a progressively detailed and nuanced understanding of the extraordinary vessels. We will next examine how these concepts are tangibly expressed in the sections of the work dealing specifically with acupuncture and herbal medicine.

Li Shi-Zhen's Extraordinary Vessel Acupuncture

Much as Chinese landscape painting is characterized by what it omits, Li Shi-Zhen's approach to extraordinary vessel acupuncture is similarly defined by what it leaves out. This is particularly evident in his failure to mention the eight confluent holes of the extraordinary vessels *(ba mai jiao hui xue* 八脈交會穴*)* anywhere in his discussion. These holes, often called the 'master-couple' holes in modern English language discussions, have been a defining characteristic of extraordinary vessel therapeutics since their appearance in Xu Feng's (徐鳳) *Comprehensive Compendium of Acupuncture and Moxibustion (Zhen jiu da quan* 針灸大全, 1439), more than 130 years prior to the publication of Li's book on the subject.

The eight (confluent) holes were first identified by Dou Han-Qing (竇漢卿) in his *Guidebook to Acupuncture Classics (Zhen jing zhi nan* 針經指南, 1295) where he also established the extraordinary vessel hole pairings we know today. Inner Pass (PC-6) is paired with Yellow Emperor (SP-4), Outer Pass (TW-5) with Close to Tears (GB-41), Broken Sequence (LU-7) with Shining Sea (KI-6), and Extending Vessel (BL-62) with Back Ravine (SI-3). Although some view Dou as the father of extraordinary vessel therapuantics based on the eight confluent holes, the link to them in his book is tenuous at best.[1] Dou simply observes, "The eight holes where two or more channels intersect are the essentials of acupuncture [practice]."[2] For Dou, the efficacy of these holes is a consequence of their influence on multiple primary channels, not on the extraordinary vessels.

One-hundred-and-forty-four years later, Xu Feng's *Comprehensive Compendium of Acupuncture and Moxibustion* explicitly linked the eight holes to the extraordinary vessels through a system of calendrical correspondences known as the 'eight methods of the divine tortoise' *(ling gui ba fa* 靈龜八法). Configured around a heaven-based arrangement of trigrams, this method assigns an extraordinary vessel and one of the eight confluence holes to each trigram. Each of the eight holes is deemed open or available to activation at a particular time of the day based on its numerological correspondences with a number of other divinatory systems, including the Water Wheel map *(he che tu* 河車圖) and the nine palaces *(jiu gong* 九宮). A similar system known as the 'soaring eightfold method' *(fei teng ba fa* 飛騰八法) is also based on a heaven-based arrangement of trigrams. The soaring eightfold method is believed to be derived from ideas presented in *The Token for the Agreement of the Three According to the Changes of Zhou (Zhou yi can tong qi* 周易參同契, 142 BCE), a seminal text of internal alchemy that figures prominently in Li Shi-Zhen's *Exposition on the Eight Extraordinary Vessels.*

By the time of Gao Wu's *Gathering of the Blossoms of Acupuncture* in 1529, the use of the eight confluent holes of the extraordinary vessels and their pairings had expanded beyond chronologically based acupuncture, and they were being combined with other holes to treat specific conditions. They have continued to be used in both ways and are unquestionably a convenient and effective means of organizing eight vessel treatments. Despite their obvious utility and their original affiliation with the *Classic of Change (Yi jing 易經)*, the eight holes are conspicuous by their absence from Li's *Exposition.* If from no other source, Li was almost certainly aware of the eight confluence holes from *Gathering of the Blossoms of Acupuncture.* His selection of holes on the trajectories of the *wei* and *qiao* vessels so closely matches those described in this text that it is difficult to imagine that he was unfamiliar with it. Yet Li makes no mention of the eight holes or their pairings, nor does he appear to give particular recognition to any of these holes in his discussion of extraordinary vessel trajectories. Shining Sea (KI-6), the confluent hole of the *yin qiao*, is granted no more importance than any other hole on that channel, and in fact, Li pointedly begins its trajectory more distally with Burning Valley (KI-2). It is simply another hole on the trajectory of the *yin qiao*.[3]

Given Li's involvement with interior alchemy, we might expect to see the eight access holes referenced indirectly in his use of trigram symbolism, yet this is not the case. The trigram attributions in his discourse conform to neither the later heaven-based arrangement of the divine tortoise method nor the earlier heaven-based arrangement of the soaring method. His use of the terminology of the *Classic of Change* in the *Exposition* provides no clear link to Dou's eight confluent holes.

The *Exposition*'s description of extraordinary vessel trajectories is largely consistent with those presented in Hua Shou's (滑壽, also known as Hua Bo-Ren 滑伯仁) *Comprehensive Elucidation of the Fourteen Channels (Shi si jing fa hui he cuan 十四經發揮合篡, 1341)* and Gao Wu's *Gathering of the Blossoms of Acupuncture.* Li's hole locations are based, for the most part, on those of the *Systematic Classic of Acupuncture and Moxibustion.* That said, Li occasionally departs slightly but significantly from these texts. The most notable instance of such a diversion is his description of the *ren*, *du*, and *chong* vessels all arising from Meeting of Yin (CV-1), an arrangement that bears directly on Li's understanding of the use of the eight vessels in interior alchemy. In the practice of interior alchemy, Meeting of Yin is a pivotal area for both the circulation of qi within the body and for its communication with the qi of the macrocosm. As the three core vessels in the eight vessel system, the *ren*, *du*, and *chong* must all have direct access to this crucial nexus of qi. He tinkered with the other end of the *ren* vessel as well. Where most sources terminate the *ren* at Sauce Receptacle (CV-24), Li terminates the *ren* at Tear Container (ST-1). The rationale for this change is less clear.

Does This Text Take Acupuncture Seriously?

An Herbalist's Acupuncture?

The absence of the eight confluent holes from Li's *Exposition* has led some commentators to conclude that the book does not really concern acupuncture at all and that Li Shi-Zhen's only real treatment modality is herbal medicine.[4] This 'herbalist's acupuncture' perspective gains some currency when one considers that the acupuncture material in the *Exposition* is invariably embedded in discussions focusing on the various pathodynamics of the extraordinary vessels. One can argue that references to specific treatment holes are largely incidental to his primary interest in the manifestations of extraordinary vessel disease, as expressed in symptoms and pulse presentations.

In his discussion of diseases of the *chong* vessel, Li uses a passage on atrophy from Ch. 44 of *Basic Questions* to advance his discussion on the importance of the yang brightness channels in *chong* pathology. This passage concludes with the recommendation that one should "tonify at the spring holes and promote flow at the transport holes [of the yang brightness channels] to regulate deficiency and excess, harmonize abnormal and normal [flow of qi] so that the sinews, vessels, bones and flesh will each recover from disease in their prevailing months."[5]

Passages such as this repeatedly confront us with the question of what to make of these acupuncture prescriptions. In this case, is the well-known spring-transport hole treatment strategy intended as a viable approach for *chong* disorders presenting as atrophy, or does it exemplify a strategy for treating all *chong* pathologies? Then again, perhaps this piece of information is completely spurious. Perhaps the thrust of the passage in the *Exposition* concerns the disease itself and not the therapy.

The herbalist's acupuncture interpretation certainly simplifies our understanding of the *Exposition on the Eight Extraordinary Vessels.* From this point of view, the text is a treatise presenting theoretical material pertinent to herbalists and practitioners of interior alchemy. The acupuncture material is of interest purely for its value in illuminating various aspects of pathological and physiological function. That is precisely why Li did not bother to include the significant body of extraordinary vessel therapies presented in the *Great Compendium* and *Gathering of the Blossoms of Acupuncture.* Yet, despite its appeal, this hypothesis leaves a number of unanswered questions.

Acupuncture in the *Exposition*

If Li Shi-Zhen was fundamentally disinterested in acupuncture, then why does he attend to it in the detail he does? His descriptions of extraordinary vessel trajectories are more detailed and precise than any that had preceded it. If he had merely wished to include a comprehensive description of their trajectories for the sake of thoroughness, then why did he go to such lengths to alter those presented in previous books, adding a hole here and omitting a hole there? This question also extends to his location of the acupuncture holes themselves. Why would he go to the trouble of painstakingly describing hole locations that are often at variance with existing sources if his book was not actually intended specifically for acupuncturists? That level of descriptive precision is of little use to either herbalists or alchemists. What difference can it possibly make to an herbalist whether the *ren* vessel terminates as Sauce Receptacle (CV-24) or Tear Container (ST-1)? The symptoms that Li attributes to the *ren* have no bearing on the head at all, much less this area of the face. For that matter, we might also ask why, if Li's interest was actually limited to herbal medicine, is the depth of this information so spotty? He goes on at length regarding herbal formulas for the *chong* vessel and yet remains completely silent concerning the herbal therapies for the *yin qiao*. This is a topic we will take up again in the next chapter on herbal medicine in the *Exposition*.

If these objections are not sufficient to dissuade us from fully embracing the herbalist's acupuncture interpretation, then there is really nothing left to say regarding the acupuncture material in the *Exposition*. From this perspective, Li Shi-Zhen was undeniably an accomplished herbalist and alchemist, and he had a finely honed sense of theoretical matters pertaining to the extraordinary vessels, but he was not an acupuncturist. To be sure, the broad pathodynamics suggested by these passages are by no means limited to herbal applications. They have a direct bearing on the range of symptoms that eight confluent hole methods may address, but we need not trouble ourselves too much with the details.

It is worth considering that, however one chooses to interpret the book as a whole, the contents that have proven to be the most influential over the course of medical history concern acupuncture, not herbal therapy or alchemy. The irony of the herbalist's acupuncture hypothesis is that it leaves five centuries of acupuncture commentators quoting from a book that is not actually about acupuncture at all.

Yet there is another lens through which to interpret the *Exposition*. Perhaps Li Shi-Zhen actually took the acupuncture therapeutics in his book seriously. Perhaps the acupuncture passages in the *Exposition* are indeed intended to suggest a viable approach to acupuncture. If so, then it behooves us to engage this material on its own terms and see where it leads. To be sure, the therapeutic model it suggests is much less tidy than that offered by the eight confluence hole methods, and it poses some challenging questions of its own. Despite its difficulties, the model of extraordinary vessel therapy presented in the *Exposition* encourages the reader to think about eight vessel acupuncture in a fresh way.

In contrast to the eight hole treatment strategies advanced by Dou Han-Qing, Xu Feng, and Gao Wu, the earliest and simplest approaches to extraordinary vessel treatment focused on the use of holes situated along their trajectories.[6] This methodology, originally presented in the *Inner Classic* and *Pulse Classic*, is the approach promoted by Li throughout his *Exposition on the Eight Extraordinary Vessels*. A symptom or complex of signs and symptoms is identified as pertaining to a particular extraordinary vessel, and a hole on the trajectory of that vessel is appointed to treat the condition. Li's citation of *Divine Pivot* in treating eye problems exemplifies this approach.

"When the eye is red and painful, beginning at the inner canthus, then select the *yin qiao* [the Intersection Reach (KI-8) hole]."

As with all channels, the trajectory of the extraordinary vessels has a significant influence on their pathology. The *yin qiao* treats ophthalmological problems in part because it terminates at the inner canthus. To Li Shi-Zhen's way of thinking, the converse must also be true: the physiology and the pathology of an extraordinary vessel must similarly influence its trajectory. He develops this principle in a number of innovative ways.

In paragraph 24 of its chapter on diseases of the greater yang, the *Discussion on Cold Damage* contains an instruction to needle Wind Pond (GB-20) and Wind House (GV-16) in the event of a failure to induce a sweat. According to Li, this choice of holes can be explained in terms of their location on the *yang wei* vessel. For Li, the chills and fever indicative of improper regulation of the protective and nutritive qi are a *yang wei* disorder. This is a curious line of reasoning for him since elsewhere he fails to include Wind Mansion on the trajectory of the *yang wei*, despite its inclusion in both the *Comprehensive Elucidation of the Fourteen Channels* and *Gathering of the Blossoms of Acupuncture*. Perhaps this omission was unintentional. Li's description of the *dai* vessel is another example of his willingness to sculpt a trajectory to accommodate the demands of theory. With the exception of the *Pulse Classic*, acupuncture texts did not include Camphorwood Gate (LR-13), the front alarm hole of the spleen, in the trajectory of the *dai*, yet Li is careful to incorporate it into his own description. His reasons for this inclusion become immediately apparent in his subsequent presentation of *dai* vessel pathology, where spleen disharmonies are the preeminent pathodynamic occurring in that vessel.

Nontrajectory Treatment Strategies

The use of non-trajectory holes as a means of activating the extraordinary vessels did not begin with eight confluence holes and Dou Han-Qing; it originated in the *Inner Classic* and *Pulse Classic*. This approach to extraordinary vessel treatment figures prominently in the *Exposition*. Li cites Wang Shu-He as advocating the use of Guest Host (GB-3) in the treatment of *yang wei* symptoms, including obstruction-itching of the muscle and flesh, skin pain, and paralysis in the lower extremities, and fainting and loss of voice. The rationale for the use of this hole to treat this syndrome is unclear. It is simply presented as one part of a pulse-symptom-treatment complex identified as an extraordinary vessel pattern. This type of treatment strategy also appears in Ch. 23 of *Divine Pivot*, which states, "For wind spasm and arched-back rigidity, first select the greater yang in the popliteal fossa at a blood network and let out blood. If the attack is due to a cold pathogen, select the *yin qiao* above the Three Hairs at the blood networks and let blood out there."[7]

Once again, we see a very specific symptom presentation that is ostensibly treated by an extraordinary vessel using a hole not on its trajectory. In the case above, the three hairs refers to the acupuncture hole Large Pile (LR-1). The *Exposition* contains many passages similar to these, and they reflect a fundamental principle that may be applied to the interpretation of the medical literature at large: Symptoms and signs consistent with eight-vessel pathology are extraordinary vessel pathologies regardless of whether or not they are explicitly identified as such. Li applies this principle most fully with regard to herbal therapy, which we will discuss in the following chapter.

In his acupuncture discourses, Li does not stray far from authoritative classical texts that explicitly mention the eight vessels. Still, his juxtaposition of somewhat obscure references to the extraordinary vessels alongside more familiar passages is informative in itself. In his discussion of diseases of the *qiao* vessel, he mentions that the abundant yang vessel *(chang yang mai* 昌陽脈) causes people to experience "low back pain, which radiates to the breast along with blurred vision, and in serious [cases], arched-backed rigidity and a curled tongue with an inability to speak."

Although this passage from *Basic Questions* does not say so directly, most commentators concur that the abundant yang vessel is the *yin qiao*, hence its inclusion in Li's *Exposition*. Li Shi-Zhen's contribution to extraordinary vessel acupuncture is characterized less by innovation than by synthesis. In bringing these disparate references together in one place, he helps to more clearly define the tools available to acupuncturists in accessing the eight vessels.

Another passage in the *Exposition* that only indirectly concerns the extraordinary vessels also presents a fairly intricate model of acupuncture treatment, combining trajectory holes with nontrajectory holes. Early in his discussion of diseases of the *chong* vessel, Li presents a passage from Ch. 26 of *Divine Pivot* addressing the treatment of qi counterflow into the chest. Here we are instructed, "when there is a counterflow ascent of qi, prick the depression below the breast and at the pulsing vessel below the chest." The passage goes on to state that, "If there is abdominal pain, prick the pulsing vessels to the left or right of the umbilicus," and, "If [the pain] does not stop, then prick Qi Thoroughfare (ST-30)." To Li's way of thinking, the symptoms of qi counterflow into the chest and abdominal pain suggest a *chong* pathodynamic. In addition, Qi Thoroughfare (ST-30) is an influential hole on the pathway of the *chong* vessl. *Divine Pivot* is vague with regard to the other holes that should be needled. Various commentators have proposed Breast Window (ST-16), Roof (ST-15), Central Treasury (LU-1), and Chest Center (CV-17) as possible candidates, the first three of which apparently influence this vessel by virtue of their capacity for treating symptoms characteristic of *chong* pathologies. Chest Center is on the trajectory of the *chong*.[8]

The approaches to acupuncture therapeutics that emerge from the *Exposition* allow for a number of treatment strategies. Treatment holes may be located on or off the trajectories of the extraordinary vessels, and these two classes of holes may be combined. At least in theory, these approaches offer a flexible means of organizing extraordinary vessel treatments responsive to a wide range of clinical presentations.

One disadvantage of relying too heavily on eight confluence hole methods of extraordinary vessel treatment is that they have the insidious tendency of distancing the practitioner from the extraordinary vessels themselves. It becomes very easy to needle Shining Sea (KI-6) and Broken Sequence (LU-7) and to think, "There! I've accessed the *yin qiao*," without having to give much thought to its trajectory or the state of qi within it. This method fosters a more abstract relationship with the eight vessels. They are easily relegated to functional entities, lurking somewhere beneath the primary channels that are more amenable to direct experience. This is taken to its extreme in some of the Japanese styles of extraordinary vessel practice where these vessels are conceptualized as functional pairs. In needling Shining Sea (KI-6) and Broken Sequence (LU-7), we no longer access the *ren* vessel so much as the *ren/yin qiao* pair.[9]

At the very least, the acupuncture methodologies presented in the *Exposition* are a potential antidote to this tendency. To be of any use whatsoever, they require a much more comprehensive understanding of extraordinary vessel trajectories and intersection holes than that demanded by the eight confluence hole methods. Because there are always multiple holes to choose from, these techniques also require a more finely tuned appreciation of extraordinary vessel pathology and hole indications. Finally, the necessity of discriminating among a potentially wide range of treatment options demands more palpatory skills of the practitioner than relying on fixed rules of hole selection.

Of course, such a system has its drawbacks. In contrast to the eight hole extraordinary vessel techniques, the methods advocated by Li Shi-Zhen are messy and potentially unwieldy. Moreover, it must be admitted that the approach advocated by Li raises more questions than it answers. We are left to wonder whether a hole described in the *Pulse Classic* or *Divine Pivot* as treating a certain extraordinary vessel treats only the symptoms with which it is associated or whether it is meant to exemplify a larger therapeutic principle. When we needle Yang Assistance (GB-38), is its influence limited to the treatment of obstruction, generalized rigidity, and seizures, or does this address all pathologies of the *yang qiao*? This question becomes even more pertinent when we move to treatment holes located off the established trajectories of the eight vessels. Does Guest Host (GB-3) treat all *yang wei* disorders, or is its influence limited to those described by Wang Shu-He?

It is highly unlikely that we will ever know precisely how Li Shi-Zhen meant for readers to interpret the quotations he includes in his *Exposition*, much less how Wang Shu-He and the original authors of the *Inner Classic* meant for us to understand them. That does not mean that the questions posed above are not worth asking. The clinical ferment engendered by such inquiry is potentially as useful as any quasi-authoritative answer.

What, then, are some of the issues facing a modern clinician interested in the practical application of these ideas? Any attempt to evaluate an acupuncture treatment strategy requires some basis for comparison with other strategies, and this is a particularly tricky proposition when it comes to the extraordinary vessels. Because they are embedded within the 12 primary channels, it can be very difficult in practice to distinguish one from the other. Regardless of whether one elects to use Dou's eight confluence holes, the holes on the trajectories of the extraordinary vessels, or any other method of engaging the eight vessels, one is still left with the question of how one knows that one has activated the extraordinary vessels as opposed to some other aspect of the channel system. This question is particularly pertinent given the diffuse nature of the acupuncture methodologies presented in the *Exposition*. When we needle the 'straight yang' portion of the *yang qiao* at Support (BL-36), Bend Center (BL-40), Sinew Support (BL-56), Mountain Support (BL-57), or Taking Flight (BL-58), how do we know we are not just activating the bladder channel? The question of feedback is especially germane to extraordinary vessel therapies.

An amelioration of the symptoms we are attempting to treat is a good indicator that we have had some beneficial influence on the channel system, but it still does not tell us precisely how. Through which vector did the relief occur? Did a patient's chest pain improve after needling Inner Pass (PC-6) because of its influence on the pericardium channel or the *yin wei*? Far from clarifying matters, combining Inner Pass with Yellow Emperor (SP-4) merely adds another variable to the equation. By their very nature, extraordinary vessel presentations are complex and multifaceted. Each of the eight vessels casts its net broadly to encompass a wide spectrum of symptoms. When we combine these two holes, how do we really know that the efficacy of this combination has anything to do with the extraordinary vessels? Pulse diagnosis, a fundamental tool of Chinese medicine, bears directly on this question.[10]

Clinicians typically rely on changes in the strength and quality of the radial pulse to assess their influence on the channel system, but the degree to which the extraordinary vessels are reflected in the pulse is less clear. The majority of the extraordinary vessel pulses described by Li are derived from the *Pulse Classic*, and they occupy a prominent role in the overall structure of his discourse. This is a topic we will address in some depth in subsequent chapters on the pulse. For now, it is sufficient to understand that these pulses appear in both the *Pulse Classic* and *Exposition on the Eight Extraordinary Vessels* as constituents of clearly defined symptom-pulse-treatment complexes.

To be sure, when we attempt to influence the extraordinary vessels, we can reasonably expect to see some positive change in the pulse. The question is, how much and what should it look like? One problem posed by the extraordinary vessel pulses is whether they are applicable to other forms of extraordinary vessel acupuncture, or whether they are limited to the syndromes presented in the *Pulse Classic*. Li's descriptions of the extraordinary vessel pulses elsewhere in his writings suggest the former.[11] Curiously, this system of pulse diagnosis is much better represented in the herbal literature than in the acupuncture tradition, though it is prominent in neither. Case histories employing extraordinary vessel pulse diagnosis are few and far between, and they are almost completely absent from the premodern acupuncture literature. Moreover, we have not been able to document their premodern use in conjunction with the eight confluent holes. The application of the extraordinary vessel pulses in this context appears to be an entirely modern phenomenon.

In the past 50 years, Yoshio Manaka and Kazuto Miyawaki have identified patterns of abdominal tension and flaccidity reflecting extraordinary vessel imbalances. Administration of the proper pair of the eight confluence holes in the proper way will release abdominal tension in the associated diagnostic area.[12] In our experience, Manaka's extraordinary vessel treatments using ion-pumping cords are very effective for normalizing abdominal tension but are not particularly useful in balancing the pulse. Moreover, although each system is internally consistent, their respective abdominal maps often contradict one another. Such incongruities suggest that one system of treating the extraordinary vessels cannot necessarily be evaluated using the measures of another; each must be assessed on its own terms.

The acupuncture material in Li's book is inextricably bound to the pulse material. We may not fully understand what to do with the package he presents, but there is little doubt that he tied it together with considerable forethought. Separating one of its components from another clearly challenges the integrity of the whole. This is not to suggest that the pulse qualities described in *Exposition on the Eight Extraordinary Vessels* cannot or should not be applied in acupuncture or herbal practice outside their original scope of use, only that such innovations require a careful and critical assessment on the part of the clinician.

Herbal Considerations

The application of extraordinary vessel strategies in the modern practice of herbal medicine has developed along a number of different lines, two of which will be discussed here. The simplest approach has been to identify individual medicinals as influencing specific extraordinary vessels. Angelicae sinensis Radix *(dang gui)*, for instance, is believed to influence the *chong* vessel. The affiliation of individual herbs with the extraordinary vessels is well-established in the medical literature, and Li Shi-Zhen's *Comprehensive Outline of the Materia Medica* contains many such references. In that text, Li's primary source of information is Wang Hao-Gu (王好古, 1200–1308), an authority he also cites extensively in his *Exposition on the Eight Extraordinary Vessels.* Yet in attributing extraordinary vessel functions to specific drugs, Li was not simply parroting the opinions of others. He was himself the source of numerous statements linking the individual drugs to the extraordinary vessels, suggesting that he actively endorsed such a treatment approach. It is therefore curious that discussions of individual drugs are almost totally absent from his book on the extraordinary vessels themselves.

Another major approach to extraordinary vessel therapeutics has been to link entire formulas to the pathodynamics characteristic of each extraordinary vessel. As we have already mentioned, each extraordinary vessel is linked to one or more key identifying pathodynamic. Formulas that treat those pathodynamics are presumed to treat their associated extraordinary vessel. Cinnamon Twig Decoction *(gui zhi tang)*, for instance, is known to treat disharmonies between the nutritive and protective layers, which are the province of the *yang wei* vessel. Hence, Cinnamon Twig Decoction *(gui zhi tang)* treats the *yang wei* (see Fig. E-1).

This strategy was probably pioneered by Zhang Yuan-Su (1151–1234), although it is most fully articulated in Li's *Exposition on the Eight Extraordinary Vessels,* which concerns itself almost exclusively with herbal formulas as opposed to individual drugs.

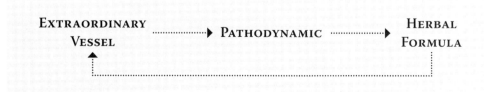

Fig. E-1   Relationship between extraordinary vessels and formulas

By and large, the drugs mentioned in Li's *Comprehensive Outline of the Materia Medica* as having an influence on the extraordinary vessels (see Table E-1 below) are not especially common in the herbal formulas cited in Li's *Exposition*. The formulas in the *Exposition* are not simply amalgams of individual drugs that have been attributed to the extraordinary vessels. They are extraordinary vessel formulas by virtue of their capacity to rectify certain key pathodynamics. For instance, although Cinnamon Twig Decoction *(gui zhi tang)* treats the diseases of the *yang wei*, Cinnamomi Ramulus *(gui zhi)* is not mentioned in the *Comprehensive Outline of the Materia Medica* as having any influence on this vessel at all. The only ingredient in that formula linked directly to the *yang wei* is Paeoniae Radix albae *(bai shao)*.

With one notable exception that will be discussed later, Li's *Exposition* is concerned exclusively with the administration of compound formulas, not single ingredients. This is hardly surprising in light of the fact that most texts of its kind, at least since the time of Zhang Zhong-Jing (ca. 200 CE), have emphasized herbal formulas as opposed to individual drugs. Yet Li's prescriptions are notable for their emphasis on the pathodynamics underlying extraordinary vessel pathologies. For instance, according to Li's logic, any formula that treats counterflow, particularly if abdominal pain and stagnation are involved, may be considered a *chong* vessel formula.

Between his *Comprehensive Outline of the Materia Medica* and *Exposition on the Eight Extraordinary Vessels*, Li appears to have embraced both methods of extraordinary vessel treatment, stressing individual drugs in the former and compound prescriptions in the latter. Both share the same principles of application in that they must both be matched to the specific expression of any extraordinary vessel pathology. For instance, although Tonify the Middle and Augment the Qi Decoction *(bu zhong yi qi tang)* treats counterflow, it is only appropriate for *chong* pathologies presenting as heat arising out of spleen deficiency. Similarly, although Angelica Sinensis Radix *(dang gui)* treats counterflow and blood stagnation in the abdomen, it is too warming for many *chong* vessel disorders and should not be used indiscriminately. As always, the specific pathological presentation determines the choice of both individual ingredients and herbal formula.

Few of the physicians who subsequently adopted extraordinary vessel strategies in their herbal prescriptions (see Part IV) actually used the formulas recommended in the *Exposition*, yet its principles of practice are evident to one degree or another in nearly all of their case records. They recognized that the central message of the *Exposition's* herbal material was that simply addressing the specific expression of their core pathodynamics produced effective extraordinary vessel treatment strategies.

The 17th century master clinician Ye Tian-Shi (1665–1745) is by far the most accomplished exponent of this approach. Ye developed an extremely versatile range of methods to address extraordinary vessel pathologies. Although he built many of his extraordinary vessel prescriptions around established formulas, his emphasis on determining the appropriate treatment strategy for a particular presentation found its clearest expression in his choice of individual drugs. His case records have been among the most influential medical writings of the past 300 years. That individual ingredients have largely eclipsed the importance of formulas in the subsequent development of extraordinary vessel therapies is due, at least in part, to Ye's approach to herbal prescriptions. In modern practice, it is the particular ingredients, and not the particular formulas, that determine extraordinary vessel therapies.

Although Ye's methods appear to have diverged greatly from Li's extraordinary vessel treatment, the versatility of his prescriptions clearly echoes Li's concern for the variety of ways in which eight vessel pathologies may present themselves. In this, even the modern predilection for writing extraordinary vessel prescriptions in terms of individual ingredients has its basis in the principles established by Li Shi-Zhen.

If the fundamental principles of using simple drugs in extraordinary vessel prescriptions are the same as those for selecting herbal formulas, and Li apparently subscribed to both methods, it is curious that he omitted individual drugs from nearly all of the *Exposition.* It may simply be that he believed he had already adequately addressed their role in extraordinary vessel treatment in *Comprehensive Outline of the Materia Medica.* Whatever his reasons, an emphasis on formulas as opposed to individual ingredients is nevertheless consistent with the larger themes of his book on the eight vessels. As already discussed, what differentiates an extraordinary vessel pattern from a primary channel or a visceral pattern is that eight vessel patterns almost invariably involve multiple systems. Extraordinary vessel pathologies are by their very nature complex and are expressed in multifaceted symptom presentations. Li's discussion of the eight vessels evidences a much greater concern for their overall pathodynamics than for any single sign or symptom. This predilection is similarly expressed in his herbal prescriptions where we again see intricate symptom presentations addressed under a common extraordinary vessel rubric directed at a root pathodynamic.

Where acupuncture treatment in the *Exposition* is centered on the trajectories of the extraordinary vessels, its herbal therapy is concerned primarily with their physiological and pathological characteristics. The influence of Cinnamon Twig Decoction (*gui zhi tang*) has little bearing on the trajectory of the *yang wei* per se, but it has a direct effect on one of its key symptoms, chills and fever. The links between formulas such as Ailanthus Decoction *(chun gen tang)* to the trajectory of the *chong* vessel are tenuous at best, yet this prescription exerts an unmistakable influence on the counterflow pathology characteristic of the *chong* vessel.

The integration of acupuncture, herbal, and alchemical perspectives is a central theme of Li's *Exposition.* By emphasizing herbal formulas over individual medicinals, Li further reinforces the integrative message of the book. The formulas themselves are emblematic of a perspective on the extraordinary vessels that engages them in the broadest possible context. For instance, Li recommends Cinnamon Twig Decoction (*gui zhi tang*), Ephedra Decoction *(ma huang tang),* and a modification of Minor Bupleurum [Decoction] *(xiao chai hu tang)* for *yang wei* disorders. All of these formulas treat chills and fever of one sort or another, but what makes them *yang wei* formulas is their capacity for harmonizing the protective and nutritive qi.

Herbs Attributed to the Vessel

Aside from a few modifications of herbal formulas, the only discussion of individual herbs in the *Exposition* occurs in the chapter on diseases of the *du*. This apparent incongruity tells us as much about Li's overall understanding of *du* vessel pathology as it does about his approach to therapy. The *Exposition* attributes 11 medicinals to the *du*. These include Notopterygii Rhizoma seu Radix *(qiang huo)*, Angelicae pubescentis Radix *(du huo)*, Saposhnikovia Radix *(fang feng)*, Schizonepetae Herba *(jing jie)*, Asari Radix et Rhizoma *(xi xin)*, Ligustici Rhizoma *(gao ben)*, Coptidis Rhizoma *(huang lian)*, Rhei Radix et Rhizoma *(da huang)*, Aconiti Radix lateralis preparata *(fu zi)*, Aconti Radix *(wu tou)*, and Xanthii Fructus *(cang er zi)*. Li's criteria for inclusion in this list are not immediately clear. *Comprehensive Outline of the Materia Medica* mentions the *du* in association with some, but by no means all, of these herbs. A number of them, including Notopterygii Rhizoma seu Radix *(qiang huo)*, Saposhnikovia Radix *(fang feng)*, and Schizonepetae Herba *(jing jie)*, are linked to the *du* only indirectly in a chapter of that book concerning wind spasm *(jing feng* 痙風*)*, which Li identifies in general terms as an affliction of the greater yang and *du* vessel. Coptidis Rhizoma *(huang lian)*, Rhei Radix et Rhizoma *(da huang)*, and Xanthii Fructus *(cang er zi)* do not appear to be affiliated at all with the *du* vessel in *Comprehensive Outline of the Materia Medica*.

More remarkable is the omission from this list of many other drugs that are explicitly identified in his *Comprehensive Outline of the Materia Medica* as influencing the *du*. They include animal products long associated with the *du* vessel such as tortoise, mutton, and the various preparations of deer antler, Cornu Cervi Pantotrichum *(lu rong)*. One-hundred-and-forty years after the publication of *Comprehensive Outline of the Materia Medica* , Ye Gui, clearly influenced by this book, redefined extraordinary vessel therapeutics with his advocacy of essence-nourishing animal products such as those in his *Case Records as a Guide to Clinical Practice (Lin zheng zhi nan yi an* 臨證 指南醫案, 1746). Yet Li has conspicuously avoided discussing this class of medicinals in his own *Exposition*.[1]

The *du* vessel is unique among the eight vessels in that its core pathodynamic is focused squarely on the trajectory of the vessel itself, which traverses the length of the spine. Li summarizes his understanding of the *du* with a line from the 29th Difficult Issue of the *Classic of Difficulties*: "When the *du* vessel becomes diseased, there is spinal rigidity and reversal." His interest in the therapeutic applications of both acupuncture and herbal medicine in treating this vessel is, for the most part, limited to musculoskeletal symptoms. In light of this, Li's list of herbs for the *du* vessel makes sense. Where Li's other extraordinary vessel formulas are keyed to the functional aspects of their associated vessel, his choice of herbs for the *du* vessel focuses on medicinals that have a localized effect along its trajectory traversing the head and spine. Coptidis Rhizoma *(huang lian)*, Rhei Radix et Rhizoma *(da huang)*, and Aconiti Radix lateralis preparata *(fu zi)* are not *du* vessel herbs per se, yet their relatively extreme thermic qualities may be interpreted as focusing the influence of the other medicinals

Drug	Disease treated	Chapter in *Comprehensive Outline of the Materia Medica*	Originally cited by
Astragali Radix (*huang qi*)	Disease of the *yang wei* where the patient suffers from cold and fever	Astragali Radix (*huang qi*)	Wang Hao-Gu
Paeoniae Radix alba (*bai shao*)	Disease of the *yang wei* where the patient suffers from cold and fever	Paeoniae Radix Alba (*bai shao*)	Wang Hao-Gu
Rehmannia Radix preparata (*shu di huang*)	Lurking heat in the *chong* and *ren*	Menstrual disorders	
Lycii Fructus (*gou qi zi*)	Debilitation of the *chong* and *ren*	Leukorrhea	
Testudinis Plastrum (*gui ban*)	Diseases of the *du*	Testudinis Plastrum (*gui ban*)	Li Shi-Zhen
Ovis Carnis (*yang*)	Diseases of the *du*	Ovis Carnis (*yang*)	Li Shi-Zhen
Ovis Carnis Spinae (*yang ji gu*)	Diseases of the *du*	Ovis Carnis Spinae (*yang ji gu*)	Li Shi-Zhen
Cervi Cornu pantotrichum (*lu rong*)	Diseases of the *du*	Cervi Cornu pantotrichum (*lu rong*)	Li Shi-Zhen
Notopterygii Rhizoma seu Radix (*qiang huo*)	Diseases of the *du*	Indirectly mentioned under wind spasms	Li Shi-Zhen
Angelicae pubescentis Radix (*du huo*)	Diseases of the *du*	Angelicae pubescentis Radix (*du huo*)	Liu Wan-Su
Saposhnikovia Radix (*fang feng*)	Diseases of the *du*	Indirectly mentioned under wind spasms	Li Shi-Zhen
Schizonepetae Herba (*jing jie*)	Diseases of the *du*	Indirectly mentioned under wind spasms	Li Shi-Zhen
Asari Radix et Rhizoma (*xi xin*)	Diseases of the *du*	Indirectly mentioned under wind spasms	Wang Hao-Gu
Ligustici Rhizoma (*gao ben*)	Diseases of the *du*	Ligustici Rhizoma (*gao ben*)	Wang Hao-Gu
Aconiti Radix lateralis preparata (*fu zi*)	Diseases of the *du*	Aconiti Radix lateralis preparata (*fu zi*)	Wang Hao-Gu
Aconti Radix (*wu tou*)	Diseases of the *du*	Indirectly mentioned under wind spasms	Li Shi-Zhen
Xanthii Fructus (*cang er zi*)	Diseases of the *du*	No mention of its association with the *du*	Li Shi-Zhen

Table E-1   Drugs affiliated with the extraordinary vessels in *Comprehensive Outline of the Materia Medica* in treating decidedly hot or cold conditions. The hot nature of Aconiti Radix lateralis preparata *(fu zi)*, in particular, also functions to open the yang, a desirable quality in treating *du* vessel pathologies that are frequently characterized by stagnation and cold.

The near absence of supplementing medicinals from Li's list of *du* vessel herbs is amplified by the complete omission of any herbal recommendation for the *ren*. Li again sculpts his message as much by omission as inclusion. As far as the *Exposition* is concerned, *ren* and *du* pathologies characterized by deep debilitation of essence and source qi are not the province of herbal therapy. Although he acknowledges the role of the *ren* vessel in maturation and development, he suggests no treatment for problems of this nature. Similarly, Li's acupuncture recommendations for the *ren* and *du* avoid this level of treatment as well. For Li, this deepest level of extraordinary vessel function lies in the realm of alchemical techniques, not acupuncture or herbal medicine.

Source Qi and Essence

Even though the *Exposition* offers little in the way of herbal therapy for deep pathologies of the *ren* and *du* vessels, the herbal strata of the book is by no means devoid of herbs that influence source or essence qi. On the contrary, the formulas in the *Exposition* contain many of the medicinals mentioned in Li's *Comprehensive Outline of the Materia Medica* as tonifying source qi and augmenting essence qi. Ginseng Radix *(ren shen)*, Astragali Radix *(huang qi)*, Cinnamomi Cortex *(rou gui)*, Aconiti Radix lateralis preparata *(fu zi)*, Schizandrae Fructus *(wu wei zi)*, Phellodendri Cortex *huang bai)*, Atractylodes macrocephelae Rhizoma *(bai zhu)*, and Glycyrrhizae Radix *(gan cao)* are among the common herbs identified by Li Shi-Zhen as tonifying the source qi. Those that specifically augment the essence qi include Polygalae Radix *(yuan zhi)*, Asari Radix et Rhizoma *(xi xin)*, Rehmanniae Radix *(sheng di)*, Ophiopogonis Radix *(mai men dong)*, Acori tatarinowii Rhizoma *(shi chang pu)*, Cinnamomi Cortex *(rou gui)*, Magnolia officianalis Cortex *(hou po)*, and Corni Fructus *(shan yu rou)*. Nearly every herbal formula in the *Exposition* contains one or more of these ingredients.

In reviewing Li's choice of extraordinary vessel herbal formulas and their constituents, it is evident that source qi plays an important, if background, role in his understanding of extraordinary vessel function. While acknowledging that an insufficiency of source qi may play a potential role in extraordinary vessel pathology, his attention remained focused on the immediate expression of the disease. This is in contrast to later physicians who chose to more directly tonify the eight vessels through the kidneys. The absence of animal products and cloying kidney tonics in his extraordinary vessel formulas is reminiscent of the treatment style of Li Dong-Yuan (李東垣, 1180–1251), who advocated the treatment of source qi through the postnatal qi of the stomach and spleen. Perhaps not surprisingly, Li Shi-Zhen's *Comprehensive Outline of the Materia Medica* contains a section devoted specifically to Li Dong-Yuan's use of medicinals according to symptom (*Li Dong-Yuan sui zheng yong yao fan li* 李東垣 隨證用藥凡例).

Expanding on Earlier Efforts and Categorizing Formulas

The arrangement of the herbal material in the *Exposition* is less than systematic in that Li links some form of herbal therapy to only six of the eight vessels. Notwithstanding the substantial potential for overlap in attributing herbal prescriptions to the extraordinary vessels, each formula mentioned in the *Exposition* is attributed to a single vessel. Prescriptions within each extraordinary vessel category are frequently further subdivided according to a variety of different schemes. Distinctions are made between *yin wei* prescriptions that address reverting yin patterns and those that address lesser yin patterns. Within each of these categories, formulas are described as addressing either cold or heat conditions. Similarly, some *yang wei* formulas are identified as treating greater yang conditions, while others address lesser yang conditions. More often than not, however, extraordinary vessel subcategorizations are implied rather than explicit. The *chong* vessel formulas in the *Exposition* are generally characterized by their treatment of counterflow conditions. They are further distinguished by the type of counterflow they address, and, for some, by the location of the aortic pulsing that they treat.

Where Li relied heavily on the authority of earlier sources for his acupuncture material, there are few sources in the herbal literature from which he could draw. Zhang Jie-Gu evidently wrote on the topic of the extraordinary vessels, but with the exception of the quotations that appear in the *Exposition*, Zhang's works concerning extraordinary vessel therapy have been lost. Another text that directly addresses the herbal treatment of the extraordinary vessels is Li Dong-Yuan's *Discussion of the Spleen and Stomach (Pi wei lun* 脾胃論*)*, and Li Shi-Zhen also quotes extensively from this book. Li Dong-Yuan's attention to the relationship between the *chong* vessel, counterflow patterns, and the yang brightness channels is one reason why formulas for this vessel are so well represented in the *Exposition*. Unfortunately, Li Dong-Yuan's interest in the extraordinary vessels did not extend far beyond the *chong*. Aside from these authors, the literature appears to have provided Li Shi-Zhen with little material to reference.

Without an existing body of literature on the herbal treatment of the extraordinary vessels, Li was evidently compelled to identify his own set of extraordinary vessel formulas. Nevertheless, those few passages by Zhang Yuan-Su and Li Dong-Yuan provided Li Shi-Zhen with a well-established methodology for linking herbal formulas to the extraordinary vessels. It was Zhang Yuan-Su, referred to by Li Shi-Zhen as Zhang Jie-Gu, who associated Cinnamon Twig Decoction *(gui zhi tang)* with the *yang wei* by virtue of its capacity to regulate the protective and nutritive qi. Li Dong-Yuan used precisely the same reasoning in his discussion of *chong* vessel patterns. Li Shi-Zhen expanded this principle to include all the extraordinary vessels. He identified a fundamental set of pathodynamics associated with each vessel and selected herbal formulas that treated similar conditions

In prescribing herbal formulas for the extraordinary vessels, Li focused on their most general pathological characteristics. Tonify the Middle and Augment the Qi Decoction *(bu zhong yi qi tang)* addresses a wide range of symptoms, but the characteristic that identifies this formula with the *chong* vessel is its fundamental capacity to treat counterflow. Li's attention to the broadest aspects of extraordinary vessel pathology allowed him to bring a wide range of sources to bear on herbal prescriptions. He found extraordinary vessel patterns and formulas in texts ranging from *Basic Questions* and Zhang Zhong-Jing's *Discussion of Cold Damage* to Sun Si-Miao's *Important Formulas Worth a Thousand Gold Pieces for any Emergency* and Chao Yuan-Fang's *Discussion of the Origins of the Symptoms of Disease*.

The distribution of herbal material throughout the *Exposition* is inconsistent. Despite the latitude that his broad perspective afforded him, Li was much more inclined to attribute herbal formulas to some vessels rather than others. Expanding on the precedents established by Li Dong-Yuan, Li Shi-Zhen identified 17 herbal formulas for the *chong* vessel. Though he acknowledged Zhang Yuan-Su's contribution of three formulas that address the *yin wei*, Li claimed that Zhang was too narrow in his vision and then went on to identify ten more prescriptions of his own. Li apparently had little to say regarding the herbal treatment of the *qiao* vessels, despite his interest in their relevance to interior alchemy and the wealth of *qiao*-related acupuncture material in the *Exposition*. Inexplicably, he mentions only one formula for the *yang qiao* and none at all for the *yin qiao*. Even more remarkable is his failure to mention even a single herbal formula influencing the *ren* vessel. This fact argues against interpreting the *Exposition* as primarily an herbal text.

Extraordinary Vessel Formulas as Organizing Principles

An extraordinary vessel diagnosis does not eliminate the need for other, more specific diagnostic criteria. Most often, it is insufficient in and of itself to guide one to an effective treatment strategy. Because it does not eliminate the need to use standard diagnostic methods, it is reasonable to wonder why one should even bother with an extraordinary vessel perspective in formulating one's herbal prescriptions. It might be argued that such an approach is at best irrelevant and at worst only serves to muddy the diagnostic waters.

The strongest argument to be made for adopting an extraordinary vessel methodology in formulating herbal prescriptions is that it is a useful means of integrating all aspects of a treatment. When skillfully applied, the extraordinary vessel model holds the potential for simplifying one's approach to the patient, peeling away secondary and tertiary issues to expose the root of the problem. This approach to herbal medicine compels us to ask, "What is the overall pathodynamic at work in this patient?" Shao Lan Sun's (邵蘭蓀, 1855–1910) case record of his treatment of the *chong* vessel is a good example of this principle at work. A translation of a case of Shao's appears in Ch. 37 of Part IV.

To be sure, Li's presentation of herbal material pertaining to the extraordinary vessels is more successful in some areas than in others. It can, in many instances, be very helpful to conceptualize counterflow conditions accompanied by abdominal pain and accumulation as disorders of the *chong* vessel. Similarly, modeling disharmonies of the nutritive and protective qi as *yang wei* patterns has the potential for tying together a wide range of disparate physical and emotional symptoms into a manageable diagnostic package.

By contrast, Li Shi-Zhen attributes no less than 14 prescriptions to *yin wei* disharmonies. He makes it clear that one must further differentiate them based on their six channel influence and according to whether the condition is hot or cold in nature. They are all *yin wei* prescriptions by virtue of their effect on heart pain, which here includes generalized epigastric discomfort. In the case of the *yin wei* vessel, an extraordinary vessel diagnosis appears to be more of a theoretical exercise than an essential tool for structuring an herbal therapy. Nevertheless, even in situations where such a model seems redundant, an extraordinary vessel diagnosis may still have some value in organizing a coherent overall treatment strategy. At the very least, working within the conceptual framework of a *yin wei* disharmony has the potential for coordinating acupuncture and herbal modalities.

If Li published any of his own case records illustrating the use of the extraordinary vessels, none has survived. His contribution to the literature of the extraordinary vessels is almost purely theoretical in nature. We must turn to the writings of others if we hope to gain some sense of how the eight vessels have actually been applied in the clinic. Indeed, to truly appreciate the perspective advanced by Li, it must be contrasted with the writings of Shen Jin-Ao and Ye Tian-Shi. These two influential physicians are the heirs to the line of thought represented in the *Exposition on the Eight Extraordinary Vessels*. In subsequent chapters, we will examine the writings of both these physicians as a means of understanding how Li Shi-Zhen's ideas on the extraordinary vessels were developed by later generations of physicians.

Of the physicians who incorporated extraordinary vessel strategies into their herbal therapies, Shen Jin-Ao adhered most closely to the methodology advanced in the *Exposition*. He also filled in some of the gaps left by Li. Most notably, Shen Jin-Ao suggested 27 new formulas for 'bulging' (*shan* 疝) disorders, which he associated with *ren* vessel pathologies, a category Li left untouched. Although he was clearly working from the basic principles laid out by Li Shi-Zhen, Ye Tian-Shi took extraordinary vessel therapeutics in entirely new directions. As already mentioned, he is responsible for identifying extraordinary vessel treatment with tonifying the liver and kidneys, and for promoting the use of animal products as a means of influencing the extraordinary vessels. Where Shen was purely a theorist, Ye's greatest contribution to the medical literature was his extensive case records. Ch. 35 in Part IV of this book presents a more thoroughgoing discussion of Ye Tian-Shi's approach to the extraordinary vessels and a selection of his case records.

The writings of Shen, Ye, and other thinkers provide the reader with a greater sense of how an extraordinary vessel diagnosis might be used to organize a treatment strategy. Ch. 37 in Part IV contains case records illustrating four different applications of a *chong* vessel diagnosis in herbal therapy. Appendix 2 summarizes the formulas and drugs appearing in the *Exposition* and their key indications. Finally, as a reference to those interested in the use of individual drugs in extraordinary vessel therapy, Appendix 3 presents a comprehensive list of individual herbs that have been associated with the extraordinary vessels, drawn from a variety of sources.

Keeping to the One: Internal Alchemy in
Exposition on the Eight Extraordinary Vessels

Daoist techniques of internal cultivation, also known as internal alchemy *(nei dan* 內 丹*)*, are closely, if often indirectly, associated with the extraordinary vessels. These sensibilities subtly but profoundly shade the conceptual picture of the extraordinary vessels painted by the *Inner Classic* and *Classic of Difficulties.* Making sense of the much more explicitly alchemical material in Li's *Exposition* is one of the greatest challenges to a full understanding of his work. In expanding the scope of extraordinary vessel function beyond a purely medical realm, Li Shi-Zhen's incorporation of material from a closely related, but fundamentally different discipline adds an entirely new dimension to our understanding of these vessels. His use of an arcane terminology largely foreign to the medical reader requires us to move in the worlds of both the physician and the Daoist adept.

Despite the importance of alchemical material to the integration of medical and alchemical perspectives on the extraordinary vessel models, Li Shi-Zhen doles out these insights in a sparing manner. His target audience probably had some familiarity with all of this material, and he needed only allude to it to make his point.[1] The philosophical and alchemical passages in *Exposition on the Eight Extraordinary Vessels* consist, at best, of just a few pages of text. Li includes just enough alchemical lore that it cannot be ignored, but he leaves it to his readers to decide for themselves how it relates to the medical material. The stratum of the *Exposition* dealing with internal alchemy is a subtle spice added to an already complex blend of flavors. Yet Li demands in no uncertain terms that we do indeed engage the extraordinary vessels from the perspective of internal alchemy as well as medicine. He closes both of his introductory chapters with an admonition to physicians and cultivators alike that each group must become conversant with both medical and alchemical perspectives on the extraordinary vessels. Competency in both these aspects of the extraordinary vessels will allow physicians to "comprehend the great purpose of the 12 channels and 15 networks." Li warns that by remaining ignorant of the larger scope of extraordinary vessel lore, physicians will "remain in the dark as to the cause of disease." Similarly, longevity seekers ignorant of the medical applications of the extraordinary vessels will find it "difficult to tame the cauldron's heat."

The alchemical material in the *Exposition* requires that we first define the bounds of internal alchemy. It will also be helpful to briefly review the alchemical texts appearing in the *Exposition* and their place in the development of internal alchemy. Along the way, we must consider the scope of Li's personal involvement with Daoism and inner alchemy, an association that was extensive, multifaceted, and nuanced. We will here treat inner alchemy as a subset of Daoism, recognizing, however, its highly syncretic use of certain Buddhist concepts and its complex relationship with religious Daoism. We will examine the major alchemical themes in the *Exposition* and consider their implications for the application of the extraordinary vessels in medicine.

It is difficult to overstate the open nature of the terminology of internal alchemy. Each term possesses a complex sphere of meaning that shifts continually with the context in which it is used and the level of accomplishment of the reader. We will examine the key alchemical terms used in Li's *Exposition* and how they shade our understanding of more familiar medical material.

Modern commentators tend to refer to the passages concerning internal alchemy in the *Exposition* as *qigong*, but this is something of an oversimplification.[2] Developing slowly over centuries as a uniquely Chinese method of personal cultivation, the term 'internal alchemy' refers to more than breathing practices or exercise. Although such practices are an integral part of internal alchemy, the goals and techniques of internal alchemy are much more far-reaching. Isabelle Robinet defines internal alchemy as a "technique of enlightenment including a method of controlling both the world and oneself and a means of fashioning (*zao hua* 造化) and hence understanding in the sense of an existential and intellectual integration."[3] Others define the goal somewhat more simply as a quest to transcend space and time that often takes the form of the pursuit of physical or spiritual transcendence. Livia Kohn has described this quest for transcendence as a progressive "lightening and brightening" wherein the corporeal body becomes ever buoyant and more luminous until the adept is finally able to soar away on the clouds.[4]

According to Robinet, internal alchemy has three distinguishing components:

1. There is a concern for mental and physiological training, with an emphasis on the mental aspects. In addition, internal alchemy strives toward a synthesis of various Daoist aspects (breathing exercises, visualization, alchemy), certain Buddhist speculations, and references to Confucian texts.

2. There is a systematized use of the trigrams and hexagrams of the *Classic of Change,* already used metaphorically in the laboratory rituals of external alchemy.

3. Finally, internal alchemy invariably involves references to metallurgical practices of a purely metaphorical nature.[5]

All of these components are plainly evident in the *Exposition's* references to internal alchemy.

It is worth noting that although they fall within the scope of internal alchemy, breathing practices and exercise are not inherently Daoist pursuits per se. Other groups, including Confucians, also claimed these practices as their own. Daniel Burton-Rose has argued that by the late Ming dynasty, internal alchemy had become so syncretic in its integration of Buddhist and Confucian principles that it could no longer be considered as uniquely Daoist at all.[6] What defines the discipline of internal alchemy is the synthesis of all three of the above-mentioned characteristics, and these components are present in all texts on the subject.

Internal alchemy is nevertheless a pivotal part of a larger set of practices and beliefs of the Daoist religion with which it shares the common aims of a transcendence of space and time. The more immediate concern for physical and mental health is an obvious corollary of such pursuits. It was understood that the techniques of transcendence often required many years to mature, and it was therefore necessary to live a long time just to complete the work. Hence adepts put a premium on maintaining their physical form.[7] Over the course of centuries, practitioners of the Daoist arts developed a variety of tools in addition to internal alchemy to achieve these ends. These include diet, chemical and laboratory technologies known as 'external alchemy' (*wai dan* 外丹), hygienic exercises known as 'stretching and guiding' (*dao yin* 導引), and practices, including the use of religious charms, talismans, and magic spells. Daoist religion maintains relationships with practices that are both contained within the scope of traditional Chinese medicine and those that are vastly different from it. Most of these practices are interpreted in relation to the philosophy expounded in the *Lao zi* (老子, 5th century BCE) and the *Zhuang zi* (莊子, 3rd century BCE). Despite the fact that they occasionally appear to stand in direct opposition to the quest for immortality, Daoist cultivators interpret them as coded instructions for precisely such practices. At the very least, these texts describe the frame of the Daoist understanding of the universe, whether expressed through ritual internal alchemical practice or medicine. Li Shi-Zhen's writings refer directly to many of the disciplines characteristic of Daoist religion.

Paul Unschuld has demonstrated the omnipresent influence of Confucian thought throughout the development of medicine in China.[8] Be that as it may, the fundamental worldview and many of the philosophical principles expressed in the *Lao zi* and *Zhuang zi* are also evident to one degree or another in most Chinese medical writings. Yet, although these values form the conceptual foundation of the medicine of China, they tend to remain in the background, typically overshadowed by other ideological threads. With its persistent references to putatively Daoist practices of internal alchemy, *Exposition on the Eight Extraordinary Vessels* is a notable exception to this rule.

Li's *Exposition* is among the most Daoist texts in the mainstream Chinese medical literature and ranks on par with Sun Si-Miao's *Important Formulas Worth a Thousand Gold Pieces [for any Emergency]* as a merger of secular Chinese medical principles and the often heterogeneous practices of Daoist religion. Li Shi-Zhen's *Comprehensive Outline of the Materia Medica* also draws heavily, though often critically, from Daoist lore.

By the time Li Shi-Zhen was writing in the 16th century, the basic technologies of internal alchemy were already well-established, and Daoist influences of all sorts were prevalent in the cultural milieu. Unschuld observes that, "Although Confucianism had 'conquered' the competing philosophies of Taoism and Buddhism since the Sung period, Taoist and Buddhist concepts, under a more or less intended disguise of Confucianism, had influenced Chinese thought to a greater degree than ever before."[9] There is no question that, regardless of their professed philosophical leanings, educated physicians during the Ming dynasty had more than a passing familiarity with the alchemical literature. This broad cultural trend is especially apparent throughout Li's work, which contains many references to the philosophical underpinnings of Daoism. Notable among these is a concern for the consequences of diverging from the virtue of the way. In *Comprehensive Outline of the Materia Medica*, Li states: "When the way and the virtue of the ancients declines even slightly, the age of evil appears." (中古道 德稍衰邪氣時至[10])

Allusions to the *Lao zi* and *Zhuang zi* are especially apparent in Li's *Exposition*. In his *Comprehensive Outline of the Materia Medica*, however, philosophical references are often overshadowed by some of the more arcane concerns of Daoist religion. Demonology was a matter of great interest to Daoists but was officially considered to be superstition by proper Confucians. Nevertheless, like many physicians of his time, Li accepts the presence of demons as etiological factors in disease as self-evident. Such concerns figure prominently in Li's writing. In this regard, his views more closely resemble those of shamans (*wu* 巫) or Daoist priests than those of a Confucian scholar. The list of herbs in *Comprehensive Outline of the Materia Medica* said to combat demons is lengthy; Li is particularly intrigued with the uses of Persica Semen (*tao ren*) in the treatment of all manner of ghostly or demonic influences (*gui qi* 鬼氣). One of the few case records in his *Exposition on the Eight Extraordinary Vessels* concerns a malevolent spirit that has taken up residence at a particular acupuncture hole. It is treated both with moxibustion and offerings of food and wine, and the condition is resolved.

The influence of Daoist herbal lore and philosophy on *Comprehensive Outline of the Materia Medica* is profound and frequently fosters innovative interpretations concerning the use of medicinals. In one case, Li invokes *Lao zi* to explain a novel use of an herb. Fraxini Cortex *(qin pi)* is generally used to treat the eyes and stop pain. Li believed that this medicinal was "also able to treat lack of male essence and augment the essence to promote fertility because it both astringes and tonifies. This is because, as Lao [zi] stated: 'the heavenly *dao* values astringing.'" (又能治男子少精益精有子皆 取其澀而補也故老云天道貴澀[11])

In another instance, Li's discussion of Acori tatarinowii Rhizoma (*shi chang pu*) draws from a text appearing in the *Daoist Canon (Dao Zang* 道藏, compiled 1445) to again expand its scope of application. Acori tatarinowii Rhizoma (*shi chang pu*) is generally regarded as a phlegm-transforming, spirit-calming medicinal, yet *On the Transcendent's Consumption of Ganoderma and Acorus (Shen xian fu shi ling cao chang pu* 神仙服食靈草菖蒲) views Acori tatarinowii Rhizoma (*shi chang pu*) as a tonifying medicinal. According to Li,

The qi of Acori tatarinowii Rhizoma (*shi chang pu*) is warm, its flavor is acrid, and it is a medicinal of the hand lesser yin and foot reversing yin. When there is an insufficiency of heat qi, both [the heart and liver channels] are employed, so that one tonifies the mother. When one suffers from an urgency of the liver, use acridity to tonify it.[12]

Critical Evaluation

Though Li Shi-Zhen was undeniably well-read in a broad range of Daoist lore, he was by no means an uncritical cheerleader of the Daoist cause. One of the major contributions of *Comprehensive Outline of the Materia Medica* was its concern with correcting inaccuracies in the existing literature of the materia medica. Many of the entries in *Comprehensive Outline of the Materia Medica* contain a section entitled "Correction of Errors" *(zheng wu* 正誤) in which Li often took issue with Daoist claims. This aspect of *Comprehensive Outline of the Materia Medica* most definitely evidences a willingness to contradict many Daoist claims regarding the uses and functions of medicinals. Li was particularly critical of the practice of ingesting mercury for the purposes of achieving alchemical transmutation and immortality. In discussing cinnabar, he states:

> *Grand Encyclopedia [of the Song People]* claims that it is nontoxic and *[Divine Husbandman's] Materia Medica* says that long-term ingestion makes one a transcendent. Zhen Quan (甄權)[13] claims that it returns one to the maternal cinnabar source and Ge Hong's (葛洪) *The Master Who Embraces Simplicity (Bao Pu-Zi* 抱朴子, 343) says that it is a medicinal of longevity. Who knows how many since the Six Dynasties have cravenly consumed [mercury] in a quest for life only to lose consciousness and their bodies. The prognosticators [i.e., early alchemists] certainly had insufficient skill, and so their materia medica contains wild talk.[14]

The *Exposition* cites the seminal text of both external and internal alchemy, *The Token for the Agreement of the Three According to the Changes of Zhou (Zhou yi can tong qi* 周易參同契, 142 BCE), in a number of places, yet in his *Comprehensive Outline of the Materia Medica*, Li takes issue with this book's assessment of the therapeutic value of sesame seed, which was commonly held to be a Daoist panacea. He refers to this medicinal by one of its alternate names, Grand Victory (*ju sheng* 巨勝): "[According to *Agreement of the Three,*] Grand Victory can prolong life, yet can be made into pills and taken orally." Li points out that," Today [this medicinal] is rarely used, and is not very effective. When taken long-term, however, it has some benefit but that is all."[15]

Li Shi-Zhen's criticisms are not limited to those medicinals that claim to confer immortality or profound longevity. He is frequently of the opinion that the claims of the Daoists are simply overblown. His discussion of Acanthopanis Cortex (*wu jia pi*) conveys a similar sentiment.

Acanthopanis Cortex *(wu jia pi)* treats painful obstruction and fortifies the sinews and bones. Its effects are good and profound. While those who engage in immortality practices go overboard in describing it and their words brim with praise, it is still commonly [well-] regarded.[16]

Li Shi-Zhen and Alchemy

From his various references to matters related to Daoism, a picture emerges of an extremely well-informed individual bent on rectifying what he perceives to be inaccuracies and superstitions in a body of knowledge he deeply respects. During his extensive travels while researching *Comprehensive Outline of the Materia Medica*, he undoubtedly interacted with a great many Daoist adepts, yet the only definitive record we have of his association with any Daoist whatsoever occurs during his time at the imperial court when he is believed to have come into conflict with them over matters of medical praxis. Once again, we see Li taking a position in opposition to the Daoist orthodoxy. This leaves one to wonder about the nature and extent of Li's personal involvement with Daoist practice.

Like many prominent figures living in an officially Confucian society, Li's personal interest in Daoism and Daoist cultivation is rather shadowy. His biographies contain no mention of an affiliation with any school or teacher. Because the texts mentioned in the *Exposition* are the common heritage of all internal cultivators, these are unhelpful in definitively associating him with a particular strain of Daoist thought. He appears to have been something of a generalist, although his fondness for citing Zhang Bo-Duan (張伯端) implies a close affinity with Zhang's approach to cultivation. Nevertheless, Gu Jing-Xing's (顧景星, 1621–1687) *Biography of Li Shi-Zhen (Li Shi-Zhen zhuan 李時珍傳)* suggests that Li was more than just a scholar, and was indeed an avid practitioner of internal alchemy.

> In my youth, I heard an anecdote about Mister [Li Shi-Zhen], who was kind to his friends and concealed his virtues. In the evening, in addition to coming to the household of my paternal grandfather to study texts from the time the sun rose, he would sit throughout the night, as if he were a divine transcendent. Is it any accident that he became such an accomplished [adept]?[17]

"Sitting throughout the night" *(ye ji duan zuo 夜即端坐)* is a reference to the Daoist longevity practices of quiet sitting, and "divine transcendent" *(shen xian 神仙)* is a common term for high-level Daoist adepts. A similar story appears in *White Thatched Hut Collection (Bai mao tang ji 白茅堂集*, ca. 1736–1792) recounting how little Li slept. In this account, he apparently saw patients by day while practicing internal alchemy through the night.[18]

Li's personal involvement in internal alchemy may have tempered his well-established willingness to critique the Daoist literature in his *Exposition*. Then again, unlike the *Comprehensive Outline of the Materia Medica* with its active concern for correcting the mistakes in earlier literature, Li's *Exposition on the Eight Extraordinary Vessels* is largely limited to material he believed was immediately useful. It is therefore likely that he simply omitted any pertinent information with which he took issue, just as he failed to mention the eight confluence holes of the extraordinary vessels. Like the rest of the material in his book on the extraordinary vessels, Li's critical assessment of this material is defined as much by what he omits as what he includes. Though couched in difficult terminology, Li appears to have striven to keep the central points of his message regarding alchemy and extraordinary vessels simple and universal.

Exposition on the Eight Extraordinary Vessels meets all of Robinet's criteria for qualification as a text of internal alchemy. It contains ample references to exercise, the symbolism of the *Classic of Change*, and chemical transmutation, often occurring in the same sentence. The alchemical passages in Li's book may be further grouped into three broad, overlapping categories. First, there are references to stillness, quietude, and emptiness as the ground from which activity in the extraordinary vessels springs. Quietude appears to be a prerequisite for any engagement of the extraordinary vessels. Next, there are references to specific methodologies involving the activation of the extraordinary vessels. These tend to center around the practice of the microcosmic orbit. Finally, chemical metaphors and the symbolism of the *Classic of Change* are used in the *Exposition* specifically to define the topographic and physiological terrain of the extraordinary vessels. Each of these topics is germane to a medical understanding of the extraordinary vessels, and we will explore them in some detail.

Treatises on Internal Alchemy Appearing in the *Exposition*

Aside from his references to the *Lao zi* and *Zhuang zi,* Li's source material rarely appears in medical texts, and readers trained exclusively in medicine may find it helpful to have some introduction to this genre of Daoist literature. This will establish the conceptual milieu from which he drew his material.

Lao zi and *Zhuang zi*

The Way and Its Virtue (Dao de jing 道德經), otherwise known as *Lao zi* (老子) after its putative author, and the *Zhuang zi* (莊子) exert an immense influence on all forms of Daoist philosophy, mysticism, religion, and practice. Their collective philosophy, as distinct from religious practice, is known as *Lao-Zhuang* thought. Whether the original intent of the material in *Lao zi* included physiospiritual cultivation is debatable; however, there is no question that *Lao zi* was subsequently used as a cultivation guide. Although some of its chapters appear to have little bearing on mystical practice, others seem difficult to interpret otherwise.

Lao zi was composed during the Warring States period (433–221 BCE) as an antidote to the social and political unrest of the time. It is unlikely that Lao zi was an historical figure, and his involvement in the compilation of the book that bears his name is uncertain at best. A brief text of 5,000 characters, the book is a collection of sayings that either seeks to correct some common assumption or recommend a certain regimen of self-cultivation.[19] Its message is directed primarily at the political and cosmological role of the sage.

Concrete descriptions of mystical techniques, physical or otherwise, are conspicuously absent from *Lao zi*, although later traditions consider it a mystical text of the first order. Much of the language used in *Lao zi* is quite similar to that found in *Inward Training* (*Nei ye* 內業), a chapter of the collection known as the *Guan Zi* (管子, 26 BCE). *Inward Training* itself is a text that is believed to predate *Lao zi* and contains unambiguous descriptions of meditation and cultivation practices.

One of the central themes of *Lao zi,* and of particular interest in the study of the extraordinary vessels, is the role of emptiness as the progenitor of all things. This is expressed on a human scale in the values of simplicity, stillness, and effortless action (*wu wei* 無為).

Where *Lao zi's* message is both personal and political, *Zhuang zi's* is focused purely on the individual. Its message is also considerably more extreme than that of *Lao zi*. Zhuang zi may indeed have been an historical figure, although this is still a topic of debate.[20] Nevertheless, the current scholarly consensus is that he is responsible for at least some of the work that bears his name. Composed during the 3rd century BCE, *Zhuang zi* is often viewed as an exposition on the principles advocated by *Lao zi*, although it presents many new ideas of its own.

Where effortless action in *Lao zi* is a means of dealing with the things of this world, in *Zhuang zi*, it is a state of consciousness. Effortless action is the quality of a perfected person's mind.

As Livia Kohn puts it, "While the *Dao de jing* seeks to remedy an unsatisfactory situation socially and through simplicity, the *Zhuang zi* much more radically encourages a revolution of people's very minds."[21] These topics also form the basis of Li's alchemical interpretation of the extraordinary vessels. His choice of Daoist material stresses the fundamental principles of emptiness, stillness, and effortless action in the realms of both internal alchemy and medicine.

Li closes his second chapter by equating the extraordinary vessels with the perception of the Mysterious Female, a common theme in *Lao zi* that first appears in Ch. 6 of that book. The Mysterious Female is synonymous with the primordial stillness that gives rise to the phenomenal world. It is a principle that Li will return to throughout the *Exposition* and we will take it up again later in greater depth. Identification with the Mysterious Female in *Lao zi* is achieved by techniques such as "keeping the mind empty and the belly full,"[22] and admonitions to "extend your utmost emptiness as far as you can, and do your best to preserve your tranquility."[23]

The fourth chapter of *Zhuang zi* contains a similar passage concerning the fasting of the mind that exemplifies the significance of stillness in Daoist thinking, mischievously using Confucius and a disciple as its advocate. In linking a quiet mind with the inherent intelligence of the primal breath (*yuan qi* 元氣), to use Victor Mair's translation of the term, this story also speaks to conditions necessary for attentive listening in the diagnostic process. To perceive things clearly, the listener must listen without the preconceptions of discursive thought.

"I venture to ask what fasting of the mind is," said Hui.

"Maintaining the unity of your will," said Confucius, "listen not with your ears but with your mind. Listen not with your mind but with your primal breath. The ears are limited to listening, the mind is limited to tallying. The primal breath, however, awaits things emptily. It is only through the Way that one can gather emptiness, and emptiness is fasting of the mind."

"Before I am able to exercise fasting of the mind," said Yan Hui, "I truly have an identity. But after I am able to exercise it, I will no longer have an identity. Can this be called emptiness?

"Precisely," said Confucius.[24]

In Ch. 6 of the *Zhuang zi*, 'sitting and forgetting' is linked to identification with the Transformational Thoroughfare (*da tong* 大通), which here is synonymous with the Great Way (*da dao* 大道), the primordial source from which all things arise.[25]

"I sit and forget."

"What do you mean, sit and forget?" Confucius asked with surprise.

"I slough off my limbs and trunk," said Yan Hui, "dim my intelligence and depart from my form, leave knowledge behind and become identical with the Transformational Thoroughfare. This is what I mean by 'sit and forget.'"[26]

The retention of essence and qi is a fundamental principle for ensuring health and longevity in Chinese medicine, and this is accomplished in a variety of ways, not the least of which involves quieting one's mind and spirit. In its introductory remarks, Ch. 1 of *Basic Questions* discusses the importance of retaining a tranquil mind in preventing illness.[27] In addition, a quiet and attentive mind is essential to effective needling. Ch. 9 of *Divine Pivot* illustrates this concept beautifully, pointing out that this practice requires that one close the "doors and windows" of one's senses.

Whenever administering needling techniques, one should … retire to a quiet place and commune with his spirit with doors and windows shut, his mind attentive and his essence and qi undivided. Undistracted by human sounds, he must marshal his essence, concentrate his mind, and direct his will entirely toward needling.[28]

With these associations so deeply ingrained in the bedrock of Chinese medicine, Li scarcely needed to resort to more arcane sources to illustrate his point. Yet later texts of internal alchemy involve the extraordinary vessels largely to the exclusion of the primary channels. The earliest of the alchemical texts mentioned in the *Exposition*, and, in many ways, the progenitor of them all, is *The Token for the Agreement of the Three According to the Changes of Zhou*. The Lao-Zhuang principles of stillness and emptiness are immediately apparent in *The Token for the Agreement of the Three*, and they are progressively developed in subsequent texts.

Wei Bo-Yang (魏伯陽) and *The Token for the Agreement of the Three*

The Token for the Agreement of the Three According to the Changes of Zhou (or simply *The Token for the Agreement of the Three*) is a seminal text of the internal alchemy tradition and the one that establishes the defining synthesis of exercise, breathing, and esoteric symbolism of internal alchemy. It ranks, along with *Lao zi, The Scriptures of the Exterior Landscape of the Yellow Court* (*Huang ting wai jing jing* 黃庭外景經), and *On the [Immediate] Awakening to Truth* (*Wu zhen pian* 悟真篇), as one of the four great classics of Daoist cultivation. A work that is concerned with the principles as opposed to the mechanics of internal alchemy, *The Token for the Agreement of the Three* explicitly endorses a life of quietism as a means of achieving immortality. The quest for immortality by internal means was historically preceded by an alchemical methodology that advocated the ingestion of elixirs blended from often-toxic substances such as lead and mercury, a practice Li vehemently opposed.[29] *The Token for the Agreement of the Three* makes extensive use of the language of external alchemy, and its putative author, Wei Bo-Yang, is presented in later works as an alchemist in both senses of the word: he was engaged in transformation by chemical and internal means. Nevertheless, this treatise is generally recognized as the text that marked the transition toward an emphasis on techniques of internal transformation. In addition, it blends the philosophy of the *Classic of Change* with that of *Lao Zi* to form the theoretical basis for the practice of internal alchemy. The symbolic language of *The Token for the Agreement of the Three*—combining symbolism from the *Classic of Change*, metaphorical use of chemical transmutation, and a variety of other fantastic imagery—defines the terminology used throughout the literature of internal alchemy.

There is some question as to whether Wei Bo-Yang was actually an historical figure. He is traditionally believed to have been an alchemist and philosopher of the 2nd century BCE who declined an appointment to court, preferring a life of personal cultivation. His involvement in external alchemy spawned an account in *Comprehensive Biographies of the Transcendents* (*Lie xian quan zhuan* 列仙全傳, 1368–1643) in which he tested two students whom he believed lacked complete faith in his skills. In what appeared to be a fatal bid to achieve alchemical immortality, he poisoned a dog, another disciple, and finally himself. Upon witnessing this carnage, his doubting students departed the scene. Wei thereupon revived himself, his faithful disciple, and even the dog, and these three went the way of the immortals. Wei paints a more prosaic description of himself and his motivations in Ch. 18 of *The Token for the Agreement of the Three.*

> A lowly man from the country of Kuai, who has no love for worldly power, glory, fame, or gains, who wastes his days leading a simple, quiet, leisurely, and peaceful life in a retreat in an unfrequented valley—such a one is the author of the present writing. The writings on the *I* [Change] by the three sages have a common goal, which is to propound according to the *Li* [Reason] and to cause the spirit to shine forth.[30]

The process of internal alchemy is described metaphorically in *The Token for the Agreement of the Three* as the preparation of a Golden Elixir (*jin dan* 金丹) that is formulated in a cauldron (*ding* 鼎) and furnace (*lu* 爐) by refining *(lian* 煉) lead and mercury using a precise methodology. The timing of the firing process is described in terms of the hexagrams of the *Classic of Change.* In practical terms, this transmutation is a protracted process requiring a variety of techniques that invariably involves stilling the mind and directing it inward. An early passage in *The Token for the Agreement of the Three* contains a typical statement of this essential principle:

> Attention should be turned to the well-being of the inner self so as to attain a state of perfect calmness and freedom from matter. The primordial substance, shining forth unseen, will illuminate the insides of the body.[31]

Yu Yan's (俞琰) *Elucidations on the Token for the Agreement of the Three According to the Changes of Zhou (Zhou yi can tong qi fa hui* 周易參同契發揮, 1284) is perhaps the most influential commentary on *The Token for the Agreement of the Three.* In remarking on the passage above, he points out its basis in Ch. 16 of *Lao Zi*: "Each one returns to its root. This is called tranquility. Tranquility, this means your life gate."[32]

Lady Wei and *The Yellow Court Scriptures*

The Yellow Court Scriptures is another of the earliest texts on internal alchemy.[33] Tradition holds that the text was transmitted to the mystic visionary Yang Xi 楊羲, 330-86) by Wei Hua-Cun (魏華存) or Lady Wei, the founder of the Great Purity Movement *(shang qing* 上清), during the 2nd century. It is paired with *The Scriptures of the Interior Landscape of the Yellow Court (Huang ting nei jing jing* 黃庭內景經), which is essentially an elaboration on the former. The book is devoted to an internal vision of the body wherein the student learns to see the form and function of the viscera as well as a variety of spirits that inhabit the body. *The Yellow Court Scriptures* attributes a spirit or divinity to each of the five viscera, six receptacles, the channel system, and the orifices. The text further assigns color, qi, form, and five phase locations to these spirits based on their function and location. In particular, it identifies a spirit of the brain and a spirit of the eyes, and it also identifies various unusual spirits within the body that are said to promote long life. It also stresses the importance of tranquility, the swallowing of pure fluids, and the accumulation of essence for the purpose of prolonging life. Li cites *The Scriptures of the Interior Landscape of the Yellow Court* in the context of the practice of conducting qi up the *du* vessel and down the *ren*.

Cui Xi-Fan (崔希范) and *Master Cui's Mirror on the Admixture of Medicines* (*Cui gong ru yao jing* 崔公入藥鏡)

Cui Xi-Fan lived during the Tang dynasty (618–906) and is best known as a Daoist adept and as the putative author of *Master Cui's Mirror on the Admixture of Medicines* in which he expounded extensively on the practice and theory of the arts of the internal elixir. The book exerted substantial influence on subsequent schools of internal alchemy through the Song and Yuan periods. Li Shi-Zhen cites this book in his chapters on the *du*.

Zhang Bo-Duan and *On the [Immediate] Awakening to Truth*

Zhang Bo-Duan (d. 1082) is the Daoist author quoted most directly by Li in the *Exposition*, whom he typically refers to by his courtesy name, Zhang Zi-Yang (張紫陽). Zhang's direct involvement with medicine is of particular interest for physicians. Trained in Daoist, Buddhist, and Confucian traditions, Zhang spent much of his life associating with Buddhists, although he did not reach realization until the age of 80 when a Daoist immortal appeared to him and instructed him in the deeper meaning of the Way. He subsequently composed *On the [Immediate] Awakening to Truth*. The text is regarded as a direct descendent of the seminal *The Token for the Agreement of the Three*, employing much of its terminology and developing its conceptual framework. Zhang's work is the basis for the Southern School (*nan zhong* 南宗) and contributed to the Complete Reality order (*quan zhen jiao* 全真教), but along with *The Token for the Agreement of the Three*, it has become a fundamental reference work for all schools of internal alchemy. Because Zhang Bo-Duan himself composed a book about the extraordinary vessels, his thoughts are particularly pertinent to Li's *Exposition*. The original manuscript of Zhang's *Eight Vessel Scripture (Ba mai jing* 八脈經) is no longer extant. The earliest surviving portion of the text first appears in *Exposition on the Eight Extraordinary Vessels*.

The alchemical texts mentioned in the *Exposition* are the basis for all schools of internal cultivation in China so it is impossible to definitively associate Li with any one strain of Daoist thought. His biographical material contains no mention of an affiliation with any specific school or teacher. The only definitive record we have of his interaction with any Daoist occurs during his time at the imperial court when he is believed to have come into conflict with them over matters of medical praxis. Yet, as already noted, Li Shi-Zhen had at least some personal experience with internal alchemy.

Internal Alchemy in *Exposition on the Eight Extraordinary Vessels*

Li Shi-Zhen's message regarding the relationship between internal alchemy and the extraordinary vessels is elegant in its simplicity. Stillness and emptiness are the ground from which the primordial yang springs, facilitating the activation of the extraordinary vessels. This opening is a phenomenon common to all the extraordinary vessels. Its focus is centered on the circulation of qi through the, *chong, ren,* and *du,* but it is dependent on the other extraordinary vessels in various ways. The *wei* vessels define the structural and energetic boundaries for this process of energetic refinement, known in alchemical terms as 'firing' *(lian* 煉). The *yin qiao* vessel connects the extraordinary vessels with the macrocosmic expression of the primal yang. The *dai* vessel regulates all of the other extraordinary vessels.

Stillness, Tranquility, and Emptiness in the *Exposition*

Stillness is not merely a prerequisite that may be dispensed with once the extraordinary vessels have been activated. It is the ongoing ground in which the extraordinary vessels are engaged. As if to drive this point home, Li's discussions of internal cultivation invariably conclude with some reference to emptiness. He establishes this pattern in his closing remarks of Ch. 2, after outlining the fundamental characteristics of the extraordinary vessels. Here, he makes his point indirectly in alluding to the Mysterious Female:

> For this reason, those who practice medicine and know of the eight vessels comprehend the great purpose of the 12 channels and 15 networks. Those who practice transcendence and know of the eight vessels miraculously attain the ascent and descent of the tiger and dragon, and the subtle aperture of the Mysterious Female.

As already noted, the Mysterious Female (*xuan pin* 玄牝 [34]) is a recurring theme in *Lao zi,* which states, "The valley spirit never dies, this is called the Mysterious Female." [35] Variously translated as Mysterious Female, [36] dark womb, [37] or mysterious femininity, there are at least two interpretations that bear on Li's use of the term. Wang Bi (王弼, 226–249), [38] among the most influential of the neo-Daoist *Lao zi* commentators, understands the Mysterious Female as an evocation of the emptiness that gives birth to all things.

> The spirit of the valley is comparable to the center of the valley, which is nothing, without form, without shadow, without opposing it and without going against it. It remains quite low and does not move. It holds on to quietude and does not decline. ... The gate is whence the subtle and profound female goes through. Following the path, which the female takes, it becomes one body with the ultimate. Therefore it is called the root of

heaven and earth. If we say it does not exist, the myriad things come into existence because of it. Therefore it is continuous and seems to be always existing.[39]

Such a perspective is later echoed by the Song dynasty commentator Su Zhe (蘇轍, 1039–1112), who observes:

> A valley is empty but has form. A valley spirit is empty but as no form. What is empty and has no form is not alive. So how can it die? Valley spirit refers to its virtue. Dark Womb [Mysterious Female] refers to its capacity. This womb gives birth to the ten thousand things and we call it dark because we see it give birth but not how it gives birth.[40]

Commentaries such as these suggest that Li Shi-Zhen's use of the term Mysterious Female may be more than a general reference to the Way. It is an explicit identification with the primordial emptiness that is a consequence of mastering regulation of yin and yang within the body. No less influential than Wang Bi, Daoist commentator He-Shang Gong (河上公, 2nd century BCE)[41] offers a more overtly cultivation-oriented yogic interpretation that also sheds light on Li's use of the term in an alchemical context:

> Dark refers to Heaven. In man, this means the nose, which links us with Heaven. Womb [female] refers to Earth. In man, this means the mouth, which links us to earth. The breath that passes through our nose and mouth should be finer than gossamer silk and barely noticeable, as if it weren't actually present. It should be relaxed and never strained or exhausted.[42]

In He-Shang Gong's interpretation, the development of breath control is the vehicle for achieving the goal of the regulation of yin and yang and is referred to in alchemical jargon as the ascent and descent of the dragon and tiger, or, alternately, the submission of the dragon and the taming of the tiger. The mysterious gate aperture *(xuan guan qiao* 玄關竅) is generally understood as having no fixed location. Practitioners identify a place within their body to rest their senses as a means of preparing the circumstances for the appearance of the mysterious gate aperture. Different traditions chose different locations for this practice, and the location typically varies from individual to individual.

Some schools place it just above the perineum. Katsuda Masayasu locates the mysterious gate aperture farther up, claiming that it is synonymous with the lower cinnabar field *(xia dan tian* 下丹田) or the acupuncture hole Stone Gate (CV-5), again placing the emphasis of the cultivation in the lower abdomen.[43] All of these interpretations are complementary reflections of one another and are consistent with the overall thrust of Li's message. They present an image of breath cultivation that promotes the regulation of yin and yang in the body and allows for a merging with the primordial emptiness. This is what Li is alluding to when he equates a familiarity with the extraordinary vessels to the "ascent and descent of the tiger and dragon, and the subtle aperture of the Mysterious Female."

The Mysterious Female appears throughout Li Shi-Zhen's *Exposition* as an allusion to the principles of stillness and quietude, yet Li stresses these ideas in a more direct manner elsewhere in the book. As we will demonstrate below, virtually every passage concerning internal alchemy explicitly mentions the role of stillness or emptiness in internal cultivation.

The Microcosmic Orbit and the *Du* Vessel

Given the prominence of the *du* vessel in many if not all methods of internal cultivation, it comes as no surprise that Li's chapter on the *du* contains the most extensive discussion on internal cultivation. Although stillness is a prerequisite to the effective manipulation of the extraordinary vessels, it is not in itself sufficient to achieve this goal. More specific means of activation are required.

Exposition on the Eight Extraordinary Vessels does not present an explicit methodology for opening the eight vessels, yet it does describe some of the general principles involved, and it alludes to some of the techniques used by adepts. Primary among these is the practice of circulating the qi up the *du* and down the *ren,* contrary to its normal flow, as a means of promoting health and longevity. This circuit is known today as the 'microcosmic orbit' *(xiao zhou tian* 小周天*)*.

In blending together passages from a wide range of alchemical texts, Li's discussion stresses the importance of activating the *ren* and the *du*, though not the actual procedure for doing so. This discourse is framed between references to the place of stillness, emptiness, and nonbeing in internal cultivation. Because it exemplifies every facet of Li's approach to inner alchemy in the extraordinary vessels, we will discuss it in some detail here. In Ch. 13, Li observes,

> Li Bin-Hu [Li Shi-Zhen] says that the two vessels of the *ren* and *du* are the human body's *zi* and *wu* [midday and midnight]. They are the elixir cultivator's pathways for the ascent and descent of the yang fire and the yin talisman. They are the place of intersection of *kun* water and *li* fire.

'Yang fire' refers to primal yang. According to Katsuda, the 'yin talisman' *(yin fu* 陰 符*)* is synonymous with another term, 'primal spirit' *(yuan shen* 元神*)*, which is the activity of conscious thought.[44] The Song dynasty commentator Gao Yi-Sun (高儀孫) equates the yin talisman to spirit in his *Classic of the Heavenly Mechanism of the Yin Talisman (Yin fu tian ji jing* 陰符天機經, Song Dynasty, 960–1341), which appears in Ding Fu-Bao's (丁福保) *Essential Flowers of the Daoist Canon (Dao zang jing hua lu* 道藏精華錄).

> In contemplating it, there is no shape, and in using it, there is no limit. The *Classic of Change* states that the unfathomable nature of yin and yang is

called spirit. "The yin talisman is an image of it." Therefore, even the sage cannot fathom this talisman. It prevails throughout the world but belongs nowhere.[45]

Li's use of alchemical imagery significantly expands the meaning of his discourse. The circulation of yin and yang within the *du* and *ren* is not limited to physiological function. It also extends to the realm of spiritual transformation and identification with the source. He develops this theme with a passage from *The Token for the Agreement of the Three*, linking specific locations on the *du* and *ren* to the process of internal cultivation:

> Therefore, Wei Bo-Yang, in *The Token for the Agreement of the Three*, states: "When the upper is closed, it is called being, and when the lower is closed, it is called nothingness. Nothingness is elevated to the upper [part or the body], and the spirit virtue resides in the upper [part of the body]. By means of this two-holed method, the golden qi also requires both [nothingness and being]."

Like all statements in the realm of inner alchemy, there are many levels of meaning associated with this passage. The most fundamental interpretation holds that when the upper is closed, the senses are sealed, shutting out external stimuli, not so much by closing one's eyes, but by directing one's gaze inward. When the lower is closed, the reproductive essence is retained. Both closures lie along the axis of the *du*.

Upper (*shang* 上) and lower (*xia* 下) may also be read as "most" and "least," slightly changing their meaning. Commentator Chen Zhi Xu (陳致虛), also known as Shang Yang-Zi (上陽子), and Chen Guan-Wu (陳觀吾, fl. 1333) added another overlay of *Classic of Change* symbolism to the passage that emphasizes the reciprocal relationship: the prenatal and postnatal world. According to Chen Zhi-Xu,

> The most obstructive is the trigram *kun*. When *kun* exerts its power, it is settled in and contracted. The being is the *wu* [earth], which lies in the central line of the trigram *kan* wherein lies the true single energy of the prenatal inner world. The least obstructive is termed nothingness. The least obstructive is the trigram *qian*. When *qian* exerts its power, it is settled, but diffused. The nothingness is the *ji* [soil], which lies in the central line of the trigram *li*, which is stored in the spontaneously arising water of the postnatal outer world.[46]

In this passage, *qian* 乾 ☰ and *kun* 坤 ☷ are atemporal or former heaven (*xian tian* 先天) representations of yin and yang, whereas *li* 離 ☲ and *kan* 坎 ☵ are temporal or latter heaven representations of yin and yang. The inner alchemist returns to the atemporal realm by "plucking [the yang line] from *kan* to fill [the yin line] of *li*" (*cai kan tian li* 採坎填離), thereby producing the atemporal *qian*. *Wu* and *ji* (戊己) are the middle heavenly branches, corresponding to the yang and yin aspects of earth in the five-phase system.

The last line of the passage from *The Token for the Agreement of the Three* is especially opaque. Richard Bertschinger translates 此兩孔穴法, 金氣亦雙須 as, "This is the law of the double entranced cave, where the gold and inner energies assist each other."[47] He notes that inner energies are the energies of "true lead," suggesting a reciprocal relationship between these alchemical substances.[48] Modern commentators Wang Luo-Zhen and Li Ding observe that the gold and qi *(jin qi* 金氣) in this passage was originally being and nothingness *(you wu* 有無) in *The Token for the Agreement of the Three,* making the line only slightly less murky. "By means of this two-holed method, the golden qi also requires both [being and nothingness]."[49]

Li continues these lines of inquiry with a passage from another influential treatise on internal alchemy by Cui Xi-Fan, which describes another aspect of the dynamic between the upper and lower aspects of the *du* vessel:

> Cui Xi-Fan in his *Mirror on the Admixture of Medicines to the Heavenly Origin (Tian yuan ru yao jing* 天元入藥鏡) states: "There is an Upper Magpie Bridge and a Lower Magpie Bridge. Heaven resonates with the stars [above], and the earth resonates with the tides [below]. [One must] restore the root aperture and return to Life Barrier, pass through the Caudal Funnel [perineum] and penetrate the Mud Ball.

This colorfully arcane imagery is a reference to the technique of reversing the qi in conducting it along the *ren* and *du*, and through the viscera. The 14th-century commentator Wang Dao-Yuan (王道淵) observes:

> In microcosmic circulation, one regards the spine of the human body as if it were the Milky Way in heaven. Since the Milky Way obstructs the two spirit bird bridge, which should meet once a year, a bridge must be built over the Milky Way. The human tongue is also called the magpie bridge. The alchemist must ask the Yellow Granny (*huang po* 黃婆) [the spleen] to beget an infant [kidney essence] and then raise this child to the mud ball [the brain] to mate with the Mythic Female *(cha nü* 姹女) [the heart]. ... From the mud ball, one lowers the kidney through the *ren* vessel down to the perineum alley, therefore this area is called the lower magpie bridge. The characters Yellow Granny and Mythic Female symbolize essence, spirit, and awareness (*yi* 意). The path of reclaiming life requires the transformation of the three gates by changing kidney essence into qi. The qi must slowly rise from the perianal region straight up to the mud ball to intersect with the spirit residing there in the base chamber.[50]

The last line of Cui's passage is reminiscent of Ch. 16 of *Lao zi,* which states: "Returning to the root is called stillness, and stillness is called reclaiming one's life."

Li next assigns a physical location for emptiness and quietude in the lower abdomen, referring to it as the Mysterious Female. *Direct Teaching of the Great Way in Three Chapters (Da dao san zhang zhi zhi* 大道三章直指, Ming era)[51] defines the boundaries of the cinnabar field in a model that orients the human body facing in a southerly direction, upon which the eight trigrams are superimposed.

> Cultivators of the elixir are possessed of a premier aperture in the body and this is called the Mysterious Female. "It is located directly below *qian*, above *kun*, to the west of *zhen* and east of *dui*, and is the place where *kan* and *li* mate. It is right in the center of the body's heaven and earth; the eight vessels, nine orifices, 12 channels, and 15 networks are all interconnected in this one grotto in the gap of emptiness and suspended in the void like pearls of barley."

This book is no longer extant, although the chapter on the Mysterious Female in the Yuan dynasty *Compass Pointer to the Principles of Contemplation (Gui zhong zhi nan* 規中指南) by Chen Xu-Bai (陳虛白) contains a similar paragraph. Li's point is that the *ren* and the *du* are extensions of this place of stillness. According to Li, again in Ch. 13:

> The two vessels of the *ren* and *du* [mentioned] in medical texts are where the primal qi is engendered, and the place from which the true breath arises. If cultivators of the elixir lack understanding of this opening, then the true breath is not engendered, and the transformation of the spirit is without foundation.

The role of the *ren* and the *du* as the active expressions of the true breath *(zhen xi* 真息) strengthens their relationship with the rest of the channel system. Li proceeds with a quotation by Yu Yan, an early and influential commentator on *The Token for the Agreement of the Three*, concerning the opening of the *ren* and the *du*, which unlocks all of the vessels in the body. It is worth noting that commentators repeatedly point out that the Mysterious Female is not a physical location or even necessarily a state of mind. It is an identification with primordial emptiness that transcends space and time. Here, the term is used in a much more limited sense.

> [T]he circulation of qi and blood within the human body ebbs and flows, day and night, without ceasing. The medical texts have the two vessels of the *du* and *ren*. "If a person can open these two vessels then all the hundreds of vessels can all be open."

Of course, the *du* and *ren* must be open to some extent simply for an individual to be alive. The opening referred to here is a deeper, more profound opening that reverberates throughout the primary channels, opening them in turn. Traditionally, however, such an opening of the *du* and *ren* does not necessarily extend to the other six extraordinary vessels. Apparently, these must be opened independently, presumably by means of other practices. Li continues in this vein with another passage that speaks to the longevity-conferring qualities of the microcosmic orbit:

> The heavenly channels are our body's Yellow Pathway, and our respiration comes and goes in relation to these. Deer movement through the Caudal Funnel enables the opening of the *du* vessel. Tortoise inhalation through one's nose enables the opening of the *ren* vessel. Hence, these two animals prolong life. These numerous theories are derived from the sublime and secret teachings of the River Vehicle[52] of the Elixir cultivators. [The lore] of herbal products and the art of firing [metals in alchemical preparation] are transmitted separately [in other texts].

The deer wags its tail and moves its yang through the spine. Hence it is associated with the *du* vessel. The deer refers to the genitals, perineum, and sacrum that are part of the alchemical process. The tortoise cannot be separated from its shell. It raises its head to breathe in through its nose, hence, it is associated with the *ren*. The deer and tortoise refer to exercises that specifically open the *du* and *ren*, although probably not the well-known 'animal frolics.' Of course, the association of the deer and the tortoise with the *du* and the *ren*, respectively, also finds expression in herbal medicine.

Li concludes his discussion of the *du* and *ren* with a passage attributed to Zhang Bo-Duan, here referred to as Ping-Shu (平叔), tying all the previous ideas together. Using the full complement of alchemical allusion, Zhang links the *du* vessel to the kidneys, primal yang, true yin, the *ren*, *chong*, and triple burner, and the primordial emptiness.

> Wang Hai-Cang says that, according to Zhang Ping-Shu, lead is the upright qi of the northern direction, which represents a drop of emerging true yang, and is a straight yang line in the middle of the trigram *kun* and is the expression of initial growth producing the Maternal Elixir; its bug is the tortoise, resulting in the two yin [lines] of [the trigram] *kan*. This [central line] is the earth's axis. This first yang line is the snake, and the root of heaven. Yang is engendered in the seed-store of the life gate, that which connects the primal qi, going and coming; thus, it functions below the umbilicus as the root of heaven and earth, the gate of the Mysterious Female flowing through the reversing yin and divided into three branches to become three vehicles. If one harbors incorrect thoughts, then it descends and leaks out. If one maintains correct thoughts, then it is stored and becomes lead. It ascends and reunites with *li*. It is further enhanced and becomes *qian*. The restoration of yin and transformation of yang is what facilitates the return to the origin. Having achieved emptiness and achieved quietude, thereby expressing the Way with spontaneity, [the adept] soars up and becomes transcendent.

The definitive source for this passage is unknown. The "upright qi of the northern direction" *(bei fang zhang qi 北方正氣)* is an allusion to the kidney qi. *Zhong [Li-Quan's] Transmission of the Dao to Lu [Dong-Bin]: A Collection (Zhong lu chuan dao ji 鍾呂 傳道集)* explains:

> Lead is that which engenders the primal yang qi within the kidneys. Within this qi is the water of the true unity. (鉛者腎中所生元陽之氣氣中有真一 之水)

The kidney essence that is the root of the entire body is called the maternal elixir *(dan mu 丹母)*.[53] The straight or yang line of the trigram *kan* reflects the initial point of yang that engenders the creation of everything. It is the yang that splits apart the undifferentiated One. Conversely, when used as an alchemical term, it refers to the coalescence of yang.

The 36th Difficult Issue of the *Classic of Difficulties* refers to the "moving qi between the kidneys below the umbilicus" as "the root of the 12 channels." Daoist meditators also refer to the "root of heaven and earth" as the "gate of the Mysterious Female." This location opens to the foot-reversing yin channel below, to the *du* vessel behind, to the *ren* vessel in front, and to the *chong* in the middle. If the qi is allowed to proceed in these channels in its normal direction, then the body matures and ages normally. However, if the flow of qi is reversed, then this promotes personal cultivation. The statement that the qi "ascends and reunites with *li* and is further enhanced to become *qian*" refers to the guiding of the heart-spirit to the head, the cultivation of the qi of pure yang and its "return to the origin."

Whatever happens in the alchemical process and regardless of the jargon used to describe it, the intended transmutation occurs in a state of emptiness and tranquility. Li's closing lines stress that the activity of the extraordinary vessels is also rooted in the stillness of the Way.

Opening the Way: Other Techniques for Activating the Extraordinary Vessels

The microcosmic orbit and its related techniques are easily integrated into the medical model of extraordinary vessel function presented in the *Inner Classic* and *Classic of Difficulties.* There is little to this aspect of alchemical praxis that challenges our existing notions of how the extraordinary vessels work. It is only in his quotations from Zhang Bo-Duan's *Eight Vessel Scripture* that Li's *Exposition* truly alters the playing field with regard to how the extraordinary vessels may be accessed. Zhang's perspective on the alchemical use of the extraordinary vessels challenges medically trained readers to view the extraordinary vessels in a new way.

Just as his quotations from the *Inner Classic* and *Classic of Difficulties* provide a theoretical rather than a practical framework for understanding the extraordinary vessels, Li's assumption appears to be that those involved in internal alchemy are already familiar with the mechanics of practice. This is, of course, consistent with much of the alchemical literature itself, which addresses the principles of transcendent practice that may be applied in whatever manner is most appropriate for a given student. The passages of *Eight Vessel Scripture* appearing in *Exposition on the Eight Extraordinary Vessels'* chapter on the *yin qiao* vessel (Ch. 6) are the earliest references to this material. All later references to *Eight Vessel Scripture* appear to draw from this, so we have no idea of the context in which the material originally appeared.[54] In light of this, one can only speculate on how Zhang Bo-Duan's perspective is meant to fit, if at all, into the more familiar model of extraordinary vessel function. Nevertheless, Zhang's model is not so unique as to be completely inaccessible, and it raises some intriguing questions for the medical use of the extraordinary vessels.

Focal Points of the Extraordinary Vessels

The key passage from *Eight Vessel Scripture* quoted by Li is concerned with specific points or areas associated with each of the extraordinary vessels.

> As for the eight vessels, the *chong* vessel is located below the Wind House (GV-16) hole, the *du* vessel is located behind the umbilicus, the *ren* vessel is located in front of the umbilicus, the *dai* vessel is located in the lumbar region, the *yin qiao* vessel is located in front of the perineum[55] below the scrotum, and the *yang qiao* vessel is located behind the perineum in the sacrococcygeal region.[56] The *yin wei* is located one *cun* and three *fen* in front of the vertex [of the skull], and the *yang wei* vessel is located one *cun* and three *fen* behind the vertex [of the skull].

These locations or focal points are the places that adepts must attend to in their efforts to open the extraordinary vessels. Rather than attending to the entire pathway of an extraordinary vessel, one's attention is directed toward a specific point or region. It is significant that all of these focal points are situated along the axis of the midline; however, the meaning of such an arrangement is unclear. Nevertheless, since the established trajectories of the *wei* and *qiao* vessels are only peripherally associated with the midline, it suggests a very different perspective on the distribution of the extraordinary vessels than Li has previously presented. A more thorough discussion of these locations appears in Ch. 7 of the present text. For now, our concern is with the larger picture suggested by Zhang Bo-Duan's perspective.

Such a model of extraordinary vessel activation is not entirely anomalous in the literature of internal alchemy. *Mind Seal of Profound Subtlety (Xuan wei xin yin* 玄微心印, Ming era),[57] a manual of sexual cultivation attributed to the Daoist Zi-Yang (紫陽), contains a chapter on the eight extraordinary vessels presenting much the same material. The only significant difference between *Mind Seal of Profound Subtlety* and

Eight Vessel Scripture is that the former locates the *dai* vessel on either side of the umbilicus.[58]

Notwithstanding the sometimes odd locations attributed to the extraordinary vessels, the basic principle of activating them as energetic entities separate from the rest of the channel system is not foreign to mainstream acupuncture practice. That is the assumption we make when we stimulate a pair of holes on the primary channels, such as Inner Pass (PC-6) and Yellow Emperor (SP-4), in an effort to mobilize the *yin wei* vessel. Zhang's interpretation of extraordinary vessel accessibility, however, is much more radical:

> People have these eight vessels, but they all remain hidden spirits because they are closed and have not yet been opened. Only divine transcendents can use the yang qi to surge through and open them so that they are able to attain the way. The eight vessels are the root of the great way of Former Heaven and the ancestor of the Unitary Qi. Only when the *yin qiao* is selected [for cultivation] first, and only when this vessel has been activated, will all the other vessels open.

In Zhang's estimation, the eight vessels are accessible only to a select few. Moreover, his reference to the surging of yang qi is understood not in the medical sense of pathological counterflow, but as an opening associated with spiritual realization. It flows not only upward, but throughout the body. Once the refining activity (*lian gong* 煉 功) of their alchemical transformation has reached a certain stage, adepts experience a warm sensation of qi movement that is referred to as "making the yang qi penetrate and open [all eight extraordinary vessels] (*yi yang qi chong kai* 以陽氣衝開)."[59] Zhang goes on to clarify that this yang qi is primal qi in the largest sense of the term. "The eight vessels are the root of the great way of Former Heaven and the ancestor of the Unitary Qi." Perhaps most remarkably, the *yin qiao* is primary in the sequence of extraordinary vessel activation.

The rationale for according the *yin qiao* such an exalted status is not immediately apparent, although the subsequent discussion suggests that the "location" of the *yin qiao* in the perineum is significant. The *yin qiao* is the axis of communication between the endogenous circulation of source qi and the universal pool of primal qi.

> Next, the three vessels of the *du*, *ren*, and *chong* [should be selected for cultivation because they] are the source of creation for all the other channels and vessels. And yet, mention of the particular vessel the *yin qiao* is scattered throughout the Cinnabar scriptures where it is variously referred to by many names. It is called Root of Heaven; it is called Death's Door; it is called Resurrection Pass; it is called Ghost Door of Feng Du; and it is called the Root of Life and Death. As the governor of the spirit, it is often called the Peach of Well-Being. Above, it penetrates the mud ball and below

it reaches down to Gushing Spring [KI-1]. If one has knowledge of [the *du, ren,* and *chong*], then one can induce the true qi to accumulate and dissipate [at will], all from these barrier orifices. Thus, the heavenly gate will be constantly open and Earth's Door will remain forever closed. The buttock vessel will flow throughout the entire body, linking and flowing freely both above and below, harmonious qi will naturally ascend to the imperial court. The yang will grow and the yin will diminish, fire will issue from the midst of water, and flowers will blossom through the snow. This is what is referred to by "When there is a languid ebb and flow between the Heavenly Root and the Moon Grotto, then the 36 officials are all spring-like."

Despite their clear association with the macrocosmic influences of primal yang, the extraordinary vessels are in many ways a closed system. The few oblique references in the medical literature to the aspects of extraordinary vessel function involving the activation of source qi require no exogenous communication. The tacit assumption is that whatever source qi one is mobilizing via the extraordinary vessels, it is coming from within the body and not from the outside. For that matter, the mainstream medical tradition offers no clear theoretical basis for explaining the means by which the source qi in the extraordinary vessels even communicates with and is reinvigorated by the true source. And yet, it is a basic assumption of internal alchemy that such communication is not only possible but essential. For Zhang and Li, the *yin qiao* provides just such a connection.

Zhang informs us that the *yin qiao* ascends to penetrate the mud ball, one of the Nine Palaces *(jiu gong* 九宮) in the head's marrow, and descends to Gushing Spring (KI-1) on the soles of the feet, and "If one has knowledge of [the *du, ren,* and *chong*], then one can induce the true qi to accumulate and dissipate [at will], all from these barrier orifices." Apparently, the *yin qiao* is crucial to the manipulation of primal qi through the barrier orifices *(guan qiong* 關竅), the sensory orifices in the upper part of the body. These sentiments are echoed in *Transcendent Mei Zhi's Odes for Collecting Medicinals (Mei Zhi xian cai yao ge ke jue* 梅志仙採藥歌口訣, probably Ming era), which states:

> The *yin qiao* is the Mud Ball, which circulates all the qi, penetrating downward to the earth's window, and issuing upward to the heavenly gate.[60]

Zhang Bo-Duan also tells us that in the literature of internal alchemy, the *yin qiao* is known by a variety of names including the Root of Heaven, Death's Door, Resurrection Pass, and Root of Life and Death. This is more than a laundry list of titles. These appellations are significant to our understanding of the role of the *yin qiao* in extraordinary vessel function.

A coalition of modern commentators known as the Japanese *Inner [Alchemy] Classic* Study Group *(Nippon Daikei Iggakukai* 日本內經醫學會) note that another text, *Instructions on Innate Nature and Lifespan (Xing ming gui zhi* 性命圭旨, 1615), contains very similar terminology. In its Chart of Reverse Illumination *(fan zhao tu* 反照圖), the *yin qiao* is given as an alternate name for a cultivator's focus on the perineum. This underlines the undesirability of conflating cultivation loci with acupuncture holes.

> The Perilous Emptiness is also called the Earth's door, or the Prohibited gate. This hole lies between the two vessels of the *ren* and *du*; above it penetrates the Heavenly Valley[61] and below it extends to Gushing Spring (KI-1). Hence, the ancient sages said: The heavenly gate should be constantly open and earth's door should remain forever closed. The accumulation and dissipation of essence qi should occur at this place.[62]

The Japanese *Inner Classic* Study Group argues that if one accepts the claim that the references to locations between the *ren* and *du* correspond to the acupuncture holes Meeting of Yin (CV-1) and Long and Strong (GV-1), then one must also accept the claim in *Eight Vessel Scripture* that the *yin qiao* is similarly located in the perineum. Given the range of names attributed to the *yin qiao* throughout the Daoist literature, it stands to reason that the reference to the mud ball and *yin qiao* in *Transcendent Mei Zhi's Odes for Collecting Medicinals* is in this case simply an allusion to the microcosmic orbit.[63]

Having outlined the fundamental relationships between the key alchemical components of the extraordinary vessels, Li tells us what to expect if they have been properly opened.

> When this is achieved, the body will become light and strong. The adept's aged countenance regains its vitality, in quiet silence he becomes recondite as if he were an imbecile or intoxicated. [Such experiences] are proof [of the effect].

A light and strong body certainly sounds appealing, a phase in the process of transcendent "lightening and brightening," as Livia Kohn describes it. But why would the adept act like a drunkard or an imbecile? This vision of the mind of the sage harkens back to *Lao zi* and *Zhuang zi*. What Roger Ames and David Hall refer to as the "unmediated potency of the child" is a common theme in *Lao zi*, where Ch. 55 informs us that "One who is vital in character *(de* 德) can be compared to a newborn baby."[64] According to Ames and Hall, "The people are able to remain childlike and to be treated as such because there is no master narrative in place that would discipline their experience and in so doing make it 'grown up'."[65] Unconditioned or unusual behavior is an essential characteristic of the sage in *Zhuang zi*, where the 'true person' *(zhen ren* 真人) acting spontaneously is free of social constraints. Zhuang zi himself laughed at his wife's funeral while another character made light of his own crippling deformities because he had undergone an internal transformation that revolutionized his perception of the world. The goal of internal alchemy is just such a transformation, and often results in behavior that appears irrational to those with a narrower perspective. Returning to more concrete matters even as he employs the symbolism of the *Classic of Change*, Zhang Bo-Duan turns our attention once again to the importance of the abdomen in alchemical transformation, a topic we will take up later.

In summarizing Zhang Bo-Duan's remarks, Li Shi-Zhen acknowledges the uniqueness of Zhang's perspective on the *yin qiao,* suggesting that its mention is more than a general reference to the microcosmic orbit. He closes with a reminder that, "In following the path along the inner landscape, only those who reverse the senses will be capable of an illuminated examination [of the eight vessels]." His mention of the "inner landscape" or "inner vistas" *(nei jing* 內景*)* refers to the practice of inwardly perceiving the physiological processes of the viscera, as described in *The Yellow Court Scriptures.*[66] Here this process is described as following a path *(sui dao* 隨道*)*, which is accompanied by a physical sensation of being conducted along an open road. The only means of accomplishing this task is by reversing the direction of the senses *(fan guan* 反觀*)*, a technique of preserving the spirit by "closing the sight and reversing the hearing *(shou shi fan ting* 收視反聽*)*." Once again, Li emphasizes the ground of quietude that is the basis of all alchemical transformation.

Trigram Symbolism Defines Extraordinary Vessel Topography

The language of internal cultivation is synonymous with the symbolism of the *Classic of Change*, metallurgical allegory, and animal imagery involving dragons, tigers, deer, and tortoises. Terminology such as this is evident in all of the passages concerning alchemy that appear in *Exposition on the Eight Extraordinary Vessels.* Li often uses the imagery of internal alchemy specifically to illustrate various aspects of extraordinary vessel topography and function.

Ch. 2 of the *Exposition* presents an overview of the general functions of each of the extraordinary vessels. Li's mention at the end of that chapter of the "ascent and descent of the tiger and dragon" is a reference to the goal of harmonizing the ascent and descent of yin and yang within the body.[67] His use of this jargon reflects more than a passing taste for the colorful imagery of internal cultivation. He is pointing out that the extraordinary vessels perform precisely this role of regulating yin and yang, and the ascending and descending functions of qi within the body.

Earlier in this chapter, Li summarizes the function of the *wei* vessels as follows: "The *yang wei* governs the exterior of the body while the *yin wei* governs the internal, and so they are referred to as *qian* and *kun.*" These two trigrams represent the fundamental yin-yang pair, and on the surface, Li's use of this symbolism appears to be little more than a passing reference to the yin-yang relationship between the two *wei* vessels. Yet these trigrams are laden with much richer imagery that is pertinent to his understanding of the extraordinary vessels, because *qian* and *kun* are the root trigrams from which the other six trigrams and the 64 hexagrams evolve. In *The Token for the*

Agreement of the Three, Wei Bo-Yang's description of these two trigrams details some of the imagery that Li is alluding to.

> *Qian* is firm and *kun* is yielding.
>
> They are fitted to embrace each other.
>
> As Yang endows, then Yin receives,
>
> The [masculine] cock and [feminine] hen depend on one other.
>
> It is this reliance that brings about creation and procreation.
>
> It is only then that the essence qi is spread afar.[68]

The Yielding and Receiving Qualities of *Qian* and *Kun*

The yielding and receiving qualities of *qian* and *kun* are expressed in the dynamic between the protective and nutritive qi in the *wei* vessels. The masculine and feminine aspects are expressed in terms of enveloping and being enveloped. Yu Yan's remarks on this speak directly to the point that Li is trying to make. The dynamic between *qian* and *kun* is one of opening and closing. According to Yu Yan, "There is a saying: As you breathe, so the firm and yielding rub against each other, so they form the very image of *qian* and *kun*, opening and closing."[69]

The relationship between the nutritive and the protective qi and the dynamic between the internal and exterior is precisely one of opening and closing. *Kun* also signifies the abdomen. Hence, the statement that *yin wei*, which is *kun*, arises from the meeting of all the yin may mean that it arises from the abdomen, the utmost internal.[70]

Qian and *kun* are also referred to as the 'cauldron' and 'furnace,' the structures within which the golden elixir of personal transformation will be refined. Such imagery is entirely consistent with the medical understanding of the *wei* vessels as the rope that draws together the net or the binding infrastructure of the channel system. Taken together, *qian* and *kun* represent the entire cosmos. Both in medicine and internal cultivation, the *wei* vessels define the bounds within which energetic activity occurs. Still, however, their influence of regulating the internal and exterior is peripheral to the deeper functions of the *chong*, *ren*, and *du*.

All of these resonances sound simultaneously in the language of internal alchemy. When Li states that the *wei* vessels are *qian* and *kun*, he is using a highly refined and richly textured set of images to evoke all of the essential physiological roles of these vessels.

In quoting a lengthy passage from the Zhang Bo-Duan's *Eight Vessel Scripture* in his chapter on the *yin qiao*, Li again employs a broad range of alchemical jargon to identify the precise physical location of primal qi within the body.

> The buttock vessel will flow throughout the entire body linking and flowing freely both above and below, harmonious qi will naturally ascend to the

imperial court. The yang will grow and the yin will diminish, fire will issue from the midst of water, flowers will blossom through the snow. This is what is referred to as the languid comings and goings of heaven's root and the moon's grotto, and the thirty-six palaces are all spring-like.

The southwest is the direction associated with the trigram *kun*, which, as previously noted, pertains to the abdomen. According to *Appended Commentaries of the Classic of the Changes of Zhou* (*Zhou yi jing xi ci* 周易經系辭, ca. 7th century BCE), the territory of *kun* is the abdominal region. Zhang Bo-Duan is elaborately defining the location of the cinnabar field, the place within the body that primal qi is engendered. Katsuda believes that it is found in front of the Caudal Funnel (*wei lü* 尾閭) or the perianal region, which is specifically a reference to the acupuncture hole Meeting of Yin (CV-1). In internal alchemy, however, the Caudal Funnel is a general region upon which one contemplates, not a specific point.

Conclusions

Despite the challenge that the alchemical strata of the *Expositions* poses for our understanding of the extraordinary vessels, this material offers a rich source of insight that bears directly on their application in medicine. Li's brief references to internal alchemy are not merely an adjunctive line of inquiry, appended as an after thought to the purely medical material. An alchemical perspective focusing on personal transformation is a defining characteristic of Li's approach to the extraordinary vessels.

The role of the eight vessels in communicating primal yang throughout the body is best facilitated in a state of stillness. The transmission of primal qi is mediated to one extent or another through all eight of the vessels, and by way of the *chong, ren,* and *du* in particular. The *yin qiao* establishes the primary axis of communication between the endogenous circulation of qi within the body and the exogenous influence that pervades all things. It primes the pump of the microcosmic orbit.

From an alchemical viewpoint, the extraordinary vessels are only 'open' when they are consciously activated by a skilled adept. Li obviously believes that the concept of whether the extraordinary vessels are open or available goes well beyond self-cultivation and bears directly on their medical applications. The ramifications of such a perspective are profound, but unclear. His integrative vision of extraordinary vessel function demands that they be engaged in some way beyond simply selecting the correct acupuncture holes and herbal formulas. Regardless of the specific technique involved, this method of activation is unequivocally grounded in quietude. One question that Li's *Exposition* does not speak to is who exactly is doing the opening in a therapeutic setting. Perhaps Li intends for us to interpret Zhang Bo-Duan's remarks in such a way that the skilled adepts are understood as opening the extraordinary vessels not only within themselves but within their patients as well. It seems unlikely that Li intended for the therapeutic use of the eight vessels to be limited to those lucky few whose channels were already open. This is poignant when one considers that those who are sickest stand to benefit most from effective extraordinary vessel treatment. The most reasonable conjecture is that both the physician and the patient play an essential role in creating the proper conditions for optimal extraordinary vessel activation.

Li's interpretation of the extraordinary vessels suggests that they may be conceptualized as having two interrelated layers of function. First, there are the aspects of extraordinary vessel physiology that have little or no bearing on the transmission of source/primal qi whatsoever. Not the least of these are the role of the *wei* and the *qiao* vessels in regulating the protective and nutritive qi, or their diurnal conduction of qi between the internal and exterior. Functions such as these, and the extraordinary vessels' capacity for receiving the overflow from the primary channels, are the foremost concern of the mainstream medical literature. For the most part, the herbal and acupuncture prescriptions in the *Exposition* are not directed at influencing source qi in the extraordinary vessels. At the same time, these capacities are embedded within a deeper and more generalized milieu of activity that is devoted to the transmission of source/primal qi throughout the body.[71] The relationship between source qi and the extraordinary vessels is most highly developed in the literature of internal alchemy. It is unclear how these two levels of function are meant to interact, yet there is little doubt that Li interprets them as working in an integrated manner.

An Overview of Extraordinary Vessel Pulse Diagnosis

Diagnosis in Chinese medicine optimally relies on both subjective and objective information. Our patients must tell us their complaints, but it is equally important that we have independent means of assessing their condition. It is difficult to have any real confidence in one's diagnosis based on subjective information alone. Hence, we rely heavily on the information gleaned from the tongue, pulse, and abdomen. In a sense, this is how we most immediately interact with a patient's qi. A variety of diagnostic techniques appear sporadically throughout *Exposition on the Eight Extraordinary Vessels.* Li Shi-Zhen discusses both abdominal palpation and the palpation of holes on the chest in the context of the *chong.* For Li, however, pulse diagnosis is the objective assessment of choice, and he discusses its role in the pathology of every extraordinary vessel. To drive this point home, he devotes a closing section specifically to the pulses of the extraordinary vessels.

We will consider the role of each individual extraordinary vessel pulse as it appears throughout Li's *Exposition,* and we will examine them in greater depth both individually and together in our commentary on the final chapter of the *Exposition.* For now, however, we will present a brief overview of the pulses attributed to the extraordinary vessels.

The majority of the pulse images described in the *Exposition* are derived from Wang Shu-He (王叔和). In describing the eight extraordinary vessel pulses, Wang's *Pulse Classic* makes use of an arcane system of pulse diagnosis known as 'The Hand Diagram of the 31 Locations' (*Shou jian tu san shi yi bu* 手檢圖三十一部). We refer to it in this text simply as the Hand Diagram. The pulses in the Hand Diagram are described in a manner that differs significantly from the standard means of pulse description. In addition to the familiar distal (*cun* 寸), middle (*guan* 關), and proximal (*chi* 尺) pulse divisions, the radial pulse is also divided longitudinally into lateral (*wai* 外), midline (*zhong* 中), and medial (*nei* 內) positions yielding a grid containing nine positions. Each position is assigned a corresponding channel. For instance, the lateral aspect of the distal position on the wrist pulse corresponds to the bladder channel and the medial aspect of the proximal position on the wrist pulse corresponds to the kidney channel (see Fig. G-1 and Table G-1).

Extraordinary vessel pulses are described in terms of their situation on this grid. In this system, extraordinary vessel pulses are distinguished from primary channel pulses in that they invariably occupy multiple grid positions. For instance, the *yang wei* pulse travels "from the [foot] lesser yin obliquely to the [foot] greater yang," covering at least three primary pulse positions.

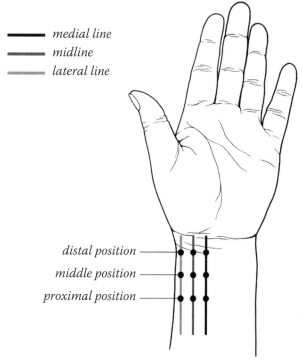

- medial line
- midline
- lateral line

distal position
middle position
proximal position

Fig. G-1 Pulse positions from the "Hand Diagram" of the *Pulse Classic*

	LATERAL	MIDLINE	MEDIAL
DISTAL	Bladder	Heart	Liver
MIDDLE	Stomach	Heart master	Spleen
PROXIMAL	Gallbladder	Lung/Large intestine	Kidney

Table G-1 Channel correspondences from the "Hand Diagram" of the *Pulse Classic*

The extraordinary vessel pulse images that originated in the *Pulse Classic* have been interpreted in a variety of ways over the centuries. In an effort to make these pulses more accessible and to eliminate many of their inherent inconsistencies, subsequent commentators have progressively simplified their interpretation of this material. Such refinements have produced a much more manageable model of pulse diagnosis, although this has been achieved at the cost of ignoring some important details. Nevertheless, for readers unfamiliar with extraordinary vessel pulse diagnosis, a simplified version of the extraordinary vessel pulses is an ideal way to begin grappling with what they might actually feel like under one's fingers. Table G-2 is such a précis. It is the interpretation of the modern extraordinary vessel pulse researcher Katsuyasu Kido, who based his material on a presentation of the extraordinary vessel pulses by Li Zhong-Zi (李中梓, 1588–1655), a contemporary of Li Shi-Zhen.[1]

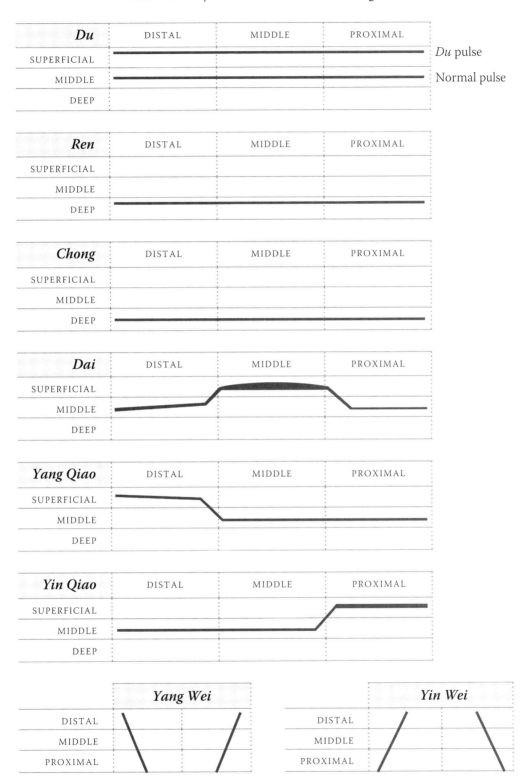

Table G-2

In the chapters that follow, it will quickly become apparent that Kido's assessment of the extraordinary vessel pulses is the product of a great deal of creative interpretation. This is a testament to the difficulty of making any practical sense of these pulses. His interpretation is far from definitive. Nevertheless, it provides an easily accessible starting point for this inquiry into the pulse images of the extraordinary vessels.

Part II

*Exposition on the Eight
Extraordinary Vessels*

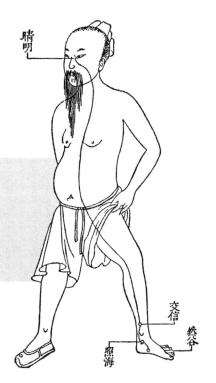

Part II presents an annotated translation of Li Shi-Zhen's *Exposition on the Eight Extraordinary Vessels,* along with the original Chinese. The annotations here are concerned primarily with different readings of the passages cited by Li, and with variations in hole locations. The chapters are arranged in the order in which they appear in the *Exposition.*

Prefaces

I. 題《奇經八脈考》 Inscription to
Exposition on the Eight Extraordinary Vessels

奇經八脈聞之久矣而不解其奧今讀瀕湖李君《八脈考》原委精詳
經絡貫徹頓覺蒙開塞決胸次豁然誠仙醫二家入室指南也然匪易牙
亦未易味之李君博極群書參討今古九流百氏鹹有撰述此特其一臠
爾因僭述其概而題之

隆慶壬申 (1572 年)，中秋日　道南　吳哲　拜題

I have heard about the eight extraordinary vessels for a long time, and yet I have not understood its profundities. Having now read Mr. Li Bin-Hu's[1] *Exposition on the Eight Vessels*, its detail and precision regarding the channels and networks has penetrated through to immediately awaken me from my ignorance and open the obstructions [in my understanding]. My chest rests easily now that there is indeed a masterful guide [uniting] the two schools of the transcendents and physicians. Unless one is [as talented as] Yi Ya, one cannot easily taste the flavor [of the extraordinary vessels].[2] Mr. Li is extremely well-read and has examined both modern and ancient literary forms and [has] written [and] expounded on all nine schools and the hundred scholars, and so this particular book is just a single slice of [his overall corpus of work]. For this reason, I have made the presumption of describing its contents and inscribing it [here].

On the *ren shen* year (1572) of the *Longqing* reign during the mid-autumn solar period,[3] in Daonan, Wu Zhe humbly inscribes this.

II. 《奇經八脈考》引 Preface to
Exposition on the Eight Extraordinary Vessels

《奇經八脈考》者李君瀕湖所撰輯以活人者也經有正有奇獨考奇
者奇經人所略故致詳焉並病原治法靡不條具若指諸掌豈惟醫學有
賴玄修之士亦因以一見身中造化真機矣用心之勤如此何其仁哉！
瀕湖世儒兼以醫鳴一門父子兄弟富有著述此特見一斑耳問不佞嘗
推其直諒多聞之益因僭識簡端以告後之君子

明萬曆丁丑 （1577 年） 小暑日　同裏　日巖　顧問　頓首書

Exposition on the Eight Extraordinary Vessels is written and edited by Mr. Li Bin-Hu for those who would vitalize people. Of channels, there are primary and extraordinary, and in considering the extraordinary, these are the extraordinary channels, of which people know little and they are therefore detailed here. Moreover, the book deals with both the origins of disease and also treatment methods. Each paragraph is as complete as all the fingers in the palm. How can one rely on medical studies alone? The practitioners of subtle cultivation have, for their part, already seen the true dynamic of creation within their bodies. In utilizing the activity of one's mind like this, how beneficial could that be! Mr. Bin-Hu is a scholar of our time, and his medical knowledge is well known.[4] Within a single household, fathers, sons, elder and younger brothers alike have produced an abundance of writings, and it is particularly apparent that they are talented. Were this humble one to be asked, [I would say that Li] had already abundantly demonstrated the virtues of uprightness, sincerity, and many have heard! For this reason, I humbly record this simple forward to inform those gentleman who follow.

Written during the the Ming dynasty in the *Wanli* reign on the *ding chou* day (July 7th, 1577) during the slight summerheat solar term, at Tongli, by Advisor Ri Yan, who respectfully writes this.

III. Preface to the Reprinting of *Pulse Studies* and *Exposition on the Eight Extraordinary Vessels*

重刻脈學奇經八脈序余奉中丞夏公教既刻《本草綱目》矣臨川令
袁君與李君時珍鄉人也復取其《脈學》與《奇經八脈考》示餘曰
李君平生學力盡在此幸並刻之為全書余

At the time I was elevated to Vice Censor-in-Chief by the Honorable Educator Xia, I had already published *Comprehensive Outline of the Materia Medica*. Mr. Yuan, the District Magistrate of Lin Chuan, and Mr. Li Shi-Zhen were from the same village. [Mr. Yuan encouraged me] to republish [Li's] *Pulse Studies* and his *Exposition on the Eight Extraordinary Vessels*, proclaiming that the entirety of the knowledge accumulated throughout Mister Li's life was contained in this [body of work]. It is fortunate that these have now been published together in a comprehensive volume.

念古良醫治疾未有不先診脈者自軒岐已然辨人鬼別男女特其粗爾
微茫呼吸之間而生死輕重系焉如濟北才人顏色不變而在死法中其
脈病也故曰無數者同之有數者異之苟不明乎脈之法則所同者多矣

I believe that when treating disease, skilled physicians of antiquity never failed to first diagnose the pulse, and it has been thus since the time of Xuan[5] and Qi [Bo]. [By means of the pulse, physicians could] distinguish man from ghost, differentiate men from women, and specify the roughness or complexity [of their constitutional predispositions]. The balance of life and death hung [in their capacity to discern] the slightest subtlety in the interval between exhalation and inhalation. For instance, [there was a case in which] the facial color of a talented man from the north of Shandong (*Ji bei* 濟北) did not change, but that he was dying was evident as his pulse was diseased. For this reason, those lacking [in the knowledge of such pulse] calculations [treat a variety of different presentations] as the same, but those who have [knowledge of such pulse] calculations treat them differently. When one [is] unclear about the methods of pulse diagnosis, there will indeed be many things that [one will erroneously treat as the] same!

脈學者專辨《脈訣》之誤也今之醫者無不誦《脈訣》而李君謂非
叔和著特條列而正之然非李君之言也宋陳無擇嘗斥為高陽生作矣
亦非無擇之言也朱晦翁嘗譏其鄙淺偽書矣《脈訣》行而《脈經》
隱《脈訣》之誤既明《脈經》其可復興乎

Pulse Studies specializes in identifying the errors in *Pulse Rhymes*. The physicians of today, without exception, recite the *Pulse Rhymes*, and Master Li asserts that [Wang] Shu-He is not its author, and moreover, lists the specific items [in *Pulse Rhymes* that are in error] and corrects them. Yet, [physicians today] deny Mr. Li's words. By the Song, Chen Wu-Ze had already rejected the opinion that Gao Yang-Sheng was the author [of *Pulse Rhymes*], and yet [physicians today] also deny Wu-Zhe's words.

Zhu Hui-Weng would have ridiculed the shallowness of such a fraudulent document [as *Pulse Rhymes*].[6] With the success [and popularity] of *Pulse Rhymes*, the *Pulse Classic* has faded into oblivion, although because the errors in *Pulse Rhymes* are so blatant, the *Pulse Classic* should be revived!

奇經八脈者其名出於《難經》而其論源於《素問》以非十二經之
正故謂之奇也昔淳於意拜受公乘陽慶脈書奇咳術即此世之醫者且
不能與其數況通其義乎

The eight extraordinary vessels get their name from the *Classic of Difficulties*, and as originally discussed in *Basic Questions*, they are not part of the 12 primary channels, and for this reason they are considered extraordinary. In former times when Chun Yu-Yi respectfully received the pulse writings of the honorable Cheng Yang-Qing, how extraordinarily marvelous that the art was as this![7] If physicians of this generation do not even know [the diagnostic] calculations [of the eight extraordinary vessels], how could they then penetrate their significance?

叔和曰瓦雨降下溝渠溢滿聖人不能圖也脈絡流溢諸經不能複復拘
也然則八脈可以不講乎八脈明而脈理盡矣脈理盡而病無不察可以
窮吾治之之方矣語云人之所病病疾多而醫之所病病道少通乎脈學
又通乎八脈之學道其患少也乎哉因並刻附於本草之後

[Wang] Shu-He said: When the rain fell down from the tiles, brimming over the irrigation canals and ditches, even sages were unable to manage this. When the vessels
and networks flow and spill over, none of the channels can again be controlled, and
thus, how could one ignore the eight vessels? But having [now] understood the eight
vessels, the principles of the vessels are complete. With the principles of the vessels
complete, there is no illness that cannot be examined, and one can exhaust [the potential scope] of methods of curing them. As the saying goes, "What people suffer from
are a multiplicity of diseases, and what physicians suffer from is a dearth of ways to
treat those diseases." When one penetrates the study of the pulse and also penetrates
the study of the eight vessels, then isn't the way of those who suffer lessened? Therefore, I have appended [these two works] to the end of this edition of *[Comprehensive
Outline of the] Materia Medica*.

癸卯秋七月上浣長洲張鼎思書

Written by Zhang Ding-Si on the *gui mao* year (1663) in the autumn of the seventh
month in Changzhou.

IV. Preface to the *Four Treasuries* Edition

提要 Summary

臣等謹案奇經八脈考一卷明李時珍撰其書謂人身經脈有正有奇手
三陰三陽足三陰三陽為十二正經陰維陽維陰蹻陽蹻衝任督帶為八
奇經正經人所共知奇經醫所易忽故特評其病源治法並枲考諸家之
說薈粹成編其原委精詳經緯貫徹洵辨脈者所不可廢又創為氣口九
道脈圖暢發內經之旨而詳其診法尤能闡前人未洩之秘

We sincerely record that *Exposition on the Eight Extraordinary Vessels* in one *juan*
by Li Shi-Zhen of the Ming dynasty states that among the channels and vessels of
the human body there are primary [channels] and extraordinary [vessels]. The three
yin [channels] on the hands and three yang [channels] on the feet are the 12 primary
channels. The *yin wei, yang wei, yin qiao, yang qiao, chong, ren, du,* and *dai* are the
eight extraordinary vessels. The primary channels are well known to many people, but
the eight extraordinary vessels are easily overlooked. For this reason, [this book] specifically reviews the origins of [extraordinary vessel] disease states and their treatment

methods, and it checks and assesses the statements of all schools [of medicine], compiling them and weaving them together. Its coverage of all the essentials and details, including its full grasp of the warp and the weft [of the channel system], indeed cannot be disregarded by those who would differentiate among the vessels. [the *Exposition*] also created a pulse diagram of the nine pathways of the qi opening, bringing forth the [original] intention of the *Inner Classic*. By detailing its diagnostic methods, it clarifies the secrets that had not been divulged by our predecessors.

考明初滑壽嘗撰十四經發揮一卷於十二經外益以督任二脈舊附刊
薛已醫案之首案薛已醫案（凡二本其一本不載此書）醫家據為繩
墨時珍此書更加精核然皆根據《靈樞》《素問》以究其委曲而得
其端緒遞推遞密雖一技亦然矣

Consider that Hua Shou of the Ming [dynasty], the author of *Elucidation of Fourteen Channels (Shi si jing fa hui)*, described the 12 major channels and the *du* and *ren* [in his book]. And in the preface to the early edition of *Xue Yi's Case Records (Xue yi yi an)*,[8] he encouraged physicians to rely on these principles. In this book, [Li] Shi-Zhen included even more careful and intensive examination, and although it is based on the *Divine Pivot* and *Basic Questions*, he studied their ins and outs in ultimate detail and figured out how to handle this information. He then transmitted and promulgated their secrets [to later generations]. Although [this was] but one branch [of his work], it was thus [that he did all things].

Editor-in-Chief Minister Ji Yun (紀昀), Minister Lu Xi-Xiong (陸錫熊), and Minister Sun Shi-Yi (孫士毅)

Chief Compiler (總校官) Minister Lu Fei-Chi (陸費墀)

乾隆四十四年三月恭校上。

Most respectfully compiled in the third month of the 44th year of the *Qianlong* reign [April/May 1779].

CHAPTER 1

奇經八脈總說

An Overview of the Eight Extraordinary Vessels

凡人一身有經脈絡脈直行曰經旁支曰絡經凡十二手之三陰三陽足
之三陰三陽是也絡凡十五乃十二經各有一別絡而脾又有一大絡並
任督二絡為十五也（難經作陰絡陽絡）共二十七氣相隨上下如泉
之流如日月之行不得休息故陰脈營於五臟陽脈營於六府陰陽相貫
如環無端莫知其紀終而復始其流溢之氣入於奇經轉相灌溉內溫臟
腑外濡腠理

People have channel vessels and network vessels throughout their bodies. Those that
travel longitudinally are called channels, while those that branch off are called networks. There are 12 channels [consisting of] three yin and three yang of the hand,
and the three yin and three yang of the foot. There are 15 networks. Each of the 12
channels has its own branching network, and the spleen also has a great network. In
addition, with the two networks of the *ren* and *du* [vessels], there are 15 [networks].
(The *Classic of Difficulties* posits a yin network and a yang network.) Combined, the
27 qi [of the channels and networks] move up and down together as if flowing from a
spring, moving like the sun and moon without rest.[1] Thus, the yin vessels manage [the
qi] in the five yin viscera while the yang vessels sustain the six yang receptacles. Yin
and yang connect with each other in an endless circuit in which there is no discernable
break. Upon reaching the end, it just starts again. The overflow of qi [from the channels and networks] enters the extraordinary vessels, providing reciprocal irrigation,
interiorly warming the yin viscera and yang receptacles, and exteriorly moistening
the interstices.

奇經凡八脈不拘制於十正經無表裡配合故謂之奇蓋正經猶夫溝渠
奇經猶夫湖澤正經之脈隆盛則溢於奇經故秦越人比之天雨降下溝
渠溢滿滂沛妄行流於湖澤此發靈素未發之秘旨也

The eight extraordinary channels are altogether eight vessels that are not controlled
by the 12 main channels, nor are they arranged in exterior-interior combinations,
and therefore they are called extraordinary. The main channels are like irrigation
ditches, and the extraordinary channels are like lakes and marshes. When the vessels

of the main channels are swollen and abundant, they overflow into the extraordinary channels. Thus it was that Qin Yue-Ren compared this to when the "rains pour down from heaven, the irrigation ditches overflow, the rain floods rush wildly, flowing into the lakes and marshes." This is the revelation of the secret meaning not presented in *Divine [Pivot]* and *Basic [Questions]*.

八脈散在群書者略而不悉醫不知此罔探病機仙不知此難安爐鼎時
珍不敏參考諸說萃集於左以備學仙醫者簽蹄之用云

[Discussions of] the eight vessels scattered throughout the masses of [medical] texts are sketchy and incomplete. If physicians are not aware [of such theories of the extraordinary channels], they will remain in the dark as to the cause of disease. If [aspiring] transcendents are not aware [of the more comprehensive theories of the extraordinary channels], it will be difficult for them to tame the furnace and the cauldron. [Although I,] Li Shi-Zhen, am not clever, I have carefully considered the statements of all [the various schools] and compiled them below to allow both transcendents and physicians to trap and snare these useful words.

CHAPTER 2

八脈

The Eight Vessels

奇經八脈者陰維也陽維也陰蹻也陽蹻也衝也任也督也帶也陽維起
於諸陽之會由外踝而上行於衛分陰維起於諸陰之交由內踝而上行
於營分所以為一身之網維也陽蹻起於跟中循外踝上行於身之左右
陰蹻起於跟中循內踝上行於身之左右所以使機關之踐捷也

The eight extraordinary vessels consist of the *yin wei, yang wei, yin qiao, yang qiao, chong, ren, du,* and *dai.* The *yang wei* arises at the meeting of all the yang and travels upward from the outer ankle in the protective aspect; the *yin wei* arises at the intersection of all the yin and travels upward from the inner ankle in the nutritive aspect, and [together] they constitute a binding network for the entire body. The *yang qiao* arises from within the heel, traversing the outer ankle and traveling upward on both sides of the body; the *yin qiao* arises from within the heel, traversing the inner ankle and moving upward on both [sides] of the body, and [together] they allow nimble springing [movement] of the organism.

督脈起於會陰循背而行於身之後為陽脈之總督故曰陽脈之海任脈
起於會陰循腹而行於身之前為陰脈之承任故曰陰脈之海衝脈起於
會陰夾臍而行直衝於上為諸脈之衝要故曰十二經脈之海帶脈則橫
圍於腰狀如束帶所以總約諸脈者也

The *du* vessel arises at the meeting of the yin, traverses the back, and proceeds along the posterior of the body such that it is the Director General [of the yang vessels]. Hence, it is called the sea of the yang vessels. The *ren* vessel [also] arises at the meeting of the yin, traverses the abdomen and proceeds along the front of the body such that it is the official controller of the yin vessels. Hence, it is called the sea of the yin vessels. The *chong* [also] arises at the meeting of the yin and travels to hug the umbilicus where it surges directly upward, constituting an essential thoroughfare for the various vessels. Hence, it is called the sea of the 12 channels. The *dai* vessel winds around the lumbar region in the form of a binding girdle, making it the overall commander of all the channels.

是故陽維主一身之表陰維主一身之裏以乾坤言也陽蹺一身左右之
陽陰蹺主一身左右之陰以東西言也督主身之陽任衝主身之陰以南
北言也帶脈橫束諸脈以六合也

Hence, the *yang wei* governs the exterior of the entire body while the *yin wei* governs the interior of the entire body, and so they are referred to as *qian* and *kun*. The *yang qiao* governs the yang [aspect] of the left and right side of the entire body while the *yin qiao* governs the yin [aspect] of the left and right side of the entire body so they are referred to as east and west. The dai vessel horizontally binds all the vessels so it is referred to as the six directions.

是故醫而知乎八脈則十二經十五絡之大旨得矣仙而知乎八脈則虎
龍升降玄牝幽微之竅妙得矣

For this reason, those who practice medicine and know of the eight vessels comprehend the great purpose of the 12 channels and 15 networks. Those who practice transcendence and know of the eight vessels miraculously attain the ascent and descent of the tiger and dragon, and the subtle aperture of the Mysterious Female.

CHAPTER 3

陰維脈
The *Yin Wei* Vessel

陰維起於諸陰之交其脈發於足少陰築賓穴為陰維之郤在內踝上五
寸腨分中上循股內廉上行入小腹合足太陰厥陰少陰陽明於府舍
（在腹結下三寸去腹中行四寸半）上會足太陰於大橫腹哀（大橫
在腹裏下三寸五分腹哀在日月下一寸五分並去腹中行四寸半）循
脅肋會足厥陰於期門（直乳下一寸半）上胸膈挾咽與任脈會於天
突廉泉上至頂前而終（天突在結喉下四寸半宛宛中。廉泉在結喉
上二寸中央是穴）凡一十四穴

The *yin wei* arises from [its places of] intersection of all the yin.[1] Its vessel issues from the foot lesser yin hole, Guest House (KI-9), which is the cleft [hole] of the *yin wei*, [and is located] five *cun* above the inner ankle in the parting of the flesh of the calf.[2] It proceeds along the inner thigh, traveling upward to enter the lower abdomen where it unites with the foot greater yin, reversing yin, lesser yin, and yang brightness at Abode (SP-13) (which is located three *cun* below the Abdominal Knot (SP-14) [hole], four-and-a-half *cun* lateral to the midline of the abdomen).[3] [The vessel] ascends to meet the foot greater yin at the Great Horizontal (SP-15) and Abdominal Lament (SP-16) holes (Great Horizontal is located one-and-a-half *cun* below Abdominal Lament, and Abdominal Lament is located one-and-a-half *cun* below Sun and Moon (GB-24); all of these holes are located four-and-a-half *cun* lateral to the midline of the abdomen).[4] [From here, the vessel] proceeds along the rib-sides to meet with the foot reversing yin at Cycle Gate (LR-14) (located one-and-a-half *cun* directly below the nipple).[5] [The *yin wei* vessel then] ascends to the chest and diaphragm and the throat to meet with the *ren* vessel at Celestial Chimney (CV-22) and Ridge Spring (CV-23). It then ascends to the front of the vertex and terminates (Celestial Chimney is in a depression four-and-a-half *cun* below the laryngeal prominence. Ridge Spring is located two *cun* above the laryngeal prominence and this hole is right in the center.[6]) There are 14 holes in all.

CHAPTER 4

陽維脈

The *Yang Wei* Vessel

陽維起於諸陽之會其脈發於足太陽金門穴在足外踝下一寸五分上
外踝七寸會足少陽於陽交為陽維之郄（在外踝上七寸斜屬二陽之
間）循膝外廉上髀厭抵少腹側會足少陽於居髎（在章門下八寸監
骨上陷中）

The *yang wei* arises from [the places it] meets with all the yang. Its vessel issues from
the foot greater yang hole, Metal Gate (BL-63), which is located one-and-a-half *cun*
below the outer ankle.[1] It ascends seven *cun* above the outer ankle to meet the foot
lesser yang [channel] at Yang Intersection (GB-35), the cleft [hole] of the *yang wei*
(located seven *cun* above the outer ankle beside the space between the two yang).[2] It
proceeds along the lateral aspect of the knee, ascending the thigh, and bores inward to
reach the sides of the lower abdomen to meet the foot lesser yang at Squatting Bone-
Hole (GB-29) (located eight *cun* below Camphorwood Gate [LR-13] in a depression
on the hip bone).[3]

循脅肋斜上肘上會手陽明手足太陽於臂臑（在肘上七寸兩筋罅陷
中肩髃下一寸）過肩前與手少陽會於臑會天髎（臑會在肩前廉去
肩端三寸宛宛中天髎在缺盆中上毖骨際陷中央）即會手足少陽足
陽明於肩井（在肩上陷中缺盆上大骨前一寸五分）

[The *yang wei* vessel] then proceeds along the rib-sides, ascending obliquely to a place
above the elbow where it meets the hand yang brightness and both hand and foot
greater yang at Upper Arm (LI-14) (located seven *cun* above the elbow in a depression
in the gap between the sinews; it is one *cun* below Shoulder Bone [LI-15]).[4] It passes in
front of the shoulder to meet with the hand lesser yang at Upper Arm Meeting (TB-
13)[5] and Celestial Bone-Hole (TB-15). (Upper Arm Meeting is located on the frontal
aspect of the shoulder in a depression three *cun* lateral to the tip of the shoulder; Celestial Bone-Hole is located in the supraclavicular fossa, at the center of the depression
above the clavicle.)[6] Next, it meets the hand and foot lesser yang and the hand yang
brightness at the Shoulder Well (GB-21) (located in a depression on the shoulder, one
cun and five *fen* above the empty basin in front of the large bone).[7]

99

入肩後會手太陽陽蹻於臑腧（在肩後大骨下胛上廉陷中）上循耳
後會手足少陽于風池（在耳後髮際陷中）上腦空（承靈後一寸半
夾玉枕骨下陷）承靈（正營後一寸半）正營（目窗後一寸）目窗
（臨泣後一寸）臨泣（在瞳人直上，入髮際五分陷中）

[Here, the *yang wei* vessel] enters behind the shoulder to meet the hand greater yang and the *yang qiao* at Upper Arm Transport (SI-10) (located behind the shoulder below the large bone in a depression above the shoulder blade).[8] It proceeds upward behind the ear to meet the hand and foot lesser yang at Wind Pond (GB-20) (located behind the ear in a depression on the hairline) and then ascends to Brain Hollow (GB-19) (located one-and-a-half *cun* behind Spirit Support in the depression below the occiptal bone), Spirit Support (GB-18) (located one-and-a-half *cun* behind Upright Construction), Upright Construction (GB-17) (located one *cun* behind Eye Window), Eye Window (GB-16) (located one *cun* behind Overlooking Tears), and Overlooking Tears (GB-15) (located directly above the pupil in a depression five *fen* within the hairline).[9]

下額與手足少陽陽明五脈會於陽白（眉上一寸直瞳人雙對）循頭
入耳上至本神而止（本神直目上入髮際中）凡三十二穴

[The *yang wei* vessel then] descends to the forehead to meet with the five vessels of the hand and foot lesser yang and yang brightness at Yang White (GB-14) (located one *cun* above the brow, directly above the pupil),[10] where it proceeds [into] the head to enter the eye. [Finally], it ascends to Spirit Root (GB-13)[11] and stops. (Spirit Root is on the hairline, directly above the eye.)[12] There are 32 holes in all.

CHAPTER 5

二維為病

Diseases of the Two *Wei*

越人曰陽維陰維者維絡於身溢蓄不能環琉灌溉諸經者也故陽維起
於諸陽之會陰維起於諸陰之交陽維維於陽陰維維於陰陰陽不能自
相維則悵然失志溶溶不能自收持（溶溶緩慢貌）

[Qin] Yue-Ren says: "The *yang wei* and *yin wei* are a binding network in the body. When they overflow from accumulation, [their contents] stagnate and they are unable to circulate and irrigate all the other [primary] channels. Therefore, the *yang wei* arises from [the places it] meets with all the yang, and the *yin wei* arises from [the places it] intersects with all the yin. The *yang wei* binds to the yang and the *yin wei* binds to the yin such that when yin and yang are unable to bind with one another, then one experiences such disappointment that one loses one's sense of purpose. One becomes sluggish and unable to support oneself. (Sluggish as in a lethargic bearing.)"

又曰陽維為病苦寒熱陰維為病苦心痛

[He] also says: "When the *yang wei* is diseased, [the patient] suffers from chills and fever; when the *yin wei* is diseased, [the patient] suffers from heart pain."

張潔古曰衛為陽主表陽維受邪為病在表故苦寒熱營為陰主裏陰維
受邪為病在裏故苦心痛陰陽相維則營衛和諧矣營衛不諧則悵然失
不能自收持矣何以知之

Zhang Jie-Gu says that the protective is yang and it governs the exterior. When the *yang wei* contracts a pathogen, it produces a disease in the exterior, and therefore [the patient] suffers from chills and fever. The nutritive is yin, and it governs the interior. When the *yin wei* contracts a pathogen, it produces a disease in the interior, and therefore [the patient] suffers from heart pain. When the yin and yang are bound together, then the nutritive and protective all work in harmony. When the nutritive and the protective do not work in harmony, then one disconsolately loses a sense of purpose and one cannot contain oneself. How would one know this?

仲景云病常自汗是衛氣不與營氣和也宜桂枝湯和之

[Zhang] Zhong-Jing says: "When a disease is characterized by frequent spontaneous sweats that are due to a lack of harmony between the protective qi and nutritive qi, one should give Cinnamon Twig Decoction (*gui zhi tang*) to harmonize it."[1]

又云服桂枝反煩不解先刺風池風府即與桂枝湯

He also says: "If one administers Cinnamon Twig Decoction (*gui zhi tang*) and on the contrary, [the patient becomes] irritable and [the condition] is unresolved, one must first prick Wind Pond (GB-20) and Wind House (GV-16) and then administer Cinnamon Twig Decoction (*gui zhi tang*) [again]."[2]

此二穴乃陽維之會也謂桂枝後尚自汗發熱惡寒其脈寸浮尺弱而反
煩為病在陽維故先針此二穴

These two holes are the meeting [holes] of the *yang wei* vessel. This means that if after [administering] Cinnamon Twig [Decoction] (*gui zhi [tang]*) the patient presents with spontaneous sweats, fever and chills, his pulse is floating in the distal position and weak in the proximal position, and yet [the patient] is irritable, then this disease is located in the *yang wei*. Therefore, one must first needle these two holes.

仲景又云臟無他病時發熱自汗出而不愈此衛氣不和也桂枝湯主之

[Zhang] Zhong-Jing also said: "[When patients] whose yin viscera have no other disease have periodic heat effusion and spontaneous sweating that does not get better, this means the protective qi is disharmonious, and Cinnamon Twig Decoction (*gui zhi tang*) masters it."[3]

又曰陰維為病苦心痛治在三陰之交太陰證則理中湯少陰證則四逆
湯厥陰證則當歸四逆揚吳茱萸湯主之

[Zhang Jie-Gu] also said: "When the *yin wei* is diseased, [the patient] suffers from heart pain" [so one must] treat the intersection of the three yin. [As for herbal treatment], for greater yin patterns, use Regulate the Middle Pill (*li zhong wan*), while for lesser yin patterns, use Frigid Extremities Decoction (*si ni tang*); reversing yin patterns are mastered by Tangkuei Decoction for Frigid Extremities (*dang gui si ni tang*) or Evodia Decoction (*wu zhu yu tang*).

李瀕湖曰陽維之脈與手足三陽相維而足太陽少陽則始終相聯附者
寒熱之證惟二經有之故陽維為病亦苦寒熱蓋衛氣晝行於陽夜行於
陰陰虛則內熱陽虛則外寒邪氣在經內與陰爭而惡寒外與陽爭而發
熱則寒熱之在表而兼太陽證者有汗當用桂枝無汗當用麻黃寒熱之
在半表半裏而兼少陽證者當用小柴胡加減治之若夫營衛慄卑而病

寒熱者黃耆建中及八物湯之類主之

Li Bin-Hu says that the vessel of the *yang wei* binds with the three yang of the hand and foot. Of these, the foot greater yang and lesser yang are in continuous contact [with the *yang wei*]. The symptoms of chills and fever belong to these two channels alone, and therefore when the *yang wei* is diseased, [the patient] also suffers from chills and fever. The protective qi moves in the yang during the day and moves in the yin at night. When the yin is deficient, there will be internal heat, and when the yang is deficient, there will be external cold. When there is pathogenic qi in the channels it internally contends with the yin, which leads to chills, and externally contends with the yang, which leads to fever. Thus, when there is cold and heat in the exterior along with a greater yang presentation that has sweating, one should administer Cinnamon Twig [Decoction] *(gui zhi [tang])*. When sweating does not occur, one should administer Ephedra Decoction *(ma huang tang)*. When chills and fever that is half in the exterior and half in the interior occurs along with a lesser yang presentation, one should use a modified form of Minor Bupleurum [Decoction] *(xiao chai hu [tang])* to treat it. Now if the nutritive and the protective are fearful and powerless and produce a disease of chills and fever, then [prescriptions] in the class of Astragalus Decoction to Construct the Middle *(huang qi jian zhong tang)* and Eight-Treasure Decoction *(ba zhen tang)* master it.

潔古獨以桂枝一證屬之陽維似未擴充至於陰維為病主心痛潔古獨
以三陰溫裏之藥治之則寒中三陰者宜矣而三陰熱厥作痛似未備矣
蓋陰維之脈雖交三陰而行實與任脈同歸故心痛多屬少陰厥陰任脈
之氣上衝而然暴痛無熱久痛無寒按之少止者為虛不可接近者為實

Jie-Gu limited his use of Cinnamon Twig [Decoction] *(gui zhi [tang])* to a single symptom that pertained to the *yang wei* [vessel], and he did not expand [its scope of application to symptoms with a] similar [pathodynamic]. Once the *yin wei* has become diseased, it governs heart pain. Jie-Gu limited himself to medicinals that [influenced] the three yin by warming the interior. Hence, these were indicated [only] once cold had struck the three yin. [For instance], in the case of heat reversal of the three yin producing pain, he did not prepare [prescriptions] such as this. Now although the *yin wei* vessel intersects with the three yin and travels [along their trajectories], in actuality, it [also] returns to the *ren* vessel. Therefore, heart pain typically pertains to an upsurge of qi in the lesser yin, reversing yin, and *ren* vessel. [This pattern presents as] sudden pain with an absence of heat or long-term pain with an absence of cold. If gentle pressure stops [the patient's pain, then this an indicator of] deficiency, and if one cannot tolerate deep pressure, this is an indicator of excess.

凡寒痛兼少陰及任脈者四逆湯兼厥陰者當歸四逆湯兼太陰者理中
湯主之凡熱病兼少陰及任脈者金鈴子散延胡索散兼厥陰者失笑散

兼太陰者承氣湯主之若營血內傷兼夫任衝手厥陰者則宜四物湯養
營湯妙香散之類因病藥之如此則陰陽虛實庶乎其不差矣

All cold pain presenting along with a lesser yin and *ren* vessel [pattern is treated by] Frigid Extremities Decoction (*si ni tang*). When presenting along with a reversing yin pattern, [the cold pain] is treated by Tangkuei Decoction for Frigid Extremities (*dang gui si ni tang*). When presenting along with greater yin pattern, Regulate the Middle Pill (*li zhong wan*) treats [the cold pain]. All heat pain presenting along with a combined lesser yin and *ren* vessel [pattern is treated by] Melia Toosendan Powder (*jin ling zi san*) or Corydalis Decoction (*yan hu suo tang*). When presenting along with a reversing yin pattern, [heat pain is treated by] Sudden Smile Powder (*shi xiao san*). When presenting along with a greater yin pattern, Order the Qi Decoction (*cheng qi tang*) masters it. If the nutritive and blood are internally damaged with combined [involvement] of the *ren*, *chong*, and hand reversing yin, then prescriptions in the class of Four-Substance Decoction (*si wu tang*), Nourish the Nutritive Decoction (*yang rong tang*), and Marvelously Fragrant Powder (*miao xiang san*) are indicated. If one administers medicinals based on the cause of the illness, attending to yin and yang, deficiency and excess, [then following these] broad outlines, one will rarely make mistakes.

王叔和脈經曰寸口脈從少陰斜至太陽是陽維脈也動苦肌肉痺癢皮
膚痛下部不仁汗出而寒又苦癲仆羊鳴手足相引甚者失音不能言宜
取客主人（在耳前起骨上廉開口有空乃手足少陽陽明之會）

Wang Shu-He in the *Pulse Classic* asserts: A wrist pulse that beats "from the [foot] lesser yin obliquely to the [foot] greater yang is a *yang wei* pulse.[4] [When the pulse is] perturbed in this way, [the patient] suffers from obstruction and itching of the muscles and flesh, skin pain, numbness in the lower parts, and sweating with chills."[5] In addition, patients will "suffer from suddenly falling down[6] where they bleat like sheep, their arms and legs will be drawn in, and in extreme [cases, suffer from] loss of voice and inability to speak. In such instances, one should select Guest Host (GB-3)." (Located above the bone in front of the ear where a hollow appears when the mouth is opened; it is the meeting of the hand and foot lesser yang and yang brightness.)[7]

又曰寸口脈從少陽斜至厥陰是陰維脈也動苦癲癇僵仆羊鳴又
苦僵仆失音肌肉痺癢應時自發汗出惡風身洗洗然也取陽白金
門（見前）僕參（見陽蹺）

[Wang Shu-He] also states: "A wrist pulse that beats obliquely from the lesser yang to the reversing yin is a *yin wei* pulse.[8] [When the pulse is] perturbed in this way, [the patient] suffers from seizures, sudden collapse, and bleating." He also says: "[the patient] will suffer from sudden collapse, loss of voice, and obstruction and itching of the muscles and flesh [and] aversion to wind accompanying spontaneous sweating and a drenching sweat." Choose Yang White (GB-14), Metal Gate (BL-63) (see above), and Subservient Visitor (BL-61) (see the *yang qiao*).

瀕湖曰王叔和以癲癇屬陰維陽維靈樞經以癲癇屬陰蹺陽蹺二說義
異旨同蓋陽維由外踝而上循陽分而至肩肘歷耳額而行於衛分諸陽
之會陰維由內踝而上循陰分而上脅至咽行於營分諸陰之交陽蹺起
於跟中循外踝上行於股外至脅肋肩膊行於一身之左右而終於目內
眥陰蹺起於跟中循內踝上行於股內陰器行於一身之左右至咽喉會
任脈而終於目內眥邪在陰維陰蹺則發癲邪在陽陽蹺循陰則發癇癲
動而屬陽陽脈主之癲靜而屬陰陰脈主之大抵二疾當取之四脈之穴
分其陰陽而已

[Li]Bin-Hu says: Wang Shu-He attributes seizure disorders to the *yin wei* and *yang wei*, and yet the *Divine Pivot* classic attributes seizure disorders to the *yin qiao* and *yang qiao*. The meanings of the two statements differ, but their intention is the same. The *yang wei* arises at the outer ankle and ascends, proceeding along the yang aspect to arrive at the shoulder and travels around the ear and cheek to travel to the protective aspect at the meeting of all the yang. The *yin wei* arises at the inner ankle, proceeding along the yin aspect, ascending to the ribs and to the throat where it travels to the nutritive aspect to intersect with all the yin. The *yang qiao* arises in the heel and proceeds upward from the outer ankle, traveling along the outer thigh to arrive at the rib-sides and shoulder, traveling along the left and right sides of the body to terminate in the inner corner of the eye. The *yin qiao* arises in the heel and proceeds upward along the inner thigh and genitals, traveling along the left and right sides of the body to arrive at the throat where it meets the *ren* vessel, terminating at the inner corner of the eye. Pathogens in the *yin wei* or *yin qiao* will produce withdrawal;[9] pathogens in the *yang wei* or *yang qiao* will produce seizures. Seizure-like perturbations pertain to yang and are governed by yang vessels. Withdrawal-like quiescence pertains to yin and is governed by yin vessels. Generally speaking, [in treating] these two illnesses, one should select the holes of these four vessels by differentiating yin and yang.

王叔和曰診得陽維脈浮者暫起目眩陽盛實者苦肩息灑灑如寒

Wang Shu-He says: "When examination reveals that the *yang wei* pulse is floating, vertigo will occur with standing. This is due to the yang being overabundant and overfull [so the patient also] suffers from raised-shoulder breathing[10] and shivering as if cold."[11]

診得陰維脈沉大而實者苦胸中痛脅下支滿心痛其脈如貫珠者男子
兩脅下實腰中痛女子陰中痛如有瘡狀

"When examination reveals that the *yin wei* pulse is deep, large, and excessive, [the patient] suffers from pain in the chest, propping fullness below the hypochondrium,[12] and heart pain. If the pulse[13] feels like a string of pearls, then in men there will be an excess below both rib-sides and lumbar pain, while in women there will be genital pain as if sores have formed."

素問腰痛論曰陽維之脈令人腰痛痛上怫然腫刺陽維之脈與太陽合
腨間去地一尺

[Ch. 41 of] *Basic Questions,* "Discourse on Lumbar Pain," states: "The vessel of the *yang wei* causes people to have lumbar pain accompanied by sudden swelling in the painful area. Prick the *yang wei* vessel where the vessel meets the greater yang vessel below the calf, one *chi* above the ground."[14]

王啓玄曰陽維起於陽則太陽之所生並行而上至腨下復與太陽合而
上也去地一尺乃承山穴也在銳腨腸下分肉間陷中可刺七分

Wang Qi-Xuan states: "The *yang wei* arises in the yang, and it is engendered by the greater yang." … "It travels parallel with [the greater yang], ascending to below the calf where it unites with the greater yang and continues its ascent. … One *chi* above the ground is the hole Mountain Support (BL-57), which is in the lower tip of the calf in a depression formed by the parting of the flesh. It may be pricked [to a depth of] seven *fen*."[15]

肉裏之脈令人腰痛不可以咳咳則筋縮急刺肉裏之脈為二痏在太陽
之外少陽絕骨之後

"The Interior Flesh vessel causes people to suffer from lumbar pain that prohibits coughing. When a patient coughs, this causes the sinew networks to tense and contract into a spasm.[16] Prick the Interior Flesh vessel with two punctures, [one] lateral to the greater yang [and the other] on the lesser yang behind the fibula."

王啓玄曰肉裏之脈少陽所生陽維脈氣所發絕骨之後陽維所過分肉
穴也在足外踝直上絕骨之端如後二分筋肉分間刺可五分

Wang Qi-Xuan states: "The Interior Flesh vessel is engendered by the lesser yang, and the *yang wei* vessel qi issues from it." "Behind the fibula, the *yang wei* travels … to the hole in the parting of the flesh. It is located on the outer ankle of the foot directly above the end of the fibula behind two sinews in the parting of the flesh. … It may be pricked to a depth of five *fen*."[17]

飛陽之脈令人腰痛痛怫怫然甚則悲以恐

"The Soaring Yang vessel causes people to have lumbar pain, producing sudden swelling in the painful area, and in extreme cases, it results in sorrow that borders on fear."

啟玄曰此陰維之脈也去內踝上五寸痛分中並少陰經而上也

[Wang] Qi-Xuan states: "This is the *yin wei* vessel that departs from the inner ankle five *cun* from the parting of the calf, where it merges with the lesser yang channel and ascends."

刺飛陽之脈在內踝上五寸少陰之前與陰維之會築賓穴也甲乙經曰
太陽之絡別走少陰者名曰飛陽

"Prick the Soaring Yang vessel five *cun* above the inner ankle in front of the lesser yin where it meets the *yin wei*." This is the Guest House (KI-9) hole. *The Systematic Classic* states: "Where the network of the greater yang diverges to travel to the lesser yin is called the Soaring Yang."

CHAPTER 6

陰蹺脈

The *Yin Qiao* Vessel

陰蹺者足少陰之別脈其脈起於跟中足少陰然谷穴之後（然谷在
內踝前下一寸陷中）同足少陰循內踝下照海穴（在內踝下五分）
上內踝之上二寸以交信為（交信在內踝骨上少陰前太陰後兼筋骨
間）直上循陰股入陰上循胸裏入缺盆上出人迎之前至咽嚨交貫衝
脈入頄內廉上行屬目內眥與手足太陽足陽明陽蹺五脈會於睛明而
上行（睛明在目內眥外一分宛宛中）凡八穴

The *yin qiao* is a branch vessel of the foot lesser yin. Its vessel arises from the center of the heel, behind the foot lesser yin hole Burning Valley (KI-2). [Burning Valley is located in a depression one *cun* in front of and below the inner heel.] It proceeds together with the foot lesser yin to the Shining Sea (KI-6) hole below the inner ankle [located five *fen* below the inner ankle] where it then ascends two *cun* above the inner ankle to Intersection Reach (KI-8). [Intersection Reach is located above the inner ankle in front to the lesser yin and behind the *tai yin* between the ridges formed by the sinew and bone.] It travels straight up, proceeding along the inner thigh to enter the perineum. From here, it proceeds upward to the interior of the chest, entering the supraclavicular fossa and emerging at Man's Prognosis (ST-9) to reach the larynx where it intersects and links with the *chong* vessel. It then enters the cheekbone and into the ridge[1] and ascends and connects to the inner canthus of the eye where it meets with the five vessels of the foot greater yang, foot yang brightness, and the *yang qiao* at Bright Eyes (BL-1). [Bright Eyes is located in a depression one *fen* outside the inner canthus of the eye.][2] In all, there are eight holes.

張紫陽八脈經云八脈者衝脈在風府穴下督脈在臍後任脈在臍前帶
脈在腰陰蹺脈在尾閭前陰裏下陽蹺脈在尾閭後二節陰維脈在頂前
一寸三分陽維脈在頂後一寸三分

Zhang Zi-Yang in his *Eight Vessel Scripture* says: "As for the eight vessels, the *chong* vessel is located below the Wind House (GV-16) hole, the *du* vessel is located behind the umbilicus, the *ren* vessel is located in front of the umbilicus, the *dai* vessel is located in the lumbar region, the *yin qiao* vessel is located in front of the perineum[3] below the scrotum, and the *yang qiao* vessel is located behind the perineum in the sacrococcygeal region.[4] The *yin wei* is located one *cun* and three *fen* in front of the vertex [of the skull], and the *yang wei* vessel is located one *cun* and three *fen* behind the vertex [of the skull]."

凡人有此八脈俱屬陰神閉而不開惟神仙以陽氣衝開故能得道八脈
者先天大道之根一氣之祖采之惟在陰蹻為先此脈才動諸脈皆通

"People have these eight vessels, but they all remain hidden spirits because they are closed and have not yet been opened. Only divine transcendents can use the yang qi to surge through and open them so that they are able to attain the way. The eight vessels are the root of the great way of Former Heaven and the ancestor of the Unitary Qi. Only when the *yin qiao* is selected [for cultivation] first and only once this vessel has been activated will all the other vessels open."

次督任衝三脈總為經脈造化之源而陰蹻一脈散在丹經其名頗多曰
天根曰死戶曰復命關曰酆都鬼戶曰死生根有神主之名曰桃康上通
泥丸下透湧泉倘能知此使真氣聚散皆從此關竅則天門常開地戶永
閉尻脈周流於一身貫通上下和氣自然上朝陽長陰消水中火發雪里
花開所謂天根月窟閒來往三十六宮都是春

"Next, the three vessels of the *du, ren,* and *chong* [should be selected for cultivation because they] are the source of creation for all the other channels and vessels. And yet, mention of this particular vessel the *yin qiao* is scattered throughout the Cinnabar scriptures where it is variously referred to by many names. It is called Root of Heaven; it is called Death's Door; it is called the Resurrection Pass; it is called the Ghost Door of Feng Du; and it is called the Root of Life and Death. As the governor of the spirit, it is often called the Peach of Well-Being. Above, it penetrates the mud ball and below it reaches down to the Gushing Spring [KI-1]. If one has knowledge of [the *du, ren,* and *chong*], then one can induce the true qi to accumulate and dissipate [at will], all from these barrier orifices. Thus, the heavenly gate will be constantly open and Earth's Door will remain forever closed. The buttock vessel will flow throughout the entire body, linking and flowing freely both above and below, harmonious qi will naturally ascend to the imperial court. The yang will grow and the yin will diminish, fire will issue from the midst of water, and flowers will blossom through the snow. This is what is referred to by 'When there is a languid ebb and flow between the Heavenly Root and the Moon Grotto, then the 36 officials are all spring-like.'"

得之者身體輕健容袁返壯昏昏默默如醉如痴此其驗也要知西南之
鄉乃坤地尾閭之前膀胱之後小腸之下靈龜之上此乃天地逐日所生
氣根產鉛之地也醫家不知有此

"When this is achieved, then the body will become light and strong. The adept's aged countenance regains its vitality; in quiet silence, he becomes recondite as if he were an imbecile or intoxicated. [Such experiences] are proof [of the effect]. It is essential to understand that the location of the southwest is in *kun* earth, in front of the perineum, behind the bladder, below the small intestine, and above the divine tortoise. This is the ground where heaven and earth day by day engender the root of the qi and give birth to lead. Physicians do not understand this."

瀕湖曰丹書論及陽精河車皆往往以任衝督脈命門三焦為說末有專
指陰蹻者而紫陽八脈經所載經脈稍與醫家之說不同然內景隧道惟
返觀者能照察之其言必不謬也

[Li] Bin-Hu says that the discussions in the alchemical texts addressing the yang essence and the Water Wheel are most often spoken of in the context of the *ren, chong,* and *du* vessels and the life gate and triple burner; the *yin qiao* is not emphasized. And yet, Zi-Yang's *Eight Vessel Scripture*, which recorded the [pathways of the] channels and vessels, differs slightly from the teachings of medical people. Therefore, in following the path along the inner landscape, only those who turn back the senses will be capable of an illuminated examination [of the eight vessels], and therefore these statements must not be misconstrued.

CHAPTER 7

陽蹺脈

The *Yang Qiao* Vessel

陽蹺者足太陽之別脈其脈起於跟中出於外踝下足太陽申脈穴（在
外踝下五分陷中容爪甲白肉際）當踝後繞跟以僕參為本（在跟骨
下陷中拱足得之）上外踝上三寸以跗陽為郄（在外踝上三寸足太
陽之穴也）直上循股外廉循脅後胛上舍手太陽陽維於臑腧（在肩
後大骨下胛上廉陷中）上行肩外廉舍手陽明於巨骨（在肩尖端上
行兩叉骨罅間陷中）會手陽明少陽于肩髃（在髆骨頭肩端上兩骨
罅陷宛宛中舉臂取之有空）

The *yang qiao* is a branch vessel of the foot greater yang. Its vessel arises in the center of the heel and emerges below the outer ankle at the foot greater yang Extending Vessel (BL-62) hole[1] (located in the depression five *fen* below the outer ankle in a depression as large as the edge of a finger nail at the border of the white flesh).[2] From behind the ankle, it encircles the heel to root at Subservient Visitor (BL-61) (located in a depression under the heel bone; find it by cupping the heel).[3] It rises above the outer ankle for three *cun* to Instep Yang (BL-59), the cleft [hole] (located three *cun* above the outer heel, it is a foot greater yang hole).[4] It ascends directly from here, proceeding along [the] outer thigh,[5] and proceeding behind the rib-sides to the scapula where it meets the hand greater yang and *yang wei* at Upper Arm Transport (SI-10) (located in a depression below the scapular crest on the upper border of the scapula).[6] [The *yang qiao*] then travels upward along the outer aspect of the shoulder to meet with the hand yang brightness at Great Bone (LI-16) (located above the tip of the shoulder in the rift that forms a depression between the two bones) and then moves on to meet the hand yang brightness and lesser yang at Shoulder Bone (LI-15) (located at the head of the humerus, at the tip of the shoulder in a rift that forms a depression between two bones; it is found in the hole that appears when the arm is raised).[7]

上入迎夾口吻會手足陽明任脈於地倉（來口吻旁四分外如近下有
微脈動處）同足陽明上而行巨窌（來鼻孔旁八分直瞳子平水溝）
復會任脈於承泣（在目下七分直瞳子陷中）至目內眥與手足太陽
足陽明陰蹺五脈會於睛明穴（見陰蹺下）從睛明上行入髮際下耳
後入風池而終（風池在耳後夾玉枕骨下發際陷中）凡二十二穴

[The *yang qiao* vessel] ascends to Man's Prognosis (ST-9) and hugs the corners of the mouth where it meets with the hand and foot yang brightness and the *ren* vessel at Earth's Granary (ST-4) (located four *fen* out from the corners of the mouth, close below which a slightly pulsing vessel can be found).[8] Together with the foot yang brightness, it ascends and travels to Great Bone-Hole (ST-3) (beside the nostrils at a distance of eight *fen*, directly [below] the eyeball, level with the philtrum).[9] From here, it returns to meet the *ren* vessel at Tear Container (ST-1) (located seven *fen* below the eye in a depression directly below the eyeball)[10] and reaches the inner canthus to meet with the five vessels of the hand and foot greater yang, foot yang brightness, and *yin qiao* at Bright Eyes (BL-1) (see the *yin qiao* [discussed] previously).[11] From Bright Eyes, [the *yang qiao*] ascends to enter the hairline and then descends behind the ear to enter Wind Pond (GB-20) where it terminates (Wind Pond is located behind the ear where it hugs the occiput; it is in a depression under the hairline).[12] In all, there are 23 holes.

難經曰蹻脈從足至目長七尺五寸會一丈五尺

The *Classic of Difficulties* states: "The *qiao* vessels extend from the feet to reach the eye. They are seven *chi* and five *cun*, ... all together, this is one *zhang* and five *chi* long."[13]

甲乙經曰蹻脈有陰陽何者當其數曰男子數其陽女子數其陰當數者
為經不當數者為絡氣之在身也如水之流如日月之行不休故陰脈營
臟而陽脈營其腑如環之無端莫知其紀終而復始其流溢之氣內溉髒
腑外濡腠理

The *Systematic Classic* states: "The *qiao* vessel has yin and yang [components], but which are counted? [Qi Bo] stated: For males, the yang is counted, and for females, the yin is counted. What is counted are the channels, and what are not counted are the networks." "The qi within the body is like flowing water, like the ceaseless movement of the sun and moon.[14] Therefore, the yin vessels nourish the yin viscera and the yang vessels nourish the yang receptacles like an endless circuit in which there is no break. Upon reaching the end, it just begins again. Its overflow of qi internally irrigates the yin viscera and yang receptacles and externally moistens the interstices."

CHAPTER 8

二蹺為病

Diseases of the Two *Qiao*

秦越人難經曰陰絡者陰蹺之絡陽絡者陽蹺之絡陰蹺為病陽緩而陰
急陽蹺為病陰緩而陽急

Qin Yue-Ren states in the *Classic of Difficulties*: "The yin networks are the networks of the *yin qiao*. The yang networks are the networks of the *yang qiao*."[1] "When the *yin qiao* is diseased, the yang is slack and the yin is tense. When the *yang qiao* is diseased, the yin is slack and the yang is tense."

王叔和脈經曰陰蹺脈急當從內踝以上急外踝以上緩陽蹺脈急當從
外踝以上急內踝以上緩

Wang Shu-He states in his *Pulse Classic*: "[When the] *yin qiao* ... vessel is tense, from the medial ankle and above, it is tense, and from the lateral ankle and above, it is slack. [When the] *yang qiao* vessel ... is tense, from the lateral ankle and above, it is tense, and from the medial ankle and above, it is slack."[2]

又曰寸口脈前部左右彈者陽蹺也動苦腰背痛又為癲癇僵仆羊鳴惡
風偏枯痞痹身體強又曰微澀為風癇並取陽蹺在外踝上三寸直絕骨
是穴（跗陽穴也）

[Wang Shu-He] also states: A wrist pulse that is "tapping in the distal left and right positions is a *yang qiao* [pulse]. [When the pulse is] perturbed in this way, [the patient] suffers from back pain." It also includes "withdrawal and seizures," and "sheep-like bleating," "aversion to wind, hemilateral withering" and "painful obstruction" and "generalized body stiffness".[3] In addition, he states: A wrist pulse that is "faint and choppy indicates wind seizures," and therefore "select the *yang qiao* [hole] (located three *cun* above the lateral ankle, directly [parallel] to the fibula" (the Instep Yang [BL-59] hole).

又曰寸口脈後部左右彈者陰蹺動苦癲癇寒熱皮膚淫痹又為少腹
痛裏急腰及髖窌下相連陰中痛男子陰疝女子漏下不止（髖，髀
骨也。窌，腰下穴也）

115

[Wang Shu-He] also states: A wrist pulse that is "tapping in the proximal left and right positions is a *yin qiao* [pulse]. [When the pulse is] perturbed in this way, [the patient] suffers from withdrawal and seizures, chills and feverishness, and stiffness and insensitivity of the skin."[4] There will also be "lower abdominal pain, abdominal urgency, and lower back and pelvis [pain] radiating into the genitals. In males, this is yin bulging,[5] and in females, there is incessant spotting"[6] (*kuan* is the hip; *liao* are the foramina below the lumbar [spine]).[7]

又曰：癲癇瘛瘲，"不知所苦，兩蹻之下．男陽女陰．"

He also states: For seizures and tonic-clonic movements [associated with the *yin qiao*], "if the patient cannot tell where the trouble is, then [treat] the two *qiao* below. In men, [treat] the *yang* [*qiao*], and in women, [treat] the *yin* [*qiao*]."[8]

張潔古曰蹻者捷疾也二脈起于足使人蹻捷也陽蹻在肌肉之上陽脈
所行通貫六腑主持諸表故名為陽蹻之絡陰蹻在肌肉之下陰脈所行
通貫五藏主持諸裏故名為陰蹻之絡陰蹻為病陰急則陰厥脛直五絡
不通表和裏痛陽蹻為病陽急則狂走目不昧表病裏和陰病則熱可灸
照海陽陵泉（在膝下一寸外廉陷中足少陽之合也筋病治此）陽病
則寒可針風池風府（風府在項後入髮際一寸大筋內宛宛中督脈太
陽陽維之會也）

Zhang Jie-Gu says that "*qiao* means nimble and fast. The two vessels arise in the foot and put a spring in the step. The *yang qiao* travels above the muscle and flesh, circulating among the yang vessels, linking the six receptacles, mastering and maintaining the exterior. It is therefore called the network of the *yang qiao*. The *yin qiao* travels below the muscle and flesh, circulating among the yin vessels, linking the five viscera, mastering and maintaining the interior. It is therefore called the network of the *yin qiao*. When the *yin qiao* is diseased the yin is tense, causing the yin channels to contract,[9] making the shins rigid, and impeding the five networks. Hence, the exterior is harmonious, but the interior is diseased. When the *yang qiao* is diseased and the yang is tense, then [the afflicted] walk about manically, never closing their eyes [to sleep]. Hence, the exterior is diseased, and the interior is harmonious. When the yin is diseased, there is heat. One may perform moxibustion on Shining Sea (KI-6) and Yang Mound Spring (GB-34) (located one *cun* below the knee in a depression on the outer aspect of the leg; it is the confluence hole of the foot lesser yang; sinew diseases are treated here). If the yang is diseased, then there is cold, and one may needle Wind Pond (GB-20) and Wind Adobe (GV-16) (located on the back of the neck, one body *cun* within the hairline, in a depression in the large sinew; it is the meeting of the governing vessel, greater yang, and *yang wei*)."

又曰在陽表者當汗之在陰裏者當下之

[Zhang Jie-Gu] also says that "[when disease is located] in the exterior yang, one must sweat it, and [when disease] is located in the interior yin, one must purge it."

又曰癲癇晝發灸陽夜發灸陰

[Zhang Jie-Gu] also says that "for diurnal seizures, one should perform moxibustion on the *yang [qiao]*, and for nocturnal [seizures], one should perform moxa on the *yin [qiao]*."

素間腰痛論曰腰痛不可舉者申脈僕參舉之（太陽之穴陽蹻之本也）

[Ch. 41 of] *Basic Questions,* "Discussion on Lower Back Pain," states: "For lumbar pain where one cannot lift [himself up out of bed, needling] Extending Vessel (BL-62) and Subservient Visitor (BL-61) will allow the patient to lift [himself up]. ([These are] holes on the greater yang channel and the root of the *yang qiao*)."

又曰會陰之脈令人腰痛痛上漯漯然汗出汗幹令人欲飲飲已欲走刺
直陽之脈上三痏在蹻上郗下五寸橫居視其盛者出血

[Ch. 41 of *Basic Questions*] also states: "The Meeting Yin vessel causes people to suffer from lower back pain that ascends [up the back] with soaking perspiration, an urge to drink after the sweat has dried, and an urge to walk after drinking. Prick the Straight Yang vessel with three punctures. This is located on the *qiao* in a cleft five body *cun* below the transverse crease [of the popliteal fossa]. If one sees [local] congestion, then let out some blood."

王啟玄云足太陽之脈循腰下會於後陰故曰會陰直陽之脈挾脊下行
貫臀至膕循腨過外踝之後條直而行者故曰直陽之脈也蹻為陽蹻所
生申脈穴也

Wang Qi-Xuan states that the vessels of the foot greater yang "traverse the lower back and meet in the area of the anus [literally, posterior yin], therefore, [this area] is called Meeting in the Yin." "The Straight Yang vessel … travels down along the spine penetrating through the buttock to the popliteal area, proceeding along the calf to behind the lateral ankle. Its trajectory is straight, and therefore it is called the straight yang vessel. [The location called] the *qiao* is the place where the *yang qiao* originates; it is the Extending Vessel (BL-62) hole."

蹻上郗下乃承筋穴也即腨中央如外陷看中也太陽脈氣所發禁針刺
但視其兩腨中央有血絡盛滿者乃刺之出血

Above the *qiao* and below the cleft is the Supporting Sinew (BL-56), "which is located in a depression on the outer side of the center of the calf. What issues from there is the qi of the greater yang vessel. It is contraindicated to pricking with a needle ... . However, if one observes that there are engorged blood vessels in the center of both calves, then prick them to let blood out."

又曰昌陽之脈令人腰痛痛引膺目然甚則反折舌卷不能言刺內筋為
三痏在內踝上大筋前太陰後上踝二寸所

[Ch. 41 of *Basic Questions*] also states: "The Abundant Yang vessel causes people to experience low back pain, which radiates to the breast, along with blurred vision, and in serious [cases], arched-back rigidity and a curled tongue with an inability to speak. Prick the inner sinew three times, [or more exactly, this hole that is located] above the medial ankle in front of the large sinew and behind the greater yin [vessel], two body *cun* or so above the ankle."

王啟玄云陰蹻起於然谷之後上內踝之上循陰股入陰而循腹入胸裏
缺盆上出人迎之前入頄內廉屬目內眥會於太陽陽蹻而上行故病狀
如此內筋即陰蹻之郄交信穴也

Wang Qi-Xuan states: "The *yin qiao* ... arises from behind Burning Valley (KI-2) and ascends to above the medial ankle, proceeding along the yin aspect of the thigh to enter the yin [genitals. From here it] proceeds along the abdomen to enter the interior of the chest, moving to the Empty Basin (ST-12) and ascending to emerge in front of Man's Prognosis (ST-9). It then enters the corner of the cheekbone [10] and joins up to the inner canthus of the eye, unites with the greater yang and *yang qiao,* and goes upward. Hence, the presentation of illness is like this." "The inner sinew ... is the cleft of the *yin qiao*, the Intersection Reach (KI-8) hole."

素問繆刺論曰邪客於足陽蹻之脈令人目痛從內眥始刺外踝之下半
寸所各二痏（即申脈也）左刺右右刺左如人行十里頃而已

[Ch. 63 of] *Basic Questions*, "Discussion of Cross Needling," states: "When pathogens visit the foot *yang qiao* vessel, this causes people to suffer from eye pain that begins from the inner canthus. Prick [the hole] one half *cun* below the lateral ankle with two punctures (at the Extending Vessel [BL-62] hole). [If the affliction is] on the left, then prick the right, and [if the affliction is] on the right, then prick the left, and it will be cured in the time it takes a person to walk ten *li*." [11]

靈樞經曰目中赤痛從內眥始取之陰蹻（交信穴也）

[Ch. 23 of] *Divine Pivot* classic states: "When the eye is red and painful, beginning at the inner canthus, then select the *yin qiao* (the Intersection Reach [KI-8] hole)."

又曰風痙反折先取足太陽及膕中及血結出血若中有寒邪取陰蹻及
三毛上及血絡出血

[Ch. 23 of] *Divine Pivot* also states: "For wind spasm and arched-back rigidity, first select the greater yang in the popliteal fossa at a blood network and let out blood. If the attack is due to a cold pathogen, select … the *yin qiao* above the Three Hairs at the blood networks and let blood out there."

李瀕湖曰足太陽京骨穴也在足外側小指本節後大骨下赤白際陷中
針三分灸七壯膕中委中穴也在曲膝後橫文中針三分陰蹻取交信穴
見前三毛大敦穴也在足大指外側三毛中肝脈之井也針三分灸三壯
血絡者視其處有始脈盛滿者出其血也

Li Bin-Hu says that the foot greater yang is the Capital Bone (BL-64) hole. It is located on the lateral side of the foot behind the joint of the small toe, below the large bone in the depression at the border of the red and white flesh. Needle to a depth of three *fen* and moxa seven cones. The popliteal fossa is the Bend Center (BL-40) hole. It is located in the horizontal crease in the crook behind the knee. Needle to a depth of three *fen*. For the *yin qiao*, select Intersection Reach (KI-8) (see above). The Three Hairs is the Large Pile (LR-1). It is located on the large toe of the foot on the lateral side of the three hairs and is the well [hole] of the liver vessel. Needle to a depth of three *fen* and moxa three times. As for the blood networks, observe the place where the blood vessels are engorged, and let out blood there.

又曰陰蹻陽蹻陰陽相交陽入陰陰出陽交於目銳眥陽氣盛則瞋目陰
氣盛則瞑目熱厥取足太陽少陽

[Ch. 21 of *Divine Pivot*] also states: "The *yin qiao* and *yang qiao* are the intersection of the yin and yang. The yang enters the yin and the yin emerges from the yang. They intersect at the outer corner of the eye. When the yang qi is overly full, then the eyes will stare, and when the yin qi is overly full, then the eyes will be closed.[12] With heat reversal, select the foot greater yang and lesser yang."[13]

甲乙經曰人病目閉不得視者衛氣留於陰不得行於陽留於陰則陰氣
盛陰氣盛則陰蹻滿不得入於陽則陽氣虛故目閉也

The Systematic Classic states: "When a patient's eyes are shut and they cannot see…, this is due to protective qi being lodged in the yin and unable to travel to the yang. When it is lodged in the yin, then the yin qi is overly full, and when the yin qi is overly full, then the *yin qiao* is full. [When the protective qi] cannot enter the yang, then the yang qi is deficient and, hence, the eyes are shut."[14]

病目不得瞑者衛氣不得入於陰常留於陽留於陽則陽氣滿陽氣滿則
陽蹺盛不得入於陰則陰氣虛故目不瞑也

"When a patient's eyes cannot close … , the protective qi cannot enter the yin and constantly lodges in the yang. If [the protective qi] lodges in the yang, then the yang qi is full. If the yang qi is full, then the *yang qiao* is overly full. [If the protective qi] cannot enter the yin, then the yin qi is deficient, hence, the eyes cannot close." [15]

靈樞曰五穀入於胃也其糟粕津液宗氣為三隧故宗氣積於胸中出於
喉嚨以貫心肺而行呼吸焉營氣者泌其津液注之於脈化而為血以營
四末內注五藏六腑以應刻數焉衛氣者出其悍氣之慓疾而先於四末
分肉皮膚之間而不休焉晝日行於陽夜行於陰常從足少陰分間行於
五藏六腑

[Ch. 71 of] *Divine Pivot* states: "The five grains enter the stomach and are divided into three pathways of dregs, fluids, and the gathering qi. Thus, gathering qi accumulates in the chest and emerges in the throat to link with the heart and lungs and propel respiration there. The nutritive qi secretes the fluids and pours into the vessels. It transforms and becomes blood to nourish the four extremities. Internally, it pours into the five viscera and six receptacles in accordance with the time of the day.[16]

Protective qi emerges with an impetuous ferocity, first in the four extremities in the partings between the flesh and skin, and it does so in a ceaseless manner. During the daytime, it circulates in the yang, and at night, it circulates in the yin from the level of the foot lesser yin, traveling to the five viscera and six receptacles."

今厥氣客於五藏六腑則衛氣獨衛其外行於陽不得入於陰行於陽則
陽氣盛陽氣盛則陽蹺陷不得入於陰則陰氣虛故目不瞑也

"When a reversal qi visits the five viscera and six receptacles, then the protective qi alone protects the outside. It travels in the yang but cannot enter the yin. By traveling [only] in the yang, the yang qi becomes overly full, and when the yang qi is overly full, then the *yang qiao* caves in. When [the yang qi] cannot enter the yin, then the yin qi is deficient and the eyes cannot close."

治當補其不足瀉其有余以通其道而去其邪飲以半夏湯一劑陰陽已
通其臥立至

"[Such a condition should] be treated by tonifying what is insufficient and draining what has a surplus, … to open the pathways and expel the pathogen. One need only drink one packet of Pinellia [and Sorghum] Decoction *(ban xia [shu mi] tang)*, and the yin and yang will communicate and the patient will immediately be able to lie down."

其方用流水千里以外者八升揚之萬遍取其清五升煮之炊以葦薪火
沸置秫米一升治半夏五合徐炊令至一升半去其滓飲汁一小杯日三
稍益以知為度故其病新發者覆杯則臥汗出則已久者三飲而已

"This prescription employs eight *sheng* of [water] dipped many times from a ten-thousand *li* source. Select five *sheng* of the clearest [liquid] for cooking, make a reed-fueled fire and bring it to a boil. Obtain one *sheng* of husked sorghum and [decoct this] and five *he* of Pinellia Rhizoma *(ban xia)* over a slow fire down to one-and-a-half *sheng*. Remove the dregs, and drink one small cup three times a day or increasing slowly until the effect is apparent. If the illness is recent, the person will be able to go to bed after downing one cup, and once they sweat, [the problem] will be over. Chronic cases will be cured after having taken three doses."

李瀕湖云靈樞有云足太陽之筋為目上綱足陽明之筋為目下綱寒則
筋急目不合熱則筋縱目不開

Li Bin-Hu says, [Ch. 13] of *Divine Pivot* has a statement: "The sinew of the foot greater yang forms the upper ocular network, and the sinew of the foot yang brightness forms the lower ocular network.[17] When cold tenses the sinews, the eye [lids] will not close. When heat loosens the sinews, the eye [lids] will not open."

又云壯者血氣盛肌肉滑營衛不失其常故晝精而夜瞑老人氣血衰氣
道澀衛氣內伐故晝不精而夜不瞑

[Ch. 18 of *Divine Pivot*] also states: "Those who are strong are brimming with qi and blood, have supple muscle and flesh, and the nutritive and protective … have not lost their normalcy. Hence, they are energetic by day and shut [their eyes] at night. The elderly have depleted qi and blood, … the qi pathways do not flow smoothly, … [and therefore] the protective qi is cut off in the inside. Hence, their days are not energetic, and they cannot shut [their eyes] at night."

又云多臥者腸胃大而皮膚澀分肉不解衛氣行遲故也

[Ch. 80 of *Divine Pivot*] also states: "In those who spend their time lying down, the intestines and stomach [become] enlarged, the skin is rough, and it is not separated from the partings of the flesh. For this reason, the protective qi moves slowly."

張子和云思氣所至為不眠為嗜臥

Zhang Zi-He states: "[Excessive] pensiveness will result in either insomnia or a propensity to lie down."[18]

巢元方云脾病困倦而嗜臥膽病多煩而不眠

Chao Yuan-Fang says that spleen diseases cause fatigue and a propensity to lie down, while gallbladder diseases cause frequent bouts of irritability and insomnia.[19]

王叔和脈經云水流夜疾有聲者土休故也人亦應之人夜臥則脾不動
搖脈為之數疾也

Wang Shu-He in his *Pulse Classic* says that water flows more swiftly at night and with [a rippling] sound. This is because earth is at rest. Humans are analogous to this.[20] When humans lie down at night, their spleens do not stir and their pulse beats more rapidly [than during the day].

一云脾之候在瞼瞼動則知脾能消化也脾病則瞼澀嗜臥矣

It is also said that the spleen's indicators are the eyelids. If the eyelids are mobile, one knows that the spleen is able to perform its digestive function. If the spleen is diseased, then the eyelids do not move smoothly, and the patient has a propensity to lie down.

數說皆論目閉目不瞑雖不言及二蹻蓋亦不離乎陰陽營衛虛實之理
可互考者也

All of these many statements discuss the closure of the eyes and eyes that will not close, [and] although they make no mention of the two *qiao*, they do not diverge from the principles of yin and yang, nutritive and protective, deficiency and excess, all of which should be considered.

CHAPTER 9

衝脈

The *Chong* Vessel

衝為經脈之海又曰血海其脈与任脈皆起於少腹之內胞中其浮而外
者起於氣衝（一名氣街在少腹毛中兩旁各二寸橫骨兩端動脈宛宛
中足陽明穴也）并足陽明少陰二經之間循腹上行至橫骨（足陽明
去腹中行二寸少陰去腹中行五分衝脈行于二經之間也橫骨在陰上
橫骨中宛如偃月去腹中行一寸半）挾臍左右各五分上行瀝大赫（
模骨上一寸去腹中行一寸半）氣穴（即胞門一名子戶大赫上一寸
去腹中行一寸半少陰衝脈之會）四滿（氣穴上一寸）中注（四滿
上一寸）育腧（中往上一寸）商曲（育腧上二寸）石關（商曲上
一寸）陰都（石關上一寸）通谷（陰都上一寸）幽門（通谷上一
寸夾巨厥兩旁各五分陷中）至胸中而散凡二十四穴

The *chong* is the sea of the channels and vessels. It is also called the sea of blood. This vessel and the *ren* vessel both arise from within the gestational membranes in the lower abdomen. Surfacing and externalizing, it arises at Qi Thoroughfare (ST-30). (Also called the qi avenue, this hole is located two *cun* on either side of the midline in the [pubic hair] of the lower abdomen, on the pubic bone in the depression of the pulsing vessel; it is a hole on the foot yang brightness.)[1] Here, it travels alongside and between the two channels of the foot yang brightness and lesser yin[2] and proceeds along the abdomen, traveling upward to the pubic bone. (The foot yang brightness [channel] is located two *cun* from the midline of the abdomen; the foot lesser yin [channel] is located five *fen* from the midline of the abdomen; the trajectory of the *chong* vessel travels between these two vessels; the Pubic Bone (KI-11) is located above the genitals on the pubic bone, [in a depression] like a crescent moon, one-and-a-half *cun* from the midline of the abdomen.) Traveling five *fen* to the left and right sides of the navel, it ascends to Great Manifestation (KI-12) (located one-and-a-half *cun* above Horizontal Bone), Qi Hole (KI-13) (whose other name is Womb Door, which is located one *cun* above great manifestation, one-and-a-half *cun* out from the midline on the abdomen; it is a meeting [hole] of the lesser yin and *chong* vessels), Fourfold Fullness (KI-14) (located one *cun* above Qi Hole), Central Flow (KI-15) (located one *cun* above Fourfold Fullness), Huang Transport (KI-16) (located one *cun* above Central Flow),[3] *Shang* Bend (KI-17) (located one *cun* above Huang Transport), Stone Pass

(KI-18) (located one *cun* above *Shang* Bend), Yin Metropolis (KI-19) (located one *cun* above Stone Pass), Open Valley (KI-20) (located one *cun* above Yin Metropolis), and Dark Gate (KI-21) (located one *cun* above Open Valley, on either side of Great Tower Gate [CV-14]; each is in a depression five *fen* deep). From here, it reaches to penetrate the chest and spreads. There are 24 holes in all.

靈樞經曰任皆超於胞中上循背裏為經絡之海其浮而外者循腹右上行會於咽喉別而絡唇口血氣盛則充膚熱肉血獨盛則澹滲皮膚生毫毛婦人有余於氣不足於血月下數脫血任衝并傷脈不榮其口唇故髭須不生宦者去其宗筋傷其衝任血寫不復皮膚內結唇口不榮故須亦不生天宦不脫於血而任衝不盛宗筋不強有氣無血唇口不榮故須亦不生

[Ch. 65 of] *Divine Pivot* classic states: "The *chong* and *ren* both arise from the gestational membranes and proceed upward along the interior of the back, constituting the sea of the channels and networks. Surfacing and externalizing, [these vessels] proceed along the right side of the abdomen in an upward trajectory to meet the throat. They then diverge and connect to the lips and mouth. When there is an exuberance of both qi and blood, it replenishes the skin and heats up the flesh. When only the blood is overly abundant, then it gently infiltrates the skin and produces hair. Women have a surplus of qi and an insufficiency of blood, and the repeated loss of blood during their menstrual flow impairs their *ren* and *chong* vessels.[4] Since these vessels do not nourish the mouth and lips, neither beards nor moustaches grow [on women]." "Because eunuchs have been deprived of their genitals, this damage to the *chong* and *ren* causes the blood to drain and not return, the skin clumps internally, and the lips and mouth are not nourished, and therefore they cannot grow beards or moustaches. Males born without genitals do not experience a monthly shedding of blood, yet their *chong* and *ren*, too, are not exuberant and their gathering sinew cannot become strong. They have qi but lack blood, and therefore their beards also cannot grow."

素問水熱穴論曰三陰之所交結於腳也踝上各一行者此腎脈之下行也名曰太衝

[Ch. 61 of] *Basic Questions*, "Discourse on Holes for Water and Heat [Diseases]," states: "The intersection of the three yin fastens [them to one another] at the leg. Each [channel] travels [separately] above the ankle. … This [intersection is located] on the lower aspect of the kidney channel. It is called the Great Thoroughfare."

王啟玄曰腎脈与衝脈并下行循足合而盛大故曰太衝

Wang Qi-Xuan states: "The kidney vessel and the *chong* vessel merge and descend, proceeding to the foot where they unite and there is a great exuberance [of qi]. Hence, it is called the Great Thoroughfare."

一云衝脈超於氣衝衝直而通故謂之衝

Someone else has said the *chong* vessel arises at the Qi Thoroughfare, where it surges directly and freely, therefore, it is called the *chong* (thoroughfare) [vessel].

素問陰陽離合論曰賢人南面而立前曰廣明後曰太衝太衝之地名曰
少陰其衝在下名曰太衝

[Ch. 6 of] *Basic Questions*, "Discourse on the Places of Unification and Separation of Yin and Yang," states: "The sage faces south and stands erect. What is before him is called Vast Illumination, and what is behind him is called the Great Thoroughfare. The place of the Great Thoroughfare is called the lesser yin. … The thoroughfare that is below is called the Great Thoroughfare."[5]

王啟玄曰心藏在南故前曰廣明衝脈在北故後曰太衝足少陰腎脈与
衝脈合而盛大故曰太衝兩脈相合為表裏也衝脈在脾之下故曰其衝
在下名曰太陰

[Wang] Qi-Xuan said: "The heart viscera is located in the south, and therefore what is ahead is called Vast Illumination. The *chong* vessel is located in the north, and therefore what is behind is called the Great Thoroughfare. There is a great abundance at the confluence of the foot lesser yin kidney vessel and the *chong* vessel, and so it is called the Great Thoroughfare. The confluence of both vessels is [a confluence] of the interior with the exterior." "Because the *chong* vessel lies beneath the spleen [channel], it is said that the *chong* is located beneath," and it is called Greater Yin.

靈樞經曰帝曰少陰之脈獨下行何也

[Ch. 38 of] *Divine Pivot* classic states: "The Yellow Emperor said: Only the lesser yin vessel travels downward, why is this?"

岐伯曰不然夫衝脈者五藏六腑之海也其上者出於頏顙滲諸陽灌諸
精其下者注於少陰之大絡起於腎下出於氣街循陰股內廉斜入膕中
伏行骺骨內廉并少陰之經下入內踝之后入足下其別者并於少陰滲
三陰斜入踝伏行出屬跗屬下循跗上入大指之間滲諸絡而溫足脛肌
肉故其脈常動別絡結則跗上不動不動則厥厥則寒矣

Qi Bo said: "It is not so [i.e., it is not the lesser yin that goes downward, it is the *chong*]. The *chong* vessel is the sea of the five yin viscera and the six yang receptacles. … Its upward [trajectory] emerges at the juncture of the hard and soft palates,[6] percolating into all of the yang [channels] and irrigating the various essences. Its downward [trajectory] pours into the great network of the lesser yin, arising below the kidneys to emerge at the Qi Thoroughfare. It continues along the posterior medial aspect of the thigh and obliquely enters the popliteal fossa. It then travels concealed along the medial aspect of the tibia to adhere to the lesser yin channel. From here, it descends to penetrate behind the inner ankle and penetrate to the bottom of the foot. A diverging branch [of the network vessel] adheres to the lesser yin and percolates into the three yin; obliquely entering the ankle and traveling concealed through the instep, it continues downward along the instep to enter into the big toe. From here, it percolates into the network vessels and warms the flesh [of the leg], so therefore this vessel normally pulsates. If the diverging network is bound up, the pulsing on the dorsum of the foot ceases. If there is no pulsing, then there is reversal, and when there is reversal, it will become cold."

王海藏曰手少陽三焦相火為一府右腎命門為相火心包主亦名相火
其脈同診腎為生氣之門出而治臍下分三歧上衝夾臍過天樞上至膻
中兩乳間元氣所系焉

Wang Hai-Cang said that the hand lesser yang triple burner is one dwelling place of the ministerial fire, the right kidney life gate is the ministerial fire, and the heart envelope master[7] is also called the ministerial fire. These vessels are all diagnosed in the same manner. The kidney is the gate of qi generation.[8] It emerges from and governs [the area] below the umbilicus, and it is divided into three forks surging upward through the umbilicus via the Celestial Pivot (ST-25), ascending to reach the Chest Center (CV-17) beside both breasts. This is where the primal qi is tied in.

又足三焦太陽之別并足太陽正路入絡膀胱約下焦

There are also diverging branches of the foot triple burner and greater yang that adhere to the main pathway of the foot greater yang to enter and network with the bladder in the lower burner.

三焦者從頭至心心至臍臍至足為上中下三焦其實真元一氣也故曰
有藏無府

The triple burner extends from the head to reach the heart, from the heart to reach the umbilicus, and from the umbilicus to reach the foot, constituting the three upper, middle, and lower burners that are actually the true primal unitary qi. Hence, it is said that it stores but has no dwelling place.

脈訣云三焦無狀空有名寄在胸中膈相應

Pulse Rhymes[6] states: "The triple burner lacks form; it is empty but has a name. It takes shelter in the chest, and the diaphragm stands in relation to it."

一云其府在氣街中上焦在胃上口治在膻中中焦在胃管治在臍旁下
焦在臍下膀胱上口治在臍

Others say that it stores and accumulates [its qi] within the Qi Thoroughfare. The upper burner is located above the upper opening of the stomach, [and disorders of this burner] are treated at Chest Center. The middle burner is located in the passageways of the stomach, [and disorders of this burner] are treated beside the umbilicus. The lower burner is located below the umbilicus and at the upper opening of the urinary bladder, and [disorders of this burner are treated] at the umbilicus.

經曰原氣者三焦之別使也腎間動氣者真元一氣分為三路人之生命
也十二經之根本也

The *Classic [of Difficulties]* states: "The source qi is the triple burner's director of separation. The moving qi between the kidneys is the true primal unitary qi that divides into three routes. It is the life force of a person, and the root of the 12 channels."

李瀕湖曰三焦即命門之用与衝任督根通者故附著于此

Li Bin-Hu says that the triple burner performs life gate's function of communicating with the *chong, ren,* and *du,* and therefore [a discussion of it] is appended here.

CHAPTER 10

衝脈為病

Diseases of the *Chong* Vessel

越人難經曰衝脈為病逆氣而裡急靈樞經曰氣逆上刺膺中陷下者
與下胸動脈腹痛刺臍左右動脈按之立已不已刺氣街按之立已

[Qin] Yue-Ren in his *Classic of Difficulties* states: "When the *chong* vessel is diseased, there is a counterflow of qi and abdominal urgency."[1] [Ch. 26 of] *Divine Pivot Classic* states: "When there is a counterflow ascent of qi, prick the depression below the breast and at the pulsing vessel below the chest. If there is abdominal pain, prick the pulsing vessels to the left or right of the umbilicus. … [After needling, one should] massage [this area, and the pain] should immediately stop. If [the pain] does not stop, then prick the Qi Thoroughfare (ST-30). … [After removing the needle,] massaging [this area] should stop [the pain]."

李東垣曰秋冬之月胃脈四道為衝脈所逆脅下少陽脈二道而反上行
名曰厥逆其證氣上衝咽不得息而喘息有音不得臥宜調中益氣湯加
吳茱萸五分隨氣多少用之脾胃論夏月有此乃大熱之證用黃連黃柏
知母各等分酒洗炒為末白湯和丸每服一二百丸空心自湯下即以美
膳壓之不令停留胃中直至下元以瀉衝脈之邪也蓋此病隨四時寒熱
溫涼治之

[Li Dong-yuan] says that if during the autumn and winter months the four pathways of the stomach vessel are made to counterflow by the *chong* vessel and the two pathways of the *shao yang* vessel below the rib-sides reverse and move upward, this is called reversal counterflow. This pattern [is characterized by symptoms of] qi surging into the throat such that one cannot catch one's breath and sounds of wheezy respiration such that one cannot lie down.[2] [In this case,] one should add five *fen* of Evodia Fructus *(wu zh yu)* to Regulate the Middle to Augment the Qi Decoction *(tiao zhong yi qi tang)*, but the dose of this medicinal is dependent on the seasonal qi (*On the Spleen and Stomach*). When this condition occurs during the summer months, it is then a pattern of great heat; use equal amounts of Coptidis Rhizoma *(huang lian)*, Phellodendron Cortex *(huang bai)*, and Anemarrhena Rhizoma *(zhi mu)* that are soaked in wine, fried, powdered, and mixed with boiled hot water into pills. Each day, take one- or two-hundred pills. This preparation is administered on an empty stomach with hot boiled water and followed by a good meal to press it [into the lower warmer]. [Hence, the medication] will not become lodged in the stomach but will pass directly to the lower base to drain the pathogen from the *chong* vessel. In treating diseases of this kind, [physicians] must account for the influence of the four seasons, [treating accordingly with] cold, hot, warm, or cool [medicinals].

又曰凡逆氣上衝或兼裡急或作躁熱皆衝脈逆也若內傷病此宜補中
益氣湯加炒黃柏炒連知母以泄衝脈凡腎火旺及任督衝三脈盛者則
宜用酒炒黃柏知母亦不可久服恐妨胃也或腹中刺痛或裡急宜多用
甘草或虛坐而大便不得者皆屬血虛血虛則裡急宜用當歸逆氣裡急
隔咽不通大便不行者宜昇陽瀉熱湯主之方見（蘭室秘藏）麻木厥
氣上衝逆氣上行妄聞妄見者宜神功丸主之方見（蘭室秘藏）

[Li Dong-Yuan] also says that whenever there is qi counterflow and a surging ascension [of qi] that may be accompanied by abdominal urgency or agitation and heat, this is invariably due to a counterflow of the *chong* vessel. If such diseases are due to internal damage, then Tonify the Middle to Augment the Qi Decoction (*bu zhong yi qi tang*) with the addition of dry-fried Phellodendron Cortex (*chao huang bai*), dry-fried Coptidis Rhizoma (*chao huang lian*), and Anemarrhena Rhizoma (*zhi mu*) is indicated to drain the *chong* vessel. Whenever there is an exuberance of kidney fire leading to an overabundance of the three vessels of the *ren, du,* and *chong*, then it is appropriate to use wine-fried Phellodendron Cortex (*chao huang bai*) and Anemarrhena Rhizoma (*zhi mu*), but one may not administer these long-term for fear that they may harm the stomach. If there is a stabbing pain in the stomach or abdominal urgency, it is appropriate to use more Glycyrrhizae Radix (*gan cao*). When one sits in vain and the stool will not come, this indicates blood deficiency, and blood deficiency causes abdominal urgency, so it is appropriate to use Angelica Sinensis Radix (*dang gui*). For counterflow of qi and abdominal urgency such that there is obstruction in the diaphragm and throat, and inability to move one's bowels, then it is appropriate to use Raise the Yang and Drain Heat Decoction (*sheng yang xie re tang*) to master [the condition] (*Secrets from the Orchid Chamber*). For numbness, qi inversion, and a surging ascension of qi, this upward movement of counterflow qi causes loss of hearing and loss of sight, so it is appropriate to administer Miraculously Effective Pill (*shen gong wan*) to master [the condition][3] (*Secrets from the Orchid Chamber*).

孫真人千金方云咳唾手足厥逆氣從小腹上衝胸口咽其面翕熱如醉
因復下流陰股小便難時復冒者寸脈沉尺脈微宜茯苓五味子湯以治
其氣衝其方用茯苓五味子二錢桂心甘草一錢水煎服胸滿者去桂

In his [*Important*] *Formulas Worth a Thousand Gold Pieces*, the True Man Sun [Si-Miao] says that when there is a cough that causes one to spit up saliva accompanied by frigidly cold extremities, qi from the lower abdomen surges upward into the chest, mouth, and throat, [and] the face will be flushed and boiling hot as if one were intoxicated. [The patient feels] as if she will experience either urinary or fecal incontinence that will flow down the inner thigh, [and] there will be urinary difficulty [although the patient] remains anxious about the possible return of these symptoms. The distal pulse will be deep, and the proximal pulse will be faint. It is appropriate to use Poria and Schisandra Decoction *(ling wu wei zi tang)* to treat this surging of qi. The formula contains Poria *(fu ling)* and Schizandrae Fructus *(wu wei zi)*, 2 *qian* [each], Cinnamon Cortex *(rou xin)* and Glycyrrhizae Radix *(gan cao)*, 1 *qian* [each]. This is decocted in water and administered. If there is chest fullness, omit the Cinnamon Cortex *(rou gui)*.

程筺墩曰太平侯病膻腥中痛喘嘔吞酸臍上一點氣上至咽喉如冰每
子後申時輒發醫以為大寒不效

Cheng Huang-Dun reports that Lord Tai Ping suffered from pain in the area of Chest Center (CV-17), asthmatic breathing with vomiting, and acid regurgitation. From a single point above the umbilicus, qi would ascend to reach the throat with an icy sensation. Episodes of this kind would recur nightly between 11 P.M. and 1 A.M., and [between] 3 P.M. and 5 P.M. The physicians took this to be intense cold, and therefore the [therapy was] ineffective.

祝橘泉曰此得之大醉及厚味過多子後申時相火自下騰上故作痛也
以二陳加芩連梔子蒼術數飲而愈

[Commenting on this case], Zhu Ju-Quan says that [because the patient] drank too much and ate too much rich food, then between 11 P.M. and 1 A.M. and between 3 P.M. and 5 P.M., the ministerial fire that naturally descends galloped upward, resulting in pain. He was then given many draughts of Two-Aged [Herb] Decoction *(er chen tang)* with the addition of Scutellaria Radix *(huang qin)*, Coptidis Rhizoma *(huang lian)*, Gardenia Fructus *(zhi zi)*, and Atractylodes Rhizoma *(cang zhu)*, and the condition was cured after drinking [the decoction] numerous times.

素問痿論曰治痿獨取陽明者何也曰陽明者五臟六腑之海也主潤宗
筋宗筋主束骨而利機關衝脈者經脈之海主滲灌溪谷與陽明合於宗
筋會於氣街而陽明為之長皆屬於帶脈而絡於督脈故陽明虛則宗筋
縱帶脈不引故足痿不用治之當各補其營而通其腧調其虛實和其逆
順筋脈骨肉各以其時受月則病已（謂肝甲乙心丙丁脾戊己主氣法
時月也）

[Ch. 44 of] *Basic Questions,* "Treatise on Atrophy," [4] states: "Why is it that in treating atrophy one need only select the yang brightness channels?" It says: "The yang brightness is the sea of the five viscera and the six receptacles. It governs the moistening of the gathering sinews, and the gathering sinews bind the bones and provide mobility for the joints. The *chong* vessel is the sea of the channels and vessels, governing the permeation and irrigation of the valleys and streams. It unites with the yang brightness at the gathering sinew. ... It meets at the Qi Thoroughfare, and the yang brightness is the leader [of them all]. They are all ascribed to the *dai* vessel and linked to the *du* vessel. Hence, when the yang brightness is deficient, the gathering sinews become slack and the *dai* vessel is no longer able to lead it. This results in atrophy and loss of use of the feet." To treat this, "one should supplement at the spring holes and promote flow at the transport holes [of the yang brightness channels] to regulate deficiency and excess, harmonize abnormal and normal [flow of qi] so that the sinews, vessels, bones, and flesh will each recover from disease in their prevailing months (it is said that the prevailing months that govern the qi are liver *jia yi*, heart *bing ding*, and spleen *wu ji*)." [5]

李東垣曰暑月病甚則傳腎肝為痿厥痿乃四肢痿軟厥乃四肢如火或
如冰心煩衝脈氣逆上甚則火逆名曰厥逆故痿厥二病多相須也

Li Dong-Yuan stated that when this disease worsens during the months of summer-heat, it will be transmitted to the kidneys and liver, producing atrophy and reversal. The atrophy causes the four extremities to become atrophied and soft while the reversal causes the four extremities to be either [hot] as if on fire or [cold] as if frozen. There will be irritability of the heart, and the qi of the *chong* vessel counterflows upward, which in extreme cases will result in counterflow of fire. This is called reversal counterflow. Hence, the two diseases of wilting and reversal are usually interrelated.

經曰下氣不足則痿厥心悗宜以清燥去濕熱之藥或生脈散合四苓散
加酒洗黃柏知母以泄其濕熱

[*On the Spleen and Stomach*] classic states: "When the lower [burner] qi is insufficient, this results in atrophy, reversal, and flusteredness. [In such instances,] it is appropriate to use clearing and drying medicinals that get rid of dampness and heat, or Generate the Pulse Powder (*sheng mai san*) combined with Four-Ingredient Powder with Poria (*si ling san*) with the addition of wine-soaked Phellodendron Cortex (*huang bai*) and Anemarrhena Rhizoma (*zhi mu*) to drain the damp-heat."

李瀕湖曰濕熱成痿乃不足中有餘也宜滲泄之藥若精血枯涸成痿乃
不足中之不足也全要峻補之藥

Li *Bin-Hu* states: "When damp-heat produces atrophy, this is surplus within an insufficiency, and [it] is appropriate to use percolating and draining medicinals. When a desiccation of essence and blood produces atrophy, this is an insufficiency within an insufficiency, and it is essential to administer extremely tonifying medicinals."

靈樞經曰胸氣有街腹氣有街頭氣有街脛氣有街故氣在頭者上之於
腦氣在胸者止之膺與背腧氣在腹者上之背腧與衝脈於臍之左右之
動脈氣在脛者上之於氣街與承山踝上以下取此者用毫針先按在上
久應手乃刺而與之所治者頭痛眩僕腹痛中滿暴脹及有新積作痛

[Ch. 52 of] *Divine Pivot* classic states: "The chest qi has a thoroughfare, the abdominal qi has a thoroughfare, the head qi has a thoroughfare, and the qi of the shin area has a thoroughfare. Hence, when qi [accumulates] in the head, it ascends to the brain. When qi [accumulates] in the chest, it stops at the breast and back transport [holes]. When qi [accumulates] in the abdomen, it ascends to the back transport [holes] and *chong* vessel at the pulsing vessels on the left and right of the abdomen. When qi accumulates in the shin area, it ascends to the Qi Thoroughfare (ST-30) and Mountain Support (BL-57) from above the ankle to below. In selecting these [holes], use a filiform needle, first locating [the hole to be needled] and leaving [one's hand there] for a long time [until the qi arrives] in response to the hand; one may then needle. This treats headache, dizziness leading to fainting and syncope, abdominal pain with fullness in the middle and sudden distention, and recent accumulations producing pain."

素問舉痛論曰寒氣客於衝脈衝脈起於關元隨腹直上寒氣客則脈不
通脈不通則氣因之故喘動應手

[Ch. 39 of] *Basic Questions,* "A Comprehensive Discourse on Pain," states: "Cold qi lodges in the *chong* vessel. The *chong* vessel arises from the Origin Pass (CV-4), traveling directly upward along the abdomen. When cold qi lodges [in it], this vessel does not flow freely. Since the [*chong*] vessel does not flow freely, the qi follows it, resulting in wheezing and movements [of the abdomen] that can be felt with the hand."

王叔和脈經曰兩手脈浮之俱有陽沉之俱有陰陰陽皆盛此衝督之脈
也衝督之脈為十二經之道路也衝督用事則十二經不復朝於寸口其
人若恍惚狂癡

In his *Pulse Classic,* Wang Shu-He states: "As for the pulses on both arms, when those that are floating all have yang, and the submerged ones all have yin, then yin and yang are both exuberant and this is the pulse of the *chong* and *du* [vessels].[6] The vessels of the *chong* and *du* are the major pathways of the 12 channels, and if the *chong* and *du* overreach themselves, [the qi of the] 12 channels will not be able to return to the wrist pulse and a person may appear to be disoriented, manic, and dull witted."

又曰脈來中央堅實徑至關者衝脈也動苦少腹痛上搶心有瘕疝遺溺
脅支滿煩女子絕孕

He also states: "A pulse that arrives hard and excessive on the midline position to reach the middle position is the [pulse of the] *chong* vessel. [When the pulse is] perturbed in this way, [the patient] suffers from lower abdominal pain and qi rushing into the heart, mobile bulging, enuresis, distressing propping fullness of the rib-sides, and infertility."[7]

又曰尺寸俱牢直上直下乃衝脈胸中有寒疝痛也

He also states: "If from the proximal to the distal positions the pulse is confined, beating straight up and down, then there is cold bulging pain in the chest part of the *chong* vessel."

張仲景曰傷寒動氣在右不可發汗汗之則衄而渴心苦煩飲水即吐
（先以五苓散次以竹葉湯）不可下下之則津液內竭頭眩咽燥鼻
干心悸（竹葉湯）

Zhang Zhong-Jing states that for cold damage "accompanied by a pulsing qi on the right [side of the abdomen], one cannot induce sweating. If sweating is induced, there will be nosebleeds and thirst, the heart will suffer from irritability, and vomiting [will occur] immediately after drinking." (First use Five-Ingredient Powder with Poria *[wu ling san]*, and then, [if there is no improvement], use Bamboo Leaf Decoction *[zhu ye tang]*.) "This condition cannot be purged. Purgation will result in the fluids being spent, with dizziness, dry throat, dry nose, and heart palpitations" (Phyllostachis Decoction *[zhu ye tang]*).

動氣在左不可發汗汗之則頭眩汗不止筋惕肉瞤此為難治（或先用
防風白朮牡妨湯次用小建中湯）不可下下之則腹裡拘急不止動氣
反劇身雖有熱反欲拳（先服甘草干姜湯次服小建中湯）

"[When cold damage is accompanied by] a pulsing qi on the left [side of the abdomen], sweating must not be induced. If sweating is induced, there will be dizziness, the sweating will not stop, the sinews will jerk and the flesh will twitch." This is a difficult condition to treat. (First use Saposhnikovia, White Atractylodes, and Oyster Shell Decoction *[fang feng bai zhu mu li tang]*, and then use Minor Construct the Middle Decoction *[xiao jian zhong tang]*.) "[This condition] cannot be purged. Purgation will result in an urgent gripping in the interior of the abdomen that will not stop. The pulsing of qi will only intensify, and although the patient is feverish, they only desire to curl up." (First administer Licorice and Ginger Decoction *[gan cao gan jiang tang]*, and then use Minor Construct the Middle Decoction *[xiao jian zhong tang]*.)

動氣在上不可發汗汗之則氣上衝正在心端（椿根湯）不可下下之
則心中熱煩身熱汗泄欲水自灌（竹葉湯）

"[When cold damage is accompanied by] a pulsing qi above [the umbilicus], sweating must not be induced. If sweating is induced, the qi will surge upward to strike the apex of the heart" (Ailanthus Decoction *[chun gen tang]*). "[This condition] cannot be purged. Purgation will cause heat and irritability in the heart region, generalized feverishness with draining sweat, and a [thirst so intense that one] desires to pour water into oneself" (Phyllostachis Decoction *[zhu ye tang]*).

動氣在下不可發汗汗之則無汗心中大煩骨節疼頭痛目運惡寒吐谷
（先服大陳皮湯次服小建中湯）不可下下之則腹滿卒起頭眩食則
下清谷心下痞堅（甘草瀉心湯）

"[When cold damage is accompanied by] a pulsing qi below [the abdomen], sweating must not be induced. If sweating is induced, there will be no sweating, intense irritability in the heart, soreness in the bones and joints, headaches and vertigo, aversion to cold and vomiting of foodstuffs." (First administer Major Orange Peel Decoction *[da chen pi tang]*, and then use Minor Construct the Middle Decoction *[xiao jian zhong tang]*.) "[This condition] cannot be purged. Purgation will result in abdominal fullness, dizziness after getting up suddenly, diarrhea with undigested food after eating, and a firm focal distention under the heart" (Licorice Decoction to Drain the Epigastrium *[gan cao xie xin tang]*).

李瀕湖曰此乃臍之左右上下有氣築築然牢而痛正衝任足少陰太陰
四經病也成無己註文以為左肝右肺上心下脾蓋未審四臟乃兼邪耳

Li Bin-Hu states: This refers to [pulsing] to the left, right, above, and below the umbilicus that is due to stagnation so severe that it is quite painful.[8] It is actually a disease of the four channels of the *chong*, *ren*, foot lesser yin, and [foot] greater yin. The annotations by Cheng Wu-Ji that posit the left as the liver, right as the lung, above as the heart, and below as the spleen show that he failed to understand the four yin viscera, and [his comments] only confuse the reader.

歧伯曰海有東西南北人亦有四海以應之胃者水谷之海其輸上在氣
街下至三里衝脈為十二經之海其輸上在於大抒下出於巨虛之上下
廉膻中者為氣之海其輸上在於柱骨之上下前在人迎腦為髓之海其
輸上在於蓋下在風府

[In Ch. 33 of *Divine Pivot*], Qi Bo says that just as there are Northern, Southern, Eastern, and Western Seas, so [too do] humans have four seas that correspond to them. "The stomach is the sea of water and grains. Its transport [holes] include Qi Thoroughfare (ST-30) above and Three Li (ST-36) below. The *chong* vessel is the sea of the 12 channels. Its transport [holes] include Great Shuttle (BL-11) above and below it issues from both Upper and Lower Great Hollow (ST-37 and ST-39). The center of the chest is the sea of qi. Its transport [holes] are above and below the neck bone,[9] and at Man's Prognosis (ST-9) in front. The brain is the sea of marrow. Its transport [holes] are on top of the head above[10] and at Wind Pool (GV-16) below."

氣海有餘氣滿胸中急息面赤氣海不足則氣少不足以言血海有餘則
常想其身大怫然不知其所病血海不足亦常想其身小狹然不知其所
病水谷之海有餘則腹滿水谷之海不足則飢不受食髓海有餘則輕勁
多力自過其度髓海不足則腦轉耳鳴脛痠眩冒目無所見懈怠安臥

"When there is a surplus in the sea of qi, there will be qi fullness in the chest, rapid breathing, and a red face. When there is an insufficiency of the sea of qi, the breath is reduced and insufficient for speech. When there is a surplus in the sea of blood, commonly there will be the illusion [that] one's body is enlarged, depression and peevishness, and an inability to tell exactly where one feels sick. When there is an insufficiency in the sea of blood, commonly there will be the illusion that one's body is small and cramped and there will be an inability to tell exactly where one feels sick. When there is a surplus in the sea of water and grains, there will be abdominal fullness. When there is an insufficiency in the sea of water and grains, there will be hunger with an inability to ingest food. When there is a surplus in the sea of marrow, [the body] will be light, agile, possessed of great strength, and one will have the ability to accomplish what is normally beyond oneself. When there is an insufficiency in the sea of marrow, the brain will spin, the ears will ring, there will be aching pain in the lower legs, dizziness, and loss of vision, indolence, and somnolence."

CHAPTER 11

任脈

The *Ren* Vessel

任為陰脈之海其脈起于中極之下少腹之內會陰之分（在兩陰之
間）上行而外出循曲骨（橫骨上毛際陷中）上毛際至中極（臍下
四寸膀胱之募）同足厥陰太陰少陰並行腹裏循關元（臍下三寸小
腸之募三陰任脈之會）歷石門（即丹田一名命門在臍下二寸三焦
募也）氣海（臍下一寸半宛宛中男子生氣之海）會足少陰衝脈於
陰交（臍下一寸當膀胱上口三焦之募）

The *ren* vessel is the sea of the yin vessels. Its vessel arises below Central Pole (CV-3) from within the lower abdomen; it divides [from the *chong* and *du* vessels] at the Meeting of Yin (CV-1) (between the two yin [orifices]).[1] It ascends and emerges, proceeding to the Curved Bone (CV-2) (in a depression above the border of the [pubic] hair on the pubic bone),[2] ascending from the border of the pubic hair to arrive at Central Pole (CV-3) (four *cun* below the umbilicus; it is the alarm [hole] of the urinary bladder), where it meets with the foot reversing yin, greater yin and lesser yin inside the abdomen. [From here it] travels to Origin Pass (CV-4) (three *cun* below the umbilicus, it is the alarm [hole] of the small intestine and the meeting of the three yin with the *ren* vessel),[3] passing Stone Gate (CV-5) (the cinnabar field, also known as gate of vitality, is two *cun* below the umbilicus, and the alarm [hole] of the triple burner), and Sea of Qi (CV-6) (in a circular weakness one-and-a-half *cun* below the umbilicus, the sea of vitality for men), to meet with the foot lesser yin, and the *chong* vessel at Yin Intersection (CV-7) (one *cun* below the umbilicus, it is located at the upper orifice of the bladder).[4]

循神闕（臍中央）水分（臍上一寸當小腸下口）會足太陰於下脘
（臍上二寸當胃下口）歷建裏（臍上三寸）會手太陰少陽足陽明
於中脘（臍上四寸胃之募也）上上脘（臍上五寸）巨闕（臍上
三寸）會手太陰少陽足陽明於中脘（臍上四寸胃之募也）上上
脘（臍上五寸）巨闕（鳩尾下一寸心之募也）鳩尾（蔽骨下五
分）中庭（膻中下一寸六分陷中）膻中（玉堂下一寸六分直兩乳
中間）玉堂（紫宮下一寸六分）紫宮（華蓋下一寸六分）華蓋

（璇璣下一寸）璇璣（天突下一寸）上喉嚨會陰維于天突廉泉
（天突在結喉下四寸宛宛中廉泉在結喉舌下中央）

[The *ren* vessel continues,] proceeding to Spirit Gate Tower (CV-8) (the center of the umbilicus), Water Divide (CV-9) (one *cun* above the umbilicus, the lower aperture of the small intestine) to meet with the foot greater yin at Lower Duct (CV-10)[5] (two *cun* above the umbilicus, the lower aperture of the stomach), passing Interior Strengthening (CV-11) (three *cun* above the umbilicus), to meet with the hand greater yin, lesser yang and foot yang brightness at Central Duct (CV-12) (four *cun* above the umbilicus, the alarm [hole] of the stomach).[6] It travels upward to Upper Duct (CV-13) (five *cun* above the umbilicus)[7] to Great Tower Gate (CV-14) (one *cun* below Turtledove Tail [CV-15], the alarm [hole] of the heart), Turtledove Tail (CV-15)[8] (five *fen* below the sternum), Center Palace (CV-16) (in a depression one *cun* and six *fen* below Chest Center [CV-17]), Chest Center (CV-17) (one *cun* and six *fen* below Jade Hall [CV-18] and directly between the two nipples),[9] Jade Hall (CV-18) (one *cun* and six *fen* below Purple Palace [CV-19]), Purple Palace (CV-19) (one *cun* and six *fen* below Florid Canopy [CV-20]), Florid Canopy (CV-20) (one *cun* and six *fen* below Jade Swivel [CV-21]), and Jade Swivel (CV-21) (one *cun* below Celestial Chimney [CV-22]). From here, it ascends to the throat to meet the *yin wei* [vessel] at Celestial Chimney (CV-22) and Ridge Spring (CV-23). (Celestial Chimney [CV-22] is located in a weakness four *cun* below the laryngeal prominence, and Ridge Spring [CV-23] is located above the laryngeal prominence and below the tongue on the centerline.)[10]

上頤循承將與手足陽明督脈會（唇下陷中）環唇上一至下齦交復
出分行循面系兩目下之中央至承泣而終（目下七分直瞳子陷中一
二穴）凡二十七穴難經甲乙經并無循面以下之說

[The *ren* vessel] ascends to the jaw and proceeds to Sauce Receptacle (CV-24) where it meets with the hand and foot yang brightness and the *du* vessel (located in the depression below the lip).[11] It encircles the lips and reaches downward to Gum Intersection (GV-26). From here, it emerges and its trajectory splits, traversing the face and linking to the center [line] below both eyes to reach Tear Container (ST-1)[12] and terminates (located seven *fen* below the eye in a depression directly [below] the eyeball, there are two holes). In all, there are 27 holes. Neither the *Classic of Difficulties* nor *The Systematic Classic* asserts that [the *ren* vessel] "traverses the face."

任脈之別絡名曰尾翳下鳩尾散於腹實則腹皮痛虛則痒搔

"The branching network of the *ren* vessel is named Tail Screen. It descends from the xiphoid process and disperses throughout the abdomen. When it is excessive, the skin of the abdomen is painful, and when it is deficient, there is itching and scratching."[13]

靈樞經曰缺盆之中任脈也名曰天突其側動脈人迎足陽明也

[Ch. 2 of] *Divine Pivot* classic states: "Between the supraclavicular fossae is the *ren* vessel. [Its hole here] is called Celestial Chimney (CV-22)." "It [moves to] the pulsing vessel on the sides [of the throat] at Man's Prognosis (ST-9) on the foot yang brightness."[14]

CHAPTER 12

任脈為病

Diseases of the *Ren* Vessel

素問曰任脈為病男子內結七疝女子帶下瘕聚

[Ch. 60 of] *Basic Questions* states: "When the *ren* vessel is diseased, men develop internal clumping and the seven kinds of bulging, while women develop vaginal discharge and mobile abdominal masses and gatherings."

又曰女子二七而天癸至任脈通太衝脈盛月事以時下七七任脈虛太衝脈衰天癸竭地道不通故形壞而無子

[Ch. 1 of *Basic Questions*] also states that: "Women at the age of two times seven [years] attain their heavenly dew; [during this time,] the *ren* vessel flows freely and the great thoroughfare vessel fills, the menses come according to their time. At the age of seven times seven [years,] the *ren* vessel is empty and the great thoroughfare vessel weakens and heavenly dew is exhausted. The passages of earth are obstructed, the body deteriorates, and [a woman] can no longer bear children."[1]

又曰上氣有音者治其缺盆中（謂天突穴也陰維任脈之會刺一寸灸三壯）

[Ch. 60 of *Basic Questions*] also states: "When there is an audible ascent [of counterflowing] qi, then treat it between the supraclavicular fossae." (This is referring to the Celestial Chimney [CV-22], which is the meeting hole of the *yin wei* and *ren* vessels. It is pricked to a depth of one *cun*, and moxa is applied three times.)

脈經曰寸口脈來緊細實長至關者任脈也動苦少腹繞臍引橫骨陰中切痛取關元治之

The *Pulse Classic* states: When the wrist pulse is "tight, fine, and excessive, and [also] long arriving at the middle position, this is a *ren* pulse. [When the pulse] is perturbed in this way, [the patient] suffers from pain in the lower abdomen and around the umbilicus that radiates to the pubic bone and a stabbing pain in the genitals. Select Origin Pass (CV-4) to treat it."

又曰橫寸口邊脈丸丸者住脈也苦腹中有氣如指上搶心不得俯仰拘
急

It also states: "Forcefully striking across the qi opening pulse with a pill-like hardness to the vessel is the *ren* pulse. [When the pulse] is perturbed in this way, [the patient] suffers from a finger-shaped mass of qi in the abdomen that may surge into the heart such that there may be an inability to bend either forward or backward, and gripping urgency [in the chest]."

CHAPTER 13

督脈
The *Du* Vessel

督乃陽脈之海其脈起於腎下胞中至於少腹乃下行於腰橫骨圍之中
央系溺孔之端男子循莖下至篡女子絡陰器合篡間俱繞篡後屏翳穴
（前陰後陰之間也）

The *du* is the sea of yang vessels. Its vessel originates from within the gestational membranes below the kidneys and reaches the lower abdomen where it travels downward to the lumbar area and circles the pubic bone, where it links with the end of the urethral opening. In men, it proceeds to the penis and then descends to reach the perineum. In women, a network travels to the genital organs and unites in the perineum. All [of these various pathways] encircle the perineum behind the Barrier Screen (CV-1) hole (between the anterior yin [urethra] and posterior yin [anus]).

別繞臀至少陰與太陽中絡者合少陰上股內廉由會陽（在陰尾尻骨
兩旁凡二穴）貫脊會於長強穴在骶骨端與少陰會並脊裏上行歷腰
腧（二十一椎下）陽關（十六椎下）命門（十四椎下）懸樞（十
三椎下）脊中（十一椎下）中樞（十椎下）筋縮（九椎下）至陽
（七椎下）靈臺（六椎下）神道（五椎下）身柱（三椎下）陶道
（大椎下）大椎（一椎下）與手足三陽會合上啞門（項後入發際
五分）會陽維入系舌本上至風府（項後入發際一寸大筋內宛宛
中）會足太陽陽維同入腦中循腦戶（在枕骨上）強間（百會後三
寸）後項（百會後一寸半）上巔歷百會（項中央旋毛中）前項
（百會前一寸半）囟會（百舍前三寸即囟門）上星（囟會前一
寸）至神庭（囟會前二寸直鼻上入發際五分）為足太陽督脈之會
循額中至鼻柱經素髎（鼻準也）水溝（即人中）合手足陽明至兌
端（在唇上端）入齦交（上齒逢中）与任脈足陽明交會而終凡三
十一穴

A diverging branch encircles the buttocks to reach the lesser yin; along with the middle networks of the greater yang,[1] it then unites with the lesser yin and ascends the inner thigh. From the Meeting of Yang (BL-35) (on either side of the yin side of the coccyx, two holes) it links with the spine to meet the Long Strong (GV-1) hole at the tip of the coccyx[2] where it meets with the lesser yin, merging into the spine, and travels upward.[3] [It passes through] Lumbar Transport (GV-2) (below the 21st vertebrae), Lumbar Yang Pass (GV-3) (below the 16th vertebrae), Life Gate (GV-4) (below the 14th vertebrae), Suspended Pivot (GV-5) (below the 13th vertebrae), Spinal Center (GV-6) (below the 11th vertebrae), Central Pivot (GV-7) (below the 10th vertebrae), Sinew Contraction (GV-8) (below the 9th vertebrae), Extremity of Yang (GV-9) (below the 7th vertebrae), Spirit Tower (GV-10) (below the 6th vertebrae), Spirit Path (GV-11) (below the 5th vertebrae), Body Pillar (GV-12) (below the 3rd vertebrae),[4] Kiln Path (GV-13) (below the large vertebrae),[5] and Great Hammer (GV-14) (below the 1st vertebrae) where it meets with the three yang [channels] of both the hands and feet.[6] From here, it ascends to Mute's Gate (GV-15) (on the nape of the neck, 5 *fen* inside the hairline), where it meets with the *yang wei* and enters [the head] to link with the root of the tongue. It then ascends to Wind House (GV-16) (on the nape of the neck, one *cun* within the hairline, in a depression within the large sinews) where it meets with the greater yang and *yang wei,* and together, they all enter into the brain.[7] [The *du* vessel] then passes to Brain's Door (GV-17) (just above the occipital bone),[8] Unyielding Space (GV-18) (three *cun* behind Hundred Convergences [GV-20]), Behind the Vertex (GV-19) (one-and-a-half *cun* behind Hundred Convergences), and ascends to the vertex and Hundred Convergences (GV-20),[9] Before the Vertex, (GV-21) (one and a half *cun* in front of Hundred Convergences), Fontanel Meeting (GV-22) (three *cun* in front of Hundred Convergences; this is also called Fontanel Door), Upper Star (GV-23) (one *cun* in front of Fontanel Meeting) to arrive at Spirit Court (GV-24) (two *cun* in front of Fontanel Meeting, directly above the nose, five *fen* inside the hairline) where the foot greater yang and the *du* vessel meet.[10] It then traverses the forehead to the bridge of the nose to connect with White Bone (GV-25) hole and Water Trough (GV-26) (also called Human Center)[11] where it meets with the hand and foot yang brightness to reach Extremity of the Mouth (GV-27) (at the margin of the upper lip) and finally enters Gum Intersection (GV-28) (on the upper gum line) where it intersects with the *ren* vessel and the foot yang brightness and terminates.[12] In all, there are 31 holes.

督脈別絡自長強走任脈者由少腹直上貫臍中央上貫心入喉上頤環
唇上系兩目之下中央會太陽於目內眥睛明穴（見陰蹻下）上額與
足厥陰同陰於巔入絡於腦

A branching network of the *du* vessel that travels from Long Strong (GV-1) to the *ren* vessel goes straight up from the lower abdomen and links with the center of the umbilicus, ascending to link with the heart. From here, it enters the pharynx, ascends to the cheek, and encircles the lips. It then ascends and connects to below the eyes on their midlines. It meets with the greater yang at the inner canthus at the Bright Eyes (BL-1) hole (see the end of the *yin qiao* [trajectory]).[13] From here, it ascends to the forehead and meets at the foot reversing yin at the vertex where it enters and networks with the brain.

又別自腦下項循肩胛與手足太陽少陽會於大杼（第一椎下兩旁去
脊中一寸五分陷中）內挾脊抵腰中入循脊絡腎

Another branch from the brain goes down to the nape, proceeds along the scapula to meet the hand and foot greater yang and the lesser yin at Large Pillow (BL-11) (on either side of the 1st vertebrae in a depression one *cun* and five *fen* out from the middle of the spine). [From here,] it moves inside, hugging the spine to support the lower back, and proceeds along the backbone to network with the kidneys.

難經曰督脈住脈四尺五寸會共九尺

The *Classic of Difficulties* states: "The *du* and *ren* [vessels] are four *chi* and five *cun* [long] … and altogether they make nine *chi*."[14]

靈樞經曰頸中央之脈督脈也名曰風府

[Ch. 2 of] *Divine Pivot* states: "The vessel on the midline of the neck is the *du* vessel. It is called Wind Adobe (GV-16)."

張潔古曰督者都也為陽脈之都網任者妊也為陰脈之妊養

Zhang Jie-Gu says that the *du* is the capital and ties together all the yang vessels. The *ren* is the pregnant female and nurtures all of the yin vessels.[15]

王海藏曰陰蹻陽蹻同起跟中乃氣並而相連任脈督脈同起中極之下
乃水溝而相接

Wang Hai-Cang says that the *yin qiao* and *yang qiao* arise together from the heel. Their qi has merged [together] and is mutually connected. The *ren* vessel and *du* vessel arise from below the Central Pivot (GV-7) at the Water Ditch (GV-26) and connect with one another there.[16]

滑伯仁曰任督二脈一源而二歧一行於身之前一行於身之後人身之
有任督猶天地之有子午可以分可以合分之以見陰陽之不離合之以
見渾淪之無間一而二二而一者也

Hua Bo-Ren states: "The two vessels of the *ren* and *du* are but two branches with a single source. One travels along the front of the body and another travels along the back of the body. A person's body has the *ren* and *du*, just as heaven and earth have *zi* and *wu* [midday and midnight], which may be perceived as divided or united. Divide them and it is apparent that their yin and yang [aspects] cannot be separated. Unite them [and] it is apparent that they are coalesced without differentiation. The singular is plural, and the plural is singular." [17]

李瀕湖曰任督二脈人身之子午也乃丹家陽火陰符升降之道坎水離
火交媾之鄉故魏伯陽參同契雲上閉則稱有下閉則稱無無者以奉上
上有神德居此兩孔穴法金氣亦雙須

Li Bin-Hu says that the two vessels of the *ren* and *du* are the human body's *zi* and *wu* [midday and midnight]. They are the elixir cultivator's pathways for the ascent and descent of the yang fire and the yin talisman. [18] They are the place of intersection of *kun* water and *li* fire. Therefore, Wei Bo-Yang, in his *Token for the Agreement of the Three*, states: "When the upper is closed, [19] it is called being, and when the lower is closed, it is called nothingness. Nothingness is elevated to the upper [part or the body], and the spirit virtue resides in the upper [part of the body]. By means of this two-holed method, the golden qi also requires both [being and nothingness]."

崔希范天元入藥镜雲上鵲橋下鵲橋天應星地應潮當根竅復命關貫
尾閭通泥九

Cui Xi-Fan in his *Mirror on the Admixture of Medicines to the Heavenly Origin* states: "There is an Upper Magpie Bridge and a Lower Magpie Bridge. Heaven resonates with the stars [above], and the earth resonates with the tides [below]. [One must] restore the root aperture and return to the Life Barrier, pass through the Caudal Funnel, and penetrate the Mud Ball."

大道三享直指雲修丹之士身中一竅名曰玄牝正在乾之下坤之上震
之西兌之東坎寓交媾之地在人身天地之正中八脈九竅十二經十五
絡聯轄虛間一穴空懸黍珠

The Direct Teaching of the Great Way in Three Chapters states that the cultivators of the elixir are possessed of a premier aperture in the body, and this is called the Mysterious Female. "It is located directly below *qian*, above *kun*, to the west of *zhen*, and east of *dui*, and is the place where *kan* and *li* mate. It is right in the center of the body's heaven and earth; the eight vessels, nine orifices, 12 channels, and 15 networks are all interconnected in this one grotto in the gap of emptiness and suspended in the void like pearls of barley."

醫書之任督二脈此元氣之所由生真息之所由超修丹之士不明此竅
則真息不生神化無基也

The two vessels of the *ren* and *du* [mentioned] in medical texts are where the primal qi is engendered, and the place from which the true breath arises. If cultivators of the elixir lack understanding of this opening, then the true breath is not engendered, and the transformation of the spirit is without foundation.

俞琰註參同契雲人身血氣往來循環晝夜不停醫書有住督二脈人能通此二脈則百脈皆通

Yu Yan's annotations to *Token to the Agreement of the Three* states that the circulation of qi and blood within the human body ebbs and flows day and night without ceasing. The medical texts have the two vessels of the *du* and *ren*. "If a person can open these two vessels, then all the hundreds of vessels can be open."

黃庭經言皆在心內運天經晝夜存之自長生

Scripture of the Yellow Court states: "Whoever circulates these heavenly channels within one's mind, protecting himself night and day, will extend one's life."[20]

天經乃吾身之黃道呼吸往來於此也鹿運尾閭能通督脈龜納鼻息能通任脈故二物皆長壽此數說皆丹家河車妙旨也而藥物火候自有別傳

"The heavenly channels are our body's Yellow Pathway, and our respiration comes and goes in relation to these. Deer movement through the Caudal Funnel enables the opening of the *du vessel*. Tortoise inhalation through one's nose enables the opening of the *ren* vessel. Hence, these two animals prolong life.[21] These numerous theories are derived from the sublime and secret teachings of the River Vehicle[22] of the elixir cultivators. [The lore] of herbal products and the art of firing [metals in alchemical preparation] are transmitted separately [in other texts]."[23]

王海藏曰張平叔言鉛乃北方正氣一點初生之真陽為丹母其蟲為龜即坎之二陰也地軸也一陽為蛇天根也陽生於子藏之命門元氣之所系出入於此其用在臍下為天地之根玄牝之門通厥陰分三峻為三車一念之非降而為漏一念之是守而成鉛升而接離補而成乾陰歸養化是以還元至虛至靜道法自然飛升而仙

Wang Hai-Cang says that: According to Zhang Ping-Shu, lead is the upright qi of the northern direction that represents a drop of emerging true yang, [and is a straight] yang line in the middle of the trigram *kan* and is the expression of initial growth producing the Maternal Elixir; its bug is the tortoise, resulting in the two yin [lines] of [the trigram] *kan*. This [central line] is the earth's axis. This first yang line is the snake and the root of heaven. Yang is engendered in the seed-store of the life gate, that which connects the primal qi; going and coming thus, it functions below the umbilicus as the root of heaven and earth, the gate of the Mysterious Female flowing through the reversing yin, and dividing into three branches to become three vehicles. If one harbors incorrect thoughts, then it descends and leaks out. If one maintains correct thoughts, then it is stored and becomes lead. It ascends and reunites with *li*. It is further enhanced and becomes *qian*. The restoration of yin and transformation of yang is what facilitates the return to the origin. Having achieved emptiness and achieved quietude, thereby expressing the Way with spontaneity, [the adept] soars up and becomes transcendent.[24]

CHAPTER 14

督脈為病
Diseases of the *Du* Vessel

素問骨空論雲督脈生疾從少腹上衝心而痛不得前後為衝疝女子為
不孕癃閉遺溺嗌乾治在骨上（謂腰橫骨上毛際中曲骨穴也）甚者
在臍下營（臍下一寸，陰交穴也）

[Ch. 60 of] *Basic Questions,* "The Discourse on the Bones and Holes," states: "When the *du* vessel is afflicted,[1] [qi] surges upward from the lower abdomen to the heart and produces pain. One cannot urinate or defecate. This is surging bulging.[2] In women, this presents as infertility,[3] dribbling urinary blockage, urinary frequency, and a dry throat … treat this above the bone (this refers to the Curved Bone (CV-2) hole that is located at the midline of the hair line above the pubic bone). In severe cases, treat the barracks below the umbilicus (one *cun* below the umbilicus is the Yin Intersection [CV-7] hole)."[4]

王啟玄曰此乃任衝二脈之病不知何以屬之督脈

Wang Qi-Xuan says, "This is a disease of the two vessels of the *ren* and *chong*. I do not know how this could pertain to the *du* vessel."

李瀕湖曰督脈雖行於背而別絡自長強走任脈者則由少腹直上貫臍
中貫心入喉上頤環唇而入於目之內眥故顯此諸證啟玄蓋未深考爾

Li Bin-Hu says, although the *du* vessel traverses the spine, a diverging network vessel issues from Long Strong (GV-1) to the *ren* vessel, [so the *du* channel] travels from the lower abdomen directly upward, linking with the center of the umbilicus, linking with the heart and entering the pharynx, ascending to the cheeks, encircling the lips and entering the inner canthus of the eye.[5] Hence, [the cause of] all of the above symptoms is obvious. [Wang] Qi-Xuan has not considered this issue very deeply.

素問曰督脈實則脊強反折虛則頭重高搖之挾脊之有過者取之所別
也

[Ch. 60 of] *Basic Questions* states: "The *du* vessel [...] when excessive, presents with

149

arched-back rigidity. When deficient, it presents with heavy-headedness such that one wobbles one's head [in an attempt to hold it up], and if there is pathological change [in the diverging network of the *du* vessel] that hugs the spine, select the diverging [hole]." [6]

秦越人難經曰督脈為病脊強而厥

Qin Yue-Ren, in his *Classic of Difficulties,* states: "When the *du* vessel becomes diseased, there is spinal rigidity and reversal." [7]

王海藏曰此病宜用羌活獨活防風荊芥細辛藁本黃連大黃附子烏頭蒼耳之類

Wang Hai-Cang says that, for this disease, it is appropriate to use medicinals in the class of Notopterygii Rhizoma seu Radix *(qiang huo),* Angelicae pubescentis Radix *(du huo),* Saposhnikovia Radix *(fang feng),* Schizonepetae Herba *(jing jie),* Asari Radix et Rhizoma *(xi xin),* Ligustici Rhizoma *(gao ben),* Coptidis Rhizoma *(huang lian),* Rhei Radix et Rhizoma *(da huang),* Aconiti Radix lateralis preparata *(fu zi),* Aconti Radix *(wu tou),* and Xanthii Fructus *(cang er zi).*[8]

張仲景金匱云脊強者五痙之總名其證卒口噤背反張而瘛瘲諸藥不巳可灸身柱大椎陶道穴

Zhang Zhong-Jing, in his *[Essentials from the] Golden Cabinet,* says that spinal rigidity is the general appellation for the five [types of] rigidity. Its symptoms include trismus, arched-back rigidity, and contractures. When medicinals are ineffective for these [symptoms] one may perform moxa on the Body Pillar (GV-12), Great Hammer (GV-14), and Kiln Path (GV-13) holes.

又曰痙家脈築築而弦直上下行

[Zhang Zhong-Jing] also states: "The pulse of those with rigidity is disturbed and wiry; its movement beats straight up and down."

王叔和脈經曰尺寸俱浮直上直下此為督脈腰背強痛不得俯仰大人癲病小兒風癇

Wang Shu-He in his *Pulse Classic* states: "When the pulses from the proximal to the distal positions are all floating [beating] straight up and straight down, this is the *du* pulse. [When the pulse is] perturbed in this way, [the patient] suffers from rigidity and pain of the entire back and will be unable to bend forward or backward. Adults will have seizures, and children will have wind seizures." [9]

又曰脈來中央浮直上下動者督脈也動苦腰背膝寒大人癲小兒癇宜
灸頂上三壯

[Wang Shu-He] also states: "A pulse that arrives as floating in the middle positions pulsing directly up and down is the *du* pulse. [When the pulse is] perturbed in this way, [the patient] suffers from cold of the back and knees, adults will have seizures, and children will have wind seizures. In such cases, it is appropriate to administer three cones of moxibustion to the vertex." [10]

素問風論曰風氣循風府而上則為腦風風入系頭則為目風眼寒

[Ch. 42 of] *Basic Questions,* "The Discourse on Wind," states: "Wind qi proceeds to the Wind House (GV-16) and ascends, which then becomes brain wind. Wind may [also] enter and link to the head, which then becomes eye wind and eye cold." [11]

王啟玄云腦戶乃督脈足太陽之會故也

Wang Qi-Xuan states: "Brain's Door (GV-17) is the meeting [hole] of the *du* vessel and the foot greater yang … ."

CHAPTER 15

帶脈

The *Dai* Vessel

帶脈者同足少陽循帶脈穴（章門足厥陰少陽之合在季肋骨端肘尖
盡處是穴帶脈穴屬足少陽經在季脅下一寸八分陷中）圍身一周如
束帶然又與足少陽會於五樞（帶脈下三寸）維道（章門下五寸三
分）凡八穴

The *dai* vessel arises at the tip of the free ribs at the foot reversing yin hole Camphor-wood Gate (LR-13). Together with the foot lesser yang, it travels to the Girdle Vessel (GB-26) hole. (Camphorwood Gate [LR-13] is the confluence of the foot reversing yin and lesser yang, and is located at the tip of the free rib bone. The hole is where the tip of the elbow [touches the side of the thorax]; the Girdle Vessel [GB-26] hole is on the foot lesser yang channel in the depression one *cun* and eight *fen* below the tip of the free ribs.) [This vessel] encircles the entire body like a girdle. [Traveling] with the foot lesser yang, it meets with Fifth Pivot (GB-27) (located three *cun* below Girdle Vessel [GB-26]) and Linking Path GB-28 (located five *cun* and three *fen* below Camphorwood Gate [LR-13]). There are eight holes in all.

靈樞經曰足少陰之正至膕中別走太陽而合上至腎當十四椎出屬帶
脈

[Ch. 11 of] *Divine Pivot* classic states: "The primary [channel] of the foot lesser yin reaches the popliteal fossa and, diverging, travels to the greater yang to unite with it. It ascends to reach the kidney, and at the 14th vertebra, emerges to home to the *dai* vessel."

揚氏曰使不妄如人束帶而前垂故名婦人惡露隨帶脈而下故謂之帶
下

Mr. Yang says that the *dai* vessel binds together all of the vessels, preventing them [from] being misaligned, like a man who ties together a belt which he hangs in front; hence the name. A woman's lochia follows the *dai* vessel and is discharged. Therefore, [similar vaginal discharges] are called *dai*.

CHAPTER 16

帶之為病

Diseases of the *Dai* Vessel

越人帶之為病腹滿腰溶溶如坐水中（溶溶緩慢貌）

[Qin] Yue-Ren states: "When the *dai* is diseased, there is abdominal fullness, and there will be [a sense of structural] dissolution in the low back as if sitting in water (dissolution, as in seeming to be lax or sluggish)."[1]

明堂曰帶脈二穴主腰腹縱溶溶如囊水之狀婦人少腹痛裏急後重瘕瘕月事不調赤白帶下可針六分灸七壯

Luminous Court[2] states: The *dai* vessel has two holes; "it masters low back and abdominal dissolution, [lacking structure] like a bag of water. In women, there will be lower abdominal pain and tenesmus, contractures, menstrual irregularity, and red and white vaginal discharge." [These holes] may be needled to a depth of six *fen,* and moxibustion can be applied seven times.

張潔古曰帶脈之病太陰主之宜灸章門二穴三壯

Zhang Jie-Gu says that for diseases of the *dai* vessel, the greater yin masters them. One should moxa both Camphorwood Gate (LR-13) holes three times.[3]

素問曰邪客于太陰之絡令人腰痛引小腹控不可以養息（胁謂季脅下之空軟處）

[Ch. 63 of] *Basic Questions* states: "When pathogens invade the networks of the greater yin, this causes a person to experience lumbar pain radiating to the lower abdomen and up to below the free ribs such that one cannot catch one's breath." ([The word] *chao* refers to the soft hollow spot below the free ribs.)[4]

張仲景曰大病瘥後腰以下有水氣牡蠣澤瀉散主之若不已灸章門穴

Zhang Zhong-Jing states: "If after a severe illness there is water qi from the lumbar region down, Oyster Shell and Alisma Powder (*mu li ze xie san*) masters it."[5] If it does not stop, then perform moxibustion at Camphorwood Gate (LR-13).

王叔和曰帶脈為病左右繞臍膘脊痛衝陰股也

Wang Shu-He states: Diseases of the *dai* vessel "extend to the left and right encircling the umbilicus [and the entire torso] with pain in the lumbar spine that surges down the inside of the thighs."[6]

王海藏曰小兒癩疝可灸章門三壯而愈以其與帶脈行於厥陰之分而
太陰主之

Wang Hai-Cang says that for pediatric protuberant bulging, one may moxa Camphorwood Gate (LR-13) three times, and this will effect a cure because the *dai* vessel passes through the region of terminal yin, and the greater yin masters it.

又曰女子經病血崩久而成枯者宜澀之益之血閉久而成竭者宜益之
破之破血有三治始則四物入紅花調黃蓍肉桂次則四物入紅花調鯪
鯉甲桃仁桂童子小便利酒煎服末則四物入紅花調易老沒藥散

He also says: "For women's menstrual diseases such as heavy uterine bleeding that becomes chronic and causes withering, one should bind [the blood] and augment [the qi]. For blood obstruction that becomes chronic and cause exhaustion, one should augment [the qi] and break up [blood stasis]. There are three treatments that break up blood [stasis]. Initially, one may use Four-Substance Decoction *(si wu tang)* with the addition of Carthami Flos *(hong hua)* and suitable amounts of Astragali Radix *(huang qi)* and Cinnamoni Cortex *(rou gui)*. Next, one may use Four-Substance Decoction *(si wu tang)* with the addition of Carthami Flos *(hong hua)*, suitable amounts of Persica Semen *(tao [ren])*, Cinnamoni Cortex *(rou [gui])*, and Urinae Hominis *(tong zi xiao bian)*, which are decocted in wine and administered. Finally, one may use Four-Substance Decoction *(si wu tang)* with the addition of Carthami Flos *(hong hua)* and suitable amounts of Myrrha Powder for Easy Aging *(yi lao mo yao san)*.[7]

張子和曰十二經與奇經七脈皆上下周流惟帶脈起少腹之側季脅之
下環身一周絡腰而過如束帶之狀而衝任二脈循腹脅夾臍旁傳流于
氣衝屬于帶脈絡于督脈衝任督三脈同起而異行一源而三岐皆絡帶
脈因諸經上下往來遺熱于帶脈之間客熱鬱抑白物滿溢隨溲而下綿
綿不絕是為白帶

Zhang Zi-He says that the 12 channels and seven of the extraordinary vessels all flow up and down. Only the *dai* vessel arises from the sides of the lateral abdomen below the free ribs and encircles the body, networking with the lumbar region and passing on like a tightly tied belt. The two vessels of the *chong* and *ren* travel along the abdomen, hugging the umbilicus and flowing from the Qi Thoroughfare [hole], which belongs to the *dai* vessel, and networking with the *du* vessel. The three vessels of the *chong*, *ren*, and *du* have the same origins but their trajectories differ. They are of a single source but have three branches and all network with the *dai* vessel. Since all of the [other] channels move upward and downward, when heat is left in the *dai* vessel, this lodged heat becomes constrained and oppressed, causing white substances to become full to overflowing. They follow the urine and are discharged in a continuous and unbroken manner [known as] white *dai* [disease in women].[8]

内經云思想無窮所願不得意淫于外入房太甚發為筋痿及為白淫

[Ch. 44 of] *Inner Classic's [Basic Questions]* says: "When obsessive thoughts persist indefinitely, when one fails to attain what one aspires to, when one engages in wanton thoughts or when one engages in excessive bedroom activity, … this causes a withering of the [ancestral] sinew [penis] leading to white excess [in men]."[9]

白淫者白物淫衍如精之狀男子因溲而下女子綿綿而下也皆從濕熱
治之與治痢同法赤白痢乃邪熱侍於大腸赤白帶乃邪熱傳於小腸後
世皆以赤為熱白為寒流誤千載是醫誤之矣

This excess emission of white is the excess emission of white substances, which take the form of semen. In men, it is discharged with the urine, and in women there will be a continuous [vaginal] discharge.[10] All of these [conditions] are treated as damp-heat and are addressed using the same methods that one would apply in treating dysentery. Red and white dysentery is [an expression of] pathogenic heat being transmitted to the large intestine, while red and white vaginal discharge is an expression of pathogenic heat being transmitted to the small intestine [channel]. In later times, everyone attributes redness to heat and whiteness to cold. This error has been perpetuated in thousands of writings, and this is a mistake that doctors make.

又曰資生絞載一婦人患赤白帶下有人為灸氣海未效次日為灸帶脈
穴有鬼附耳云昨日灸亦好只灸我不著今灸著我我去矣可為酒食祭
我其家如其言祭之遂愈

[Zhang Zi-He] also says that in *Classic of Nourishing Life* there was a woman who suffered from red and white *dai* [disease] and someone applied moxibustion to the Sea of Qi (CV-6) [hole], which proved ineffective, so the next day I [Zhang] did moxa on the Girdling Vessel (GB-26) hole. A ghost attached itself to my ear and said, "Yesterday's moxibustion [on the Sea of Qi (CV-6)] was good, but it did not get to me [and] cleave to me, but today's moxibustion [where I am residing] did cleave to me so I will leave now. You may offer wine and food to propitiate me." [The patient's] family did the propitiation as instructed, and she thereupon recovered.

予初怪其事因思晉景公膏育二鬼之事乃虛勞已甚鬼得乘虛居之此
婦亦或勞心虛損故鬼居之灸既著穴不得不去

At first, I [Li Shi-Zhen] was taken aback by this affair as I was reminded of the two ghosts who resided in the Gao Huang [BL-43 holes] of Duke Jing of Jin [during the Warring States period]. That is to say, [the prince was suffering from] such severe exhaustion that the ghosts were able take advantage of this deficiency and take up residence there. This woman [with red and white *dai* disease] may also have suffered deficiency and harm from overexertion by the heart, hence, ghosts could have taken up residence in the Girdling Vessel (GB-26) [hole]. Once moxibustion had cleaved to [the ghost] in the hole, it could not help but depart.

自是凡有病此者每為之按此穴莫不應手酸痛令歸灸之無有不愈其
穴在兩脅季肋之下一寸八分若更灸百合穴尤佳內經云上有病下取
之下有病上取之又曰上者下之下者上之是矣

Since this [experience], whenever a patient has a disease such as this, I always palpate these holes and they are invariably sore when pressed. I have them return to apply moxibustion over [this hole], and they are invariably cured. The hole is one *cun* and eight *fen* below the tip of both free ribs. [Also] if one applies moxibustion to the Hundred Convergences (GV-20) hole, this [will] yield an even better [result].[11] The reason [I also added Hundred Convergences (GV-20) to treat this condition] is that [Ch. 9 of] *Inner Classic's [Divine Pivot]* states: "When the upper [part of the body] is diseased, then select [holes] in the lower [part of the body to treat it]; when the lower [part of the body] is diseased, then select [holes] to treat [it in the upper part of the body]." It also says for that which is above, cause it to descend, and for that which is below, raise it.

劉宗厚曰帶下多本於陰虛陽竭營氣不升經脈凝澀衛氣下陷精氣積
滯下焦奇經之分蘊釀而成以帶脈為病得名亦以病形而名白者屬氣
赤者屬血多因醉飽房勞服食燥熱所致亦有濕痰流注下焦者腎肝陰
淫濕勝者或驚恐而木乘土位濁液下流或思慕無窮發為筋痿所謂二
陽之病發心脾也或余經濕熱屈滯於少腹之下或下元虛冷子宮濕淫
治之之法或下或吐或發中兼補補中兼利燥中兼升發潤中兼溫養或
溫樸或收澀諸例不同亦病機之活法也

Liu Zong-Hou[12] says that vaginal discharge is most often due to yin deficiency and yang exhaustion. The nutritive qi does not ascend, and the channels and vessels become congealed and bound up; the protective qi collapses; [and] the essence qi accumulates and stagnates in the lower burner in the area of the extraordinary channels with accumulation and fermentation that leads [to this problem]. It gets its name because the *dai* vessel becomes diseased and also because of the form it takes. The white type pertains to the qi while the red type pertains to the blood. These are most often caused by drunkenness, overeating, exhaustion from sexual excess, and the consumption of drying and hot foods. There are also cases due to damp-phlegm pouring into the lower burner, or the kidney and liver yin being overwhelmed by excessive dampness. In other instances, [one may experience] fear and fright such that wood overwhelms the seat of earth, and turbid fluids flow downward; or persistent lamentation[13] may produce a withering of the [ancestral] sinew, and this is what is referred to as diseases of the two yang developing in the heart and spleen; or the other channels have damp-heat that concentrates and stagnates in the inferior aspect of the lower abdomen. In other instances, the primal [qi] of the lower [burner] may be deficient and chilled, causing the womb to become excessively damp. The methods for treating [these conditions] include purgation, or emesis, or simultaneously supplementing while discharging, simultaneously promoting [urination] while supplementing the middle, simultaneously raising and discharging while drying, simultaneously warming and nourishing while moistening, or warming and tonifying, or restraining and binding. All cases require different [treatment techniques] as well as their flexible application based on the [particular expression] of the pathodynamic.

巢元方病源曰腎著病膘痛冷如冰身重腰如帶五千錢不渴小便利因
勞汗出衣裏冷濕而得久則變為水也

Chao Yuan-Fang, in his *[Discussion of the] Origins of the Symptoms of Disease,* says that [in the case of] fixed kidney disease, the lower back is painful and as cold as ice, generalized heaviness, a feeling like one's back is weighed down by a belt containing five-thousand coins, absence of thirst, and uninhibited urination due to profuse sweating after exertion such that one has become cold and damp inside one's clothes. When this has lasted a long time, then it turns into a water [disease].[14]

千金用腎著湯三因用滲濕湯東垣用獨活湯主之

Thousand Gold uses Kidney Fixity Decoction *(shen zhuo tang)*,[15] *Three Etiologies* uses Dampness Leeching Decoction *(shen shi tang)*,[16] and [Li] Dong-Yuan uses Pubescent Angelica Decoction *(du huo tang)* to master it.[17]

CHAPTER 17

氣口九道脈

The Pulses of the Nine Pathways of the Qi Opening

手檢圖曰肺為五藏華蓋上以應天解理萬物主行精氣法五行應四時
知五昧氣口之中陰陽交會中有五部前後左右各有所主上下中央分
為九道診之則知病邪所在也

The Hand Diagram [of the 31 Locations] states: "The lung is the canopy of the five viscera, analogous to heaven above, which manages the ten-thousand things, masters the
movement of the essence and qi, serves as a model for the five phases, in accordance
with the four seasons, and allows for the perception of the five flavors. Within the qi
opening [on the wrist], the yin and yang intersect, and it is divided into five positions,
front and back, left and right, [and the middle], each of which has its master. The upper, lower, and middle positions are then divided into the nine pathways. When [the
pulse is] examined in this manner, one may know where the disease pathogen lies."[1]

李瀕湖曰氣口一脈分為九道總統十二經並奇經八脈各出診法乃岐
伯秘援黃帝之訣也扁鵲惟之獨取寸口以訣死生蓋氣口為百脈流註
朝會之始故也三部雖傳而九道淪隱放奇經之脈世無人知今撰為圖
並附其說於後以泄千古之秘藏云

Li Bin-Hu states: "The radial wrist pulse is divided into the nine pathways and provides an overall system, merging the 12 [primary] channels with the eight extraordinary vessels. Each [position] has its own diagnostic presentation according to Qi Bo's
secret teaching of the *Yellow Emperor's Rhyme*. Bian Que promoted [the principle]
that one need only refer to the qi opening pulse to decide whether one will die or live.
The qi opening is the starting place where the hundred vessels flow and converge in
the morning. Although they pass through the three [standard] positions, the nine
pathways are submerged [within it]. Because nobody in the world knows the pulses
for the eight extraordinary vessels, I have now decided to draw a diagram [of this pulse
diagnosis system] and append an explanation after it to transmit the secrets that have
remained unknown throughout the ages."

岐伯曰前部如外者足太陽膀胱也動苦目眩頭項腰背強痛男子陰下
濕癢女子少腹痛引命門陰中痛子臟閉月水不利浮為風濇為寒滑為
勞熱緊宿食

Qi Bo states: "On the lateral side of the distal position is the foot greater yang bladder.[2] [The patient] suffers from visual dizziness and rigidity and pain in the head, neck, low back, and back. In men, the genitals will be damp and itchy. In women, there will be lesser abdominal pain radiating to the gate of vitality, genital pain, genital obstruction, and disordered menses. A floating [pulse in the anterior position] means wind, a choppy [pulse] means cold, a slippery [pulse][3] means heat from exhaustion, and a tight pulse means retained food."[4]

中部如外者足陽明胃也動苦頭痛面赤滑為飲浮為大便不利濇為嗜
臥腸鳴不能食足脛痹

On the lateral side of the middle position is the foot yang brightness stomach. [When the pulse is] perturbed in this way, [the patient] suffers from headache and a red face. A slippery [pulse in this position] means thin mucus, a floating [pulse] means that there is difficulty with bowel movements,[5] [and] a choppy [pulse] means that there is somnolence and intestinal rumbling, inability to eat, and painful obstruction of the legs and shins.

後部如外者足少陽膽也動苦腰背胇肢肢節痛浮為氣濇為風急為轉
筋為勞

On the lateral side of the proximal position is the foot lesser yang gallbladder. [When the pulse is] perturbed in this way, [the patient] suffers from pain in the low back, [mid]back, legs, thighs, and joints of the extremities. A floating [pulse in this position] means qi [stagnation],[6] a choppy [pulse] means wind, and an urgent [pulse] means there is twisting of the sinews and exhaustion from overwork.

前部如內者足膽陰肝也動苦少腹痛引腰大便不利男子莖中痛小便
難疝氣兩丸上入女子月水不利陰中寒子戶閉少腹急

On the medial side of the distal position is the foot reversing yin liver. [When the pulse is] perturbed in this way, [the patient] suffers from lower abdominal pain radiating to the low back and irregular bowel movements. In men, there will be pain in the penis, difficult urination, and bulging qi in both testicles that enters from above. In women, there will be disordered menstruation, a sense of cold in the vagina, vaginal obstruction, and lesser abdominal urgency.[7]

中部如內看足太陰脾也動苦腹滿胃中痛上管有寒食不下腰上狀如

居水中沈澀為身重足脛寒痛煩滿不能臥時咳唾有血泄利食不化

On the medial side of the middle position is the foot greater yin spleen. [When the pulse is] perturbed in this way, [the patient] suffers from abdominal fullness and pain in the stomach, esophageal cold, an inability to get food down, and a sensation in the low back like one is standing in water. A sunken and choppy [pulse in this position] means that there is bodily heaviness and cold and pain in the feet and shins, irritability and fullness such that one is unable to lie down, episodic cough where one hacks up blood, and diarrhea with undigested food.

後部如內看足少陰腎也動苦少腹痛與心相引背痛小便淋女人月水
來上搶心胸脅滿股裏拘急

On the medial side of the proximal position is the foot lesser yin kidney. [When the pulse is] perturbed in this way, [the patient] suffers from lesser abdominal pain that reciprocally radiates to and from the heart, back pain, urinary dribbling. In women during menstruation, there will be a piercing sensation ascending to the chest and heart, fullness in the rib-sides, and gripping spasms inside the thigh.

前部中央直者手少陰心手太陽小腸也動苦心下堅痛腹脅急實急者
為感忤虛者為下利腸鳴女子陰中癢痛滑為有娠

Directly on the midline of the distal position is the hand lesser yin heart and hand greater yang small intestine. [When the pulse is] perturbed in this way, [the patient] suffers from firmness and pain below the heart, [and] abdominal and rib-side urgency. If [the pulse] is excessive and urgent, [the patient] will experience frustration. If [the pulse] is deficient, then there will be diarrhea, rumbling intestines, and itching, and women will experience itching and pain in the genitals. A slippery [pulse in this position] means pregnancy.

中部中央直中看手厥陰心主也動苦心痛面赤多喜怒食苦咽微浮苦
悲傷恍惚澀為心下寒沈為恐怖如人將捕之狀時寒熱有血氣

Directly on the midline of the middle position is the hand reversing yin heart master. [When the pulse is] perturbed in this way, [the patient] suffers from heart pain, a red face, frequent [excesses] of joy and anger, and food tasting bitter in the throat.[8] A slightly floating [pulse in this position] means that one will suffer from sadness and disorientation. A choppy [pulse] means that there will be cold below the heart. A sunken [pulse] means that there will be apprehension as if [one was] about to be arrested. Even if there are periodic chills and fever, they have [some] qi and blood.

後部中央直者手太陰肺手陽明大腸也動苦咳逆氣不得息浮為風沈
為熱緊為胸中積熱澀為時咳血

[A pulse that is located] directly on the midline in the proximal position is the hand greater yin lung and hand yang brightness large intestine. [When the pulse is] perturbed in this way, [the patient] suffers from cough and a counterflow of qi such that they cannot catch their breath. A floating [pulse in this position] means wind. A sunken [pulse] means heat. A tight [pulse] means that heat accumulates in the chest, and a choppy [pulse] means there will be periodic coughing of blood.[9]

前部橫於寸口丸丸者住脈也動苦少腹痛逆氣搶心胸拘急不得俯仰

[A pulse that is] pill-like across all of the distal positions is a *ren* pulse. [When the pulse is] perturbed in this way, [the patient] suffers from lesser abdominal pain and counterflow qi that pierces the heart. There will be a sense of gripping urgency in the thorax that prevents forward or backward bending.

脈經曰寸口脈緊細實長下至關者任脈也動苦少腹繞臍病男子七疝
女子瘕聚

The *Pulse Classic* states that when the radial pulse is tight, fine, excessive, and long that reaches from below [the proximal position] to the middle position, this is a *ren* pulse. [When the pulse is] perturbed in this way, [the patient] suffers from lesser abdominal pain and periumbilical pain.[10] Men will suffer from the seven types of bulging, and women will suffer from accumulations and masses.

三部俱浮直上直下著督脈也動苦腰脊強痛不得俯仰大人癲小兒癇

[A pulse that is] floating in all three positions [and beats] perpendicularly up and down is a *du* pulse. [When the pulse is] perturbed in this way, [the patient] suffers from rigidity and pain in the lumbar spine with an inability to bend forward or backward. Adults will have withdrawal, [and] children will have seizures.

三部俱牢直上直下者衝脈也苦胸中有寒疝

[A pulse that is] confined in all three positions [and beats] perpendicularly up and down is a *chong* pulse. [When the pulse is] perturbed in this way, [the patient] suffers from cold bulging in the chest.

脈經曰脈來中央堅實徑至關者衝脈也動苦少腹痛上搶心有瘕疝遺
溺女子絕孕

The *Pulse Classic* states that a pulse that arrives hard and excessive on the midline position to reach the middle position is a *chong* pulse. [When the pulse is] perturbed in this way, [the patient] suffers from lower abdominal pain and piercing pain ascending to the heart with accumulations and bulging, urinary incontinence, and female infertility.

前部左右彈者陽蹺也動苦腰背痛癲癇僵僕羊鳴偏枯癮頑痺身休強

[A pulse that is] tapping in the distal left and right positions is a *yang qiao* [pulse]. [When the pulse is] perturbed in this way, [the patient] suffers from low back and [mid]back pain, seizures with falling down, and sheep-like bleating, hemilateral withering, recalcitrant obstruction,[11] and generalized rigidity.

中部左右彈者帶脈也動苦少腹痛引命門女子月事不來絕繼復下令
人無子男子少腹拘急或失精也

[A pulse that is] tapping in the middle left and right positions is a *dai* pulse. [When the pulse is] perturbed in this way, [the patient] suffers lesser abdominal pain radiating to the gate of vitality. In women, the menses are absent or cease and resume again, rendering them infertile.[12] In men, there is hypertonicity in the lesser abdomen and perhaps loss of semen.

後部左右彈者陰蹺也動苦癲癇寒熱皮膚強痺少腹痛里急腰胯相連
痛男子陰疝女子漏下不止

[A pulse that is] tapping in the proximal left and right positions is a *yin qiao* [pulse]. [When the pulse is] perturbed in this way, [the patient] suffers from seizures and falling down, fever and chills, stiffness and insensitivity of the skin, lesser abdominal pain, abdominal urgency, [and pain] that links the low back to the groin.[13] In males, there is yin bulging,[14] and in females, there is unremitting spotting.[15]

從少陰斜至太陽者陽維也動苦顛仆羊鳴手足相引甚者失音不能言
肌肉痺癢

[A pulse] that goes obliquely from the [foot] lesser yin to the [foot] greater yang is a *yang wei* [pulse]. [The patient] tends to fall down with sheep-like bleating and draws up their hands and feet. In extreme cases, there will be loss of voice with an inability to speak and obstruction and itching of the muscles and flesh.

從少陽斜至厥陰者陰維也動苦癲癇僵仆羊鳴失音肌肉痺癢汗出惡
風

From the [foot] lesser yang obliquely to the [foot] reversing yin is a *yin wei* [pulse]. [When the pulse is] perturbed in this way, [the patient] suffers from seizures with sudden collapse, sheep-like bleating, loss of voice, [and] obstruction and itching of the muscles and flesh.[16] There will be sweating with an aversion to wind.

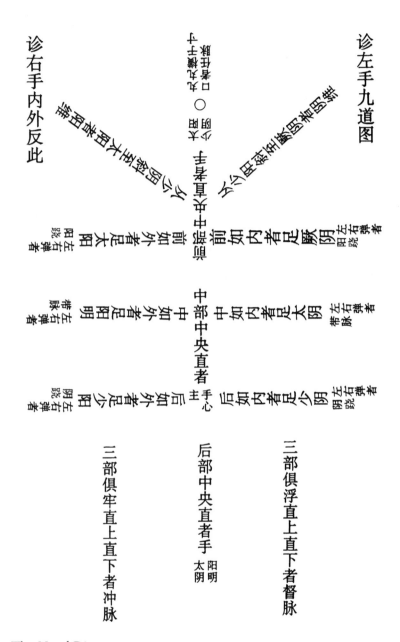

Fig. 17-1   The Hand Diagram

CHAPTER 18

釋音

An Explanation of Pronunciation

蹻腳卻喬蹻四音舉足高也又蹻捷也

The word 蹻 may be pronounced in four ways: *jiāo*, *què*, *qiáo*, or *qiāo*. It means to raise the foot high, and also means quick and nimble.

跗音膚足背也

The word 跗 is pronounced *fū*, and means the instep.

跟音根足踵也

The word 跟 is pronounced *gēn*, and means the heel of the foot.

踝花上聲足螺螄骨也

The word 踝 *huái* [is pronounced with] an indistinct rising tone, and means the malleolus (literally, the spiral bones) of the foot.

嗌音益喉也

The word 嗌 is pronounced *yì*, and means the larynx.

噤音禁口閉也

The word 噤 is pronounced *jìn*, and means oral obstruction.

齦音銀齒根肉也

The word 齦 is pronounced *yín*, and means the flesh at the base of the teeth.

臑濡嫩二音軟肉也

The word 臑 is pronounced either *rú* or *nèn,* and means the soft flesh [in the region of the upper arm].[1]

眇音杪季肋下也

The word 眇 is pronounced *miǎo,* and means the area below the ribs.

腨音喘脚肚也

The word 腨 is pronounced *chuǎn,* and means the belly of the [lower] leg.

膕音國曲膝腕中也

The word 膕 is pronounced *gúo,* and means the crease in the crook of the knee.

膻音亶胸中也

The word 膻 is pronounced *dǎn,* and means the center of the chest.

腧音戌五臟腧也

The word 腧 is pronounced *shù,* and means the transport holes of the five viscera.

脘音管胃脘也

The word 脘 is pronounced *guǎn,* and means the gastric cavity.

胛音甲背兩旁骨也

The word 胛 is pronounced *jiǎ,* and means the bones on either side of the upper back.

膂音旅夾脊肉也

The word 膂 is pronounced *lü,* and means the flesh that hugs the spine.

臀髀股也

The word 臀 means the buttocks or thighs.

瞤音犉目動也

The word 瞤 is pronounced *rún,* and means twitching of the eyes.

昧音妹目不明也

The word 昧 is pronounced *mèi,* and means that the vision is dim.

瞋音嗔怒目張也

The word 瞋 is pronounced *chēn,* and means fierce glaring.

瞑音眠寐也

The word 瞑 is pronounced *mián,* and means sleep.

瞼音檢眼弦也

The word 瞼 is pronounced *jiǎn,* and means the rim of the eyelid.

髆音博肩胛骨也

The word 髆 is pronounced *bó,* and means the scapula.

髖音寬髀上也

The word 髖 is pronounced *kuān,* and means the upper part of the thigh.

胻音行臁骨也

The word 胻 is pronounced *xíng,* and means the shank.

髃虞偶二音肩前也

The word 髃 is pronounced either *yú* or *oǔ,* and means the front of the shoulder.

骭音幹脛骨也

The word 骭 is pronounced *gàn,* and means the shin bone.

骶音氐尾脊骨也

The word 骶 is pronounced *dǐ,* and means the coccyx.

髎音寥骨空處也

The word 髎 is pronounced *liáo,* and means the bony foramina.

窌與髎同說文音皰窖也

The word 窌 is the same as 寥. According to *Elucidations of the Signs,* it is pronounced *pào* or *jiào.*

癲音顛仆病也

The word 癲 is pronounced *diān*, and means falling-down disease.

癇音閑驚病也

The word 癇 is pronounced *xián*, and means fright disease.

痙音頸風強病也

The word 痙 is pronounced *jǐng*, and means a pathogenic wind disease.

瘛瘲去聲乍前乍後病也

The word 瘛 [is pronounced] *chì* with a falling tone; it is a disease where one suddenly moves forward and suddenly moves backward [meaning that the patient is in spasm].[2]

癱音頑，痺也

The word (wán) is pronounced *wán*, and means obstruction.

痿音委肢軟也

The word 痿 is pronounced *wěi*, and means weak extremities.

瘕音賈積病也

The word 瘕 is pronounced *jiǎ*, and is an accumulation disease.

疝山訕二音寒痛病也

The word 疝 is pronounced either *shān* or *shàn*, and is a disease characterized by cold pain.

癃音隆小便淋也

The word 癃 is pronounced *lóng*, and means dribbling urination.

癲音頹陰腫也

The word 癲 is pronounced *tuí*, and means swelling of the genitalia.

瘂與啞同

The word 瘂 is the same as *yǎ* (啞) [which here means mute or dumb].

痠與酸同

The word 痠 is the same as *suān* (酸) [which here means sore].

痏音洧針瘢也

The word 痏 is pronounced *wěi*, and means a scar left from a needle.

瘥楚懈切楚嫁切病除也

The word 瘥 is pronounced *chìe* or *chài*, and means the disease has been eliminated.[3]

輳音湊輻輳也

The word 輳 is pronounced *còu*, and means the convergence at a hub.

俠古文俠挾通用

The word 俠 is *xía* in the ancient literature and *xíe* in current usage [meaning to coerce, to hug, or to hold under the arm].

俛音免俯也

The word 俛 is pronounced *miǎn*, and means to lower one's head.

仆音赴顛倒也

The word 仆 is pronounced *fù*, and means to fall down.

溉音概灌也

The word 溉 is pronounced *gài*, and means to irrigate.

泌音筆別水也

The word 泌 is pronounced *bǐ*, and means to expel water.

溺音尿小便也

The word 溺 is pronounced *niào*, and means urine.

溲音搜小便也

The word 溲 is pronounced *sōu*, and means urine.

澀音嗇不滑也

The word 澀 is pronounced *sè*, and means [rough or] not smooth.

怫音佛怫郁也

The word 怫 is pronounced *fó*, and means angry and sullen.

悍音汗猛也

The word 悍 is pronounced *hàn*, and means ferocious.

慓音漂疾也

The word 慓 is pronounced *piāo*, and means quick [or urgent].

悗音悶同義又音瞞惑

The word 悗 is pronounced *mèn*, and has the same meaning [as that word, i.e., a stifling sensation]. It is also pronounced *mán*, and means confused.

惕音狄心動也

The word 惕 is pronounced *dì*, and means agitation [or the sense of one's heartbeat].

頏音杭頸也

The word 頏 is pronounced *háng*, and means the neck.

頄音求面顴也

The word 頄 is pronounced *qiú*, and means the cheek bones on the face.

顙桑上聲額也

The word 顙 [is pronounced] *sāng*, with a rising tone, and means the forehead.

郄與隙同孔郄也

The word 郄 is the same as *xì* 隙, and means a hole or small cleft.

罅呼訝切孔罅也

The word 罅 is pronounced *xià*, and means hole or crack.

擴音郭引長之意

The word 擴 is pronounced *kuò*, and means stretched out.

隧音遂小路也

The word 隧 is pronounced *suì*, and means a path or trail.

篡初患切陰下縫間也

The word 篡 is pronounced *chuàn*, and is the perineal crease.

募與膜同

The word 募 is the same as *mó* [which means membrane].

毖音琵

The word 毖 is pronounced *pí*.

椎音縋脊之骨節也

The word 椎 is pronounced *zhuī*, and means the bony articulations of the back.

髀厭音箪掩股後骨即環跳也

The word 髀厭 is pronounced *pái yǎn*. It means the bone in the back of the hip, that is, the Circular Jump (GB-30) [hole].

瘈瘲瘛瘲並音治縱手足舒縮也

The words 瘈瘲 and 瘛瘲 are pronounced *zhì zòng*, and mean extension and contraction [i.e., convulsions] of the arms and the legs.[4]

膏肓音高荒心上鬲下也

The word 膏肓 is pronounced *gāo huāng*, and means the [membranous tissues in the entire thoracic and abdominal area] from above the heart to below the diaphragm.

慄卑音蝶怯弱也

The word 慄卑 is pronounced *dié qìe*, and means feebleness.[5]

漐漐音踏汗應時出之貌

The word 漐漐 is pronounced *tà [tà]*, and refers to one's appearance when sweating.

（目+荒）音荒目不明也

The word 目+荒 is pronounced *huāng*, and means the vision is dim.

築築氣痛如筑也

The word 築築 [is pronounced] *zhù zhù*, and means a pounding qi pain.

丸丸脈如珠丸也

The word 丸丸 [is pronounced] *wán wán*, and means the pulse is round like a pearl.

洗洗音璽皮毛淒滄惡寒之貌

The word 洗洗 is pronounced *xǐ xǐ*, and means the skin and the hair are pale blue, [and that] the patient appears to have an aversion to cold.

洒洒音洗同義

The word 洒洒 is pronounced *xǐ xǐ*, and has the same meaning [as in the entry above].

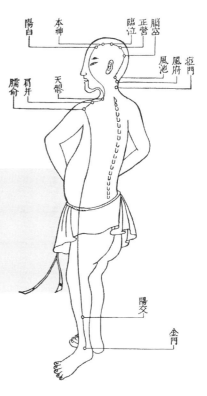

Part III

COMMENTARY ON
Exposition on the Eight Extraordinary Vessels

Part III contains full commentaries on each chapter of *Exposition on the Eight Ex-traordinary Vessels*. The yin and yang *wei* vessels and the yin and yang *qiao* vessels are each discussed together, rather than in separate chapters, because they are most readily understood in relation to one another. The chapters are arranged in the same order as the material is presented in the *Exposition*.

CHAPTER 19

On the Overview of the Eight Extraordinary Vessels

Li Shi-Zhen begins his exposition on the eight extraordinary vessels by establishing their place in the overall scheme of the channels and networks: "People have channel vessels and network vessels throughout their body. Those that travel longitudinally are called channels, while those that branch off are called networks." Here Li introduces a technique that he uses throughout the book, juxtaposing passages from earlier texts in a way that expands their meaning. Li's opening statement glosses a line from Ch. 17 of *Divine Pivot* that compares the channels and networks and states: "The channels and vessels are the interior and those that branch from it and travel horizontally are networks."[1]

The modern commentator Wang Luo-Zhen notes that the original meaning of the graph 經 *(jing,* 'channel') is a vertical or longitudinal line, whereas the original meaning of the graph 絡 *(luo,* 'network') indicates a connecting net. Thus, the channels and vessels are the trunk and their trajectories are typically deep, while the network vessels are the branches and these are disseminated superficially.[2] Li develops this theme, elaborating on Ch. 1 of *Divine Pivot*:

> There are 12 channels [consisting of the] three yin and three yang of the hand, and the three yin and three yang of the foot. There are 15 networks. Each of the 12 channels has its own branching network, and the spleen also has a great network. In addition, with the two networks of the *ren* and *du* [vessels], there are 15 [networks]. (The *Classic of Difficulties* posits a yin network and a yang network.) Combined, the 27 qi [of the channels and networks] move up and down together as if flowing from a spring, moving like the sun and moon without rest.

The original passage from Ch. 1 of *Divine Pivot* is considerably less detailed. "There are 12 channel vessels, and 15 network vessels. Altogether these make 27 [channels], and the qi thus ascends and descends [through them]."[3] Ch. 1 of *Divine Pivot* makes no mention of the great network of the spleen, nor does it include the networks of the *ren* and *du*.

In an annotation of his own, Li mentions that the *Classic of Difficulties* omits the *yin* and *yang qiao* in its count of the networks, tacitly pointing out that these vessels have been substituted for the *ren* and *du*. Although this appears to be a passing comment, the relationship of the *qiao* vessels to the networks is central to Li's understanding of extraordinary vessel physiology. Li makes no mention of the *Classic of Difficulties* as the source of the great network of the spleen.

In *Discerning the Truth Regarding Pulse Theory* (*Mai li qiu zhen* 脈理求真, 1769), Huang Gong-Xiu (黃宮繡) takes this idea a step farther. Huang identifies the *qiao* vessels not only as constituents of the networks, but as their primary controllers. The *yang qiao* masters the yang networks and the *yin qiao* masters the yin networks.[4] At least one modern commentary goes so far as to claim that the *qiao* vessels are synonymous with yin and yang networks.[5] These interpretations echo Li's own perspective on the extraordinary vessels, which will be developed in subsequent chapters of *Exposition on the Eight Extraordinary Vessels*. Here in the introduction, Li lays the groundwork for his development of this idea in later chapters. For him, the *qiao* vessels are intimately related to the networks while the *ren* and *du* have a much more generalized function in regulating yin and yang.

Li next presents his own explanation of the flow of qi between the channels and networks and the extraordinary vessels.

> Thus, the yin vessels manage [the qi] in the five yin viscera while the yang vessels sustain the six yang receptacles. Yin and yang connect with each other in an endless circuit in which there is no discernable break. Upon reaching the end, it just starts again. The overflow of qi [from the channels and networks] enters the extraordinary vessels, providing reciprocal irrigation, interiorly warming the yin viscera and yang receptacles, and exteriorly moistening the interstices.

Although it is regarded as part of the bedrock understanding of the extraordinary vessels today, the notion of a reciprocal flow of qi between the extraordinary vessels and the rest of the channel system is an innovation of Li's. In the *Inner Classic (Nei jing)*, the relationship between the flow of qi in the primary channels and extraordinary vessels is unclear. Li reframes the meaning of a passage from Ch. 17 of *Divine Pivot* to fit his own more versatile interpretation. The original passage reads:

> At no time does the qi not circulate. It is like the flow of water, like the ceaseless movement of the sun and moon. Therefore, the yin vessels nourish the viscera while the yang vessels nourish the receptacles, like an endless circuit in which there is no discernable break. The overflow of qi internally irrigates the viscera and receptacles and externally moistens the interstices.[6]

This passage appears in the context of a discussion of the trajectory of the *qiao* vessels and their transmission of qi to the eyes and interstices in the exterior, and to the yin viscera and yang receptacles in the interior. Li has taken a statement pertaining to the physiology of a specific extraordinary vessel and extrapolated it to include all the extraordinary vessels as a whole. Li asserts that the overflow of *all* the extraordinary vessels irrigates the viscera and receptacles. By contrast, the 27th and 28th Difficult Issues of the *Classic of Difficulties* posit a much different dynamic between the primary channels and the extraordinary vessels. In this scheme, the networks receive the overflow from the primary channels, and the extraordinary vessels in turn receive the overflow from the networks. The extraordinary vessels of the *Classic of Difficulties* clearly do not flow back into the primary channels or their networks.

> When they are filled to overflowing, they stagnate and they cannot return to the circulating [qi] by drainage into the [primary] channels … they are no longer part of the circulation because the 12 channels cannot seize this [surplus].[7]

Similarly, the symptoms associated with the extraordinary vessels in the *Classic of Difficulties* tend to reflect conditions most commonly associated with excesses such as lower back stiffness, chest pain, abdominal urgency, and accumulations and masses. The only treatment strategy mentioned in the *Classic of Difficulties* is to "pierce [the respective vessel] with a sharp stone" *(bian she zhi* 砭射之) to relieve swelling and heat resulting from the stagnation of pathogenic heat within it."[8]

Li's proposal that the flow of qi between the extraordinary vessels and the rest of the channel system is reciprocal (*chuan xiang guan gai* 傳相灌溉) skillfully reconciles this apparent contradiction. According to Katsuda Masayasu, "When the circulating qi is in excess, it flows into the extraordinary vessels. It also flows back to the 12 primary channels to nourish the viscera and receptacles and the interstices."[9] This interpretation has become the standard understanding of the relationship between the extraordinary vessels and the rest of the channel system. Having established this key piece of extraordinary vessel physiology, Li then returns to the 27th Difficult Issue to explain what is so extraordinary about the extraordinary (*qi* 奇) vessels. "The eight extraordinary channels are eight vessels that are not controlled by the 12 main channels, nor are they are arranged in exterior-interior combinations. Therefore, they are called extraordinary."

This is not the only interpretation of the word *qi* 奇. According to the Tang dynasty commentator Yang Xuan-Cao (楊玄操),

> *Qi* 奇 means 'odd or unpaired' *(yi* 異). These eight vessels are not part of the [system of] mutual seizure regulation [of contents] among the 12 conduits; they constitute passageways proceeding separately. They are different from the main conduits. Hence, they are called extraordinary channels.[10]

However, during the Song dynasty, Yu Shu (虞庶) took issue with Xuan-Cao's interpretation:

> *Qi* 奇 is to be read as 'fundamental' *(ji* 基); it stands for 'slanted, oblique' *(xie* 斜), 'odd' *(ling* 零); it means 'singular'*(bu ou* 不偶). That is to say, the eight vessels are not regulated by the main channels, there are no interior-exterior combinations between yin and yang [vessels], and they constitute

separate pathways with unusual circulations, therefore they are called the extraordinary vessels. [Thus] Master Yang's statement that *qi* means odd is incorrect.[11]

Katsuda points out that there may be another shade of meaning to Yu Shu's association of 'odd' with the extraordinary vessels. He claims that *ling* (零) often refers to small things like the falling of leaves or the dripping of water and so evokes an image of the extraordinary vessels as branching off of or falling away from the major channels.[12]

The Qing dynasty physician Xu Da-Chun (徐大椿, 1693–1771) noted that "[The word] *qi* 奇 should be read as 'odd or singular' (*ji ou* 奇偶). That is to say, in contrast to the 12 channels, there are no pairs of foot or hand [channels] in the case [of the extraordinary vessels]."[13]

As previously mentioned, the extraordinary vessels are not arranged in hand and foot pairings but in interior-exterior pairings, such as the *yin* and *yang qiao* and the *yin* and *yang wei*. The *ren* and *du* are also a functional pair, and, as we will see, there is even a tacit pairing of the *chong* and the *dai*.

> The main channels are like irrigation ditches, and the extraordinary channels are like lakes and marshes. When the vessels of the main channels are swollen and abundant, they overflow into the extraordinary channels. Thus it was that Qin Yue-Ren compared this to when the "rains pour down from heaven, the irrigation ditches overflow, the rain floods rush wildly, flowing into the lakes and marshes." This is the revelation of the secret meaning not presented in the *Divine* [*Pivot*] and *Basic* [*Questions*].

Qin Yue-Ren is also known as Bian Que (扁鵲), the apocryphal author of the *Classic of Difficulties*. The above passage is a synthesis of the 27th and 28th Difficult Issues, which state:

> The sages constructed irrigation ditches and kept the waterways open so that they would be prepared for any extraordinary situation. When the rains poured down from heaven, the irrigation ditches overflowed. In times such as that when the rain rushed recklessly, even the sages could not make plans again [and therefore they had to be prepared].[14]

The 28th Difficult Issue continues:

> This is comparable to the sages planning and constructing irrigation ditches. When these irrigation ditches were full to overflowing, [this excess water] flowed into deep lakes because even the sages were unable to [find other means to] seize [this overflow] and ensure the continuation of a circulatory flow.[15]

This passage again emphasizes the one-way flow of qi from the channels to the extraordinary vessels. It suggests that once the networks overflow with qi and blood, the 12 channels cannot further add more qi and blood. Because this statement does not actually appear in the *Inner Classic*, Li considers it to be "a revelation of the secret meaning of the *Divine* [*Pivot*] and *Basic* [*Questions*]."[16] Li Shi-Zhen evidently has a low opinion of the existing literature concerning the extraordinary vessels. His goal was to compile the information he considered most relevant to their study and to present it in a coherent manner so that those involved in internal alchemy could benefit from his synthesis of these materials.

> [Discussions of] the eight vessels scattered throughout the masses of [medical] texts are sketchy and incomplete. If physicians are not aware [of the theories of the extraordinary channels], they will remain in the dark as to the cause of disease. If [aspiring] transcendents are not aware of [the more comprehensive theories of the extraordinary channels] it will be difficult for them to tame the furnace and the cauldron. [Although I,] Li Shi-Zhen, am not clever, I have carefully considered the statements of all [the various schools] and compiled them below to allow both transcendents and physicians to trap and snare these useful words.

The "transcendents" (仙 *xian*) mentioned here refer to practitioners of internal alchemy concerned with longevity practices. In the lexicon of Daoist alchemy, the "furnace and the cauldron" (*lu ding* 爐鼎) is the elixir of immortality. The 50th hexagram of the *Classic of Change* is also called *ding* or cauldron. Li concludes his introduction with an allusion to *Zhuang zi*, establishing the Daoist thread that runs through his *Exposition*. His reference to a "trap" (*quan* 筌) is a bamboo fish trap and the "snare" (*ti* 蹄) is a snare for catching rabbits. The phrase is from *Zhuang zi*, Ch. 2, titled "On External Things" (*wai wu* 外物), which says:

> Nets exist for catching fish; once a fish is caught, the net is forgotten. Traps exist for catching rabbits; once a rabbit is caught, the trap is forgotten. Words exist for expressing ideas; once the ideas are expressed, the words are forgotten. I would like to find someone who forgets words and have a talk with him![17]

Li is making it clear that he understands the limitations of the written word. He intends his book to be a snare for capturing the meaning of the extraordinary vessels, but once the reader has grasped their meaning, the words can be discarded.

CHAPTER 20

On the Eight Vessels

Where Ch. 1 was concerned with the relationship between the extraordinary vessels and the rest of the channel system, Li-Shi-Zhen's second chapter in *Exposition on the Eight Extraordinary Vessels*, simply titled "The Eight Vessels," focuses on the rough trajectories and general characteristics of each of the extraordinary vessels as well as their relationships with one another. Before embarking on a more comprehensive discussion of pathology, Li first devotes this chapter to describing the normal physiological functioning of the extraordinary vessels as large-scale regulators of yin and yang within the body. He begins with an amalgam of material culled from passages appearing in the 27th and 28th Difficult Issues in the *Classic of Difficulties.*

> The eight extraordinary vessels consist of the *yin wei, yang wei, yin qiao, yang qiao, chong, ren, du,* and *dai.* The *yang wei* arises at the meeting of all the yang and travels upward from the outer ankle in the protective aspect; the *yin wei* arises at the intersection of all the yin and travels upward from the inner ankle in the nutritive aspect, and [together] they constitute a binding network for the entire body. The *yang qiao* arises from within the heel, traversing the outer ankle and traveling upward on both sides of the body; the *yin qiao* arises from within the heel, traversing the inner ankle and moving upward on both [sides] of the body, and [together] they allow nimble springing [movement] of the organism.

In this concise introductory statement, Li skillfully blends his own ideas into these passages, first interjecting a relationship between the *wei* vessels and the protective and nutritive aspects that does not appear in the *Classic of Difficulties.* The original lines from the 28th Difficult Issue read:

> The *yang wei* and *yin wei* are the binding network of the entire body. When they overflow, [their qi] cannot return to the circulation of all the [primary] channels. Hence, the *yang wei* arises at the meeting of all the yang, and the *yin wei* arises at the meeting of all the yin." [1]

The concept of the *wei* vessels as overseers of the protective and nutritive aspects is central to Li's subsequent development of treatment strategies pertaining to these vessels, and he has insinuated this idea into the bedrock principles of *wei* vessel activity presented in the *Classic of Difficulties.* Similarly, the original passage in the 28th Difficult Issue of the *Classic of Difficulties* makes no mention of the "nimble springing" movement initiated by the *qiao* vessels, limiting itself to a rudimentary description of their trajectories. According to that text:

> The *yang qiao* vessel arises at the heel; it proceeds along the outer ankle, ascends upward and enters the wind pond [hole]. The *yin qiao* vessel arises at the heel; it proceeds along the inner ankle, ascends upward, and reaches the throat where it intersects and links with the *chong* vessel.[2]

Li's intial statements establish an essential dynamic between the *wei* and *qiao* vessels. While the *wei* vessels constitute the gross energetic structure of the extraordinary vessels and the infrastructure of qi that defines the body, the two *qiao* vessels mobilize qi in the body, allowing for physical movement. Having established the boundaries and the motivating force of the extraordinary vessels, Li continues his recitation of eight vessel function, alluding to passages from the *Classic of Difficulties*, quietly inserting his own innovations into this orthodox material:

> The *du* vessel arises at the meeting of the yi, traverses the back, and proceeds along the posterior of the body such that it is the Director General [of the yang vessels]. Hence, it is called the sea of the yang vessels. The *ren* vessel [also] arises at the meeting of the yin, traverses the abdomen, and proceeds along the front of the body such that it is the official controller of the yin vessels. Hence, it is called the sea of the yin vessels.

The 28th Difficult Issue identifies the beginning of the *du* vessel less specifically as "the transport [hole] at the [body's] lower end."[3] In his subsequent discussion of the trajectory of the *du* vessel, Li clarifies this point by stating that "Its vessel arises from within the gestational membranes below the kidneys." He attributes the imperial title of Director General (*zong du* 總督) to the *du* vessel, a term in use since the Western Han (206 BCE–24 CE), denoting one who is generally in charge, typically of regional clusters of two or more provinces. By Li's time, in the Ming dynasty (1368–1644), the title was also associated with executive officials such as ministers or vice ministers delegated to deal with military problems in a region overlapping provincial jurisdiction.[4]

The terms "sea of yang vessels" (*yang mai zhi hai* 陽脈之海) and "sea of yin vessels" (*yin mai zhi hai* 陰脈之海) do not appear in the *Classic of Difficulties.* They first appear in the *Pulse Classic* in the chapter titled "On Treating Diseases of the Eight Extraordinary Vessels" (*Ping qi jing ba mai bing* 平奇經八脈病).[5] They also appear in a commentary by Lu Guang (呂廣) who asserts that the *chong* vessel was originally designated as the sea of yin. However, according to Yang Xuan-Cao, "The classic states: The *chong* vessel is the sea of [all] 12 channels. The *chong* vessel is not only the sea of the yin vessels. I'm afraid that Mr. Lu is in error."[6]

Yang Xuan-Cao's argument is based on the statement in Ch. 33 of *Divine Pivot* that the *chong* vessel is "the sea of the 12 channels."[7] This is the interpretation Li subscribes to in his description of the *chong* vessel.

> The *chong* [also] arises at the meeting of the yin and travels to hug the umbilicus where it surges directly upward, constituting an essential thoroughfare for the various vessels. Hence, it is called the sea of the 12 channels. The *dai* vessel winds around the lumbar region in the form of a binding girdle, making it the overall commander of all the channels.

All of the extraordinary vessels regulate yin and yang; however, the *du* and *ren* vessels are the most comprehensive and overarching regulators of yin and yang within the body, and they serve to regulate the rest of the extraordinary vessels as well. The *chong* shares the same origins as the *ren* and the *du,* but its role is very different. In this context, the *chong* is more akin to the *dai* vessel in its function. According to Yang Xuan-Cao, "*Dai* means to bind. This refers to the overall binding of all the vessels to regulate them. It [begins] at the 11th and 12th ribs, below the costal margins, and descends to connect between the hips, returning [to its beginning] and coiling. It coils around the entire body like a binding belt."[8,9]

While the *dai* vessel provides a restrictive boundary for the trajectory of all the channels, the *chong* defines an axis or thoroughfare along which all of the channels are aligned. Hence, it is the sea of the 12 channels. If we think of the *dai* as exerting regulatory control inward from the outside, then the *chong* may be understood as exerting its influence outward from the core. As the sea of the 12 channels, the *chong* may be perturbed by an imbalance in virtually any channel.

Next, Li summarizes these topological resonances in a manner that lays the groundwork for the chapters that follow:

> Hence, the *yang wei* governs the exterior of the entire body while the *yin wei* governs the interior of the entire body, and so they are referred to as *qian* and *kun.* The *yang qiao* governs the yang [aspect] of the left and right side of the entire body while the *yin qiao* governs the yin [aspect] of the left and right side of the entire body, so they are referred to as east and west. The *dai* vessel horizontally binds all the vessels so it is referred to as the six directions.

The *wei* and *qiao* vessels both regulate yin and yang as it pertains to day-to-day structure and function. They have distinct but complementary roles. The *wei* vessels regulate the communication of qi between the protective and nutritive levels, the two aspects of qi that most immediately define human interaction with the environment. The nutritive and protective are the day-to-day qi that allow us to move effectively and safely in the world. Proper communication between the exterior and the interior ensures an 'organizational binding' *(gang wei* 網維*)* of the channels and vessels, providing an energetic superstructure to the body.

The idea that the *qiao* vessels govern the sides is an innovation of Li's based on an inference. The 28th Difficult Issue traces the trajectory of the *qiao* vessels roughly up the sides. The 29th Difficult Issue describes *qiao* pathology in terms of tension and flaccidity, which are generally interpreted as referring to musculoskeletal disorders. This prompts Li to conclude that the *qiao* vessels govern the sides.

Li's reference to the trigrams *qian* ☰ and *kun* ☷ from the *Classic of Change* further expands the resonances attributed to the *wei* vessels. The *yang wei* governs the exterior, and its influence is analogous to the attributes of heaven, maleness, and the trigram *qian*. The *yin wei* governs the interior, and its influence is analogous to earth, femininity, and the trigram *kun*.[10] The *yin* and *yang qiao* vessels govern the yin and yang channels on the sides of the body, respectively, and taken together, this influence is analogous to the east and west directions. The *chong, ren,* and *du* govern the core vertical axis of the body, the influence of which is analagous to north and south. The *dai* vessel links the entire body together such that its influence is analogous to the six confluences. The six directions or confluences (*liu he* 六合) include the compass points plus up and down, and they organize the perception of space. Just as the six confluences provide a unifying concept for all spatial relations, the *dai* vessel organizes all of the extraordinary vessels into a coherent whole.

If the *dai* vessel defines the ultimate boundaries of the extraordinary vessels, the extraordinary vessels themselves define the spatial boundaries of the channel system as a whole. In governing the yin and yang on the sides, the structural periphery of the body, the emphasis of the *qiao* vessel lies more in the physicality of the body. The *qiao* vessels concern themselves with the healthy ascent and descent of yin and yang through the relatively superficial aspects of the body, allowing movement in the world. The *Classic of Difficulties* makes no mention of the role of the *qiao* vessels in diurnal and nocturnal circulation of protective qi between the interior and exterior. In Li's discussion of diseases of the *qiao*, this circulatory function appears only after his presentation of material pertaining to tension and slackness of the exterior, suggesting that he considers it secondary to these structural resonances.

While not ignoring their other functions, Li organizes his material in a manner that emphasizes the role of the *wei* vessels in governing the interior-exterior dynamic of yin and yang, and the role of the *qiao* vessels in governing the sides of the body. He concludes his overview by recapitulating the relevance of this material to both physicians and those involved in spiritual practice.

> For this reason, those who practice medicine and know of the eight vessels comprehend the great purpose of the 12 channels and 15 networks. Those who practice transcendence and know of the eight vessels miraculously attain the ascent and descent of the tiger and dragon, and the subtle aperture of the Mysterious Female.

The implication is that the alchemical resonances of the eight vessels will deepen a physician's understanding not only of the extraordinary vessels, but of the channel system at large, while spiritual cultivators will equally benefit from the medically oriented material. Once again, Li's final statement on the topic makes plain his alchemical influences.

The ascent and descent of the dragon and tiger *(long hu sheng jiang* 龍虎升降*)* is alchemical jargon laden with many layers of meaning. In its most basic meaning here, the dragon connotes yang qi and the tiger connotes yin qi. The goal of alchemical cultivation is to promote the optimal interpenetration of yin and yang. Another common resonance of the dragon and tiger concerns the necessity of subduing the dragon of the intellect and taming the tiger of sexual desire, both of which are accomplished through contemplative practice.

Where Ch. 1 finishes with an allusion to the *Zhuang zi*, Ch. 2 concludes with a reference to the *Lao zi*. The term Mysterious Female (*xuan pin* 玄牝) appears in Ch. 6 of the *Lao zi:* "The valley spirit never dies, this is called the Mysterious Female" (*gu shen bu si, shi wei xuan pin* 谷神不死是為玄牝).[11] As previously discussed, Mysterious Female is an evocation of emptiness that gives birth to all things, and it is an allusion to the development of breath control as the vehicle for achieving the goal of regulating the ascent and descent of the dragon and tiger.

His interest in spiritual cultivation notwithstanding, Li's *Exposition* is, nevertheless, primarily a medical text, and the challenge for physicians is to make some practical use of the alchemical material he believes is so important. In subsequent chapters, we will address in some detail how this stratum of the book holds the potential for enriching the practical application of the extraordinary vessels.

CHAPTER 21

On the *Wei* Vessels

Origins

The chapters in Li Shi-Zhen's *Exposition on the Eight Extraordinary Vessels* are divided into two broad categories, those that cover physiological function, trajectory, and other background information pertaining to each extraordinary vessel, and those that concern pathology and treatment strategies. General information regarding the paired *wei* vessels appears in consecutive chapters followed by a single chapter on their pathology and treatment. This format is repeated for the *qiao* vessels as well. The amount of information contained in these overview chapters varies greatly from one extraordinary vessel to another. The section on the *chong* vessel, for instance, is quite elaborate and contains detailed information on its physiology, its role as the sea of blood and sea of the 12 channels, and its relationships with the other channels in addition to the requisite description of its trajectory. By contrast, the preliminary chapters on the *wei* are exceedingly terse. They are nearly, although not quite entirely, limited to descriptions of their trajectories. Li opens his two chapters on the *yin wei* and *yang wei* with enigmatic statements from the 28th Difficult Issue of the *Classic of Difficulties* before presenting a detailed description of their trajectories.

> The *yin wei* arises from [its places of] intersection of all the yin. Its vessel issues from the foot lesser yin hole, Guest House (KI-9), which is the cleft [hole] of the *yin wei.* …
>
> The *yang wei* arises from [the places it] meets with all the yang. Its vessel issues from the foot greater yang hole, Metal Gate (BL-63) … .

Most commentators simply dismiss Li's remarks as a clarification of the original passage from the *Classic of Difficulties.* The standard reading is that the intersection of all yin is at Guest House (KI-9) and the meeting of all yang is at Metal Gate (BL-63). For instance, Matsumoto and Birch translate Li Shi-Zhen as follows: "The *yin wei* vessel starts at the crossing of the yin at Guest House (KI-9)" and "The *yang wei* vessel starts at the meeting of each yang at Metal Gate (BL-63)."[1]

Such an interpretation is attractive. There is no question that Guest House (KI-9) and Metal Gate (BL-63) are the first holes on their respective trajectories, and interpreting these holes as the intersection of all the yin and the meeting of all the yang simplifies matters greatly. A few commentators, however, believe that the *wei* vessels actually arise elsewhere and that these statements regarding their communication with all the yin and all the yang pertain exclusively to their relationships with other channels. This perspective has its basis in the 28th Difficult Issue of the *Classic of Difficulties*.

> The *yang wei* and the *yin wei* are bound like a network to the body. When they are filled to overflowing, they stagnate and cannot return to the circulating qi by drainage into the main channels. Hence the *yang wei* vessel arises from the meeting [places] of all the yang [vessels], and the *yin wei* [vessel] arises from the intersection [places] of all the yin. This can be compared to the planning and construction of ditches and reservoirs by the sages of antiquity. When the ditches and reservoirs are full, their surplus contents flow into deep lakes because [even] the sages were unable to [find other] means to seize [these contents and ensure the continuation of circulatory] flow. Similarly, when the [channels and network vessels] in people are filled [to overflowing, their surplus contents] enter the eight extraordinary vessels where they are no longer part of the circulation, because the 12 main channels cannot seize this [surplus].[2]

The 27th Difficult Issue of the *Classic of Difficulties* addresses the question of why the extraordinary vessels are not a part of the circulation of the primary channels and networks. It explains that the extraordinary vessels are extraordinary by virtue of their capacity to receive the overflow from the primary channels and networks, like ditches receiving the overflow from rivers, and it attributes this function equally to all the extraordinary vessels. The 28th Difficult Issue is concerned with the question of where the qi of the extraordinary vessels originates since it is not part of the circulation of the primary channels. It recapitulates the waterworks analogy presented in the 27th Difficult Issue but associates it specifically with the *wei* vessels. The above passage from 28th Difficult Issue identifies the *wei* vessels as being especially associated with these functions of absorbing and storage. It recognizes that the origination of the *wei* vessels in the yin and yang vessels is central to its capacity to absorb the overflow from the channels and networks. Although it traces rough trajectories for the other six extraordinary vessels, its primary interest lies in physiological dynamics suggested by their place of origin. The *du, ren,* and *chong* arise together in the uterus or cinnabar field, reflecting their functions of regulating the deepest, most fundamental aspects of the qi. The *qiao* vessels arise near the ankles, reflecting their function of pumping the qi between the interior and exterior, and the *dai* arises at the waist where it girds all of the channels in the body. The *Classic of Difficulties'* discussion of the *wei* vessels in the present chapter underlines this physiological emphasis in that no mention of their trajectories is made per se, but the focus is exclusively on their place of origin. It is as if the trajectories of the *wei* vessels were almost incidental once their physiological function of binding the body together has been established. In light of this, it seems unlikely that the author of the *Classic of Difficulties* intended to say that each of the *wei* vessels originates from a single hole.

Another seminal text in the development of the extraordinary vessels, Hua Shou's *The Elucidation of the Fourteen Channels*, reframes a number of the passages from the *Classic of Difficulties* to amplify this point:

> The *yin wei* [vessel] binds to all the yin. Its vessel arises from [the places] it intersects with all the yin. As for the *yin* [*wei*], if it is unable to bind the yin, then one becomes sluggish and unable to support oneself. The *yang wei* [vessel] binds to all the yang. Its vessel arises from [the places it] meets with all the yang. Together with the *yin wei,* they all bind with the networks in the body. As for the *yang* [*wei*], if it is unable to bind the yang, then one experiences such disappointment that one loses one's sense of purpose.[3]

It is evident that the discussions regarding the wellspring of the *wei* vessels in both the *Classic of Difficulties* and *The Elucidation of the Fourteen Channels* were originally intended to illustrate the fundamental physiological relationship between the *wei* and the network vessels, and the consequences of a breakdown of that affiliation. The *wei* vessels originate in the yin and yang because they constitute a structural matrix that develops from the very networks they bind. In modern terms, they may be understood as an emergent system or systems arising out of the network vessels themselves. Though the *wei* vessels represent a distinct pair of channels, their existence would be spurious if divorced from their relationship to the primary channels and their networks.

Wang Luo-Zhen is of the opinion that Li Shi-Zhen's reference to the intersection of all the yin refers to "the meeting of the *yin wei* with the yin channels in the abdominal region."[4] In this interpretation, the meeting of all the yin refers specifically to the intersection of the *yin wei* with the three foot yin channels at Receptacle Abode (SP-13), Great Horizontal (SP-15), Abdominal Lament (SP-16), and Cycle Gate (LR-14). *The Systematic Classic of Acupuncture and Moxibustion* identifies Receptacle Abode (SP-13) as:

> The meeting of the foot greater yin, *yin wei*, and terminal yin [channels]. This vessel's ascent and descent enters the abdomen and envelops the chest, binding to the heart and lungs. From the rib-sides, it ascends to the shoulder. This is the cleft of the greater yin, the three yin, and branching [network] of the yang brightness.[5]

Thus, the *yin wei*'s passage through Receptacle Abode (SP-13) alone ensures that it communicates with the liver, spleen, and kidney channels, as well as the heart and lungs, but Wang fails to provide any accounting of the three yin channels of the upper extremity. Nevertheless, Wang stretches this reasoning farther, citing a well-known passage from the appended commentaries to the *Zhou Classic of Change*: "[The trigram] *kun* is earth, and ... *kun* is the abdomen."[6]

Because *kun* is the abdomen and the *yin wei* arises from the abdomen, Wang goes so far as to conclude that the use of the word *kun* is an oblique reference to the *yin wei* vessel in medical texts throughout early Chinese medical history.[7]

Wang similarly interprets the origination of the *yang wei* at "the meeting [places] of all the yang" as a reference to the intersection of the *yang wei* vessel with holes on each of the yang channels on the shoulder and head. This interpretation is more inclusive than his reading of the intersection of all of the yin. The combination of Upper Arm (LI-14), Upper Arm Meeting (TB-14), Celestial Hole (TB-15), Shoulder Well (GB-21), Upper Arm Transport (SI-10), Wind Pond (GB-20), Brain Hollow (GB-19), Upright Construction (GB-17), Eye Window (GB-16), and Overlooking Tears (GB-15) accounts for all of the yang channels with the exception of the foot greater yang bladder channel.

Again citing the *Classic of Change*, "[The trigram] *qian* is heaven, ... and *qian* is the head," Wang Luo-Zhen applies the same logic to the *yang wei* and concludes that the use of the term *qian* in early medical texts was a reference to this extraordinary vessel.[8] Katsuda Masayasu recapitulates Wang's fundamental interpretation of both the intersection of the yin and the meeting of the yang in his own commentary, although he does not comment on their possible connection to the *Classic of Change*.[9]

The proposition that these terms from the *Classic of Change* carry broad extraordinary vessel resonances in other medical texts is difficult to substantiate. However, as we have already seen, the basic premise that the *wei* vessels originate in the network vessels does have some historical basis. In addition to the *Classic of Difficulties* and the *Elucidations of the Fourteen Channels*, the *Golden Mirror of the Medical Tradition* comments that "the intersection of all the yin means that the binding networks of all the yin [channels] meet at the *ren* [vessel]."[10] This curious interpretation leaves us with the *yin wei* arising in the vicinity of the acupuncture holes Celestial Chimney (CV-22) and Ridge Spring (CV-23) on the neck, nowhere near the abdomen favored by Wang and Katsuda. Still, it has the obvious merit of actually accounting for the *yin wei's* intersection with *all* the yin because the intersection occurs on the *ren* vessel, the sea of all the yin channels.

Of course, the origination of the *wei* vessels need not have a single fixed location at all. Because they bind all the yin and yang throughout the body, they cannot really be said to originate anywhere in particular. It is for this reason that we have translated *qi* (起) as 'arise' rather than 'originates' in the context of the *wei* vessels. Their wellspring is best understood as a global phenomenon occurring in every place that the *wei* vessels contact the networks, which is, quite literally, everywhere. From this perspective, the holes assigned to the trajectories of the *wei* vessels are really only the central nodes of a seamless web of communication with the network vessels.

A final argument for a broader interpretation of the terms 'intersection' and 'meeting' lies in the structure of the *Exposition* itself. If the intersection of all the yin and the meeting of all the yang are indeed references to the initial holes on the trajectories of the *wei* vessels, then the content of Li's two chapters on the *yin* and *yang wei* is limited exclusively to their trajectories. This would make them unique insofar as the content of all the other introductory chapters in the *Exposition* include something, however brief, regarding physiology or some other characteristic of each extraordinary vessel in addition to their trajectories. The organization of the *Exposition* as a whole suggests that these phrases pertain to something more than an anatomical referent for the beginning of their respective trajectories.

The intimate relationship between the network and *wei* vessels is central to Li Shi-Zhen's vision of the extraordinary vessels. This theme is framed between his opening statements concerning the intersection and meeting of the yin and yang and his final remarks concerning diseases of the *wei* vessels where he identifies the ancillary networks of the interior flesh and soaring yang vessels as synonymous with the *wei*.

Wei Vessel Trajectories

The trajectory for the *yin wei* vessel described by Li Shi-Zhen is more elaborate than that described in *Comprehensive Recording of Sagely Beneficence from the Zhenghe Era* or *The Elucidation of the Fourteen Channels*, the first two texts to trace the trajectory of these vessels hole by hole. Though all three texts locate the same holes along the trajectory of the *yin wei*, each counts them differently. The *Comprehensive Recording* claims 11 holes, *The Elucidation* claims 12 holes, and Li's *Exposition* attributes 14 holes to the *yin wei* vessel. Guest House (KI-9), Receptacle Abode (SP-13), Great Horizontal (SP-15), Abdominal Lament (SP-16), and Cycle Gate (LR-14) account for 10 holes bilaterally. Celestial Chimney (CV-22) and Ridge Spring (CV-23) bring the tally to 12 holes, not the 14 he mentions. Wang Luo-Zhen and Katsuda Masayasu both believe that Thoroughfare Gate (SP-12) must be included in the *yin wei* count, bringing the total to 14 holes. They base their view on a statement in *Arcane Essentials of the Imperial Library*, which describes this hole as "the meeting of the foot greater yin and the *yin wei*."[11] A much simpler and more likely explanation is that the number 14 in the text is a typographical error and should be read as 12.

Li carefully specifies the locations of each hole on every extraordinary vessel, including the *yin wei*, typically employing the wording used in *The Systematic Classic*, though his locations are sometimes somewhat idiosyncratic. For instance, *The Systematic Classic* locates Receptacle Abode (SP-13) three-and-a-half *cun* lateral to the midline of the abdomen, as opposed to the four-and-a-half *cun* lateral to the midline specified by Li. It also describes Great Horizontal (SP-15) as being located "three *cun* below Abdominal Lament (SP-16) directly lateral to the umbilicus," whereas Li locates this hole one-and-a-half *cun* below Abdominal Lament (SP-16).[12]

According to Li Shi-Zhen, subsequent to its intersection with Celestial Chimney (CV-22) and Ridge Spring (CV-23), the *yin wei* vessel "then ascends to the front of the vertex and terminates." This is an innovation that appears in none of the earlier descriptions of the *yin wei* trajectory, nor is it adopted in subsequent descriptions. He offers no explanation for why the *yin wei* should terminate anterior to the vertex, although such a trajectory suggests that the *yin wei* penetrates the brain. In the descriptions of the extraordinary vessels from the *Inner Classic* and *Classic of Difficulties,* the only vessel that is described as explicitly traversing the brain is the *du* vessel. According to the 28th Difficult Issue of the *Classic of Difficulties,* "The *du* vessel arises from the transport [hole] at the body's lower end where it moves upward along the interior to reach Wind House (GV-16) and enter the brain." [13]

Yet after tracing the orthodox trajectory of the *yin qiao,* Li quotes from Wei Bo-Yang's *The Token for the Agreement of the Three According to the Changes of Zhou,* which states that this vessel "penetrates the mud ball," a euphemism for the brain. Li's assertion that the *yin wei* ascends to the vertex may be based on Zhang Bo-Duan's idea that the area anterior to the vertex corresponds to the *yin wei.* A discussion of this appears in Li's chapter on the *yin qiao.* It may then be that Li Shi-Zhen's alchemical influences prompt him to explicitly link the extraordinary vessels directly to the brain in a way that other authors do not.

The *Yang Wei* Hole Count

Whether by accident or design, Li Shi-Zhen introduces some innovations to the trajectory of the *yang wei* vessel. He includes some new holes on the trajectory that do not appear on the trajectories described in earlier texts, and he also omits some holes that those texts commonly included. For instance, *The Systematic Classic* does not include Squatting Bone-Hole (GB-29), Upper Arm (LI-14), and Upper Arm Meeting (TB-13) on the trajectory of the *yang wei* vessel. Most notably, Li omits the two holes Mute Gate (GV-15) and Wind Pond (GB-20), which *The Systematic Classic* considers to be "meeting [holes] of the *du* and *yang wei* [vessels]." [14] Wang Luo-Zhen and Katsuda are both of the opinion that this is an oversight on Li's part. [15] Wang Luo-Zhen observes that Celestial Chimney (CV-22) and Ridge Spring (CV-23) on the anterior aspect of the throat are the meeting holes of the *ren* and *yin wei,* and Mute Gate (GV-15) and Wind Pond (GB-20) are their anatomical correlates on the posterior aspect of the neck. He suggests that this is why these two holes should be included on the trajectory of the *yang wei* vessel. One of Li's primary sources, *The Elucidations of the Fourteen Channels,* also includes Mute Gate (GV-15) and Wind House (GV-16) along the trajectory of the *yang wei.*

Although Li fails to include Wind House (GV-16) in his description of the *yang wei* trajectory, he explains its use with Wind Pond (GB-20) in the *Discussion of Cold Damage* as relating specifically to a *yang wei* pathodynamic. This suggests that Li probably considered both of these holes to be associated with the trajectory of the *yang wei.*

Wang Bing's commentary on Ch. 58 of *Basic Questions* has the *yang wei* issuing from another hole:

The Division of the Flesh (GB-38) is located three *fen* from the edge of the fibulae above the external malleolus where the flesh divides. It is the place where the qi of the *yang wei* vessel issues.[16]

The Systematic Classic refers to this hole by its alternate name Yang Assistance (GB-38). Whatever its name, this hole is conspicuously absent from Li's *yang wei* trajectory. Because he has already designated the meeting of all the yang, or arguably Metal Gate (BL-63), as the place from whence the vessel issues, there is no reason to place Yang Assistance (GB-38) on the course of the *yang wei*.

Conclusion

Li Shi-Zhen's view of the *wei* vessels as simultaneously arising from and forming the structural framework for the network vessels has a sound basis in the literature of the extraordinary vessels, and yet prior to Li, no known author understood them in quite this way. His innovations permeate even what appear to be most straightforward discussions of extraordinary vessel function and structure. In the following chapter on extraordinary vessel pathology, Li becomes much more adventuresome in shaping the extraordinary vessel literature to produce a new perspective.

CHAPTER 22

On Diseases of the Two *Wei*

A Binding Network

The name '*wei* vessel' *(wei mai* 維脈) is closely linked to its physiological functions and pathological expressions. *Wei* (維) originally meant thick ropes such as those used to bind poles to construct a house. From this comes the meaning of holding together or connecting, and in turn, the meaning of maintaining or communicating. *Wei* appeared in a medical context very early in Chinese history. *Records of the Grand Historian (Shi Ji* 史記, 91 BCE) uses *wei,* in addition to *zhong jing* (中經, central thread) and *luo* (絡, network), to describe various aspects of the human physical and energetic anatomy. The *Inner Classic* discusses both the binding vessels (維脈 *wei mai)* and the binding sinews *(wei jin* 維筋), conveying this same idea of binding.[1]

The 28th Difficult Issue of the *Classic of Difficulties* describes the *wei* vessels as "bound like a network to the body" *(wei luo yu shen* 維絡於身). This characteristic defines one of their primary functions of binding the body into an integrated whole. Yet their influence is not absolute. The *du* and *ren* are the ultimate executors of this function, but the *wei* vessels are second in command.[2] Li Shi-Zhen's discussion of *wei* vessel pathology begins with a gloss of a line from the 28th Difficult Issue of the *Classic of Difficulties* that bears strongly on these meanings:

> [Qin] Yue-Ren says: "The *yang wei* and *yin wei* are a binding network in the body. When they overflow from accumulation, [their contents] stagnate and they are unable to circulate and irrigate all the other [primary] channels. Therefore, the *yang wei* arises from the [places it] meets with all the yang, and the *yin wei* arises from [the places it] intersects with all of the yin.

The perspective presented here differs from the view presented in Ch. 1. The rough trajectory outlined in the first chapter describes the normal physiological flow of qi through the *wei* vessels whereas this chapter is concerned with pathological presentations. Here the contents of the yin and yang *wei* are stagnating, and once full, they cannot recycle their qi back to the channels. This interpretation is echoed by Zhang Shi-Xian (張世賢, fl. 1506–1521) in his *Illustrated and Annotated Classic of Difficulties (Tu zhu nan jing* 圖註難經), which states:

[These vessels] bind and manage the channels and networks of the body; when these two channels are filled to overflowing [and the qi within them] accumulates and builds up, then [this qi] is unable to circulate and irrigate within the 12 channels. Hence, the *yang wei* arises in the meeting of the yang and the *yin wei* arises at the place of intersection of all the yin.

Zhang's point is that, under normal circumstances, the qi in the extraordinary vessels does not return to the circulation of the primary channels. As is the case with all of the extraordinary vessel pathology discussed in the *Classic of Difficulties*, the pathological process at work here is one of excess. At this relatively early stage in the development of extraordinary vessel theory, no mention is made of deficiency patterns. As we have already discussed, the location of the meeting of the yin and intersection of the yang is open to debate.

The second part of this passage is concerned with the pathological unbinding of the *wei* vessels, and is a quotation from the 29th Difficult Issue of the *Classic of Difficulties*:

The *yang wei* binds to the yang and the *yin wei* binds to the yin such that when yin and yang are unable to bind with one another, then one experiences such disappointment that one loses one's sense of purpose. One becomes sluggish and unable to support oneself.

At Loose Ends

Wei vessel pathology presents on both psychoemotional and physical levels. This passage has been interpreted in a number of ways, not least of which by Li Shi-Zhen himself who defines the presentation as "sluggish, as in a lethargic bearing." "Abstraction" *(huang hu* 恍惚*)* denotes an inattention to present objects or surroundings, or poor mental concentration. *Elucidations of the Signs and Explications of the Graphs (Shuo wen jie zi* 說文解字*)* states: "*Chang* means one's hopes and aspirations *(Chang wang hen ye* 悵望恨也*)*."[3] Lu Guang comments:

悵然者其人驚驚即維脈緩故今人身驚則失志善忘恍惚

Chang ran means the person is frightened. Fright causes the binding tension in the vessels to loosen. Therefore, a person is unable to hold things together. Fright also produces a loss of will, tendency to forgetfulness, and abstraction."[4]

The Song-dynasty commentator Ding De-Yong (丁德用, fl. 1056-1063) observes:

陽維者是陰陽之網維也而主持陰陽之脈今不能相為者是陽不能註持諸
陽陰不能注註持諸陰故言悵然失志也溶溶者緩慢所以不能收持也

The *yang wei* is the binding of the yin and the yang and manages the yin
and the yang vessels. If it is unable to bind them, then the yang will be unable to manage all the yang and the yin will be unable to manage all the
yin. Hence, this is referred to as disappointment such that one is unable
to hold things together. 溶溶 *(rong rong)* means lethargy such that one is
unable to control [oneself].[5]

Two of the current English translations of this passage have significantly different
emphases. The interpretation of Larre and Rochat de la Valee again stresses the psychoemotional state of falling apart: "One is without strength and no longer has a hold
on oneself."[6] By contrast, Unschuld's translation of the *Classic of Difficulties* interprets
this passage in a more structural or musculoskeletal vein: "One is weak and cannot
support one's [stature]."[7]

The psychophysical despondency and falling apart mentioned in the *Classic of
Difficulties* is not a symptom of either the *yang wei* or the *yin wei* per se. Instead it
results from a failure of the both the *yang wei* and *yin wei* to work together in binding
the yin and yang. In describing emotional symptoms before physical symptoms, the
Classic of Difficulties may be interpreted as giving tacit priority to these psychological
states. On the other hand, the text may be interpreted simply as presenting the more
general symptoms before discussing the indicators of more specific disorders, which
just happen to be more physical in nature. "[He] also says: 'When the *yang wei* is
diseased, [the patient] suffers from chills and fever; when the *yin wei* is diseased, [the
patient] suffers from heart pain.'"

According to Lu Guang:

陽為衛故寒熱陰為榮榮為血血者心故心痛也

The yang is the protective, hence, there will be chills and fever. The yin
is the nutritive, and the nutritive is the blood. Blood pertains to the heart,
hence, heart pain [is associated with the *yin wei*.][8]

Chills and fever *(han re* 寒熱) refers to simultaneous chills and feverishness, with or
without an elevation in basal body temperature. Because the periodicity of the alterna-
tion between sensations of cold and heat is undetermined, the term is best understood
as a generalized thermoregulatory disorder that may express itself in a variety of ways.
The premodern use of the term 'heart pain' *(xin tong* 心痛) is rather vague, encompassing pain in the pit of the stomach or heart region. It might be more accurately
translated as epigastric pain.[9] For instance, Ye Tian-Shi adopts this interpretation in
a case record of his treatment of a *yin wei* disorder. (The case appears later in this
book in Part IV, Ch. 35.)

In the early 13th century, Zhang Yuan-Su (1151–1234) was the first to link the *yin
wei* to nutritive qi in the interior, and the *yang wei* to protective qi in the exterior.

The protective is the yang, and it governs the exterior. When the *yang wei* contracts a pathogen, it produces a disease in the exterior, and therefore [the patient] suffers from chills and fever. The nutritive is in the yin, and it governs the interior. When the *yin wei* contracts a pathogen, it produces a disease in the interior, and therefore [the patient] suffers from heart pain.

Zhang Yuan-Su provides Li with a crucial link between the different types of material. Though the pathology presented in the acupuncture classics is quite obviously specific to the *wei* vessels, it fails to suggest a treatment strategy. Zhang's insight allows this information to be integrated into a much broader field of literature, most notably, the *Discussion of Cold Damage.*

Zhang's original writings on this subject have been lost. The above passage is a gloss of a statement by Hua Shou, which reads:

The *yang wei* encompasses all the yang and masters the protective. The protective is the qi, and the qi resides in the exterior. Hence, one suffers from chills and fever. The *yin wei* encompasses all the yin and masters the nutritive. The nutritive is the blood, and blood pertains to the heart. Hence, one suffers from heart pain.[10]

Following Zhang Yuan-Su's lead, Li rehearses some of the seminal passages in the *Discussion on Cold Damage* pertaining to Cinnamon Twig Decoction's *(gui zhi tang)* function of regulating the nutritive and the protective, establishing Cinnamon Twig Decoction *(gui zhi tang)* as a formula for addressing the *yang wei* vessel. Li also offers the novel explanation as to why the *Discussion on Cold Damage* instructs us to needle Wind Pond (GB -20) and Wind House (GV-16) in the event of a failure to induce a sweat utilizing apparently appropriate medicinals. According to Li, both holes are located on the trajectory of the *yang wei* vessel.

These two holes are the meeting [holes] of the *yang wei* vessel. This means that if, after [administering] Cinnamon Twig [Decoction] *(gui zhi [tang])*, the patient presents with spontaneous sweats, fever and chills, his pulse is floating in the distal position and weak in the proximal position, and yet [the patient] is irritable, then this disease is located in the *yang wei*. Therefore, one must first needle these two holes.

This is an especially curious statement coming from Li Shi-Zhen, who, in describing the trajectory of the *yang wei* vessel just two chapters previously, makes no mention of Wind House. It is apparently an *ad hoc* inclusion to the trajectory of the *yang wei* vessel.

Zhang Yuan-Su's Treatment Strategies for the *Yin Wei*

Zhang Jie-Gu [Zhang Yuan-Su] also said: "When the *yin wei* is diseased, [the patient] suffers from heart pain" [so one must] treat the intersection of the three yin. [As for herbal treatment], for greater yin patterns, use Regulate the Middle Pill *(li zhong wan)* while for lesser yin patterns, use Frigid Extremities Decoction *(si ni tang)*; reversing yin patterns are mastered by Tangkuei Decoction for Frigid Extremities *(dang gui si ni tang)* or Evodia Decoction *(wu zhu yu tang)*.

Having established the basis for his herbal prescriptions with quotations from orthodox sources, Li then begins extrapolating on these principles, expanding their scope of application.

Li Bin-Hu says that the vessel of the *yang wei* binds with the three yang of the hand and foot. Of these, the foot greater yang and lesser yang are in continuous contact [with the *yang wei*]. The symptoms of chills and fever belong to these two channels alone, and therefore when the *yang wei* is diseased, [the patient] also suffers from chills and fever. The protective qi moves in the yang during the day and moves in the yin at night. When the yin is deficient, there will be internal heat, and when the yang is deficient, there will be external cold. When there is pathogenic qi in the channels, it internally contends with the yin, leading to chills, and externally contends with the yang, leading to fever. Thus, when there is cold and heat in the exterior along with a greater yang presentation that has sweating, one should administer Cinnamon Twig [Decoction] *(gui zhi [tang])*. When sweating does not occur, one should administer Ephedra Decoction *(ma huang tang)*. When chills and fever that is half in the exterior and half in the interior occurs along with a lesser yang presentation, one should use a modified form of Minor Bupleurum [Decoction] *(xiao chai hu [tang])* to treat it.

Citing a passage from a chapter that is probably a later addendum to the *Discussion on Cold Damage* titled "Pulse Balancing Methods *(Ping mai fa* 平脈法)," Li further links *wei* vessel pathology to the nutritive and protective qi.

Now if the nutritive and the protective are fearful and powerless and produce a disease of chills and fever, then [prescriptions] in the class of Astragalus Decoction to Construct the Middle *(huang qi jian zhong tang)* and Eight-Treasure Decoction *(ba zhen tang)* master it.

Opinions range widely as to the meaning of "fearful" and "powerless" in this passage; however, it is clear that they are associated with deficiencies of the protective and nutritive qi. The original passage states:

衛氣弱名曰慄蓉氣弱名曰卑慄卑相搏名曰損

When the protective qi is weak, this is called fearfulness, and when the
constructive qi is weak, this is called shameful timidity. When the fearful
and the powerless combine, this is called detriment.[11]

Li appears to be making a simple statement that when both the nutritive and protective qi are weak, this produces cold and heat disease, however his use of these two
words suggests that he may have been thinking in broader terms. Fearful and powerless are not only synonymous with deficiencies of the protective and nutritive qi, they
also refer to the signs and symptoms that express these deficiencies. Cheng Wu-Ji (成
無己, 1056–1166), an early *Cold Damage* commentator, gives this passage a distinctly
psychological slant in his *Annotation and Explanation of the Discussion of Cold Damage (Zhu jie shang han lun* 註解傷寒論, 1144):

慄者心中氣勤迫怯街出上焦弱則上虛而心中氣勤迫怯也卑者心中常知
羞愧針經曰血者神氣也血弱則神弱故常自羞愧損者五臟六腑之虛假也

Fearfullness is a stirring of qi in the mind characterized by oppressive timidity. The protective emerges from the upper burner. When it is weakened,
the upper [burner] is deficient, and this causes the mind to stir, causing
oppressive timidity. Powerlessness is a [stirring of qi] in the mind characterized by an awareness of shame. The *Needle Classic* [also known as the
Divine Pivot] states: The blood is the spirit qi. When the blood is weakened
the spirit is weakened, therefore one is ashamed of oneself. Detriment is a
deficiency of both the five viscera and the six yang receptacles.[12]

Here, fearfulness and powerlessness are more than flowery synonyms for deficiencies of protective and nutritive qi; they refer to specific expressions of weakness.
Cold Damage scholars occasionally recapitulate Cheng's psychiatric interpretation,
however most commentators believe that what we have translated as fearfulness and
powerlessness are actually pulse qualities. The lines in question are part of a lengthy
discussion of how excess and deficiency of the protective and nutritive qi are reflected
in the pulse. Specific pulse qualities are attributed to each permutation of excess or
deficient protective or nutritive qi. For instance, the passage opens with a similar discussion concerning excess pulses:

When the protective qi at the wrist pulse is exuberant, this is called elevated
(elevated [*gao* 高] means violently chaotic and robust [*bao kuang er fei* 暴狂
而肥]). When the nutritive qi is exuberant, this is called structured (structured [*zhang* 章] means violently lustrous and smooth [*bao ze er guang* 暴
澤而光]).[13]

Wang Ken-Tang (王肯堂), a near-contemporary of Li Shi-Zhen, exemplifies the pre-vailing perspective that fearfulness and powerlessness are indeed pulse qualities. In *Cold Damage Criterion (Shang han zhun sheng* 傷寒準繩, 1604), Wang states:

舉之濡弱懷惚故憏營主血為陰按以候之其脈深而無力故為卑

[The pulse pertaining to the protective qi] is soggy, weak, and indistinct when [palpated] lightly; therefore, it is [called] fearful. The nutritive, which masters the blood, is yin, and is felt when the pulse is pressed deeply. The pulse is deep and lacks strength; therefore, it is called powerless.[14]

Consensus only goes so far, however, and while most commentators agree that fearful-ness and powerlessness are pulse qualities, each has a different interpretation of what those qualities might be. For example, Wu Qian (吳謙, 1736–1793) suggests a very different set of pulse images in the *Golden Mirror of the Medical Tradition.*

脈隨指無力上來衛氣弱也謂之憏脈隨指無力下去營氣弱也謂之卑憏者
恍惚也卑者縮下也

A pulse that lacks strength on arrival means that the protective qi is weak. This is called fearfulness. A pulse that lacks strength in departing means that the nutritive qi is weak. This is called powerlessness. Those with fearfulness are abstracted, and those with powerlessness have shrinkage below.

In his aptly titled *Precision in the Four Examinations (Si zhen jue wei* 四診抉微, 1723), Lin Zhi-Han (林之瀚, fl. 1723) proposes a particularly comprehensive and exacting set of criteria for these pulse qualities.

衛氣弱名曰憏憏者寸口微滑而按之軟弱舉之瞥瞥似數而仍力微以衛氣
主表表虛不能勝邪故有似乎心中怵惕之狀

When the protective qi is weak, it is called fearfulness. Fearfulness means that the wrist pulse is slightly slippery and soft and weak when pressed. The pulse is glancing with light pressure, as if rapid, and the strength is still slight. The protective qi masters the exterior, and when the exterior is deficient, it is unable to overcome pathogens; therefore, it is similar to the mental state of apprehension.

When the nutritive qi is weak, it is called powerlessness. Powerlessness means that none of the pulses respond to the fingers. This is commonly accompanied by deep and choppy pulse forms, which are felt very deeply. They are similar to a hidden pulse and difficult [to palpate].

營氣弱名曰卑卑者諸脈皆不應指常兼沈澀之形而按之隱隱似伏而且澀

難以營氣主裡裡虛則陽氣不振故脈不顯有似妾婦之甲屑不能自主故以
卑字譬之

> Nutritive qi masters the interior. When the interior is deficient, the yang
> qi cannot rise, and so the pulse is not evident. This is akin to a concubine's
> inability to restrain herself from paring her nails. Hence, the image of pow-
> erlessness.[15]

Finally, Zhang Nan (章楠, fl. 1835) attempts to explain fearfulness as a specific weakness of the muscles and flesh that is like fearfulness and timidity (肌肉松薄故名慄猶
怯也).[16]

It is evident that the words fearful and powerless are laden with meaning. They
hint at a clinical picture that is far more nuanced and complex than fever and chills,
expanding both the scope of *wei* vessel pathology and applications of Astragalus Decoction to Construct the Middle *(huang qi jian zhong tang)* and Eight-Treasure Decoction *(ba zhen tang)*.

The variety of these opinions remind us that pulse findings in Chinese medicine
are simply echoes of larger health dynamics at play within an individual. In clinical
practice, it is common to observe that people with urgent (*ji* 急) pulses tend to have
a tense or urgent bearing. The above discussion is an apt illustration of this principle.
The phenomena of fearfulness and powerlessness as expressions of disharmony in the
protective and nutritive qi may potentially manifest on every level.[17]

From Li's perspective, despite the breadth of Zhang Yuan-Su's interpretative approach, Zhang failed to take his own principles to their logical conclusion. According
to Li, "Jie-Gu limited his use of Cinnamon Twig [Decoction] *(gui zhi [tang])* to a single
symptom that pertained to the *yang wei* [vessel], and he did not expand [its scope of
application to symptoms with a] similar [pathodynamic]."

Li then takes Zhang's basic idea and runs with it, listing an impressive array of
herbal formulas that ostensibly address *yin wei* pathologies. These formulas influence
the *yin wei* only by virtue of the fact that they treat various types of abdominal pain.

> Jie-Gu limited his use of Cinnamon Twig [Decoction] *(gui zhi [tang])* to a
> single symptom that pertained to the *yang wei* [vessel], and he did not ex-
> pand [its scope of application to symptoms with a] similar [pathodynamic].
> Once the *yin wei* has become diseased, it governs heart pain. Jie-Gu limited
> himself to medicinals that [influenced] the three yin by warming the inte-
> rior. Hence, these were indicated [only] once cold had struck the three yin.
> [For instance], in the case of heat reversal of the three yin producing pain,
> he did not prepare [prescriptions] such as this. Now although the *yin wei*
> vessel intersects with the three yin and travels [along their trajectories], in
> actuality, it [also] returns to the *ren* vessel. Therefore, heart pain typically
> pertains to an upsurge of qi in the lesser yin, reversing yin, and *ren* vessel.
> [This pattern presents as] sudden pain with an absence of heat or long-term

pain with an absence or cold. If gentle pressure stops [the patient's pain, then this an indicator of] deficiency, and if one cannot tolerate deep pressure, this is an indicator of excess.

All cold pain presenting along with a lesser yin and *ren* vessel [pattern is treated by] Frigid Extremities Decoction *(si ni tang)*. When presenting along with a reversing yin pattern, [the cold pain] is treated by Tangkuei Decoction for Frigid Extremities *(dang gui si ni tang)*. When presenting along with a greater yin pattern, Regulate the Middle Pill *(li zhong wan)* treats [the cold pain]. All heat pain presenting along with a combined lesser yin and *ren* vessel [pattern is treated by] Melia Toosendan Powder *(jin ling zi san)* or Corydalis Decoction *(yan hu suo tang)*. When presenting along with a reversing yin pattern, [heat pain is treated by] Sudden Smile Powder *(shi xiao san)*. When presenting along with a greater yin pattern, Order the Qi Decoctions *(cheng qi tang)* master it. If the nutritive and blood are internally damaged with combined [involvement] of the *ren*, *chong*, and hand reversing yin, then prescriptions in the class of Four-Substance Decoction *(si wu tang)*, Nourish the Nutritive Decoction *(yang rong tang)*, and Marvelously Fragrant Powder *(miao xiang san)* are indicated.

According to Li, despite the fact that all of these prescriptions influence the *yin wei* vessel, the appropriate prescription must be selected with care. "If one administers medicinals based on the cause of the illness, attending to yin and yang, deficiency and excess, [then following these] broad outlines, one will rarely make mistakes." Of all the herbal discussions in *Exposition on the Eight Extraordinary Vessels*, this passage most begs the question of why we should bother with an extraordinary vessel diagnosis at all. Here such a perspective appears to offer little in the way of conceptual and diagnostic clarification, despite its lengthy recitation of herbal formulas for the *yin wei*.[18]

Wei Vessel Pulses

Li next shifts his discussion to the pulse patterns of the *wei* vessels, quoting exclusively from the *Pulse Classic*.

Wang Shu-He in the *Pulse Classic* asserts: A wrist pulse that beats "from the [foot] lesser yin obliquely to the [foot] greater yang is a *yang wei* pulse. [When the pulse is] perturbed in this way, [the patient] suffers from obstruction and itching of the muscles and flesh, skin pain, numbness in the lower parts, and sweating with chills." In addition, patients will "suffer from suddenly falling down where they bleat like sheep, their arms and legs will be drawn in, and in extreme [cases, suffer from] loss of voice and inability to speak. In such instances, one should select Guest Host (GB-3)" (located above the bone in front of the ear where a hollow appears when the mouth is opened; it is the meeting of the hand and foot lesser yang and yang brightness).

[Wang Shu-He] also states: "A wrist pulse that beats obliquely from the lesser yang to the reversing yin is a *yin wei* pulse. [When the pulse is] perturbed in this way, [the patient] suffers from seizures, sudden collapse, and bleating." He also says: "[The patient] will suffer from sudden collapse, loss of voice, and obstruction and itching of the muscles and flesh," and "aversion to wind accompanying spontaneous sweating and a drenching sweat." Choose Yang White (GB-14), Metal Gate (BL-63) (see above), and Subservient Visitor (BL-61) (see the *yang qiao*).

	OUTSIDE (RADIAL)	MIDDLE	INSIDE (ULNAR)
DISTAL			
MIDDLE			
PROXIMAL			
	DISTAL	MIDDLE	PROXIMAL
SUPERFICIAL			
MIDDLE			
DEEP			

Fig. 22-1 *Yang wei* pulse

While subsequent authors, including Li Zhong-Zi and Shen Jin-Ao, have divorced these pulse images from their accompanying symptoms and acupuncture treatments, it is clear that they were originally presented together as a diagnostic package. The final chapter of *Exposition on the Eight Extraordinary Vessels* recapitulates "The Hand Diagram of the Thirty-One Locations," the final chapter in the *Pulse Classic*, which consolidates much of the extraordinary vessel pulse material scattered elsewhere throughout the *Pulse Classic*, while also adding some new material of its own. Here too, the pulse descriptions not only reflect a *yin wei* or *yang wei* disorder, but an accompanying symptom complex. It is unclear whether one should infer that Guest Host (GB-3) influences all *yang wei* conditions or just presentations with those specific symptoms. Equally vague is what we are to make of Yang White (GB-14), Metal Gate (BL-63), and Subservient Visitor (BL-61) as treatment holes for *yin wei* disorders.

The symptom of "obstruction and itching of the muscles and flesh, skin pain, numbness in the lower parts" appears in Volume 10 of the *Pulse Classic* in association with the disorders of the yang networks *(yang luo* 陽絡*)* and not the *yang wei* vessel.[19] Li has merged the two pathologies. In his interpretation, disorders of the yang networks are synonymous with those of the *yang wei*. This is an idea that would be developed further by later physicians, particularly Ye Tian-Shi.

The Interrelationship of the *Wei* and *Qiao* Vessels

Somewhat incongruously, Li uses the references to seizure disorders in the above passages to make a point about the intimate relationship between the *wei* and *qiao* vessels. He reconciles the apparent incongruity between the seizure pathodynamics presented by Wang Shu-He and those appearing in the *Divine Pivot* by asserting that both interpretations basically address the same pathology. They are two sides of the same coin.

> [Li] Bin-Hu says: Wang Shu-He attributes seizure disorders to the *yin wei* and *yang wei*, and yet the *Divine Pivot* classic attributes seizure disorders to the *yin qiao* and *yang qiao*. The meaning of the two statements differs, but their intention is the same. The *yang wei* arises at the outer ankle and ascends, proceeding along the yang aspect to arrive at the shoulder, and travels around the ear and cheek to travel to the protective aspect at the meeting of all the yang. The *yin wei* arises at the inner ankle, proceeding along the yin aspect, ascending to the ribs and to the throat where it travels to the nutritive aspect to intersect with all the yin. The *yang qiao* arises in the heel and proceeds upward from the outer ankle, traveling along the outer thigh to arrive at the rib-sides and the shoulder, traveling along the left and right sides of the body to terminate in the inner corner of the eye. The *yin qiao* arises in the heel and proceeds upward along the inner thigh and genitals, traveling along the left and right sides of the body to arrive at the throat where it meets the *ren* vessel, terminating at the inner corner of the eye. Pathogens in the *yin wei* or *yin qiao* will produce withdrawal. Pathogens in the *yang wei* or *yang qiao* will produce seizures. Seizure-like perturbations pertain to yang and are governed by yang vessels. Withdrawal-like quiescence pertains to yin and is governed by yin vessels. Generally speaking, [in treating] these two illnesses, one should select the holes of these four vessels by differentiating yin and yang.

Adjunctive Qualities Associated with the *Wei* Pulses

Wang Shu-He's extraordinary vessel pulse scheme not only allows multiple pulse images to be attributed to each extraordinary vessel, it also allows for an extraordinary vessel pulse to have other concurrent qualities. These adjunctive qualities are also predictors of specific symptoms.

> Wang Shu-He says: "When examination reveals that the *yang wei* pulse is floating, vertigo will occur with standing. This is due to the yang being overabundant and overfull [so the patient also] suffers from raised-shoulder breathing and shivering, as if cold."

"When examination reveals that the *yin wei* pulse is deep, large, and excessive, [the patient] suffers from pain in the chest, propping fullness below the hypochondria, and heart pain. If the pulse feels like a string of pearls, then in men there will be an excess below both rib-sides and lumbar pain, while in women there will be genital pain as if sores have formed."

Low Back Pain and Acupuncture Strategies Involving the *Wei* Vessels

The final section of the chapter on diseases of the *wei* vessels is concerned specifically with acupuncture treatments for lumbar pain. Li rarely mentions any of the eight master holes of the extraordinary vessels. For example, here Outer Pass (TW-5) and Inner Pass (PC-6), the well-known master holes of the *yang* and *yin wei*, respectively, are absent from his discussion. He cites *Basic Questions* and Wang Qi-Xuan, which access the *yang wei* via its cleft hole, Yang Intersection (GB-35), and possibly Mountain Support (BL-57). The latter may be an error since it is not actually on the trajectory of the *yang wei*. Li quotes Wang Qi-Xuan for locating the hole: "One *chi* above the ground is the hole Mountain Support (BL-57), which is in the lower tip of the calf in a depression formed by the parting of the flesh." However, in his commentary to Ch. 10 of the *Yellow Emperor's Inner Classic: Grand Essentials*, Yang Shang-Shan uses nearly identical wording to describe Yang Intersection: "Below the calf about one qi from the ground is Yang Intersection, the *yang wei* cleft [hole]."[20]

In the passages that follow, Li equates two ancillary network vessels with the *wei* vessels, each of which is associated with a single acupuncture hole. Li's inclusion of these vessels in his discussion of diseases of the *wei* further amplifies the intimate relationship between the *wei* and network vessels. The Interior Flesh Vessel issues from the *yang wei* and is accessed at Yang Assistance (GB-38), and the *yin wei* issues from the Soaring Yang vessel and is accessed at Guest House (KI-9). Both holes can be used to treat lumbar pain.

The Interior Flesh vessel causes people to suffer from lumbar pain that prohibits coughing. When a patient coughs, this causes the sinew networks to tense and contract into a spasm. Prick the Interior Flesh vessel with two punctures, [one] lateral to the greater yang [and the other] on the lesser yang behind the fibula.

The Soaring Yang vessel causes people to have lumbar pain, producing sudden swelling in the painful area, and in extreme cases, it results in sorrow that borders on fear. Li bases the relationship between the *yang wei* and the Interior Flesh vessel on Wang Qi-Xuan:

Wang Qi-Xuan states: "The Interior Flesh vessel is engendered by the lesser yang, and the *yang wei* vessel qi issues from it." "Behind the fibula, the *yang wei* travels to the hole in the parting of the flesh. … It is located on the outer ankle of the foot directly above the end of the fibula behind two sinews in the parting of the flesh. … It may be pricked to a depth of five *fen*.

Wang Qi-Xuan, *Basic Questions*, and *The Systematic Classic of Acupuncture and Moxibustion* all confirm the connection between the *yin wei* vessel and the Soaring Yang vessel.

[Wang] Qi-Xuan states: "This is the *yin wei* vessel that departs from the inner ankle five *cun* from the parting of the calf, where it merges with the lesser yang channel and ascends.

"Prick the Soaring Yang vessel five *cun* above the inner ankle in front of the lesser yin where it meets the *yin wei*." This is the Guest House (KI-9) hole. *The Systematic Classic* states: Where the network of the greater yang diverges to travel to the lesser yin is called the Soaring Yang.

The original passage in *Basic Question*s locates Guest House (KI-9) five *cun* above the inner ankle and identifies it as Guest House. Both *The Systematic Classic* and the *Yellow Emperor's Inner Classic: Grand Essentials* locate the hole seven *cun* above the inner ankle. Li's location of just one *cun* above the ankle suggests that the hole in question is actually Recover Flow (KI-7). The general consensus, however, is that Recover Flow (KI-7) is an unlikely candidate because it is not recognized as having a *yin wei* influence. Hence, Li's location is probably simply an error.

Conclusion

In this chapter on *wei* vessel pathology, Li expands his inferential approach to textual interpretation and in the process develops the scope of *wei* vessel influence and treatment. Li's presentation of pulse and acupuncture material establishes the structure that he will use throughout the book. In discussing the relationship between the *wei* and *qiao* vessels, he prepares the way for his subsequent presentation of the *qiao*. His emphasis in this chapter on the similarities between the two sets of vessels in addressing seizure disorders contrasts with the very different way that he approaches the *qiao* vessels in the chapters that follow.

CHAPTER 23

On the *Qiao* Vessels

Yin Qiao Trajectory

It is apparent from Li Shi-Zhen's opening remarks regarding the *qiao* vessels that his understanding of these vessels differs significantly from that of the *wei*, which arise from their diffuse intersections with all the yin and yang and cannot be pegged to a specific channel. By contrast, the *yin* and *yang qiao* vessels are unequivocally recognized as branch vessels of the foot lesser yin and foot greater yang, respectively. Their function of conveying qi between the exterior and the deepest reaches of the interior is defined by their relationship with these two primary vessels. Li again cobbles together a detailed description of the *qiao* trajectories based on earlier sources. He follows Ch. 17 of *Divine Pivot* in identifying the origin of the *yin qiao* as being somewhere behind Burning Valley (KI-2) prior to traveling the short distance to Shining Sea (KI-6).[1] Nowhere is Burning Valley (KI-2) explicitly mentioned as an intersection hole of the *yin qiao* per se; however, by including the location for this hole in his own annotations, he tacitly includes it in its trajectory. The original editions of *Exposition on the Eight Extraordinary Vessels* contained no drawings, however the earliest edition of *Elucidations on the Fourteen Channels*, one of Li's primary sources, shows that the vessel proceeds from the inner angle and ascends to reach the throat sources, clearly depicting the *yin qiao* as beginning at Shining Sea (KI-6).

> The *yin qiao* is a branch vessel of the foot lesser yin. Its vessel arises from the center of the heel, behind the foot lesser yin hole Burning Valley (KI-2). (Burning Valley is located in a depression one *cun* in front of and below the inner heel.) It proceeds together with the foot lesser yin to the Shining Sea (KI-6) hole below the inner ankle (located five *fen* below the inner ankle) where it then ascends two *cun* above the inner ankle to Intersection Reach (KI-8). (Intersection Reach is located above the inner ankle in front of the lesser yin and behind the greater yin between the ridges formed by the sinew and bone.)

This description is more specific than the trajectory recorded in the 28th Difficult Issue, which has the *yin qiao* simply arising from the center of the heel and proceeding to the inner ankle. *The Systematic Classic of Acupuncture and Moxibustion*, by contrast, further simplifies the *yin qiao*'s initial trajectory by skipping the heel altogether and asserting that Shining Sea (KI-6) "[is the place] from which the *yin qiao* vessel is engendered."[2]

Continuing with the overall trajectory originally described in Ch. 17 of *Divine Pivot*, Li then traces the *yin qiao* upward to its terminus at the inner canthus.

> It travels straight up, proceeding along the inner thigh to enter the genitals. From here, it proceeds upward to the interior of the chest, entering the supraclavicular fossa and emerging at Man's Prognosis (ST-9) to reach the larynx where it intersects and links with the *chong* vessel. It then enters the ridge on the cheek bone and ascends and connects to the inner canthus of the eye where it meets with the five vessels of the foot greater yang, foot yang brightness, and the *yang qiao* at Bright Eyes (BL-1). (Bright Eyes is located in a depression one *fen* outside the inner canthus of the eye.) In all, there are eight holes.

Ch. 17 of *Divine Pivot* describes the *yin qiao*'s trajectory thusly: "Entering the sides of the nose and homing to the inner canthus to unite with the ascending trajectories of the hand greater yang and *yang qiao*" 入頄, 屬目內眥, 合手太陽, 陽蹺二上行.[3] Wang Bing observes that this means that both the *yin qiao* and *yang qiao* join at the [inner] canthus (是因蹺脈同向目眥而言).[4]

The Extraordinary Vessels in the *Eight Vessel Scripture* (*Ba mai jing* 八脈經)

The *yin qiao*'s intersection with the vessel is consistent with the trajectory presented in the 28th Difficult Issue of the *Classic of Difficulties*. The trajectory described in Ch. 17 of *Divine Pivot* makes no mention of this, simply stating that it "issues from Man's Prognosis."[5] Although Li begins his discussion of the *yin qiao* predictably enough with a description of its trajectory, he also expresses his interest in internal cultivation. He contrasts his initial description of the orthodox trajectory of the *yin qiao* with the unique perspective outlined by Zhang Bo-Duan in the *Eight Vessel Scripture*:

> As for the eight vessels, the *chong* vessel is located below the Wind House (GV-16) hole, the *du* vessel is located behind the umbilicus, the *ren* vessel is located in front of the umbilicus, the *dai* vessel is located in the lumbar region, the *yin qiao* vessel is located in front of the perineum below the scrotum, and the *yang qiao* vessel is located behind the perineum in the sacrococcygeal region. The *yin wei* is located one *cun* and three *fen* in front of the vertex [of the skull], and the *yang wei* vessel is located one *cun* and three *fen* behind the vertex [of the skull].

Zhang Zi-Yang's family name was Bo Duan (伯端), and his literary name was Ping Shu (平叔). He was a Daoist adept of the Southern Song dynasty. *Eight Vessel Scrip-*

ture is no longer extant, and *Exposition on the Eight Extraordinary Vessels* contains the earliest remaining fragments of the text; therefore, the sole context we have for interpreting these fragments is the one given to them by Li himself. The passage from *Eight Vessel Scripture* cited by Li identifies each vessel in the context of a particular area to be activated rather than in terms of a specific trajectory.

Zhang Zi Yang's Extraordinary Vessel Loci

Some of Zhang's extraordinary vessel loci are more comprehensible than others. For instance, because it girds the waist, the *dai* is located in the lumbar region. The location of the *ren* vessel in front of the umbilicus is consistent with what is arguably the most important and defining aspect of its trajectory. Taken on its own, the location of the *du* vessel behind the umbilicus is more problematic. The *du* vessel is certainly located behind the umbilicus, but it would be much more accurately described as being located behind the spine. Zhang's location of the *du* vessel only makes sense when it is considered together with the *ren* vessel. Zhang's reference to the umbilicus (*ji* 臍) must be more than a superficial anatomical referent. It is synonymous with the sea of qi (*qi hai* 氣海) and the cinnabar field (*dan tian* 丹田), the center of qi in the pelvis. Thus, the *ren* and *du* may indeed be understood as located in front of and behind the umbilicus, and as the functional extensions of the cinnabar field.

The trajectory of the *chong* vessel is described as dispersing in the chest with no direct relationship to the head or neck. Yet, in the beginning of his chapter on the *yin qiao*, he follows the description in the 28th Difficult Issue of the *Classic of Difficulties* that states that the *chong* communicates with the *yin qiao* at Man's Prognosis (ST-9). Zhang Zi-Yang also places the *chong* roughly in this vicinity, somewhere "below the Wind Mansion." This location may be an oblique reference to Great Shuttle (BL-11). According to Ch. 33 of *Divine Pivot*: "The *chong* vessel is the sea of the 12 channels, its transporting hole above is Great Shuttle (BL-11), and Upper and Lower Great Hollow (ST-37 and ST-39, respectively) below."[6] With these inferences, Li expands the scope of the *chong's* influence into the neck and head.

The *yin qiao* is located anterior to the perineum, and the *yang qiao* is located in the sacral area posterior to the perineum. The orthodox trajectories of these two vessels pass nowhere near these regions. According to Zhang, the *yin wei* and *yang wei* vessels are located anterior and posterior to the vertex. Zhang's descriptions of the *yin wei* and *yang wei* may well have influenced Li's interpretations of these vessel trajectories, as "ascending to reach to the front of the crown and terminate."

He explains the location of the *yang wei* in a similar manner, as "ascending to the Spirit Root hole and terminates" 上本神而止.[7] This explanation is less than satisfying since Spirit Root (GB-13) is traditionally located one *cun* and five *fen* to the side of Bend Center (BL-40), directly above the ears, four *fen* within the hairline, a position nowhere near the posterior vertex.

Qiao and *Wei* Vessel Relationships

The *qiao* and *wei* vessels perform similar but distinct functions within the channel system. The *wei* vessels provide a coherent and enveloping structure for their respective yin and yang channels. According to Li, the *qiao* vessels govern the sides of the body, which also suggests a crucial influence on the exterior structural aspects of yin and yang regulation. The *wei* vessels regulate communication between the protective and nutritive qi while the *qiao* vessels are responsible for the transmission of yin and yang on a larger scale, shuttling protective qi to the interior at night and back to the exterior during the day. In a sense, the *wei* and *qiao* may be interpreted as a single functional unit. Li's own comments in the immediately preceding chapter regarding the role of the *wei* and the *qiao* in seizure disorders support such a perspective. They address much the same pathology. Zhang's scheme also tacitly suggests a longitudinal dynamic between the *wei* vessels above and the *qiao* vessels below.

Divine Transcendents

At least as far as Li is concerned, Zhang's discussion of the extraordinary vessels is a discourse on spiritual and energetic cultivation rather than medicine. From this perspective, the eight vessels are inaccessible unless they have been deliberately activated. Wang Luo-Zhen explains that the reference to the extraordinary vessels as "hidden spirits" in this passage means that ordinary people cannot even detect their trajectories. His mention of divine transcendents *(shen xian* 神仙*)* is a reference to practitioners of Daoist internal alchemy. Once the tempering work *(lian gong* 煉功*)* of their alchemical transformation has reached a certain stage, these individuals experience a warm sensation of qi movement that is referred to as "making the yang qi penetrate and open [all eight Extraordinary Vessels]" *(yi yang qi chong kai* 以陽氣衝開*)*. Hence, the goal of this practice is the attainment of spiritual realization.[8]

The locations described in *Eight Vessel Scripture* are the places where each of the eight vessels are most amenable to conscious activation, although it provides no clue as to what that stimuli might be. Zhang informs us that the *yin qiao* must be the first of the extraordinary vessels to be activated and that the others can be opened only after the *yin qiao* has been activated.

> People have these eight vessels but they all remain hidden spirits because they are closed and have not yet been opened. Only divine transcendents can use the yang qi to surge through and open them so that they are able to attain the way. The eight vessels are the root of the great way of Former Heaven and the ancestor of the Unitary Qi. Only when the *yin qiao* is selected [for cultivation] first and only once this vessel has been activated will all the other vessels open.

According to Zhang, the *du, ren,* and *chong* vessels, the sources of all the other channels in the body, are subordinate to the *yin qiao* when it comes to their role in spiritual cultivation. He then claims that the *yin qiao* is referred to by a variety of names in Daoist manuals of qi cultivation.

> Next, the three vessels of the *du, ren,* and *chong* [should be selected for activation because they] are the source of creation for all the other channels and vessels. And yet, mention of the particular vessel the *yin qiao* is scattered throughout the *Cinnabar Scriptures* where it is variously referred to by many names. It is called Root of Heaven; it is called Death's Door; it is called the Resurrection Pass; it is called the Ghost Door of Fengdu; and it is called the Root of Life and Death. As the governor of the spirit, it is often called the Peach of Well-Being.

Cinnabar Scriptures (丹經 *dan jing*) are the texts comprising the Daoist Canon, particularly those dealing with internal alchemy and the cultivation of qi. Fengdu is a district near Sichuan said to be located near the entrance to the infernal regions. Whatever its appellation, from the Daoist perspective, the *yin qiao* links the brain above with the Gushing Spring (KI-1) below. In terms of spiritual development, it is crucial to establishing conscious control of yin and yang throughout the body.

> Above, it penetrates the mud ball, and below it reaches down to the Gushing Spring [KI-1]. If one has knowledge of [the *du, ren,* and *chong*], then one can induce the true qi to accumulate and dissipate [at will], all from these pass orifices. Thus, the heavenly gate will be constantly open, and earth's door will remain forever closed. The buttock vessel will flow throughout the entire body, linking and flowing freely both above and below, harmonious qi will naturally ascend to the imperial court. The yang will grow and the yin will diminish, fire will issue from the midst of water, and flowers will blossom through the snow.

Zhang makes heavy use of Daoist metaphors in these passages. The mud ball *(ni wan* 泥丸*)* is one of the Nine Palaces *(jiu gong* 九宮*)* in the head. By virtue of its central position, the mud ball is also regarded as the sum total of the nine palaces. Ishida Hidemi has suggested that it may allude to the round form of the brain and to the central agent soil (*ni* or mud).[9] Acccording to Henri Maspero, *ni wan* 泥丸 is a Chinese transliteration of the Sanskrit word nirvana, linking the brain directly to spiritual development.[10]

The pass orifices (*guan qiao* 關竅) are the orifices associated with the sense organs in the upper part of the body. The growth of the yang and the reduction of yin *(yang zhang yin xiao* 陽長陰消*)* is the goal of internal alchemy. He continues with references to the *Lao zi* and an arcane Daoist poem.

> When there is a languid ebb and flow between the Heavenly Root and the
> Moon Grotto, then the the 36 officials are spring-like.[11]

The root of heaven *(tian zhi gen* 天之根) is a reference to Ch. 6 of *Lao zi,* which Li had
already mentioned in Ch. 2: "The gate of the Mysterious Female is the root of heaven
and earth" 玄牝之門是謂天地根. Wang Luo-Zhen interprets the root of life as the
cinnabar field.[12] Similarly, the moon cave or grotto *(yue ku* 月窟) refers to the head
and specifically the brain, which is also known as the upper cinnabar field *(shang dan
tian*上丹田). These efforts are ultimately rewarded with a physical form that, while
less substantial, is actually lighter and stronger. More importantly, the spirit of the
adept becomes rarified. The irrelevant accoutrements of consciousness have been so
stripped away that the adept appears to be a simpleton to ordinary people.

> When this is achieved, then the body will become light and strong. The
> adept's aged countenance regains its vitality; in quiet silence, he becomes
> recondite as if he were an imbecile or intoxicated. [Such experiences] are
> proof [of the effect]. It is essential to understand that the location of the
> southwest is in *kun* earth, in front of the perineum, behind the bladder,
> below the small intestine, and above the divine tortoise. This is the ground
> where heaven and earth day by day engender the root of the qi and give
> birth to the lead. [Even] skilled physicians do not understand this.

Its emphasis on the *yin qiao* notwithstanding, the practice of internal cultivation via
the extraordinary vessels presented in *Eight Vessel Scripture* is not a matter of tracing their trajectories so much as focusing on key loci associated with them. Zhang
reiterates this point in his emphasis on the lower cinnabar field. The southwest is the
direction associated with the trigram *kun,* which also pertains to the abdomen. *Appended Commentaries of the Classic of the Changes of Zhou* states that "*Kun* denotes
earth [and] the abdominal region."

A similar and more poetic passage appears in Chen Nan's (陳楠, 13th century)
Song-dynasty manual of Daoist practice, *Emerald Emptiness (Cui xu pian* 翠虛篇):
"The moon shines brightly over the southwest road and great medicines are produced
in this place" 西南路上月華明大藥還從此處生.[13]

However, the cinnabar field is not located just anywhere in the abdomen. Zhang
specifies its location "in front of the Caudal Funnel, behind the urinary bladder, below
the small intestine and above the divine tortoise." The Caudal Funnel *(wei lü* 尾閭) is
the perianal region in the vicinity of the acupuncture hole Meeting of Yin (CV-1), and
the divine tortoise *(ling gui* 靈龜) is a euphemism for the penis. In this scheme, the *yin
qiao,* as the root of all the extraordinary vessels, is naturally located at the base of the
lower cinnabar field "in front of the Caudal Funnel, and behind the genitals."

Couched in heavy Daoist jargon, Li's summary comment articulates the larger
implications of the material he has just presented:

Bin-Hu says, the discussions in the cinnabar texts addressing the yang essence and the Water Wheel are most often spoken of in the context of *ren,*
chong, and *du* vessels, and the life gate and triple burner; the *yin qiao* is not
emphasized. And yet, Zi-Yang's *Eight Vessel Scripture,* which recorded the
[pathways of the] channels and vessels, differs slightly from the teachings
of the medical sects. Therefore, in following the path along the inner landscape, only those who return the senses will be capable of an illuminated
examination [of the eight vessels], and therefore these statements must not
be misconstrued.

Li's comment that the view of the extraordinary vessels presented in *Eight Vessel
Scripture* differs slightly from the standard medical understanding is something of an
understatement; this material represents a significant departure from the perspectives
presented in the *Inner Classic)* and *Classic of Difficulties.* Nevertheless, he is adamant
in his conviction that this material is profoundly relevant to physicians. Using terminology from the internal alchemical text *Exterior Landscape of the Yellow Court* (黃庭
外景經 *Huang ting wai jing jing),* Li goes a step farther, arguing that it is not enough
to content oneself with a theoretical knowledge of such things. If we wish to achieve
inner illumination *(nei zhao* 內照*)* through direct apprehension *(sui dao* 隨道*)* of the
physiological processes of the viscera known as the inner landscape *(nei jing* 內景*),*
then we must cultivate our own internal development by nurturing our essence spirit.
This is accomplished in part by the meditative technique of returning the senses *(fan
guan* 反觀*),* which involves the filtering out of external stimuli *(shou shi fan ting* 收視
反聽*),* literally, closing the sight and hearing.

On the whole, the *Exposition's* chapter on the *yin qiao* is concerned less with alternate perspectives on trajectories of the eight vessels than it is with the importance
of meditation in guiding clinical practice. It posits that extraordinary vessels cannot
be effectively manipulated without a firsthand experience of their activities within the
body. Though a consummate scholar himself, Li implies that book learning must be
balanced with active engagement.

Yang Qiao Trajectory

Li's presentation of the *yang qiao* is much less extensive than his discussion of the
yin qiao. He contents himself with a description of its trajectory and two concise passages that summarize the fundamental physiological function of both the *yin* and *yang
qiao.* In keeping with the pathway traced by its sister vessel, the trajectory of the *yang
qiao* "arises from the center of the heel and emerges below the outer ankle at the foot
greater yang Extending Vessel (BL-62) hole."

Where the *yin qiao* emerges slightly anterior to the heel behind Burning Valley
(KI-2), the *yang qiao* travels directly to the Extending Vessel (BL-62) hole but then
doubles back and encircles the heel before proceeding up the outer leg.

From behind the ankle, it encircles the heel to root at Subservient Visitor (BL-61) (located in a depression under the heel bone; find it by cupping the heel). It rises above the outer ankle for three *cun* to Instep Yang (BL-59), the cleft [hole] (located three *cun* above the outer heel, it is a foot greater yang hole). It ascends directly from here, proceeding along [the] outer thigh, and proceeding behind the rib-sides to the scapula where it meets the hand greater yang and *yang wei* at Upper Arm Transport (SI-10) (located in a depression below the scapular crest on the upper border of the scapula).

Oddly, Li omits Squatting Bone-Hole (GB-29) from the trajectory of the *yang qiao*, which *The Systematic Classic* describes as "the intersection hole of the *yang qiao* and the lesser yang."

[The *yang qiao*] then travels upward along the outer aspect of the shoulder to meet with the hand yang brightness at Great Bone (LI-16) (located above the tip of the shoulder in the rift that forms a depression between the two bones) and then moves on to meet the hand yang brightness and lesser yang at Shoulder Bone (LI-15) (located at the head of the humerus, at the tip of the shoulder in a rift that forms a depression between two bones; it is found in the hole that appears when the arm is raised).

[The *yang qiao* vessel] ascends to Man's Prognosis (ST-9) and hugs the corners of the mouth where it meets with the hand and foot yang brightness and the *ren* vessel at Earth's Granary (ST-4) (located four *fen* out from the corners of the mouth, close below which a slightly pulsing vessel can be found). Together with the foot yang brightness, it ascends and travels to Great Bone-Hole (ST-3) (beside the nostrils at a distance of eight *fen*, directly [below] the eyeball, level with the philtrum). From here, it returns to meet the *ren* vessel at Tear Container (ST-1) (located seven *fen* below the eye in a depression directly below the eyeball), and reaches the inner canthus to meet with the five vessels of the hand and foot greater yang, foot yang brightness, and *yin qiao* at Bright Eyes (BL-1) (see the *yin qiao* [discussed] previously). From Bright Eyes, [the *yang qiao*] ascends to enter the hairline and then descends behind the ear to enter Wind Pond (GB-20) where it terminates.

For the most part, Li Shi-Zhen follows *The Systematic Classic* in determining which acupuncture holes intersect with which extraordinary vessels. *The Systematic Classic,* however, describes Wind Pond as "the meeting of the lesser yang and the *yang wei*," making no mention of its intersection with the *yang qiao*.[14] Li's inclusion of this hole in the trajectory of the *yang qiao* is probably based on the *Classic of Difficulties,* which states that the *yang qiao* "enters Wind Pond."

What Counts as a *Qiao* Vessel?

After tracing the trajectory of the *yang qiao*, and apparently having nothing further to say regarding the *yang qiao* in particular, Li next turns his attention to the overall physiology of the *qiao* vessels. This he does in a very concise manner with a gloss of a passage from the 23rd Difficult Issue of the *Classic of Difficulties*, addressing the length of the *qiao* vessels, and a related passage from *The Systematic Classic*.

> The *Classic of Difficulties* states: "The *qiao* vessels extend from the feet to reach the eye. They are seven *chi* and five *cun*, … all together, this is one *zhang* and five *chi* long.
>
> The *Systematic Classic* states: "The *qiao* vessel has yin and yang [components], but which are counted? [Qi Bo] stated: "For males, the yang is counted, and for females, the yin is counted. What are counted are the channels, and what are not counted are the networks." "The qi within the body is like flowing water, like the ceaseless movement of the sun and moon. Therefore, the yin vessels nourish the yin viscera and the yang vessels nourish the yang receptacles like an endless circuit in which there is no break. Upon reaching the end, it just begins again. Its overflow of qi internally irrigates the yin viscera and yang receptacles and externally moistens the interstices."

The counting referred to in the latter passage concerns which channels should be included in the tally of the overall length of all the channels. All 12 channels and the *du*, *ren*, and *chong* vessels are counted, yet curiously, only one of the *qiao* vessels is included in this tally. The *yin qiao* is counted in females and *yang qiao* is counted in males. Though such matters are of concern to modern readers, Li's interest clearly extends beyond the anatomical accounting practices of the early medical literature. The issue of which *qiao* vessel should be included in the tally is merely a means of introducing the notion that, depending on the circumstances, the *qiao* vessels may be viewed as either channels or network vessels. As Yang Shang-Shan explains, "In men, the *yang qiao* is the channel and the *yin qiao* is the network. In women, the *yin qiao* is the channel and the *yang qiao* is the network."[15]

Because he fails to comment on the implications of one *qiao* vessel being a "channel" and the other a "network," Yang's interpretation is really just an elaborate way of restating what we already know: The *yin qiao* is primary in women and the *yang qiao* is primary in men.

Zhang Zhi-Cong's (張志聰, fl. 1873) explanation is that the ascent of earthly yin via the *yin qiao* to females and the descent of heavenly yang through the *yang qiao* to males are equally unhelpful.

> The vessel of the *yin qiao* resonates with the ascent of the earthly qi. Therefore, in women, it is counted as yin. The *yin qiao* pertains to the eye and

inner canthus, and by uniting with the upward movement of the *yang qiao*, the *yang qiao* receives the qi of the *yin qiao*. [This qi] returns [along the *yang qiao*] from the hairline, traveling downward to the foot, and rightly [causes the] descent of the heavenly qi; therefore, in men, it is counted as yang.[16]

Both of the above commentaries nevertheless amplify the notion of the *qiao* as a continuous yin-yang pair through which qi circulates. The reason that we may exercise the option of including only one of the *qiao* in our tally of channels is that they are simply two parts of a united whole. We are left with an impression that, for whatever reason, the *yin qiao* is simply more *apparent* in women and hence is deemed a channel, with the *yang qiao* assuming a secondary but essential role as network in facilitating a closed circulatory circuit. The converse is, of course, true in men. There is no question that in the larger context of the channel system as a whole, the *qiao* vessels are both intimately associated with the network vessels in both sexes. The notion of deeming one a channel and the other a network is merely a means of assigning the primacy of one *qiao* vessel over the other when comparing the two in a very circumscribed context.

Regardless of gender, however, the *yin qiao* facet of the pair nourishes the yin organs as it passes into the interior, while the *yang qiao* nourishes the yang organs and the striae in moving to the exterior. This function pervades the entire body. Li's quotation from *The Systematic Classic* actually originates in Ch. 17 of *Divine Pivot*, which stresses this point in prefacing its remarks by stating: "There is nowhere that this qi does not travel" (*qi zhi bu de wu xing* 氣之不得無行).[17] The perfusion of qi throughout the body is itself a characteristic of the network vessels, which reach beyond the primary channels into every nook and cranny of the energetic structure.

Whatever their differences, the *wei* and *qiao* work together to define much of the external stucture of the channel system and the body as a whole. Their close relationship to the network vessels is evidence of this role. But where the influence of the *wei* vessels is concerned primarily with the regulation of yin and yang in the relative exterior of the body, the *qiao* control the passage of yin and yang from the exterior to much deeper aspects of the body.

CHAPTER 24

On Diseases of the Two *Qiao*

The relationship between the *qiao* and *wei* vessels and the network vessels is a major theme in Li Shi-Zhen's *Exposition on the Eight Extraordinary Vessels*. His opening statement regarding diseases of the *qiao* echoes his introductory comments concerning diseases of the *wei* vessels. In quoting the 29th Difficult Issue of the *Classic of Difficulties*, Li asserts that the network vessels of the *qiao* are synonymous with the rest of the network vessel system: "The yin networks are the networks of the *yin qiao*. The yang networks are the networks of the *yang qiao*."

Before venturing any comment regarding *qiao* vessel pathology, Li first establishes a fundamental principle of their physiological function: The *qiao* are as intimately connected to the network vessel system as the *wei*. This statement frames the content of the entire chapter. To one degree or another, diseases of the *qiao* are diseases of the network vessels. For instance, the tonus of the network vessels is a key indicator of imbalance within the *qiao* vessels. His opening statement is followed by a passage from the 26th Difficult Issue of the *Classic of Difficulties*. "When the *yin qiao* is diseased, the yang is slack and the yin is tense. When the *yang qiao* is diseased, the yin is slack and the yang is tense."

Li's arrangement of these passages is not random, nor is it a chronological laundry list of quotations pertaining to the *qiao* vessels. The orthodox literature is his means of substantiating his point that the resiliency of the tissues nourished by the *qiao* vessels is a function of their physiological relationship with the network vessels. Later in this chapter, Li quotes Zhang Jie-Gu, who reinforces this perspective. Li Shi-Zhen then follows the passages from the *Classic of Difficulties* with a similar passage from Wang Shu-He's *Pulse Classic (Mai jing* 脈經), which specifies precisely where along the *qiao* vessel this tension or slackness should be evaluated.

> [When the] *yin qiao* ... vessel is tense, from the medial ankle and above it is tense, and from the lateral ankle and above it is slack. [When the] *yang qiao* vessel ... is tense, from the lateral ankle and above it is tense, and from the medial ankle and above it is slack.

Changes in the tonus of the *qiao* vessels on the lower extremities are the essential expression of an imbalance in those vessels, which is mediated through the network vessels. Ding De-Yong (丁德用, fl. 1062) interprets the pathodynamic of imbalanced tonus within the *qiao* very specifically:

221

> Diseases [of the extraordinary vessels] cannot emerge from within [the extraordinary vessels] themselves. They are caused by an influx of [surplus contents] from [primary] channels when the latter are excessive. ... Whenever the yang vessels are excessive, they distribute [their excess qi] into the *yang qiao* vessels, and as a result, the *yang qiao* vessels become diseased.[1]

According to Ding, the unaffected *qiao* vessel is only "slack" when compared to the "tension" produced by the pathogenic excess in the affected *qiao* vessel.[2] Zhang Shi-Xian (張世賢, fl. 1506–1521) explicitly associates tension with excess and slackness with deficiency, which suggests that slackness does not simply refer to an absence of pathological excess but to a relative state of pathological deficiency.[3] Regardless of which emphasis one prefers, the majority of other symptoms associated with the *qiao* may be understood in light of this pathodynamic.

Diseases of the *qiao* vessels tend to present with symptoms commonly associated with the network vessels such as seizure disorders, paralysis, and lumbar pain. As we will see, the relationship between networks and the *qiao* vessels plays an important role even in the *qiao* function of sleep regulation.

Of course, not all *qiao* pathology is as severe as the sheep-like bleating mentioned in the *Pulse Classic*. Subsequent interpretations of extraordinary vessel pathodynamics have invariably allowed for both subtle and dramatic presentations. In principle, tension and/or slackness in the *qiao* vessels referred to in the 26th Difficult Issue may also be interpreted as a simple palpatory diagnostic parameter. Here, they are necessarily relative qualities. For instance, the *yang qiao* vessel on the lower extremity may only be considered tense in relation to the perceived slackness of the *yin qiao*. Nevertheless, the extraordinary vessel pathologies described in the *Pulse Classic* and in much of *Exposition on the Eight Extraordinary Vessels* are generally severe and reflect a deep level of imbalance. This is a topic that will be addressed further in our discussion of extraordinary vessel pulse-symptom complexes in Ch. 33.

Qiao Vessel Pulses

Li himself takes no stand on which of these propositions is the most helpful or accurate, suggesting that they may all be relevant in one situation or another. Having reintroduced Wang Shu-He into his discussion, Li continues with Wang's presentation of the pulses associated with the *qiao* vessels, their symptoms, and appropriate acupuncture and moxibustion strategies.

> [Wang Shu-He] also states: A wrist pulse that is "tapping in the distal left and right positions is a *yang qiao* [pulse]. [When the pulse is] perturbed in this way, [the patient] suffers from back pain." It also includes "withdrawal and seizures," and sheep-like bleating, "aversion to wind, hemilateral withering" and "painful obstruction" and "generalized body stiffness".

A wrist pulse that is "tapping in the proximal left and right positions is a *yin qiao* [pulse]. [When the pulse is] perturbed in this way, [the patient] suffers from withdrawal and seizures, chills and feverishness, and stiffness and insensitivity of the skin."[4] There will also be "lower abdominal pain, abdominal urgency, and lower back and pelvis [pain] radiating into the genitals. In males, this is yin bulging,[5] and in females, there is incessant spotting."

Curiously, Li makes no mention of a pebble-like or tapping (*tan* 彈) pulse anywhere in his writings. Katsuda Masayasu defines this pulse as hard and bouncing laterally to the right and left, in this case, in the proximal position on the wrist.[6] (A more comprehensive discussion of this pulse quality appears in Ch. 17 below.) According to Wang Shu-He, at least one secondary pulse quality may shade the basic qualities associated with the *qiao* vessels. If the *yang qiao* pulse is "faint and choppy, this indicates wind seizures." Wang recommends Instep Yang (BL-59) only for wind seizures accompanied by a faint and choppy *yang qiao* pulse and makes no mention of how the other *yang qiao* symptoms should be addressed. Because it is evidently difficult to discriminate between which of the two *qiao* vessels to treat in seizure disorders, Wang suggests that "If the patient cannot tell where the trouble is, then [treat] the two *qiao* below. In men, [treat] the *yang* [*qiao*], and in women [treat] the *yin* [*qiao*]."[7]

According to the modern commentators Wang Luo-Zhen and Li Ding, the "two *qiao* below" are Shining Sea (KI-6) and Extending Vessel (BL-62).[8] Given the context in which this reference to the *qiao* vessels occurs, some commentators suggest that the treatment modality referred to is moxibustion.

A Pathway between the Interior and the Exterior

Having made his first point that diseases of the *qiao* are intimately linked to pathologies of the network vessels, Li moves on to the next characteristic of the *qiao*, their role in the transmission of yin and yang between the interior and the exterior. Yet he links even this characteristic to their fundamental function of regulating the networks and their pathological expression of tension and slackness.

Wang and Li note that 蹻 *(qiao)* originally meant "to walk by raising one's legs high." 蹻蹻 *(qiao qiao)* meant "to walk in a powerful manner," as in *Odes of Lu* (*Lu Song* 魯頌) in the *Canon of Poetry* (*Shi jing* 詩經, ca. 900—700 BCE), which states "its horses stride powerfully" *(qi ma qiao qiao* 其馬蹻蹻). By extension, *qiao qiao* may also mean "to be excited." Again, the *Canon of Poetry* states "the child is excited" *(xiao zi qiao qiao* 小子蹻蹻).[9] "The Record of Emperor Gao" in the *Book of Han (Han shu Gao di ji* 漢書高帝紀) contains a passage stating that one must "wait with a raised leg" *(ke qiao zu dai* 可蹻足待). Similarly, Ch. 54 of *Basic Questions* states, "[to locate the] Great Hollows (ST-37, ST-39) holes, [one must] raise (*qiao* 蹻) one's leg and find a single hole between the tibia and the fibula."[10] Wang Bing observes, "[*qiao*] means 'to raise one's leg.'"[11]

The word 蹻 *qiao* is often associated with the feet. The "Biography of Minister Yu" (*Yu qing zhuan* 虞卿傳) in the *Canon of History (Shi jing* 史經) contains the phrase 躡蹻 *(nie qiao)*, which means to wear straw shoes or clogs.[12] In his annotations to the *Classic of Difficulties,* Yang Xuan-Cao states that "蹻 *(qiao)* means to be quick and agile. They are [therefore concerned with] the mechanisms of movement and the origins of movement in the feet."

All of this complements Li's own discussion of the word *qiao.* Li attributes the idea that "*qiao* means 'agile' *(jie* 捷*)* and 'fast' *(ji* 疾*)*" to Zhang Jie-Gu; however, because his work is no longer extant, this is impossible to confirm. According to Zhang, "the two vesels arise in the foot and put a spring in the step." His discussion of the relationship between the two *qiao* is similar to that of the *wei* vessels. Like the *wei,* the *yang qiao* and *yin qiao* have an exterior-interior relationship that is closely linked to the network vessels.[13]

Zhang Jie-Gu's discussion illustrates the links between the trajectories of the *qiao,* their association with the networks, and their function of promoting communication between the interior and the exterior. It also introduces another of the key indicators of *qiao* disharmonies: eyes that are either fixed open or closed shut. Zhang Jie-Gu's remarks closely resemble those of two earlier commentators, Yang Xuan-Cao and Ding De-Yong, whose discussions make it clear that the opening or closure of the eyes is not really separate from the phenomenon of tension or slackness. The pathology associated with the eye is actually just an extension of the more fundamental pathodynamic involving tonus in the networks:

> 陰蹻為病，則陽緩而陰急，即病陰厥，足勁直二絡不通．陽蹻為病，則陰緩而陽急，即狂走不臥

> When the *yin qiao* is diseased, then the yang is slack and the yin is tense, resulting in a disease of yin reversal where the foot and shins [are involved] and the two networks are impeded. When the *yang qiao* is diseased, then the yin is slack and the yang is tense, causing [the afflicted] to walk around crazily, never lying down.[14]

Another version of this passage concludes with the death of the patient, again testifying to the overall severity of extraordinary vessel patterns in general.[15]

Li quotes Zhang Jie-Gu as clearly specifying the depth of the *qiao* vessels:

> The *yang qiao* travels above the muscle and flesh, circulating among the yang vessels, linking the six receptacles, mastering and maintaining the exterior. It is therefore called the network of the *yang qiao.* The *yin qiao* travels below the muscle and flesh, circulating among the yin vessels, linking the five viscera, mastering and maintaining the interior. It is therefore called the network of the *yin qiao.*

This idea first appears in Ding's comment on the 70th Difficult Issue of the *Classic of Difficulties* wherein he remarks, "Through the skin … is where the yang qi moves. Through the muscle and flesh below … is where the yin qi moves." 皮膚之上 … 陽氣所行肌肉之下 … 陰氣所行.[16]

The *Classic of Difficulties* itself, however, says nothing of the kind. It makes a much more general statement regarding seasonal variation in the depth of the qi:

> It is like this. In spring and summer, the yang qi is in the upper [regions], and a person's qi is also in the upper regions. Hence, one must [needle] superficially in order to remove them. In autumn and winter, the yang qi is in the deeper [regions], and a person's qi is also in the deeper [regions]. Hence, one must [needle] deeply in order to remove them.[17]

These passages reflect a progressive reframing of material from earlier texts. By substituting the word "vessel" *(mai* 脈*)* for the word "qi" (氣), Zhang, and then Li in turn, reinterprets the original meaning of the *Classic of Difficulties* to apply to the extraordinary vessels.

Needles and Moxa

Moxibustion is the treatment of choice for diseases of the *yin qiao*, whereas needling is indicated for pathologies involving the *yang qiao*. Shining Sea (KI-6) is not used here as a master hole per se, nor is it paired with Broken Sequence (LU-7). Its pairing with Yang Mound Spring (GB-34), the master point of the muscles, reflects the musculoskeletal and network vessel 'resonance' associated with the *yin qiao* described above. The *yin qiao* condition is characterized by deficiency heat whereas the *yang qiao* condition is characterized by deficiency cold. This treatment most probably originated in *The Systematic Classic of Acupuncture and Moxibustion;* however, in that text needling was the treatment of choice for both conditions.[18] The rationale for performing moxibustion in the case of deficiency heat and needling in the case of deficiency cold is unclear.

According to Zhang Jie-Gu, *yang qiao* pathology may also be due to cold, and in this case, Wind Pond (GB-20) and Wind Adobe (GV-16) should be needled. Li recommends these same holes for some types of *yang wei* pathology due to cold, again illustrating how interrelated are the *wei* and *qiao* vessel pathologies.

Although Li attributes these statements to Zhang Jie-Gu, Zhang simply tells us to treat Wind Pond (GB-20) and Wind Adobe (GV-16); he does not specify the method, nor does he mention Yang Mound Spring (GB-34). These are Li's innovations.[19] Li continues with a generalized statement regarding herbal treatment strategy, ostensibly quoting from Zhang Jie-Gu, and links it specifically to the herbal treatment of the *qiao* vessels. This is one of the few statements regarding the herbal treatment of the *qiao* vessels in the *Exposition*.

[Zhang Jie-Gu] also says that "[when disease is located] in the exterior yang, one must sweat it, and [when disease] is located in the interior yin, one must purge it."

This passage lays the groundwork for Li's subsequent prescription, later in the chapter, of Pinellia [and Sorghum] Decoction *(ban xia [shu mi] tang)* to treat insomnia due to a *yang qiao* imbalance. Diurnal seizure disorders exemplify two of the fundamental characteristics of *qiao* physiology and pathology. In terms of *qiao* pathology, seizures may be interpreted as an extreme form of the tension and slackness originally described in the *Classic of Difficulties.* As previously noted, tension or slackness in *qiao* vessel disorders may present anywhere on a continuum of severity from seizures to subtle differences in the tone of the yin and yang channels of the leg. Because the *qiao* are responsible for the transmission of protective qi between the exterior during the daytime and the interior at night, disorders that occur exclusively during the day or night are particularly amenable to treatment via the *qiao* vessels. Once the situation has become sufficiently severe that seizures are occurring, Zhang recommends moxibustion regardless of whether the problem is in the *yin qiao* or the *yang qiao*: "[Zhang Jie-Gu] also says that 'For diurnal seizures, one should perform moxibustion on the *yang [qiao]*, and for nocturnal [seizures], one should perform moxa on the *yin [qiao].*'"

The *Qiao,* Ancillary Vessels, and Back Pain

Li continues his discussion of *qiao* vessel pathology with a series of quotations from *Basic Questions* describing a number of acupuncture holes and their associated network vessels. The common thread running through these ancillary vessels is that they all treat back pain. Li posits that the ancillary vessels are all intimately related to the *qiao* vessels. The first of these passages simply cites two holes on the trajectory of the *yang qiao* that treat a specific kind of back pain.

[Ch. 41] of *Basic Questions,* the "Discussion on Lower Back Pain," states: "For lumbar pain where one cannot lift [himself up out of bed, needling] Extending Vessel (BL-62) and Subservient Visitor (BL-61) will allow the patient to lift [himself up]."

Li presents the reader with the relatively familiar association between Extending Vessel (BL-62) and the *yang qiao* before moving into the more challenging territory of the Meeting Yin vessel *(hui yin mai* 會陰脈).

[Ch. 41 of *Basic Questions*] also states: "The Meeting Yin vessel causes people to suffer from lower back pain that ascends [up the back] with soaking perspiration, an urge to drink after the sweat has dried, and an urge to walk after drinking. Prick the Straight Yang vessel with three punctures. This is located on the *qiao* in a cleft five *cun* below the transverse crease [of the popliteal fossa]. If one sees [local] congestion, then let out some blood."

The Meeting Yin vessel has been interpreted in two different ways. The first is that "meeting yin" simply refers to the main channel of the foot greater yang. In his comments to Ch. 41 of *Basic Questions*, Wang Bing observes that the Meeting Yin vessel is "the main channel of the foot greater yang. Its vessel proceeds from the lumbar region downward to meet at the anus [literally, posterior yin]. Therefore, [this area] is called Meeting in the Yin." [20]

Wang also states that the Meeting Yin vessel travels "from within the lumbar area and descends, hugging the spine" (*cong yao zhong xia xia ji* 從腰中下俠脊), meaning that it issues from the kidney transport hole and descends to the eight bone-holes and the meeting of the yang. From here, the Meeting Yin vessel then unites with the *ren* vessel at the meeting of the yin.

The second interpretation is that the Meeting Yin vessel refers to the *ren* and *du* vessels and their intersection at the Meeting Yin (CV-1) hole, hence the name Meeting Yin vessel. In his comments to Ch. 41 of *Basic Questions*, Ma Shi (馬蒔, 15th–16th century) explains:

> As for the meeting yin, this is the name of the hole of the *ren* and *du* channel. The *du* vessel arises at the meeting of [the] yin and travels along the spine, hence the Meeting Yin vessel is naturally the meeting below the lumbar region at the posterior yin.[21]

Gao Shi-Zong (高士宗, 1623–1670) adopts a similar opinion, which is also advocated by Wu Kun (吳昆, 1552–1620), Zhang Jing-Yue (張景岳, 1563–1640), and Zhang Zhi-Cong (張志聰, 1610–1682). According to Gao:

> The meeting of the yin is located in front of the anus and behind the urethra. The two vessels of the *ren* and *du* meet here between the two anterior and posterior yin [orifices] and hence, [this region] is called the meeting of the yin.[22]

Given such unanimity of opinion, Li's association of the Meeting Yin vessel with the *yin qiao* would at first seem to be somewhat anomalous. The Meeting Yin vessel is the vessel associated with the eponymous hole. Yet Li's view is much more intelligible once we recall his inclusion of Zhang Bo-Duan's remarks regarding the extraordinary vessels in the previous chapter. According to Zhang Zi-Yang, "The *yin qiao* vessel is located in front of the perineum, behind the genitals, and the *yang qiao* vessel is located in the sacrum behind the perineum." In light of this, Li would naturally consider the Meeting Yin vessel to be synonymous with the *yin qiao*.

Li next quotes Wang Qi-Xuan, whose straightforward remarks reinforce the linkage between these ancillary networks and the *qiao*:

Wang Qi-Xuan states that the vessels of the foot greater yang "traverse the lower back and meet in the area of the anus, therefore [this area] is called meeting in the yin." "The Straight Yang vessel ... travels down along the spine, penetrating through the buttock to the popliteal area, proceeding along the calf to behind the lateral ankle. Its trajectory is straight, and therefore it is called the Straight Yang vessel. [The location called] the *qiao* is the place where the *yang qiao* originates; it is the Extending Vessel (BL-62) hole."

According to Wang Bing, the Straight Yang vessel is so named because of its direct trajectory downward from the spine:

The Straight Yang vessel is a vessel of the greater yang that hugs the spine and travels downward to link with the thigh. It descends to reach the popliteal center and proceeds downward along the shins to behind the outer ankle. Its trajectory is direct. Hence, it is called the Straight Yang vessel.[23]

This describes the straight portion of the trajectory of the foot greater yang that links the thigh, the popliteal area, Support (BL-36), Bend Center (BL-40), Sinew Support (BL-56), and Mountain Support (BL-57) in a direct line. At Taking Flight (BL-58), the trajectory veers to the outer side of the lower leg. Li continues with a description of an acupuncture hole on the trajectory of the *yang qiao* that, although it is contraindicated to needling, may under certain circumstances be bled.

Above the *qiao* and below the cleft is the Supporting Sinew (BL-56), "which is located in a depression on the outer side of the center of the calf. What issues from there is the qi of the greater yang vessel. It is contraindicated to pricking with a needle. ... However, if one observes that there are engorged blood vessels in the center of both calves, then prick them to let blood out."

Because bleeding is a technique that is closely, though not exclusively, associated with the network vessels, this passage further amplifies the relationship between the *qiao* and the networks.

The next ancillary network vessel, the Abundant Yang vessel, treats symptoms closely associated with the trajectory of the *yin qiao*:

The Abundant Yang vessel causes people to experience low back pain, which radiates to the breast, along with blurred vision, and in serious [cases], arched-backed rigidity and a curled tongue with an inability to speak. Prick the inner sinew three times, [or more exactly, this hole that is located] above the medial ankle in front of the large sinew and behind the greater yin [vessel], two *cun* or so above the ankle.

Unlike the ancillary vessels mentioned thus far, the Abundant Yang vessel has no trajectory of its own, nor does it refer to a particular segment of a primary channel trajectory. The passage is best understood as a reference to an acupuncture hole that intersects the trajectory of the *qiao*. Wang Bing believes that the hole in question is the cleft hole of the *yin qiao*, Intersection Reach (KI-8).[24] According to Ma Shi and Zhang Jie-Bin, it is Return (KI-7). Ma Shi argues that this hole is chosen to treat certain symptoms because the trajectory of the *yin qiao* vessel traverses the back, penetrates the chest, emerges in front of the throat, and terminates at the inner canthus. He observes that the symptoms of low back pain that radiates to the breast with blurred vision and a curled tongue with an inability to speak are all consistent with the *yin qiao* trajectory.[25] Zhang Jie-Bin, on the other hand, attributes all of these symptoms to the foot lesser yin kidney channel and only mentions in passing that this hole is the cleft of the *yin qiao*. He observes that "The kidney vessel traverses the throat, and therefore the tongue is curled and unable to speak."[26] Zhang interprets Intersection Reach (KI-8) simply as a hole on the kidney channel that happens to intersect with the trajectory of the *yin qiao*. In the end, Li leaves it to Wang Qi-Xuan to voice his own opinion as to which hole he believes is associated with the Abundant Yang vessel:

> Wang Qi-Xuan states: "The *yin qiao* … arises from behind Burning Valley (KI-2) and ascends to above the medial ankle, proceeding along the yin aspect of the thigh to enter the yin [genitals. From here it] proceeds along the abdomen to enter the interior of the chest, moving to the Empty Basin (ST-12) and ascending to emerge in front of Man's Prognosis (ST-9). It then enters the corner of the cheekbone[27] and joins up to the inner canthus of the eye, unites with the greater yang and *yang qiao,* and goes upward. Hence, the presentation of illness is like this." "The inner sinew … is the cleft of of the *yin qiao*, the Intersection Reach (KI-8) hole."

Li follows with a series of passages, first from Ch. 63 of *Basic Questions* and then from Ch. 23 of *Divine Pivot,* detailing the use of Extending Vessel (BL-62) and Intersection Reach (KI-8) in the treatment of visual disorders, which should be pricked contralaterally.

> [Ch. 63 of] *Basic Questions*, the "Discussion of Cross Needling," states: "When pathogens visit the foot *yang qiao* vessel, this causes people to suffer from eye pain that begins from the inner canthus. Prick [the hole] one half *cun* below the lateral ankle with two punctures (at the Extending Vessel [BL-62] hole). [If the affliction is] on the left, then prick the right, and [if the affliction is] on the right, then prick the left, and it will be cured in the time it takes a person to walk ten *li*."

> [Ch. 23 of] *Divine Pivot* classic states: "When the eye is red and painful,

beginning at the inner canthus, then select the *yin qiao* (the Intersection Reach [KI-8] hole)."

Li continues his discussion with another passage from Ch. 23 of *Divine Pivot* concerning spasmodic pain that includes a hole associated with the *yin qiao* as one of its treatment points, finishing with a few comments of his own, here referring to himself as Bin-Hu ('Lakeside Master'):

> [Ch. 23 of] *Divine Pivot* also states: "For wind spasm and arched-back rigidity, first select the greater yang in the popliteal fossa at a blood network and let out blood. If the attack is due to a cold pathogen, select ... the *yin qiao* above the Three Hairs at the blood networks and let blood out there."
>
> Li Bin-Hu says that the foot greater yang is the Capital Bone (BL-64) hole. It is located on the lateral side of the foot behind the joint of the small toe, below the large bone in the depression at the border of the red and white flesh. Needle to a depth of three *fen* and moxa seven times. The popliteal fossa is the Bend Center (BL-40) hole. It is located in the horizontal crease in the crook behind the knee. Needle to a depth of three *fen*. For the *yin qiao*, select Intersection Reach (KI-8) (see above). The Three Hairs is the Large Pile (LR-1). It is located on the large toe of the foot on the lateral side of the three hairs and is the well [hole] of the liver vessel. Needle to a depth of three *fen* and moxa three times. As for the blood networks, observe the place where the blood vessels are engorged, and let out blood there.

Sleep and Sorghum

One of the defining physiological functions of the *qiao* vessels is their capacity to transmit protective qi between the interior and the exterior. Although Li's discussion of this role of the *qiao* vessels appears to be perfunctory, on close inspection it is quite nuanced. The crux of his understanding rests on a rather idiosyncratic interpretation of a passage from Ch. 80 of *Divine Pivot* as it appears in *The Systematic Classic*.

The gist of his discussion is that there are actually two pathodynamics involved in insomnia-related disorders of the *qiao* vessels. One involves an excess of the *yang qiao* vessel itself, which fails to divert yang qi to the interior at night, thus causing sleeplessness. The other involves stagnation of the networks surrounding the *yang qiao*, which fails to allow the transmission of any protective qi to it at all. In the former case, the *yang qiao* may be understood as being in a state of excess, while in the latter, it is in a state of deficiency. (A detailed discussion of this appears in Part IV, Ch. 38 below.) The sole herbal therapy indicated for either pathodynamic is Pinellia [and Sorghum] Decoction *(ban xia [shu mi] tang)*,[28] which holds the distinction of being one of the very few herbal formulas mentioned in the *Inner Classic*: "One need only drink one packet of Pinellia [and Sorghum] Decoction *(ban xia [shu mi] tang)*, and the yin and yang will communicate and the patient will immediately be able to lie down."

Regardless of how one chooses to interpret the involvement of the *qiao* vessels, it is clear that this prescription works by transforming phlegm. The patient sweats once a therapeutic dose has been reached, and this is what is referred to in the preceding paragraph as "opening the pathways." Once the phlegm has been cleared away and a healthy qi dynamic has been restored, the condition resolves quite quickly; therefore, the patient should be cured after having taken only a few doses of the remedy.

> Remove the dregs, and drink one small cup three times a day or increase slowly until the effect is apparent. If the illness is recent, the person will be able to go to bed after downing one cup, and once they sweat, [the problem] will be over. Chronic cases will be cured after having taken three doses.

In concluding his discussion of *qiao* vessel disorders, Li presents a series of passages from a variety of texts, all of which address the pathodynamics of insomnia and somnolence. His closing remarks explain why he has included them here.

> All of these many statements discuss the closure of the eyes and eyes that will not close, [and] although they make no mention of the two *qiao*, they do not diverge from the principles of yin and yang, nutritive and protective, deficiency and excess, all of which should be considered.

Li views the *qiao* vessels as the overarching regulators of yin and yang in cases of somnolence and insomnia. The viscera patterns he presents are merely specific subsets of fundamental *qiao* pathology.

> Li Bin-Hu says, [Ch. 13 of] *Divine Pivot* has a statement: "The sinew of the foot greater yang forms the upper ocular network, and the sinew of the foot yang brightness forms the lower ocular network. When cold tenses the sinews, the eye [lids] will not close. When heat loosens the sinews, the eye [lids] will not open."

The association of tension or slackness in the sinew with eyes that will not open or shut naturally suggests a disorder of the *qiao* vessels. Though not explicitly stated, these are the two key symptoms of the *qiao*. Similarly, an obstruction of protective qi resulting from an internal debilitation of qi and blood is consistent with a *yang qiao* disease.

> [Ch. 18 of *Divine Pivot*] also states: "Those who are strong are brimming with qi and blood, have supple muscle and flesh, and the nutritive and protective ... have not lost their normalcy. Hence, they are energetic by day and shut [their eyes] at night. The elderly have depleted qi and blood, the qi pathways do not flow smoothly, [and therefore] the protective qi is cut

off in the inside. Hence, their days are not energetic, and they cannot shut [their eyes] at night."

The relationship of the *qiao* vessels to the pathodyamics described in his final passages is less clear. Li appears to be making a case for the *qiao* vessels as the general rubric for understanding insomnia and somnolence regardless of the pathodynamic involved. On the other hand, the unifying factor in these final passages is that they all concern spleen deficiency. In practical terms, the scope of *qiao* vessel involvement may only extend to patterns involving the spleen and stomach. According to Li,

> [Ch. 80 of *Divine Pivot*] also states: "In those who spend their time lying down, the intestines and stomach [become] enlarged, the skin is rough, and it is not separated from the partings of the flesh. For this reason, the protective qi moves slowly."
>
> Zhang Zi-He states: "[Excessive] pensiveness will result in either insomnia or a propensity to lie down." [29]

Li then extrapolates on Chao Yuan-Fang's remarks regarding visceral pathodynamics to diseases of the *qiao* vessels: "Chao Yuan-Fang says that spleen diseases cause fatigue and a propensity to lie down, while gallbladder diseases cause frequent bouts of irritability and insomnia." [30]

Once again, the *qiao* vessels are not mentioned directly. We may assume that spleen diseases characterized by fatigue and a propensity to lie down are *yin qiao* disorders, while gallbladder diseases characterized by frequent bouts of vexation and insomnia are disorders of the *yang qiao*.

> Wang Shu-He in his *Pulse Classic* says that water flows more swiftly at night and with [a rippling] sound. This is because earth is at rest. Humans are analogous to this. [31] When humans lie down at night, their spleens do not stir and their pulse beats more rapidly [than during the day].
>
> It is also said that the spleen's indicators are the eyelids. If the eyelids are mobile, one knows that the spleen is able to perform its digestive function. If the spleen is diseased, then the eyelids do not move smoothly, and the patient has a propensity to lie down.

Conclusion

Li's discussion of *qiao* vessel pathologies covers a remarkably broad range of perspectives, and yet they are all united by two fundamental ideas. *Qiao* pathology is expressed in imbalances characterized by slackness or tension in the networks, and in disharmonies in the communication of qi between the exterior and the core of the body. Wherever these dynamics are present, they may be interpreted as *qiao* pathology.

CHAPTER 25

On the *Chong* Vessel

The *chong* is the vessel that most captures Li Shi-Zhen's interest. His chapters on this vessel are the longest in the *Exposition on the Eight Extraordinary Vessels.* They contain more on physiology and pathology, more treatment strategies, and more potential pulse presentations than any other chapter in the book. In this, Li accords the *chong* the recognition it deserves as the extraordinary vessel around which all others revolve.

The physiological functions of the extraordinary vessels are all tied, to one extent or another, to their trajectories. Nowhere is this more evident than in Li's discussion of the *chong*. His presentation of material in this chapter alternates between discussions of *chong* vessel physiology and its trajectory, weaving them tightly together.

Where the *wei* and *qiao* vessels are concerned with relatively superficial circulations of yin, yang, qi, and blood, the *chong* is the bedrock of the channel system, as evidenced by its titles as the 'sea' of the channels and vessels, and also as the 'sea' of blood. This is the starting point for Li's discussion of *chong* vessel physiology.

The Sea of the Channels and Vessels

Li opens with a reference to two different passages from the *Inner Classic.* The first is a quotation from Ch. 44 of *Basic Questions*: "The *chong* vessel is the sea of the channels and vessels."[1] To this, he adds a few words from Ch. 33 of *Divine Pivot*, which he interprets as defining the *chong* vessel as the "sea of blood."[2] This is a theme he will develop later in the chapter. Both of these functions are rooted in the gestational membranes (*bao* 胞). He then cites Ch. 65 of *Divine Pivot*, observing that "This vessel and the *ren* both arise from within the gestational membranes in the lower abdomen."[3] Yang Shang-Shan (楊上善) elaborates on this idea in his own annotations in *Yellow Emperor's Inner Classic: Grand Essentials (Huang di nei jing tai su* 黄帝内經太素*)*.

> The moving qi between the kidneys under the umbilicus is the root of human life and the 12 channels, [and] the *chong* vessel is the sea of blood [and] sea of the five viscera, six receptacles, and the 12 channels. [It] permeates [qi and blood] through all the yang [aspects of the body], irrigates [qi and blood] to all the essence [aspects of the body], [and] therefore, all the five viscera and six receptacles can receive nourishment. [This is to say that] the moving qi between the kidneys resides in the gestational membranes. [The vessel] that moves up and down is the *chong* vessel.[4]

A central tenet of Li's understanding of the *chong* is its close association with the moving qi between the kidneys, a relationship it shares with both the *ren* and the *du* vessels. All three of these vessels arise from the gestational membranes, an organ believed by some to be the locus of the moving qi.[5] The *chong* vessel is intimately linked to both the gestational membranes and to the physiological functions of the kidneys. This is a thread that runs throughout Li's discussion of the *chong* vessel.

Li follows Ch. 62 of *Divine Pivot* in describing the external trajectory of the *chong* as surfacing at Qi Thoroughfare (ST-30). Ch. 60 of *Basic Questions* describes the *chong* as traveling alongside (*bing* 并) the foot lesser yin kidney channel at this hole.[6] The 28th Difficult Issue of the *Classic of Difficulties* states that it runs alongside the foot yang brightness rather than the lesser yin.[7] Li reconciles these opposing opinions by locating the trajectory of the *chong* vessel between the two.

> Here, it travels alongside and between the two channels of the foot yang brightness and lesser yin and proceeds along the abdomen, traveling upward to the pubic bone (the foot yang brightness [channel] is located two *cun* from the midline of the abdomen; the foot lesser yin [channel] is located five *fen* from the midline of the abdomen; the trajectory of the *chong* vessel travels between these two vessels; the Pubic Bone (KI-11) is located above the genitals on the pubic bone [in a depression] like a crescent moon, one-and-a-half *cun* from the midline of the abdomen).

From the Pubic Bone (KI-11) hole onward, the *chong vessel* is superimposed on the kidney channel so that the holes of the kidney channel are effectively the holes of the *chong*. Many commentators, including Wu Qian 吳謙, compiler of the *Golden Mirror of the Medical Tradition (Yi zong jin jian* 醫宗金鑑, 1742), believe that the trajectory of the *chong* along the abdomen is a direct expression of the moving qi between the kidneys,[8] an interpretation that further links the moving qi to the pulsations of the aorta.

Li's tally of 24 holes is idiosyncratic in his inclusion of Hundred Convergences (GV-20) and Intersection Reach (KI-8) in his tally.

With its trajectory established, Li returns to the physiological mechanisms controlled by the *chong*, articulating its close relationship to the *ren* vessel. *Divine Pivot* defines the internal branch of the *chong* that ascends along the inner spine as the "sea of the channels and vessels." It is specifically this facet of the *chong*'s trajectory that communicates directly with the rest of the channel system.

> [Ch. 65 of] *Divine Pivot* classic states: "The *chong* and *ren* both arise from the gestational membranes and proceed upward along the interior of the back, constituting the sea of the channels and networks. Surfacing and externalizing, [these vessels] proceed along the right side of the abdomen in

an upward trajectory to meet the throat. They then diverge and connect to the lips and mouth."

Li makes no effort to reconcile the unilateral trajectory traced here by *Divine Pivot* with the description in his opening statement. His initial description assumes a bilateral trajectory, but it is not explicitly stated as such. The *chong* trajectory described in *Divine Pivot* does not disperse into the chest but instead continues upward in tandem with the *ren* to reach the face. This lengthier trajectory is essential to explaining a key physiological function of the *chong*.

Sea of Blood

Along with the *ren* vessel, the internal and external trajectories of the *chong* are responsible for transmitting qi and blood to the head and facilitating the growth of facial hair. Monthly menstruation creates a functional depletion of blood within the *chong* and *ren* that prohibits the growth of facial hair in women. This dynamic is also present in congenital eunuchs (*tian huan* 天宦), those born without reproductive capacity. In both cases, the problem is with the blood, not the qi.

> When only the blood is overly abundant, then it gently infiltrates the skin and produces hair. Women have a surplus of qi and an insufficiency of blood, and the repeated loss of blood during their menstrual flow impairs their *ren* and *chong* vessels. Since these vessels do not nourish the mouth and lips, neither beards nor moustaches grow [on women]. Because eunuchs have been deprived of their genitals, this damage to the *chong* and *ren* causes the blood to drain and not return, the skin clumps internally, and the lips and mouth are not nourished, and therefore they cannot grow beards or moustaches.

In the above passage, we have translated 宗筋 *(zong jin),* literally, the 'ancestral sinew' or 'gathering of sinews,' as the male genitals or penis. This is a term that can mean a number of different things in the context of *chong* vessel function and physiology. The original passage in Ch. 65 of *Divine Pivot* contains the words "remains immature" *(bu cheng* 不成) rather than "cannot become strong" *(bu qiang* 不強), though the end result remains the same: reproductive failure.[9]

The Great Thoroughfare

Li next moves on to the distal facet of the *chong* trajectory, which is closely associated with the foot lesser yin kidney channel and has its own name, the Great Thoroughfare (*tai chong* 太衝).

[Ch. 61 of] *Basic Questions,* "Discourse on Holes for Water and Heat [Diseases]," states: "The intersection of the three yin fasten [to one another] at the leg. Each [channel] travels [separately] above the ankle … . This [intersection is located] on the lower aspect of the kidney channel. It is called Great Thoroughfare."

The Great Thoroughfare defines the juncture of the kidney and *chong* vessels somewhere on the lower extremity. In the interest of clarifying his meaning, Li's version of this passage omits some relevant information. The original passage from Ch. 61 of *Basic Questions* contains the additional words "six trajectories" (*xing liu* 行六) so that the passage originally read: "As for the region above the ankle where each single trajectory has six trajectories" (踝上各一行六行者).[10] The term "six trajectories" was used to refer to six holes (*liu xue* 六穴). Wang Bing comments that these six holes consist of the "the three holes Supreme Thoroughfare (LR-3), Recover Flow (KI-7), and Yin Valley (KI-10), and the three holes on the *yin qiao* vessel, Shining Sea (KI-6), Intersection Reach (KI-8), and Guest House (KI-9)."[11] Zhang Zhi-Cong identifies the holes as Shining Sea (KI-6), Water Source (KI-5), Large Goblet (KI-4), Great Ravine (KI-3), Burning Valley (KI-2), and Gushing Spring (KI-1).[12]

This suggests that the Great Thoroughfare was not a single point, but a nexus of loci located predominantly, but perhaps not exclusively, on the kidney channel. Li's version skirts this issue and keeps our attention directed squarely on the kidney channel.

Historically, though, at least one commentator has located these six 'holes' or trajectories not on the kidney but on the spleen channel. Gao Shi-Zong identifies them as Three Yin Intersection (SP-6), Shang Hill (SP-5), Leaking Valley (SP-7), Yellow Emperor (SP-4), Supreme White (SP-3), and Great Metropolis (SP-2).[13] Similarly, the modern commentator Yasuzo Shibazaki asserts that the three foot yin channels meet at Three Yin Intersection (SP-6), and they descend to the foot along with the kidney channels.[14]

His bias toward the kidney channel notwithstanding, Li certainly acknowledged the influence of the spleen in *chong* vessel physiology. Later in the chapter, a passage from Wang Qi-Xuan expressly illustrates the relationship between the Great Thoroughfare and the spleen. There is no doubt that both channels are involved in *chong* function. What remains unclear is how precisely this nexus of qi influences the *chong* vessel, and why it has the name it does.

The first use of the term *tai chong* 太衝 originally had little to do with surging or thoroughfares; it denoted an emptiness or void, and connoted a profoundly quiet, harmonious state of mind.[15] The word first appears in *Zhuang zi*, where a Master Hu is demonstrating the "neutrality (*tai chong* 太衝) of great nonvictory."[16] (Further discussion of the role of *tai chong* in internal cultivation and the extraordinary vessels appears in Part IV, Ch. 38.)

Other translators of *Zhuang zi* have rendered *tai chong* in this passage as Absolute Emptiness,[17] Mighty Void,[18] and the Great Vastness where Nothing Wins Out,[19] all evoking images of internal and external spaciousness on a cosmic scale. The *tai chong* is the emptiness from which all things arise.

Larre and Rochat de la Vallee observe that the descending trajectory of the *chong* vessel terminates at the instep, suggesting the first hole on the kidney channel, Gushing Spring (KI-1), another name for which is 'earth thoroughfare' *(di chong* 地衝*)*. They assert: "The meaning is certainly that at this point the power of the *chong* vessel meets the power of the earth. After that there is a kind of delegation of power—the power of the *chong* vessel has joined the power of the earth, making it able to filter into the yin circulation." [20]

The notion that the descending trajectory of the *chong* vessel is the link between the internal potency of the *chong* and the power of earth fits nicely with the sense of *tai chong* as emptiness. The greater *chong* is the grounding constituent of the *chong* vessel that allows access to the void, which is attained not only by opening to heaven but through communication with earthly qi. Its association with earthly qi is also evident in its intimate relationship with the stomach channel. It is impossible to be truly open, spacious, and empty if one is not also well grounded. The *chong* vessel may be understood as the axis by which the stomach channel communicates earthly qi, and the kidney channel communicates heavenly qi, throughout the body.

The word *chong* 衝 was subsequently written as 沖 and is described in *The Elucidations of the Signs and Explications of the Graphs* (*Shuo wen jie zi* 說文解字) as an open road (*tong dao* 通道).[21] A *chong* 衝 is a wide road or a thoroughfare that facilitates the passage of heavy traffic. *Broadening of the Refined* (*Guang ya* 廣雅, 3rd century) also describes *chong* 衝 as active *(dong* 動*)* and mobile *(xing* 行*)*. The various meanings of *chong* reflect different aspects of its physiological and pathological functions.

The nominal use of the word *chong* is emblematic of the fundamental physiological function of the *chong* vessel. It is a thoroughfare, or highway, along which the primary channels pass, and it provides yet another means of organizing them. Where the *wei* and *qiao* vessels coordinate the primary channels on the exterior, the *chong* vessel provides deep structure.

Chong also denotes a vigorous rushing or colliding. There is a strong association with fluidity. To *chong* is to surge. Such violent activity is associated with the pathological manifestations of the *chong* vessel. When the *chong* vessel becomes diseased, the qi counterflows and surges upward, causing symptoms such as vomiting, asthma, and headaches. Surging is rarely healthy in the context of the *chong*.

Nevertheless, if a highway is to function properly, there must be no traffic jams. A certain amount of activity and mobility is required for the thoroughfare to remain clear, and the normal ebb and flow of qi and blood through the *chong* vessel is enough to keep it open. This is the basis for Yang Xuan-Cao's comment on the *chong* vessel in the 28th Difficult Issue of the *Classic of Difficulties*:

> *Chong* means to penetrate. It means that this vessel reaches downward to the feet and reaches upward to the head. So that when it is open, it receives

the qi and blood of the 12 channels. Therefore, it is called the Thorough-fare.[22]

Li's next passage continues this train of thought. He introduces the idea of a surging of qi that arises out of the kidneys as a localized expression of the larger concept of an extreme surge, although the word "surging" is used in the sense of simply ensuring openness and free flow within the channels. The passage again emphasizes the descending nature of the *chong* and kidney trajectories.

> Wang Qi-Xuan said: "The kidney vessel and the *chong* vessel merge and descend, proceeding to the foot where they unite and there is a great exuberance [of qi]. Hence, it is called the Great Thoroughfare. Someone else has said that the *chong* vessel arises at the Qi Thoroughfare, where it surges directly and freely; therefore, it is called the *chong* (thoroughfare) [vessel].

The first of these sentences does indeed originate with Wang Bing, although the source of the latter sentence is unknown. It may be a reference to the 28th Difficult Issue of the *Classic of Difficulties*, which states: "The *chong* vessel arises at the qi thoroughfare" (*chong mai zhe qi yu qi chong* 衝脈者起於氣衝).[23]

These statements again exemplify a fundamental aspect of *chong* vessel physiology. As the sea of the 12 channels, qi permeates the *chong*, but the qi does not travel in any particular direction. The *chong* has branches that travel in opposite directions. Yang's use of the word *tong* 通 means that the pathways of qi are open and unimpeded, although it does not imply that qi flows linearly from point A to point B. In fact, when the qi does move in one direction, this is counterflow, a benchmark of *chong* vessel pathodynamic.

Li next presents an arcane passage from Ch. 6 of *Basic Questions* that places the term Great Thoroughfare in a cosmological context:

> [Ch. 6] of *Basic Questions*, "Discourse on the Places of Unification and Separation of Yin and Yang," states: "The sage faces south and stands erect. What is before him is called Vast Illumination, and what is behind him is called the Great Thoroughfare. The place of the Great is called the lesser yin. ... The thoroughfare that is below is called the Great Thoroughfare."

Vast Illumination (*guang ming* 廣明) refers to a great exuberance of yang qi. In the natural world, the south is yang and the north is yin. On a human scale, the anterior is yang, and so it is called Vast Illumination. Also, the upper part of the body is yang, and the lower part of the body is yin, hence the name Vast Illumination.[24] The Vast Illumination of yang that resides in the upper part of the body is counterposed with the Great Thoroughfare of yin from the lower part of the body. Up to this point, Li's presentation of *chong* vessel physiology has revolved entirely around its relationship with the kidney channel.

Li next presents Wang Bing's interpretation of this passsage from Ch. 6 of *Basic Questions*.[25] It muddies the waters considerably by involving the foot greater yin spleen channel in his explanation of *chong* physiology.

> [Wang] Qi-Xuan said: "The heart viscera is located in the south, and therefore what is ahead is called Vast Illumination. The *chong* vessel is located in the north, and therefore what is behind is called the Great Thoroughfare. There is a great abundance at the confluence of the foot lesser yin kidney vessel and the *chong* vessel, and so it is called the Great Thoroughfare. The confluence of both vessels is [a confluence] of the interior with the exterior." "Because the *chong* vessel lies beneath the spleen [channel], it is said that the *chong* is located beneath," and it is called Greater Yin.

Wang prefaces his statements by recapitulating the relationship between the Great Thoroughfare and the northerly direction. The *tai* (greater) *chong* is the grounding constituent of the *chong* vessel that allows access to the void, which is attained not only by opening to heaven but through communication with earthly qi. Wang's take on the Great Thoroughfare as an intersection of kidney and *chong* vessel influences is that the *greater chong* is the uniting place of the interior and exterior. He then takes another tack entirely, explaining that the *chong* vessel is called Greater Yin by virtue of its association with the distal end of the spleen channel. This is rather incongruous given the emphasis Li has thus far placed on the relationship between the *chong* and the kidney channel. Taking this line of thought further, he cites a well-known passage from *Divine Pivot*, tying much of this material together.

> [Ch. 38 of] *Divine Pivot* classic states: "The Yellow Emperor said: Only the lesser yin vessel travels downward, why is this?"
>
> Qi Bo said: "It is not so [i.e., it is not the lesser yin that goes downward, it is the *chong*]. The *chong* vessel is the sea of the five viscera and the six receptacles. … Its upward [trajectory] emerges at the juncture of the hard and soft palates, percolating into all of the yang [channels] and irrigating the various essences. Its downward [trajectory] pours into the great network of the lesser yin, arising below the kidneys to emerge at the Qi Thoroughfare. It continues along the posterior medial aspect of the thigh and obliquely enters the popliteal fossa. It then travels concealed along the medial aspect of the tibia to adhere to the lesser yin channel. From here, it descends to penetrate behind the inner ankle and penetrate to the bottom of the foot. A diverging branch [of the network vessel] adheres to the lesser yin and percolates into the three yin; obliquely entering the ankle and traveling concealed through the instep, it continues downward along the instep to enter into the big toe. From here, it percolates into the network vessels and warms the flesh (of the leg), so therefore this vessel normally pulsates. If the diverging network is bound up, the pulsing on the dorsum

of the foot ceases. If there is no pulsing, then there is reversal, and when there is reversal, it will become cold."

Qi Bo's central point is that the *chong* vessel travels downward, and not by way of the foot lesser yin kidney channel. Yet the pertinence of this passage to Li's presentation extends beyond this. Although the descending branch of the *chong* is closely affiliated with the kidney channel, a subsidiary branch suffuses all three of the leg yin. Not only is the spleen channel involved, but so too is the liver channel. It then becomes clear how some acupuncturists might designate Yellow Emperor (SP-4) as the master hole of the *chong* vessel and why a hole on the liver channel might be called Great Thoroughfare (LR-3).

The *Chong* and Source Qi

Having established the relationship of the *chong* to the blood, the channels and vessels, and the kidney channel, Li next introduces an association between the *chong* and the triple burner. The essential function of the triple burner is the transmission of source qi. Just as the *wei* vessels are specifically associated with the nutritive and protective qi, the *chong* is inextricably linked to source/primal qi through its relationship with the triple burner.

> Wang Hai-Cang said that the hand lesser yang triple burner is one dwelling place of the ministerial fire, the right kidney life gate is the ministerial fire, and the heart envelope master is also called the ministerial fire. These vessels are all diagnosed in the same manner. The kidney is the gate of qi generation. It emerges from and governs [the area] below the umbilicus, and it is divided into three forks surging upward through the umbilicus via the Celestial Pivot (ST-25), ascending to reach the Chest Center (CV-17) beside both breasts. This is where the primal qi is tied in.

Neither this nor any of the passages that follow reference the *chong* vessel by name. The basis for Li's inclusion of these passages in this chapter is that both the *chong* and the triple burner are closely tied to kidney qi.

Adopting the same format that he uses for the extraordinary vessels, Li first outlines the anatomical boundaries of the triple burner and links these to its physiological role in disseminating the moving qi between the kidneys.

> There are also diverging branches of the foot triple burner and greater yang that adhere to the main pathway of the foot greater yang to enter and network with the bladder in the lower burner.

Li then goes on to articulate the anatomical location of the triple burner at some length.

The triple burner extends from the head to reach the heart, from the heart to reach the umbilicus, and from the umbilicus to reach the foot, constituting the three upper, middle, and lower burners that are actually the true primal unitary qi. Hence, it is said that it stores but has no dwelling place.

Pulse Rhymes states: "The triple burner lacks form; it is empty but has a name. It takes shelter in the chest, and the diaphragm stands in relation to it."

A very influential book during its time, *Pulse Rhymes* (*Mai jue* 脈訣) was composed during the Five Dynasties period (907—960) by Gao Yang-Sheng (高陽生), although it was attributed to Wang Shu-He. The book itself survives only in the wealth of publications devoted to correcting its many errors, including one by Li's father.

Others say that it stores and accumulates [its qi] within the Qi Thoroughfare. The upper burner is located above the upper opening of the stomach, [and disorders of this burner] are treated at Chest Center. The middle burner is located in the passageways of the stomach, [and disorders of this burner] are treated beside the umbilicus. The lower burner is located below the umbilicus and at the upper opening of the urinary bladder, and [disorders of this burner are treated] at the umbilicus.

This passage is a synopsis of the 31st Difficult Issue of the *Classic of Difficulties*. Li continues his presentation by again emphasizing that the moving qi between the kidneys provides a crucial link between the triple burner and the *chong*.

The source qi is the triple burner's director of separation. The moving qi between the kidneys is the true primal unitary qi that divides into three routes. It is the life force of a person, and the root of the 12 channels.

Traveling along the inside of the spine, the internal branch of the *chong* transects the anatomical location of the moving qi, thereby establishing a direct line of communication between the *chong*, the triple burner, and the moving qi. It is also this branch of the *chong* that is specifically designated as the sea of the channels and vessels. Li is simply continuing to point out relationships that are implicit, though often not explicit, in the source literature.

In his closing comment, Li extends the direct influence of the triple burner beyond the *chong* to the *du* and *ren* vessels. All three vessels may be understood as extensions of the triple burner's function of facilitating the dissemination of source/primal qi. "Li Bin-Hu says that the triple burner performs life gate's function of communicating with the *chong, ren,* and *du*, and therefore [a discussion of it] is appended here."

From Li's perspective, the triple burner's function of disseminating source qi is limited to the *chong, ren,* and *du*. Here he conspicuously fails to mention the other five extraordinary vessels as regulators of source qi. Li Shi-Zhen's understanding explicitly links the *wei* vessels with the nutritive and protective qi, and the *qiao* vessels are also concerned with this level of qi in their nocturnal and diurnal shunting of qi from the interior to the exterior. Source qi is the domain of the deeper vessels that form the core of the extraordinary vessel system. Li focuses here primarily on source (*yuan* 原) qi, the totality of all the qi in the body, including the prenatal influences we were born with. In his chapters on the *yin qiao* and *du* vessels, which are concerned more directly with internal cultivation, Li tends to use the term primal (yuan 元) qi to denote the primordial qi of the cosmos that may be engaged through the extraordinary vessels.

CHAPTER 26

On Diseases of the *Chong* Vessel

The essential physiological functions of the *chong* are the storage and dissemination of blood and source qi, yet Li Shi-Zhen's discussion of *chong* pathology only addresses these functions indirectly. It is remarkable that although Li acknowledges the intimate physiological relationship of the *chong* to maturation, reproduction, and overall gynecological function, his discussion of *chong* diseases makes no specific mention of gynecological disorders. Although many of the passages included in this chapter describe pathologies that are potentially germane to gynecological problems, they are by no means uniquely gynecological presentations.

In the previous chapter, Li described the physiological functions of the *chong* as the preeminent regulator of the channels and vessels, and in terms of its storage of blood and source qi. In this chapter, we are informed that the fundamental pathological mechanisms at work in the *chong* vessel are counterflow and abdominal urgency. Li begins with the 29th Difficult Issue:

> Yue-Ren, in his *Classic of Difficulties* states: "When the *chong* vessel is diseased there is a counterflow of qi and abdominal urgency."

Abdominal urgency *(li ji* 裏急*)*, literally, internal urgency, is part of a phrase 'abdominal urgency and rectal heaviness' *(li ji hou zhong* 裏急後重*)* that first appears in the 15th Difficult Issue of the *Classic of Difficulties*.[1] Wiseman and Feng define abdominal urgency and rectal heaviness as the urgent desire to defecate with difficulty in defecation characterized by heaviness or pressure in the rectum.[2]

Li continues with a passage from Chapter 26 of *Divine Pivot* that both illustrates this pathodynamic and also suggests a treatment. These two lines extrapolate on the basic principles presented in the 29th Difficult Issue.

> When there is a counterflow ascent of qi, prick the depression below the breast and at the pulsing vessel below the chest. If there is abdominal pain, prick the pulsing vessels to the left or right of the umbilicus ... [After needling, one should] massage [this area, and the pain] should stop. If [the pain] does not stop, then prick the Qi Thoroughfare (ST-30). ... [After removing the needle,] massaging [this area] should stop [the pain].

Chapter 26 of *Divine Pivot* is concerned with a miscellany of diseases including heart pain, throat obstruction, malaria-like diseases *(nüe* 瘧*)*, toothache, deafness, nosebleeds, pain in various locations, abdominal distention, and problems of elimination. There is no evidence that the authors of *Divine Pivot* had the *chong* vessel in mind in their above-mentioned discussion of counterflow qi ascent. Li has presumably identified these symptoms as *chong* pathologies based on the presence of a generalized qi counterflow and the use of the acupuncture hole Qi Thoroughfare (ST-30). His use of this passage subtly but significantly expands the scope of *chong* pathology. The *Classic of Difficulties* limits the range of *chong*-related symptoms to a very specific species of abdominal discomfort known as 'abdominal urgency.' With its use of the generalized term 'abdominal pain' *(fu tong* 腹痛*)*, the *Divine Pivot's* presentation of counterflow conditions allows for a much broader set of potential presentations. Zhang Zhi-Cong explains the first sentence as follows:

> When there is a counterflow ascent of qi, the qi counterflows upward and does not circulate. The vessel of the foot yang brightness channel travels between the chest and the breast, and pricking it causes the upwardly counterflowing qi to open downwardly in the channel. The [proper trajectory] of the yang brightness qi is said to be from Man's Prognosis (ST-9) traveling downward to the breast. From the breast, it moves downward to the chest, and from the chest, it moves downward to the umbilicus.

Zhang's interpretation identifies the foot yang brightness as the primary channel involved in this pathology. Given the intimate association between the *chong* and the foot yang brightness, this explanation sheds some light on why Li may have linked this passage to the *chong*. Nevertheless, one is left to wonder why Li chose the particular passage he did from Chapter 26 of *Divine Pivot*, which contains many other references to qi reversal *(jue* 厥*)* and counterflow, one of which involves the foot yang brightness channel and another the foot lesser yin. One explanation may be that the treatments described in these other passages are much less specific. We are simply told to "select the foot yang brightness" or "select the foot lesser yin." The passages from Chapter 26 cited by Li are remarkable in that they contain instructions about where to treat, though the choice of specific acupuncture holes is still open to some interpretation. Ma Shi identifies the depression below the breast as Breast Window (ST-16), but Zhang Jing-Yue (張景岳) believes it is Roof (ST-15). There are also various opinions regarding the location of this pulsing vessel below the chest. Yang Shang-Shan and Zhang Jing-Yue both agree "the pulsing vessel below the chest is Central Treasury (LU-1)," however, Ma Shi identifies it as Chest Center (CV-17). According to some commentators, the movement of qi between the chest and the umbilicus suggests the trajectory of the *ren* vessel, making this a pathology of the *ren* and not the *chong* at all. Such an interpretation is in accord with Ma Shi's idea that the hole in question is Chest Center (CV-17),[3] yet this passage is one of the bulwarks of Li's perspective on *chong* pathology. As we will see, Chest Center will appear again in this chapter in contexts that strongly suggest Li associated it with the *chong*.

Where *Classic of Difficulties* unambiguously links qi counterflow and abdominal urgency, the *Divine Pivot's* discussions of qi counterflow and abdominal distention are clearly derived from two separate, albeit sequential passages. Nevertheless, Li has linked them in such a way as to suggest that the two symptoms may occur together.

Li Shi-Zhen has complicated considerably the meaning of the second line from Chapter 26 of *Divine Pivot*. In the original text, both instances of the words "massaging it" *(an zhi 按之)* were originally "once pricked" *(yi ci 已刺)*. Hence, the original sentence reads, "Once this area is pricked, [the pain] should stop." No mention of palpation or massage is made there. According to Katsuda Masayasu, if the qi counterflows upward, then the pulsing at Breast Window (ST-16) should be needled for chest pain and muscle spasm. In the case of abdominal pain, Celestial Pivot (ST-25) next to the umbilicus should be needled. One should massage the point after removing the needle, and the pain should stop. If the pain persists, then one must needle Qi Thoroughfare (ST-30) and massage the hole immediately, and the pain will improve.[4]

With these few lines from the 29th Difficulty and Chapter 26 of *Divine Pivot*, Li establishes that counterflow is the fundamental pathodynamic of the *chong* vessel. He then expands on these principles, beginning with a passage from Li Dong-Yuan's *On the Spleen and Stomach*.

> Li Dong-Yuan says that if during the autumn and winter months the four pathways of the stomach vessel are made to counterflow by the *chong* vessel and the two pathways of the lesser yang vessel below the rib-sides reverse and move upward, this is called reversal counterflow.

Li's discussion illustrates the reciprocal relationship between the *chong* and the primary channels. Here the *chong* vessel initiates counterflow in a number of channels, including the stomach and gallbladder. The implication is that although the root of the problem may reside within the *chong* vessel, it may express itself in a myriad of ways. In subsequent passages, we will see that the *chong* may itself become disordered as a consequence of some other, more fundamental, pathology. Once the extraordinary vessels become involved, however, the pathodynamic becomes much more pervasive throughout the body and more complex. Li's mention of four pathways is a reference to the nexus of the stomach and *chong* channels at Qi Thoroughfare (ST-30). Because a thoroughfare *(chong 衝)* is traditionally understood to mean a roadway leading in four directions, the entire channel is spoken of as having four pathways. Similarly, because the gallbladder channel traverses bilaterally across the flanks, it is said to have two channels.[5] According to Li, "This pattern [is characterized by symptoms of] qi surging into the throat such that one cannot catch one's breath and sounds of wheezy respiration such that one cannot lie down."

Here Li Shi-Zhen uses a passage by Li Dong-Yuan, who in turn makes an oblique reference to a discussion of counterflow from Chapter 5 of *Basic Questions*. The original passage makes no mention of the *chong* vessel.[6] In this instance, Li is the innovator who links the *chong* to this species of counterflow. Li Shi-Zhen merely gives the passage context and develops the concept further.

Also worth noting is the seasonal nature of this disorder. It is the first mention of an association between the extraordinary vessels and seasonal influences in *Exposition on the Eight Extraordinary Vessels*. The nutritive and protective disharmonies characteristic of *yang wei* pathologies may be externally contracted, but it does not specifically mention a seasonal involvement. Cold damage and wind attack may occur in any season. Li's understanding of external pathogens was firmly grounded in the framework of *On Cold Damage*, but the pattern referred to here is not cold damage per se. The thermal nature of the pathogen here is of little interest to either Zhang Zhong-Jing or Li Shi-Zhen.

Li is primarily concerned with seasonal influences on the *chong* vessel. Yet although these pathologies manifest seasonally, they are not necessarily externally contracted. For instance, Regulate the Middle to Augment the Qi Decoction *(tiao zhong yi qi tang)*, the formula recommended for this condition, is not typically associated with acute, externally-contracted diseases.

Certainly, the *Cold Damage* model posits that unresolved contractions of external cold tend to work their way inward to lodge in the interior. But for Li, the thermal quality of the pathogen is almost irrelevant. The season determines the presentation. When counterflow qi occurs in the winter, it tends to present as a cold condition that requires warming methods, whereas in the summer, it presents as heat, requiring cooling and draining medicinals. Whatever the season, the presence of counterflow confirms that the pathogen is fundamentally lodged in the *chong*.

> [In this case,] one should add five *fen* of Evodia Fructus *(wu zh yu)* to Regulate the Middle to Augment the Qi Decoction *(tiao zhong yi qi tang)*, but the dose of this medicinal is dependent on the seasonal qi *(On the Spleen and Stomach)*. When this condition occurs during the summer months, it is then a pattern of great heat; use equal amounts of Coptidis Rhizoma *(huang lian)*, Phellodendron Cortex, *(huang bai)*, and Anemarrhena Rhizoma *(zhi mu)*, which are soaked in wine, fried, powdered, and mixed with boiled hot water into pills. Each day, take one- or two-hundred pills. This preparation is administered on an empty stomach with hot boiled water and followed by a good meal to press it [into the lower burner]. [Hence, the medication] will not become lodged in the stomach but will pass directly to the lower base to drain the pathogen from the *chong* vessel. In treating diseases of this kind, [physicians] must account for the influence of the four seasons, [treating accordingly with] cold, hot, warm, or cool [medicinals].

This passage describes a seasonal qi activating a pathogenic factor that lies dormant, lurking within the *chong*. The pathogen then expresses itself through the stomach and gallbladder channels. Although Li Shi-Zhen's language leaves open the possibility that patterns of *chong* counterflow may be due to either external or internal causes, his interest remains on more internal etiologies. He discusses these in some detail.

> [Li Dong-Yuan] also says that whenever there is qi counterflow and a surging ascension [of qi] that may be accompanied by abdominal urgency or agitation and heat, this is invariably due to a counterflow of the *chong* vessel. If such diseases are due to internal damage, then Tonify the Middle to Augment the Qi Decoction *(bu zhong yi qi tang)* with the additions of dry-fried Phellodendron Cortex *(chao huang bai)*, dry-fried Coptidis Rhizoma *(chao huang lian)*, and Anemarrhena Rhizoma *(zhi mu)* is indicated to drain the *chong* vessel. Whenever there is an exuberance of kidney fire leading to an overabundance of the three vessels of the *ren, du,* and *chong,* then it is appropriate to use wine-fried Phellodendron Cortex *(chao huang bai)* and Anemarrhena Rhizoma *(zhi mu),* but one may not administer these long-term for fear that they may harm the stomach. If there is a stabbing pain in the stomach or abdominal urgency, it is appropriate to use more Glycyrrhizae Radix *(gan cao)*. When one sits in vain and the stool will not come, this indicates blood deficiency, and blood deficiency causes abdominal urgency, so it is appropriate to use Angelica Sinensis Radix *(dang gui)*. For counterflow of qi and abdominal urgency such that there is obstruction in the diaphragm and throat, and inability to move one's bowels, then it is appropriate to use Raise the Yang and Drain Heat Decoction *(sheng yang xie re tang)* to master [the condition] (this formula appears in the *Secrets from the Orchid Pavillion)*. For numbness, qi inversion, and a surging ascension of qi, this upward movement of counterflow qi causes loss of hearing and loss of sight, so it is appropriate to administer Miraculous Feat Pill *(shen gong wan)* to master [the condition] (this formula appears in the *Secrets from the Orchid Pavillion)*.

In the passage above, Li Dong-Yuan attributes a variety of pathological presentations to the *chong* vessel. Although he acknowledges the primacy of counterflow in *chong* pathodynamics, his perspective is characterized by a strong emphasis on abdominal urgency or at least some degree of abdominal discomfort. Li Shi-Zhen takes a broader view, focusing his emphasis on the counterflow side of the equation. The *Exposition* attributes more herbal prescriptions to the *chong* vessel than any of the other extraordinary vessels, and these provide a concrete basis for understanding Li Shi-Zhen's approach to *chong* pathology. If we use the traditional indications for these formulas as our criteria, we must conclude that as far as Li Shi-Zhen is concerned, there may or may not be a subjective experience of abdominal discomfort. For instance, abdominal discomfort is clearly a component of the Poria and Schisandra Decoction *(ling wu wei zi tang)* and Minor Construct the Middle Decoction *(xiao jian zhong tang)* presentations, but not necessarily Tonify the Middle to Augment the Qi Decoction *(bu zhong yi qi tang)* or Generate the Pulse Powder *(sheng mai san)* combined with Four-Ingredient Powder with Poria *(si ling san)* with the addition of wine-soaked of Phellodendron Cortex *(huang bai)* and Anemarrhena Rhizoma *(zhi mu)*.

Li Dong-Yuan also discusses Tonify the Middle to Augment the Qi Decoction *(bu zhong yi qi tang)* in the context of *du* vessel disorders. "As for the early stages of internal heat, the fire of the *chong* vessel sticks to the interior of the two yin channels and transmits this heat to the *du* vessel. The *du* vessel originates from the twenty-first vertebrae of the spine below the Long Strong (GV-1) hole."[7]

Li Shi-Zhen apparently finds this unworthy of mention. He has already made his point. Much like the stomach and gallbladder channels mentioned above, the *du* vessel is merely the recipient of a pathogen that is fundamentally grounded in an imbalance in the *chong* vessel.

Li Shi-Zhen has thus far relied on the venerable Zhang Zhong-Jing to substantiate the principle that all counterflow patterns may be understood and treated as *chong* vessel pathologies. From this firm footing, Li Shi-Zhen now moves his presentation onto less solid ground. He next quotes a passage from Sun Si-Miao's *Important Formulas Worth a Thousand Gold Pieces [for any Emergency]* that fits Li's criteria for a *chong* vessel disorder, although, once again, it does not mention the *chong* by name.

> In his *[Important] Formulas Worth a Thousand Gold Pieces,* the True Man Sun [Si-Miao] says that when there is a cough that causes one to spit up saliva accompanied by frigidly cold extremities, qi from the lower abdomen surges upward into the chest, mouth, and throat, [and] the face will be flushed and boiling hot as if one were intoxicated. [The patient feels] as if she will experience either urinary or fecal incontinence that will flow down the inner thigh, [and] there will be difficult urination [although the patient] remains anxious about the possible return of these symptoms. The distal pulse will be deep, and the proximal pulse will be faint. It is appropriate to use Poria and Schisandra Decoction *(ling wu wei zi tang)* to treat this surging of qi. The formula contains Poria *(fu ling)*, Schizandrae Fructus *(wu wei zi)*, 2 *qian* [each], Cinnamon Cortex *(rou gui)*, and Glycyrrhizae Radix *(gan cao)*, 1 *qian* [each]. This is decocted in water and administered. If there is chest fullness, omit the Cinnamon Cortex *(rou gui)*.

Poria and Schisandra Decoction *(ling wu wei zi tang)* elegantly illustrates how the careful combination of just a few medicinals can treat a complex pattern. In addition to its well-known functions of promoting urination in the treatment of urinary difficulty or diarrhea due to the stagnation of fluids, strengthening the spleen and calming the spirit, the sovereign ingredient Poria *(fu ling)* also treats qi counterflow. This function was recognized as early as *Divine Husbandman's Classic of Materia Medica* where it is claimed to treat "rebellious qi in the chest and hypochondria."[8] This single medicinal treats the essential symptoms defining the pattern.

Schizandrae Fructus *(wu wei zi)*, the other primary ingredient in this formula, is often combined with drying or draining medicinals to treat cough and wheezing due to cold, thin phlegm. It also supplements the kidneys, binds the essence, and stops diarrhea to treat the root of the problem in the lower burner. Together, they strengthen the spleen and kidneys, regulate the fluids in both the upper and lower burners, and redirect counterflow downward.

Although Sun describes the face as flushed and hot, this is the result of an upflushing of yang qi, not pathological heat per se. The pattern is fundamentally cold. Cinnamon Cortex *(rou gui)* strengthens and warms the spleen and kidney yang, opens the blood vessels, and roots the yang back in its source in the lower burner.

Li Shi-Zhen next submits a case record that illustrates the principle he has just presented. It is one of only two case records that appear in Li's *Exposition*; the other appears in his discussion of *dai* vessel pathology. Here, Li includes both the case by Cheng Huang-Dun[9] and a commentary by Zhu Ju-Quan.[10]

> Cheng Huang-Dun reports that Lord Tai Ping suffered from pain in the area of Chest Center (CV-17), asthmatic breathing with vomiting, and acid regurgitation. From a single point above the umbilicus, qi would ascend to reach the throat with an icy sensation. Episodes of this kind would recur nightly between 11 P.M. and 1 A.M., and [between] 3 P.M. and 5 P.M. The physicians took this to be intense cold, and therefore the [therapy was] ineffective.
>
> [Commenting on this case], Zhu Ju-Quan says that [because the patient] drank too much and ate too much rich food, then between 11 P.M. and 1 A.M. and between 3 P.M. and 5 P.M. the ministerial fire that naturally descends galloped upward, resulting in pain. He was then given many draughts of Two-Aged [Herb] Decoction *(er chen tang)* with the addition of Scutellaria Radix *(huang qin)*, Coptidis Rhizoma *(huang lian)*, Gardenia Fructus *(zhi zi)*, and Atractylodes Rhizoma *(cang zhu)*, and the condition was cured after drinking [the decoction] numerous times.

Previous physicians had interpreted this condition as a species of running piglet disease *(ben tun 奔豚)* due to cold when in reality it was due to a more generalized counterflow of qi due to phlegm and heat. Li Shi-Zhen includes this case in his discussion here because it illustrates the core symptoms and pathodynamics he has so carefully laid out in this chapter. Here we see counterflow qi causing symptoms in the chest, specifically the chest center. This case also exemplifies the symptom complex described by as "qi surging into the throat such that one cannot catch one's breath and sounds of wheezy respiration such that one cannot lie down." Such a presentation fits neatly into Li's model of *chong* pathology, although neither Cheng Huang-Dun nor Zhu Ju-Quan identify it as such. It also establishes another crucial link between acupuncture theory and herbal application.

As we have seen, Li attributes these symptoms indirectly to the stomach and gallbladder channels, and the medicinals used to treat them are consistent with this interpretation. Zhu Ju-Quan describes the pathodynamic in terms of ministerial fire that is running amok, a species of qi that the previous chapter has linked closely to the *chong* via the moving qi between the kidneys.

Although the pathology described in this case is not tied to any of the seasonal influences stipulated by Li, there is nevertheless a temporal component. The problems occur between 11 P.M. and 1 A.M. and between 3 A.M. and 5 A.M. During these times, the qi in the gallbladder and lung channels is peaking. This is quite similar to the pathodynamic discussed in the preceding passages. The *chong* vessel counterflows along these channels, producing symptoms only at the time when they are at their zenith.

Ch. 44 of *Basic Questions* contains a discussion of atrophy *(wei* 痿*)* that involves the *chong* vessel, yang brightness channels, and the qi throroughfares in its pathodynamic. Li presents an abbreviated form of this passage as a means of laying the groundwork for additional material from *On the Spleen and Stomach* that involve other types of counterflow.

> [Ch. 44 of] *Basic Questions'* "Treatise on Atrophy" states: "Why is it that in treating atrophy one need only select the yang brightness channels?" It says: "The yang brightness is the sea of the five viscera and the six receptacles. It governs the moistening of the gathering of sinews,[11] and the gathering sinews bind the bones and provide mobility for the joints. The *chong* vessel is the sea of the channels and vessels, governing the permeation and irrigation of the valleys and streams. It unites with the yang brightness at the gathering of sinews. ... It meets at the qi thoroughfare, and the yang brightness is the leader [of them all]. They are all attributed to the *dai* vessel and linked to the *du* vessel."

The passages from *On the Spleen and Stomach* earlier in this chapter stressed the primacy of the *chong* over the channels in which its symptoms are expressed. Here the opposite is true. Although the *chong* plays an important role, the yang brightness is the central player. An insufficiency in the yang brightness channels will compromise the *chong, dai,* and *du* vessels, which in turn damage the gathering of sinews *(zong jin* 宗筋*)*.

The "gathering of sinews" has multiple meanings. As we have already seen, it may refer to the genitals. As Zhang Jing-Yue explains:

> The gathering of sinews accumulates at the genitals. The genitals are the place where the nine vessels of the foot three yin, yang brightness, lesser yang, and *chong, ren, du,* and *qiao* meet. Of these nine, the yang brightness is the sea of the five viscera and six receptacles, while the *chong* is the sea of the channels and vessels. Of these, one is yin and one is yang, but be-

tween them, they constitute the totality [of all the channels]. Hence, we say that the sum of yin and yang meets at the gathering of sinews. As for the meeting at the qi thoroughfare, the qi thoroughfare is the primary vessel of the yang brightness. Hence, the yang brightness alone is the chief. The *dai* vessel originates in the rib sides and encircles the entire body. The *du* vessel originates at the meeting of the yin. It branches into three, making the *ren* and *chong*, [all of which] travel up the abdomen and spine. Hence, all of the channels invariably link and home to the *dai* vessel and have branch networks with the *du* vessel.[12]

Another interpretation is that the gathering of sinews mentioned in Ch. 44 of *Basic Questions* simply refers to the sinews surrounding the lumbar spine, and that is how they influence the extremities to "bind the bones and provide mobility for the joints."[13] Wiseman and Feng describe the gathering of sinews as a bundling of muscles at the pubic bone.[14] Katsuda Masayasu has a more generalized interpretation, viewing this gathering as the plexus of deep pelvic and perineal musculature.[15] When this system becomes compromised, the entire body loses an essential component of its structural support, causing reverberations throughout the system. Still, the two meanings are somewhat related. When the structural integrity of the pelvic floor becomes impaired, this predisposes one to sexual and reproductive dysfunction. This is the context in which the present passages refer to the gathering of sinews.

Li Shi-Zhen continues his discussion about Ch. 44 of *Basic Questions*:

> "Hence, when the yang brightness is deficient, the gathering sinew becomes slack and the *dai* vessel is no longer able to lead it. This results in atrophy and loss of use of the feet." To treat this, "one should supplement at the spring holes and promote flow at the transport holes [of the yang brightness channels] to regulate deficiency and excess, harmonize abnormal and normal [flow of qi] so that the sinews, vessels, bones, and flesh will each recover from disease in their prevailing months (it is said that the prevailing months that govern the qi are liver *jia yi*, heart *bing ding*, and spleen *wu qi*)."

The acupuncture method recommended by the authors of this chapter of *Basic Questions* may well have been of only passing interest to Li Shi-Zhen, whose primary focus was on the pathodynamics of atrophy and its seasonal influences. Nevertheless, this sophisticated needling strategy is a direct response to the mechanism of disease described in Ch. 44.

The yang brightness is deficient to be sure, but this deficiency has also allowed the qi to stagnate. We are first instructed to supplement the spring *(ying* 營*)* holes. Because channel qi pools *(liu* 留*)* at the spring holes, administering a tonifying technique here marshals the qi. The qi then pours *(zhu* 注*)* through the transport *(shu* 俞*)* holes using an opening *(tong* 通*)* technique. This opening is not a draining technique, nor is it an even method. Zhang Jing-Yue explains opening simply as "the means by which one promotes movement of the qi *(suo yi xing qi 所以行氣)*."[16]

Zhang Jing-Yue believes that this passage implies that regulating the yang brightness channels is only the first step in the therapeutic process. One must examine the patient carefully to determine which other channels are affected. In his view, this is what the authors of *Basic Questions* meant by "regulating deficiency and excess, and harmonizing the abnormal and normal [flow of qi]." Therefore, if there is atrophy of the sinews, we must also select the spring and transport holes of the reversing yin channels. If there is vascular atrophy, we must also select spring and transport holes of the lesser yin, and so on, selecting the yin channels that correspond to the affected tissue.

Once the yang brightness channels are treated and the channels associated with affected tissues are regulated and harmonized, then the disease will be cured in the appropriate season. Ma Shi explains that since the liver tends to become diseased in the spring, sinew atrophy also tends to occur during this time. Similarly, vascular atrophy pertains to the heart, and so tends to occur in the summer. Atrophy of the flesh pertains to the spleen, and so tends to occur during the period known as extreme yin *(zhi yin 至陰)*, which is in the eighth month of the agricultural calendar, usually during the end of August. Dermal atrophy pertains to the lungs, so it tends to occur in the autumn, and bone atrophy pertains to the kidneys, so it tends to occur in the winter.[17] Li Shi-Zhen apparently believes that because the atrophy described in Ch. 44 of *Basic Questions* is mediated through the liver, heart, and spleen, it will be cured during the spring and summer months.

One of the reasons that we first activate the yang brightness channels is because they contain the most qi and blood and are therefore most amenable to mobilization. Having done this, we must still marshal the qi of the yin channels according to the location of the disease and season in which it appears. This strategy is consistent with Ch. 6 of *Divine Pivot*, which also mentions needling the spring and transport holes together: "When there is a disease residing within the yin of the yin, then prick the spring and transport [holes]."[18] A disease in the yin of the yin is a disease of the viscera. Atrophy is expressed on the level of the channels and bodily structure, but it is rooted in a visceral imbalance, hence the necessity for treating it on the level of the affected viscera and the yang brightness channels.

The pathodynamic of atrophy as it has been described thus far does not actually involve counterflow. Li Shi-Zhen uses this passage to illustrate the principle that the extraordinary vessels may become depleted if the primary channels do not adequately supply them, but this is merely the groundwork for his subsequent discussion. Citing Li Dong-Yuan, Li Shi-Zhen will build on this in the passages that follow, adding both a seasonal component and counterflow into the mix.

Li Shi-Zhen's inclusion of the treatment for atrophy in *Basic Questions* may have been motivated primarily by his interest in its seasonal considerations, but the needling strategy contained in this passage is also germane to his ongoing discussion of counterflow pathodynamics. In addition to being the treatment of choice for the deficiency atrophy described above, the spring transport hole combination is a hallmark of the needling strategy for treating chaotic qi *(luan qi 亂氣)*. This needling method is described in detail in Ch. 34 of *Divine Pivot.* Chaotic qi, as it is used in this context, may be understood as counterflow in multiple directions, and it is in many ways the quintessential expression of a systemic counterflow within the body.

Given the prominence of Li Dong-Yuan's thought throughout this discussion of *chong* pathology, it is worth noting that he was also responsible for articulating an acupuncture strategy specifically for treating counterflow conditions. It is a methodology that relies heavily on spring and transport hole combinations. Gao Wu, in *A Gathering of the Blossoms of Acupuncture* (1529), was the first to acknowledge the value of the acupuncture material quietly embedded in Li Dong-Yuan's *On the Spleen and Stomach,* lauding his insight and coining the term 'Dong-Yuan's acupuncture method' *(Dong-Yuan zhen fa 東垣針法)*. Much of Li Dong-Yuan's approach to herbal prescribing is an expression of his effort to emulate the principles inherent in this needling methodology.

Into these few terse lines from *Basic Questions* are packed a wealth of information that bears directly on the material that follows. This passage touches upon the essential deficiency that lies at the root of atrophy, its potential expression in the flesh, sinew, vessel, or bone, and its seasonal influences. Li Shi-Zhen employs this passage as a skillful segue into more material by Li Dong-Yuan, who next points out that atrophy may be compounded by inversion *(jue 厥)* and counterflow *(ni 逆)*.

> Li Dong-Yuan stated that when this disease worsens during the months of summerheat, it will be transmitted to the kidney and liver, producing atrophy and reversal. The atrophy causes the four extremities to become atrophied and soft while the reversal causes the four extremities to be either [hot] as if on fire or [cold] as if frozen. There will be irritability of the heart, and the qi of the *chong* vessel counterflows upward, which in extreme cases will result in counterflow of fire. This is called reversal counterflow. Hence, the two diseases of wilting and reversal are complex and interrelated.

This passage is substantially a paraphrase of the passage that appears in volume 2 of *On the Spleen and Stomach.* The original makes no mention of *chong* involvement. Li Shi-Zhen has adapted Li Dong-Yuan's remarks in a manner that expands the symptomology of the *chong* to include weakness of the extremities and either chilled or burning extremities.

Quoting Ch. 28 of *Divine Pivot,* Li continues to present the concept that an insufficiency of qi in the lower part of the body may cause a variety of symptoms, including atrophy and reversal: "[On the Spleen and Stomach] classic states: When the lower [burner] qi is insufficient, this results in atrophy, reversal, and flusteredness." Li Dong-Yuan's discussion contains no recommendations for herbal therapy so Li Shi-Zhen proposes his own treatment, reflecting an amalgam of strategies by Li Dong-Yuan and

Zhu Dan-Xi (朱丹溪): "[In such instances,] it is appropriate to use clearing and drying medicinals that get rid of dampness and heat or Generate the Pulse Powder *(sheng mai san)* combined with Four-Ingredient Powder with Poria *(si ling san)* with the addition of wine-soaked Phellodendron Cortex *(huang bai)* and Anemarrhena Rhizoma *(zhi mu)* to drain the damp-heat."

This mix of formulas suggests a relatively complex pathodynamic. Generate the Pulse Powder *(sheng mai san)* appears in another chapter of the middle volume of *On the Spleen and Stomach* titled "Concerning Diseases Occurring in Different Seasons Due to Spleen and Stomach Deficiency and Formula Composition According to Different Diseases," where it also addresses atrophy and reversal. Here, Li Dong-Yuan recommends Generate the Pulse Powder *(sheng mai san)* for "heat damaging the original qi," particularly when summerheat is involved. He remarks that "the vessels [mentioned in the title of the prescription] are the original qi" *(mai zhe yuan qi ye 脈 者,元氣也)*. According to Li Dong-Yuan, the sweetness of Ginseng *Radix (ren shen)* tonifies the primal qi, which here is synonymous with original qi, and drains heat and fire. The bitter cold of Ophiopogonis Radix *(mai men dong)* tonifies the source of water and also clears and circulates dry metal. The sourness of Schisandrae Fructus *(wu wei zi)* drains fire and supplements the large intestine and lung metal.[19]

Generate the Pulse Powder *(sheng mai san)* addresses the fundamental debility of original qi that lies at the root of *chong* vessel disorders characterized by counterflow and atrophy, but this is only half of the problem. Not only is there a deficiency in the lower burner impairing the flow of qi into the legs, there is also a concurrent accumulation of dampness and heat, further obstructing the transmission of qi into the lower extremities. The combined insufficiency of original qi and damp-heat obstruction in the lower burner results in a counterflow condition that also produces the middle and upper burner symptoms already discussed.

Li Shi-Zhen eschews the many formulas developed for treating precisely this complex in favor of a therapeutic strategy of his own. He combines Generate the Pulse Powder *(sheng mai san)* with Zhu Dan-Xi's Four-Ingredient Powder with Poria *(si ling san)*, which emphasizes the use of draining and percolating medicinals.

Four-Ingredient Powder with Poria *(si ling san)* appears in *Essential Teachings of [Zhu] Dan-Xi (Dan-Xi xin fa 丹溪心法)* as a treatment for diarrhea due to dampness. The formula contains Poria *(fu ling)*, Polyporus *(zhu ling)*, Alismatis Rhizoma *(ze xie)*, and Atractylodis macrocephalae Rhizoma *(bai zhu)*. Elsewhere in this book, Zhu Dan-Xi cites a case of a person suffering from exhuastion *(lao 勞)* complicated by summerheat in which Ginseng Radix *(ren shen)* is added to the base formula. This is probably the usage that Li Shi-Zhen had in mind, although neither atrophy nor reversal are involved.[20]

Li Shi-Zhen concisely summarizes the main points he wishes to make in his presentation of this material. Atrophy may be due to two fundamental pathodynamics, damp-heat and blood deficiency, each of which requires a specific treatment strategy. According to Li: "When damp-heat produces atrophy, this is surplus within an insufficiency, and it is appropriate to use percolating and draining medicinals. When a desiccation of essence and blood produces atrophy, this is an insufficiency within an insufficiency, and it is essential to administer extremely tonifying medicinals."

Throughout his *Exposition,* Li Shi-Zhen has repeatedly alluded to the relationship between the thoroughfares *(chong* 衝*)* and the *chong* vessel. Here, he fleshes out this relationship, using the discussion of the thoroughfares from Ch. 52 of *Divine Pivot.* In so doing, he also lays further groundwork for the idea that periumbilical pulsing is directly related to the *chong* vessel.

> [Ch. 52 of] *Divine Pivot Classic* states: "The chest qi has a thoroughfare, the abdominal qi has a thoroughfare, the head qi has a thoroughfare, and the qi of the shin area has a thoroughfare. Hence, when qi [accumulates] in the head, it ascends to the brain. When qi [accumulates] in the chest, it stops at the breast and back transport [holes]. When qi [accumulates] in the abdomen, it ascends to the back transport [holes] and *chong* vessel at the pulsing vessel on left and right of the abdomen. When qi accumulates in the shin area, it ascends to the Qi Thoroughfare (ST-30) and Mountain Support (BL-57) from above the ankle to below. In selecting these [holes], use a filiform needle, first locating [the hole to be needled] and leaving [one's hand there] for a long time [until the qi arrives] in response to the hand; one may then needle. This treats headache, dizziness leading to fainting and syncope, abdominal pain with fullness in the middle and sudden distention, and recent accumulations producing pain."

If we consider the number of lines devoted explicitly to the *chong,* it would appear that this vessel plays only a small part in this passage. It informs us that when there is qi in the posterior of the abdomen, it accumulates in the back transport holes. One modern commentator explains that these are the back transport holes of the yang organs on the level of the 11th thoracic vertebrae below the diaphragm.[21] Similarly, when there is qi in the anterior aspect of the abdomen in the *chong* vessel, it presents as a pulsing on the left or right side of the umbilicus that, according to the same commentator, is the region of Celestial Pivot (ST-25) or Huang Transport (KI-16).

If these were Li's only lines of interest, then it is curious that he took the trouble to cite the passage in its entirety. As we have already seen, he has demonstrated a willingness to abbreviate other quotations to serve his purposes. It is likely that there is something else in this passage that Li believes is germane to *chong* pathology.

The symptoms mentioned in this passage are ambiguous in that it is unclear if they pertain only to qi accumulating in the shin or to qi accumulations in all of the thoroughfares. This certainly appears to be a more generalized statement regarding the symptom presentation and treatment of all the thoroughfares.

Qi accumulation at the shin is the only thoroughfare requiring treatment at a specific hole, such as Mountain Support (BL-57) or distally at Qi Thoroughfare (ST-30). The other thoroughfares should be needled in the region where the qi stops *(zhi* 止*)*.

The symptom complex described in this passage pertains to accumulations in any or all of the thoroughfares.

If this is correct, then the systemic relationship between all the thoroughfares and the *chong* becomes clear. The symptoms of the thoroughfares conform closely to Li Shi-Zhen's theory of *chong* pathology. Headache and dizziness leading to fainting and syncope are commonly associated with counterflow. Abdominal pain, fullness in the middle and sudden distention, and recent accumulation producing pain all fit Li's expanded criteria for abdominal urgency.

Finally, the original authors of both this and the passages that follow attend closely to the palpatory experience associated with evaluating and treating the specific areas of the body. It is unlikely that this aspect of the material escaped Li's attention, particularly since he has slightly altered the punctuation in the passage above. The original passage from Ch. 52 differs from Li's version, and states: "first massaging [the hole to be needled] for a long time, and once [the qi] responds to one's hand, one may then needle" (必先按而在久應於手乃刺而與之).[22]

It is certainly possible that such a minor change is of no consequence. It may simply be an artifact of Li's imperfect memory. However, Katsuda Masayasu believes that the difference is significant. He argues that Li's punctuation changes the emphasis of the sentence from massaging the hole for a long time until the qi arrives to simply massaging the hole and waiting as long as it takes for the qi to arrive.[23] In the latter interpretation, the skilled physician does not simply rub the hole until he or she feels the qi arrive, but provides some initial stimulation and then awaits a connection with the qi in a much more passive and patient manner. Palpation also plays a role in the following passage, where the physician is instructed to palpate the abdomen to determine whether the *chong* vessel may be disordered.

> [Ch. 39 of] *Basic Questions*' chapter titled "A Comprehensive Discourse on Pain" states: "Cold qi lodges in the *chong* vessel. The *chong* vessel arises from the Origin Pass (CV-4), traveling directly upward along the abdomen. When cold qi lodges [in it], this vessel does not flow freely. Since the [*chong*] vessel does not flow freely, the qi follows it, resulting in wheezing and movements [of the abdomen] that can be felt with the hand."

The preceding passages suggest that although the *chong* vessel is the deepest of the extraordinary vessels, it is particularly amenable to palpation. These descriptions of massaging, awaiting the arrival of qi, and palpating the aortic pulse in the abdomen precede a more straightforward discussion of pulse diagnosis as it pertains to the *chong* vessel. Even here, the *Pulse Classic* provides not one, but three distinct pulse qualities for the *chong*, the first of which reflects a dual disharmony of both the *chong* and *du*.

> When the pulses of both hands are floating in all of the yang [positions] and deep in all the yin [positions], the yin and yang are both exuberant.

> This is the pulse of the *chong* and *du* [vessels]. The vessels of the *chong* and *du* are the pathways of the 12 channels, and if the *chong* and *du* overreach themselves, [the qi of the] 12 channels will not be able to return to the wrist pulse, and a person may suffer from distraction,[24] irritation, and agitation *(hu* 惚), and experience mania and dull wittedness.[25]

The pulse quality described here is simply excess in both the superficial and deep positions, reflecting an overabundance of both yin and yang. The symptoms associated with this pattern are uniformly cognitive and psychiatric. There is such a preponderance of qi that it profoundly disturbs the spirit in ways ranging from a giddy disengagement from reality to manic irritability and agitation.

	OUTSIDE (RADIAL)	MIDDLE	INSIDE (ULNAR)
DISTAL			
MIDDLE			
PROXIMAL			

	DISTAL	MIDDLE	PROXIMAL
SUPERFICIAL	███████	███████	███████
MIDDLE			
DEEP	███████	███████	███████

Fig. 26-1 Combined *du* and *chong* pulse

The next pulse is palpated only in the middle position along the midline of the pulse axis.

> If the pulse arrives hard and excessive in the midline position, popping up in the middle, this is [the pulse of the] *chong* vessel. [When the pulse is] perturbed in this manner, [the patient] suffers from lower abdominal pain and qi rushing into the heart, amassment bulging, enuresis, distressing propping fullness of the rib-sides, and infertility.

Although the hard and excessive quality is especially apparent in the middle position, it is presumably also palpable in the proximal position. No information is offered regarding the quality of the distal position, but whatever is happening there is likely to be unremarkable by comparison to the qualities of the pulse experienced in the middle and proximal positions. Given the hardness along the midline of the pulse, it might accurately be described as a wiry or bowstring pulse. It reflects the classic *chong* vessel pathodynamic of qi counterflow and abdominal urgency. Since this is fundamentally an excessive pulse, the infertility referred to here is most probably due to stagnation, as opposed to a debilitation of essence and blood.

	OUTSIDE (RADIAL)	MIDDLE	INSIDE (ULNAR)
DISTAL			
MIDDLE			
PROXIMAL			

	DISTAL	MIDDLE	PROXIMAL
SUPERFICIAL			
MIDDLE		███████████████	
DEEP			

Fig. 26-2 A hard, excessive *chong* pulse that reaches the middle position

The final pulse is also an excessive pulse that is firm and pounding throughout all three pulse positions. The stagnation here has become sufficiently entrenched that it has moved from the middle and lower burners up to the chest.

> If the pulse is firm from the proximal to the distal positions, beating straight up and down, this is [the pulse] of the *chong* vessel, [indicating] stabbing pain in the chest.

The assumption here is that while the pulse of the *du* lacks a pulse wave and is floating, the pulse of the *chong* lacks a pulse wave and is sinking to the point of being a 'confined' or 'prison' *(lao 牢)* pulse. This interpretation is evident in Kido Katsayasu's pulse graphic G-2 that appears in Part I, Ch. G of the introductory materials.

The *chong* is the only extraordinary vessel that Li associates with an abdominal finding. As the above-mentioned passage from *Basic Questions* notes, aortic pulsing is indicative of a *chong* vessel disorder. Li takes up this topic in greater detail, pointing out that the precise location of the pulsing dictates the herbal formula appropriate to the overall condition. He quotes a passage from *On Cold Damage* titled "Discriminating Pulse Patterns that Preclude the Application of Sweating Methods and Their Treatments" (*Bian bu ke fa han bing mai zheng bing zhi* 辨不可發汗病脈證並治) that is often omitted from the text. Most scholars concur that Zhang Zhong-Jing is probably not the author of this chapter and that a later editor appended it to the original text.

> Zhang Zhong-Jing states that for cold damage "accompanied by a pulsing qi on the right [side of the abdomen], one cannot induce sweating. If sweating is induced, there will be nosebleeds and thirst, the heart will suffer from irritability, and vomiting [will occur] immediately after drinking (first use Five-Ingredient Powder with Poria *[wu ling san]*, and then [if there is no improvement,] use Phyllostachis Decoction *[zhu ye tang]*). "This condition cannot be purged. Purgation will result in the fluids being spent, with dizzi-

ness, dry throat, dry nose, and heart palpitations" (Phyllostachis Decoction
[*zhu ye tang*]).

Like many of the situations described in *On Cold Damage*, the formulas mentioned
here remedy the consequences of improper treatment. Neither sweating nor purgation is permitted in any instance of pulsing qi around the abdomen. Strictly speaking,
Five-Ingredient Powder with Poria *(wu ling san)* and Phyllostachis Decoction *(zhu
ye tang)* are not indicated for pulsing on the right side of the abdomen; they treat
nosebleeds, vomiting, and a sense of vexing irritability in the heart, or dizziness, dry
throat, dry nose, and heart palpitations arising from erroneous sweating or purgation.
Abdominal pulsing is merely a diagnostic indicator. Nevertheless, Li associates the
symptoms and formulas described in this passage with the *chong* vessel. The fact that
the symptoms in question would not have occurred if the patient had not first been
mistreated is essentially irrelevant. He has clearly stretched the bounds of the relationship between right-sided abdominal pulsing and the herbal formulas discussed in this
passage, and this is true of the following passages as well. Because the original author
of these passages makes no recommendations for treatment, Li has included his own
suggestions for herbal therapy (in parentheses).

Li is quick to counter Cheng Wu-Ji's more orthodox interpretation of these passages, claiming that he only confuses the issue. As far as he is concerned, periumbilical
pulsation is primarily the result of stagnation in the *chong* vessel, with secondary *ren*,
kidney, and spleen involvement.

> Li Bin-Hu states: This refers to [pulsing] to the left, right, above, and below
> the umbilicus that is due to stagnation so severe that it is quite painful. It
> is actually a disease of the four channels of the *chong*, *ren*, foot lesser yin,
> and greater yin. The annotations by Cheng Wu-Ji that posit the left as the
> liver, right as the lung, above as the heart, and below as the spleen show
> that he failed to understand the four yin viscera, and [his comments] only
> confuse the reader.

There is scarcely a more apt expression of the *chong*'s role as the sea of blood than
a pulsing around the umbilicus. This is tangible evidence that the *chong* is somehow
linked to the cardiovascular system. The ancient Chinese, when performing dissec-
tions on human cadavers, may well have (as some writers have suggested) identified
the *chong* as the aorta and femoral arteries, and this is certainly consistent with the
Chinese medical notion of a sea of blood.[26] That said, such an association does not go
far in explaining the overall function of the *chong* in early Chinese medical thought.
The anatomical and physiological relevance of a "vascular *chong* vessel" is largely limited to identification with a physical structure. As the above passages illustrate, although
aortic pulsing is undeniably a cardiovascular phenomena, it is only indirectly linked to
blood-related pathologies. For Li Shi-Zhen, aortic pulsing is an unambiguous indicator
of qi counterflow, reminding us that the *chong* is not only the sea of blood, it is the sea

of the channels and vessels. The formulas he recommends for these conditions reflect pathologies of the qi, not of the blood.

Li concludes his discussion of the *chong* vessel pathology with a passage from Ch. 33 of *Divine Pivot* dealing with the four seas. Here the emphasis is on the *chong* as the sea of the channels and vessels.

> Qi Bo says that just as there are Northern, Southern, Eastern, and Western Seas, so [too do] humans have four seas that correspond to them. "The stomach is the sea of water and grains. Its transport [holes] are Qi Thoroughfare (ST-30) above and Three Li (ST-36) below. The *chong* vessel is the sea of the 12 channels. Its transport [holes] include Great Shuttle (BL-11) above and below it issues from both Upper and Lower Great Hollow (ST-37 and ST-39). The center of the chest is the sea of qi. Its transport [holes] are above and below the neck bone, and at the Man's Prognosis (ST-9) in front. The brain is the sea of marrow. Its transport [holes] are on top of the head above and at the Wind Pool (GV-16)."

The transport holes of the sea of qi "above and below the neck bone" are generally considered to be Mute's Gate (GV-15) and Great Hammer (GV-14), respectively. The transport hole of the sea of marrow on top of the head is Hundred Convergences (GV-20). The passage continues with a recitation of the symptoms associated with each sea.

> When there is a surplus in the sea of qi, there will be qi fullness in the chest, rapid breathing, and a red face. When there is an insufficiency of the sea of qi, the breath is reduced and insufficient for speech. When there is a surplus in the sea of blood, commonly there will be the illusion [that] one's body is enlarged, depression, and peevishness, and an inability to tell where one feels sick. When there is an insufficiency in the sea of blood, commonly there will be the illusion that one's body is small and cramped and there will be an inability to tell where one feels sick. When there is a surplus in the sea of water and grains, there will be abdominal fullness. When there is an insufficiency in the sea of water and grains, there will be hunger but an inability to ingest food. When there is a surplus in the sea of marrow, [the body] will be light, agile, possessed of great strength, and one will have the ability to accomplish what is normally beyond oneself. When there is an insufficiency in the sea of marrow, the brain will spin, the ears will ring, there will be aching pain in the lower legs, dizziness, and loss of vision, indolence, and somnolence.[27]

It is clear that all of the seas are intimately related to one another, but the *chong* and the stomach share an especially close connection. Conspicuous by its absence is any mention of pathology associated with the sea of the channels and vessels. It may be that the *chong* is so closely linked to the stomach and the yang brightness that it is virtually synonymous with the sea of water and grains. On the other hand, it may be that Li intends for us to interpret all of the pathologies mentioned above as disorders of the sea of the channels and vessels. He has gone to considerable lengths to establish the relationships between the *chong* and the yang brightness channels (the sea of water and grains); between the *chong* and the chest center (the sea of qi); and finally between the *chong*, essence, and the moving qi between the kidneys (and, therefore, the marrow with its location in the brain). In placing this passage where he has, Li provides the reader with a fitting summary of his perspectives on the overarching nature of *chong* pathologies.

CHAPTER 27

On the *Ren* Vessel

Ren the Controller

任 *(ren)* means to be in charge of (*dan ren* 担任) or to guarantee (*dan bao* 担保).[1] *Elucidations of the Signs and Explications of the Graph* states that "*Ren* means to keep or protect." In his commentary on the *Classic of Difficulties*, Yang Shang-Shan states that "*Ren* means to be pregnant; this is the root of human life and its nourishment" (任者妊也此是人之生養之本). Wang Bing's commentary on Ch. 60 of *Basic Questions* states, "The reason that the *ren vessel* is called this is because it is the means by which women become pregnant. Therefore the Classic states, '[If] this channel is diseased, women will be infertile.'" The *ren* is therefore closely linked to fertility. Moreover, as the early 19th century Japanese commentator Mototane Take (1819) points out in *Subcommentary on Patterns in the Classic of Difficulties* (*Nan gyo so shou* 難經疏証), *ren* is similar in meaning to *ren* 衽, "the front of traditional garments," also referred to as *jin* 襟. Thus the *ren* vessel travels upward from the lower abdomen along the anterior of the body, contacting the same area as the front of the clothing. Insofar as each yin channel travels along the abdomen and connects with the *ren* vessel, Yang Shang-Shan observes, "the *ren* networks with all the channels [on the front of the abdomen] and, therefore, it is called the *ren vessel*."[2] This is another reason that the *ren* is called the sea of the yin channels. Each of these ideas points to some aspect of *ren* function, some more obliquely than others.

The Sea of Yin

Given the importance of the *ren* vessel in clinical practice, it is remarkable how little Li Shi-Zhen has to say about either its physiology or its pathology. As the most basic regulator of yin within the body, the *ren* vessel is the obvious candidate for the title of "sea of yin." Yet some sources accord this honor to the *chong* by virtue of this vessel's influence on the blood. The *Pulse Classic,* in the chapter entitled "On Balancing Diseases of the Eight Extraordinary Vessels" (*Ping qi jing ba mai bing* 平奇經八脈病), and Lu Guang's comment on the 28th Difficult Issue in the *Classic of Difficulties*, both state: "The *chong* vessel is the sea of the yin vessels."[3] Li is evidently in agreement with Yang Xuan-Cao, who observes: "The Classic states that the *chong* vessel is the sea of the twelve vessels, hence it cannot only be the sea of the yin vessels. I am afraid that Mister Lu is in error."[4]

Trajectory

The trajectory described in the *Exposition* is somewhat more complex than the one sketched out in Ch. 60 of *Basic Questions,* which simply states:

> The *ren* vessel arises below Central Pole (CV-3) and ascends to the border of the [pubic] hair, proceeding along the interior of the abdomen upward to Pass Head (CV-4) arriving at the throat, ascending to the corners of the jaw and proceeding [up] the face to enter the eyes.[5]

The 28th Difficult Issue of the *Classic of Difficulties* contains the same passage; however, it does not describe the *ren* as entering the eyes. Although it too begins "below" Central Pole (CV-3), Li's trajectory first travels interiorly downward to Meeting of Yin (CV-1) where it differentiates itself from the *chong* and *du* prior to ascending via Curved Bone (CV-2) to Central Pole (CV-3).

> The *ren* vessel is the sea of the yin vessels. Its vessel arises below Central Pole (CV-3) from within the lower abdomen; it divides [from the *chong* and *du* vessels] at Meeting of Yin (CV-1) (between the two yin [orifices]). It ascends and emerges, proceeding to Curved Bone (CV-2) (in a depression above the border of the [pubic] hair on the pubic bone), ascending from the border of the pubic hair to arrive at Central Pole (CV-3) (four *cun* below the umbilicus; it is the alarm [hole] of the urinary bladder), where it meets with the foot reversing yin, greater yin, and lesser yin inside the abdomen.

As the intersection of the three leg yin channels, Central Pole (CV-3) is indeed a central axis of communication between the lower extremities and the rest of the body. Its position on the *ren* is juxtaposed with Great Hammer (GV-14) on the *du,* which is a meeting hole of all the yang channels. Whereas the yang exteriorizes at Great Hammer (GV-14), the yin moves into the abdomen and the interior at Central Pole (CV-3).

The *Systematic Classic,* one of Li's primary sources, describes a secondary network vessel as issuing from Meeting of Yin (CV-1), which hugs the *du* and meets the *chong.* "[From here] a branching network [vessel] of the *ren* vessel hugs the *du* vessel. It is a meeting hole of the *chong* vessel."[6]

Li makes no mention of this internal branch.[7] From here, the trajectory of the *ren* passes upward in the conventional manner to a slightly novel terminus on the head.

> [The *ren* vessel] ascends to the jaw and proceeds to Sauce Receptacle (CV-24) where it meets with the hand and foot yang brightness and the *du* vessel (located in the depression below the lip). It encircles the lips and reaches

downward to Gum Intersection (GV-26). From here, it emerges and its trajectory splits, traversing the face and linking to the center [line] below both eyes to reach Tear Container (ST-1) and terminates (located seven *fen* below the eye in a depression directly [below] the eyeball, there are two holes). In all, there are 27 holes. Neither the *Classic of Difficulties* nor *The Systematic Classic* asserts that [the *ren* vessel] "traverses the face."

Li's interpretation of the distal trajectory of the *ren* is as obscure as his description of its origins. *The Systematic Classic* describes Sauce Receptacle (CV-24) only as "a meeting of the foot yang brightness and *ren* vessel."[8] Yet Li identifies this hole as a point of intersection between the *ren* and *du* vessels. From here, Li's trajectory encircles the lips and communicates with Gum Intersection (GV-28) where it bifurcates to reach Tear Container (ST-1). Contrary to Li's claim, *The Systematic Classic* does indeed trace the trajectory of the *ren* across the face. Li has merely specified where the *ren* terminates. This, of course, begs the question of why the *ren* should terminate at Tear Container (ST-1) as opposed to Bright Eyes (BL-1). Were the *ren* to terminate at this hole, its trajectory would more likely have been described as "traversing the nose" (*xun bi* 循鼻). By including Gum Intersection (GV-26) and the two Tear Container (ST-1) holes on its trajectory, Li effectively increased the number of holes on the *ren* vessel from 24 to 27.

Branches

While Li ignores the network vessel associated with the Meeting of Yin (CV-1), he specifically identifies Turtledove Tail (CV-15) as such, citing a passage from Ch. 10 of the *Divine Pivot*. The word *bie* 列, 'branching', is an addition by later editors.[9] Because it scatters into the abdomen, it treats abdominal pain when excessive, and when deficient, it treats itching and scratching, presumably also occurring on the abdomen.

> The branching network of the *ren* vessel is named Tail Screen. It descends from the xiphoid process and disperses throughout the abdomen. When it is excessive, the skin of the abdomen is painful, and when it is deficient, there is itching and scratching.

In his closing statement regarding the trajectories of the *ren* vessel, Li quotes another passage from Ch. 2 of the *Divine Pivot* that enumerates what are often referred to today as the Windows of the Sky holes.[10]

> [Ch. 2 of] *Divine Pivot* classic states: "Between the supraclavicular fossae is the *ren* vessel. [Its hole here] is called Celestial Chimney (CV-22). ... It [moves to] the pulsing vessel on the sides [of the throat] at Man's Prognosis (ST-9) on the foot yang brightness."

Li's rationale for including this line is somewhat perplexing. He has already informed us that Celestial Chimney (CV-22) is on the *ren* channel in his earlier discussion of the *ren* trajectory, and there is no apparent reason for repeating this fact in a slightly different context. Li has also made a slight change in the wording of the passage that he quotes. The original text in the *Divine Pivot* reads as follows: "The first line beside it [the *ren*] is the pulsing vessel Man's Prognosis (ST-9) on the leg yang brightness [channel]."

Ch. 2 of the *Divine Pivot* then goes on to enumerate eight other holes, listing them in the order of their distance from the *ren*.[11] In this listing, the text is not suggesting that these other points have any relation to the *ren* vessel per se. For instance, Wind Abode (GV-14) on the *du* vessel is described as the seventh line posterior to the *ren*. "The seventh vessel [posterior to the *ren*], on the midline of the neck, is the *du* vessel. [The place where the vessel moves] is called Wind Abode (GV-14)."

It appears that the *ren* is merely a landmark, a topological starting point for enumerating these holes. That begs the question of why these holes are enumerated in terms of their orientation to the *ren*, or for that matter, why they are enumerated at all. Premodern commentaries on this passage offer little explanation as to what these holes are for or what this list is doing in this passage of the *Divine Pivot*. Man's Prognosis (ST-9) is the only hole that is described as a pulsing vessel, and indeed it is the only hole on the list at which a pulse can be found. It is therefore unlikely that they were all used for diagnostic purposes. Modern commentators interpret this list of holes as facilitating communication between the head and torso and often attribute esoteric qualities to them.[12] Yet none of this information sheds any light on why a reference to Man's Prognosis (ST-9) appears at the end of Li's chapter on the *ren*.

Li makes no similar reference to other holes when he cites a line from the same passage in the *Divine Pivot* in his discussion of the *du*. It makes no sense for Li to include Man's Prognosis (ST-9) in the discussion unless he believed that it had some direct relevance to the *ren*. Although there is no definitive way to answer this question, a few possibilities come to mind.

Li may be intimating that he believes Mans' Prognosis (ST-9) is actually on the *ren* channel. He clearly states that there are 27 holes on the channel. These include the standard 24 holes we recognize today, plus Gum Intersection (GV-27) and Tear Container (ST-1). So to reach a tally of 27, we must count Tear Container (ST-1) twice, or we have to add another hole, the most likely candidate being Man's Prognosis (ST-9).

It is also worth considering where the line in question is situated in the chapter, appearing as it does at its end, following Li's reference to a branching network vessel associated with the *ren*. By placing this passage where he has, Li may be associating Man's Prognosis (ST-9) with the *ren* in a manner that is purposefully vague. Still, given the well-established use of Man's Prognosis (ST-9) for pulse diagnosis in Ch. 48 of the *Divine Pivot*, and the pervasive influence of the *ren* as the sea of yin, it is not surprising that Li linked the two in some way.

Man's Prognosis (ST-9) may not rise to the level of a legitimate meeting hole of the *ren*, but it is worth noting that an alternate name for this hole is Heaven's Five Meetings (*tian wu hui* 天五會) or just Five Meetings (*wu hui* 五會). Yet the only other channel that this hole is known to communicate with is the leg yang brightness gallbladder channel. Perhaps Li knew something we do not about the meaning of this alternate name.

Finally, it is possible that this is a transcription error of sorts; Li may have inadvertently extended his quotation of the passage beyond his intended stopping point. Alternatively, he may simply have considered the reference to Man's Prognosis (ST-9) to be part of the same thought pertaining to the *ren* and therefore a part of the same sentence. These possibilities are merely conjecture. In the final analysis, the presence of these nine characters at the end of Li's chapter on the *ren* remains a conundrum.

Summary

Li Shi-Zhen's primary contribution to the *ren* lies in his refinements at both ends of its trajectory. In his discussions of the *du, chong,* and the *yin qiao,* Li repeatedly alludes to the triune relationship between *ren, du,* and *chong* as three branches of a single functional unit. It is necessary for the *ren* to communicate with Meeting of Yin (CV-1) not only because we recognize that hole as the first on its trajectory, but because it is here that it communicates with the *du* and the *chong.* There is no need to posit a separate network vessel that connects to the *du* and the *chong,* as *The Systematic Classic* has, because they are all fundamentally the same channel. It certainly makes sense to include the area around the mouth in the trajectory of the *ren* because it, along with the *chong,* is so influential in the growth of facial hair. Yet Li's reasons for including Man's Prognosis (ST-9) and Tear Container (ST-1) on the trajectory of the *ren* are less clear.

CHAPTER 28

On Diseases of the *Ren* Vessel

Bulging Disorders

Imbalances in the *ren* are characterized by internal clumping. *Basic Questions* and the *Classic of Difficulties* are in fundamental agreement on this point, although they differ slightly in their emphasis. Li Shi-Zhen begins his chapter on diseases of the *ren* with a passage from Ch. 60 of *Basic Questions* presenting this idea.[1]

> [Ch. 60 of] *Basic Questions* states: "When the *ren* vessel is diseased, men develop internal clumping and the seven types of bulging, while women develop vaginal discharge and mobile abdominal masses and gatherings."

The 29th Difficult Issue of the *Classic of Difficulties* contains a very similar passage that identifies all the *ren* symptoms as a species of internal binding: "When the *ren* becomes diseased, one will experience internal binding. Men will develop the seven types of bulging, and women will develop mobile abdominal masses and gatherings."[2]

According to Xu Da-Chun, "binding *(jie* 結) means 'taut and tense' *(jin jie* 緊結), or 'congealed' *(ning jie* 凝接). The *ren* vessel originates from the cervix and proceeds along the abdomen. Hence, [in the case of illness], internal knots will result."[3] In the *Classic of Difficulties*, bulging, leukorrhea, and masses and gatherings are simply the gender-specific expressions of internal binding. Women are not commonly diagnosed with bulging diseases, and men do not tend to suffer from masses and gatherings.

The medical literature invariably refers to seven types of bulging but the constituents of this list are not fixed. According to Yu Shu, there are seven types of bulging: "The seven bulging are called reversal bulging, plate bulging, cold bulging, amassment bulging, receptacle bulging, wolf bulging, and qi bulging" (七疝者謂厥疝盤疝寒疝癥疝附疝狼疝氣疝).[4]

Ch. 64 of *Basic Questions* identifies wind bulging *(feng shan* 風疝) and fox-like bulging *(hu shan* 狐疝) with the five viscera.[5] Ch. 49 of *Basic Questions* also mentions a protuberant bulging *(tui shan* 癩疝).[6] All of the above-mentioned diseases are characterized by pain or swelling in the abdomen or scrotum. They are typically attributed to a deficiency of qi and blood, dietary irregularity and exposure to cold, or a congealing of cold qi. (For a more comprehensive discussion of the role of bulging disorders in extraordinary vessel pathodynamics, see Part IV, Ch. 36 below.)

Mobile abdominal masses and gatherings *(jia ju* 瘕聚) are masses of indefinite form that gather and dissipate at irregular intervals and are attended by pain without a fixed location. They are attributed to disease in the qi aspect of the yang receptacles. Gatherings are commonly understood as occurring primarily in the middle burner while mobile abdominal masses occur mainly in the lower burner and are associated with gynecological diseases. Given its context here, the term 'mobile abdominal masses and gatherings' seems to be used more in a general sense to refer to masses and gatherings of any sort that are specifically gynecological in nature.

Reproduction

Abruptly changing tacks, the *Exposition* continues with a statement from Ch. 1 of *Basic Questions* regarding the role of the *ren* vessel in reproductive maturation and decline.[7] This passage could have easily appeared in the preceding chapter. By placing this material here, Li reframes the *ren* vessel's normal physiological decline in a pathological light.

> [Ch. 1 of *Basic Questions*] also states that: "Women at the age of two times seven [years] attain their heavenly dew; [during this time,] the *ren* vessel flows freely and the great thoroughfare vessel fills, the menses come according to their time. At the age of seven times seven [years,] the *ren* vessel is empty and the great thoroughfare vessel weakens and heavenly dew is exhausted. The passages of earth are obstructed, the body deteriorates, and [a woman] can no longer bear children."

In women, the development of the human body, sexual function, and the ability to produce offspring all depend on the heavenly dew. The arrival of the heavenly dew corresponds to the point at which reproductive maturation is reached, and its exhaustion corresponds to the point at which reproductive function disappears. Yang Shang-Shan observes that the "The heavenly dew is essence qi." In his view, the two terms are synonymous.[8]

Counterflow

So far, accumulations of one type or another have characterized the pathology of the *ren*. Li now introduces ascending counterflow into the mix, a pathodynamic more characteristic of the *chong* than of the *ren*.

> [Ch. 60 of *Basic Questions*] also states: "When there is an audible ascent [of counterflowing] qi, then treat it between the supraclavicular fossae." (This is referring to the Celestial Chimney [CV-22], which is the meeting hole of the *yin wei* and *ren* vessels. It is pricked to a depth of one *cun,* and moxa is applied three times).

An audible ascent of counterflowing qi refers to labored breathing that can be heard by others. The term includes, but is not limited to, asthma. Admittedly, this sounds much like a *chong* vessel presentation. Since they have so many physiological characteristics in common, the *chong* and *ren* naturally share many symptoms, yet they are distinguished by one important feature. Both vessels may be afflicted by counterflow, accumulations, and masses, yet counterflow in the *ren* channel presents exclusively in the upper burner. Counterflow in the *chong* may occur in any burner, and it tends to occur in the middle and upper burners simultaneously.

This passage originates in Ch. 60 of *Basic Questions*. Li's version alters its meaning slightly but significantly. Where Li's interest is limited exclusively to Celestial Chimney (CV-22), the original is typically interpreted as a reference to two separate treatment holes: "If there is audible qi ascent, then treat it in the center of the throat and at [the hole] in the supraclavicular fossae."[9]

The *Yellow Emperor's Inner Classic: Grand Essentials* concurs with this interpretation. The center of the throat refers to Ridge Spring (CV-23), and the center of the supraclavicular fossae refers to Celestial Chimney (CV-22).[10] Li's rationale for omitting Empty Basin (ST-12) from this sentence is consistent with his citation of *Divine Pivot* at the close of the previous chapter, where the text states, "Between the supraclavicular fossae is the *ren* vessel. [Its hole here] is called Celestial Chimney (CV-22)."

Pulse

Li Shi-Zhen concludes his brief discussion of the *ren* with two passages from the *Pulse Classic* describing the pulse-symptom complexes associated with *ren* pathology. These pulse images vividly echo the two essential pathodynamics of the *ren* vessel.

> The *Pulse Classic* states: When the wrist pulse is "tight, fine, and excessive, and [also] long arriving at the middle position, this is a *ren* pulse.[11] [When the pulse] is perturbed in this way, [the patient] suffers from pain in the lower abdomen and around the umbilicus that radiates to the pubic bone and a stabbing pain in the genitals. Select Origin Pass (CV-4) to treat it."

The first of the *ren* pulses originally appears in the *Pulse Classic's* chapter titled "On Balancing Diseases of the Eight Extraordinary Vessels." In this text, however, the location of the treatment hole is less specific than Li's version. It simply states, "Select [the hole] three *cun* below the umbilicus."[12]

Like the *chong* pulse, the text provides no information regarding the quality of the distal position. The pulse image is focused on the tense, fine, excessive, and long qualities in the middle and proximal positions. It extends only to the middle position, and it is specifically associated with pain in the lower burner. By contrast, the other *ren* pulse mentioned by Li is associated with abdominal masses and counterflow causing chest "urgency" accompanied by impaired range of motion in the torso. This pulse appears in the same chapter of the *Pulse Classic*.

	OUTSIDE (RADIAL)	MIDDLE	INSIDE (ULNAR)
DISTAL			
MIDDLE		▮	
PROXIMAL			

	DISTAL	MIDDLE	PROXIMAL
SUPERFICIAL			
MIDDLE			
DEEP			

Fig. 28-1 A tight, excessive, and long *ren* pulse

> It also states: "Forcefully striking across the qi opening pulse with a pill-like hardness to the vessel is the *ren* pulse. [When the pulse] is perturbed in this way, [the patient] suffers from a finger-shaped mass of qi in the abdomen that may surge into the heart such that there may be an inability to bend either forward or backward, and gripping urgency [in the chest]."

This second *ren* pulse is illustrated in Fig. 33-1 (p. 304). Where the first *ren* pulse is only palpable in the proximal and middle positions, the latter *ren* pulse is felt only in the distal position. The pill-like hardness in the distal position reflects the qi counterflow congesting in the chest. Both passages describe abdominal masses accompanying counterflow, however the influence of masses are not limited to this. The inability to bend forward or backward, a symptom more typically associated with the *du*, belies the close relationship between the *ren* and the *du* vessels: symptoms reminiscent of the *ren* and *chong* vessels may actually be caused by imbalances in the *du*. In the subsequent chapter on "Diseases of the *Du* Vessel," Li makes a point of correcting this misconception. Here, the opposite is true, further illustrating how inextricably tied these three channels really are.

Summary

For Li Shi-Zhen, *ren* vessel pathology is synonymous with bulging disorders of all sorts, and, to a much lesser extent, counterflow patterns into the chest. Clearly short of things to say in this chapter, Li also includes a description of the role of the *ren* in normal maturation, reproduction, and aging. Curiously though, Li makes no mention of how to address this, one of the most pivotal vessels in the entire channel system, with herbal medicine.

CHAPTER 29

On the *Du* Vessel

Trajectory

Li Shi-Zhen has considerably more to say about the *du* vessel than about the *ren*. Before tracing its primary trajectory along the outside of the spine, he begins with a quotation that appears in both the *Pulse Classic* and Lu Guang's commentary on the 28th Difficult Issue in the *Classic of Difficulties*: "The *du* vessel is the sea of the yang vessels."

Like the *chong* and the *ren*, its sister channels, the *du* also arises from the womb. Ch. 65 of *Divine Pivot* is the original source for the origination of the *chong* and *ren* vessels at this location. Li's assertion that the *du* arises from within the womb below the kidneys, giving the *chong*, *ren*, and *du* the same origin, figures prominently in his integration of Daoist and medical perspectives later in this chapter. According to Li,

> The *du* is the sea of yang vessels. Its vessel originates from within the gestational membranes below the kidneys and reaches the lower abdomen where it travels downward to the lumbar area and circles the pubic bone, where it links with the end of the urethral opening. In men, it proceeds to the penis and then descends to reach the perineum. In women, a network travels to the genital organs and unites in the perineum. All [of these various pathways] encircle the perineum behind the Barrier Screen (CV-1) hole (between the anterior yin [urethra] and posterior yin [anus]).

Ch. 60 of *Basic Questions* states:

> The *du* vessel arises in the lower abdomen in the center of the pubic bone. In women, it enters the vagina and the end of the urethral orifice. A network travels to the genital organs and unites with the area between them. … In men, it proceeds below the penis to reach the perianal region, as well as in women.[1]

Wang Bing comments: "What is referred to as 'between' means what is between the anterior and posterior yin [orifices]" (所謂間者謂在前陰後陰之間也).[2]

According to *The Yellow Emperor's Inner Classic: Grand Essentials*, the word *cuan* (篡) refers to the perianal region. *The Systematic Classic of Acupuncture and Moxi-*

bustion (Zhen jiu jia yi iing 針灸甲乙經) states that the Mountain Support (BL-57) hole masters "prolapse of the perianal region" *(cuan fan chu* 篡反出) and that the Sinew Support (BL-56) hole masters "rectal pain" *(cuan tong* 篡痛).[3] Wang Luo-Zhen interprets *jian cuan* (間篡) as "the anterior perianal region surrounding the urethra and Meeting of Yin (CV-1)," while *hou cuan* (後篡) is "the posterior perianal region surrounding Long Strong (GV-1)." *Ting kong* (廷孔) refers to the vagina and *niao kong* (溺孔) refers to the urethral orifice.[4]

Li's count of 31 holes on the *du* vessel may strike those accustomed to the World Health Organization standard of 28 holes as odd. His inclusion of Barrier Screen (CV-1) and Meeting of Yang (BL-35) has increased the number of holes associated with the *du* channel from 28 to 31.

Branches

Li Shi-Zhen next proceeds to elucidate the various branches of the *du* vessel.

> A branching network of the *du* vessel that travels from Long Strong (GV-1) to the *ren* vessel goes straight up from the lower abdomen and links with the center of the umbilicus, ascending to link with the heart. From here, it enters the pharynx, ascends to the cheek, and encircles the lips. It then ascends and connects below the eyes on their midlines. It meets with the greater yang at the inner canthus at the Bright Eyes (BL-1) hole (see the end of the *yin qiao* [trajectory]). From here, it ascends to the forehead and meets at the foot reversing yin at the vertex where it enters and networks with the brain.

Which Pathology Is It?

The influence of the *du* vessel on the heart figures prominently in the following chapter where, again quoting Ch. 41, Li describes a pattern of qi counterflow surging to the heart and producing pain. In his estimation, the symptoms associated with the internal pathways of the *du* are easily confused with those of the *chong* and *ren* vessels.

The descending branch of the *du* vessel complicates considerably the picture that is forming of its overall trajectory and function. Li then glosses a passage from Ch. 60 of *Basic Questions* that describes this branch as descending to connect with the kidneys. We cannot simply interpret the *du* vessel as the central vector along which yang qi ascends in the body. According to Li,

> Another branch from the brain goes down to the nape, proceeds along the scapula to meet the hand and foot greater yang and the lesser yin at Large Pillow (BL-11) (on either side of the first vertebrae in a depression one *cun* and five *fen* out from the middle of the spine). [From here,] it moves

inside, hugging the spine to support the lower back and proceeds along the backbone to network with the kidneys.

Like his passing mention of the length of the *yang qiao*, Li cites the *Classic of Difficulties* in describing the length of the *du*, apparently for no reason other than thoroughness: "The *Classic of Difficulties* states: 'The *du* and *ren* [vessels] are four *chi* and five *cun* [long] … and altogether they make nine *chi*.'" He continues with a similarly obscure passage that nevertheless fits more neatly into the overall picture of the *du* that he is trying to paint: "[Ch. 2 of] *Divine Pivot* states: 'The vessel on the midline of the neck is the *du* vessel. It is called Wind Adobe (GV-16).'"

   This line appears in a passage from Ch. 2 of *Divine Pivot* that describes the places where one may actually feel the movement of the vessels in the region of the neck and shoulders for the purpose of diagnosis.[5] It is reminiscent of Zhang Zi-Yang's focus on a single point or area that is particularly effective in opening each of the eight extraordinary vessels.

Relationships with Other Extraordinary Vessels

The above passage from *Divine Pivot* segues into a series of quotations defining the relationship of the *du* with other extraordinary vessels, most notably the *ren*.

> Zhang Jie-Gu says that the *du* is the capital and ties together all the yang vessels. The *ren* is the pregnant female and nurtures all of the yin vessels.
>   Wang Hai-Cang says that the *yin qiao* and *yang qiao* arise together from the heel. Their qi has merged [together] and is mutually connected. The *ren* vessel and *du* vessel arise from below the Central Pivot (GV-7) at the Water Ditch (GV-26) and connect with one another there.

Alchemical Influences

Li Shi-Zhen's exposition on the relationships of the *du* with other vessels takes on a much more Daoist bent with the inclusion of a passage from Hua Bo-Ren. Although Hua is primarily a medical author, his language has an undeniably alchemical resonance.

> Hua Bo-Ren states: "The two vessels of the *ren* and *du* are but two branches with a single source. One travels along the front of the body and another travels along the back of the body. A person's body has the *ren* and *du*, just as heaven and earth have *zi* and *wu* [midday and midnight], which may be perceived as divided or united. Divide them and it is apparent that their yin and yang [aspects] cannot be separated. Unite them [and] it is apparent that they are coalesced without differentiation. The singular is plural, and the plural is singular."

Li devotes the remainder of his chapter on the *du* vessel to an extensive exposition on the role of the *du* in alchemical practice. We have already considered this material at some length in previous chapters, so we will not review it again here. In summary, Li presents the concept of emptiness as an essential precursor for opening the extraordinary vessels. He identifies the *du* as the axis linking unifying alchemical functions in the upper and lower aspects of the body. The function of the *du* is closely tied to the primordial emptiness embodied in the lower abdomen, and activation of the *du* and the *ren* facilitates the activation of all the vessels. Using the symbolism of the *Classic of Change*, Li identifies the *du* and the lower abdomen as the source for the arousal of primordial yang. Finally, Li closes with yet another reminder that these goals may only be achieved in a state of utmost emptiness and quietude.

CHAPTER 30

On Diseases of the *Du* Vessel

Discourse on Words explains the word '*du*' (督) as follows: "The Governor judges [his people] by the middle path (*zhong dao* 中道)." According to *Zhuang zi,* "If one lives according to the *du*, he will live a long life." Wang Bing observed: "That which is referred to as the *du* vessel is the sea of that which leads the channels and vessels. The *du* vessel merits its name because it governs and controls the sea of [all] channels."[1]

Much as they linked the *ren* to clothing, Wang Luo-Zhen and Li Ding observe that the *du* or governing vessel is in the center of the human body and the center fold of a piece of cloth is also called the 'governing fold' *(du feng* 督縫).[2] Some annotators claim that *du* simply means center or middle *(zhong* 中).[3]

Record of the Rites of the Zhou by Zhou Li (周禮, 2nd century BCE) states, "The middle means *du* because the middle governs both sides." Thus, the *du* may be interpreted as a reference to the *du* vessel's control of the center of the spine and its regulation of the channels on either side of it. Master Lu expands upon this interpretation, explaining that the *du* is the sea of yang vessels because it courses directly through the center of the spine and controls not only the yang channels but also affects all the channels and vessels of the whole body.[4]

Yang Xuan-Cao's annotation in the *Classic of Difficulties (Nan jing* 難經) explains that "*du* means 'the capital' *(du* 都) and as such, it is the capital of the yang channels."[5] As already mentioned, *du* may be understood in militaristic and political terms as an allusion to the imperial title of Director General *(zong du* 總督), a term in use since the Former Han, denoting one who is generally in charge, typically of regional clusters of two or more provinces.[6] Similarly, Wang and Li attribute to the *du* the connotation of governing and observing *(shen cha* 審察), controlling and leading *(tong shuai* 統率), and being properly centered *(zheng zhong* 正中).[7]

In the previous chapter, Li Shi-Zhen described a number of branches of the *du* vessel in addition to its main trajectory, and he opens his discussion of pathology with a passage that highlights some of the symptoms that may be associated with them. He then goes on to point out that such symptoms may be erroneously attributed to the *chong* and *ren* vessels.

[Ch. 60 of] *Basic Questions,* "The Discourse on the Bones and Holes," states: "When the *du* vessel is afflicted, [qi] surges upward from the lower abdomen to the heart and produces pain. One cannot urinate or defecate. This is surging bulging. In women, this presents as infertility, dribbling urinary blockage, urinary frequency, and a dry throat ... treat this above the bone (this refers to the Curved Bone [CV-2] hole that is located at the midline of the hair line above the pubic bone[8]). In severe cases, treat the barracks below the umbilicus (one *cun* below the umbilicus is the Yin Intersection [CV-7] hole)."

This paragraph is a paraphrase of the original passage as it appears in *Basic Questions*, but it contains the salient points. The vast majority of the symptoms mentioned by Li that are associated with the *du* vessel concern pain, stiffness, and spasm along the course of the channel. Those mentioned here are among the most visceral symptoms associated with the *du*. He begins with the interior and works outward. Li is quick to respond to Wang Qi-Xuan's criticism that the above-mentioned symptoms are in fact symptoms of the *ren* and *chong*. This must have been an influential argument at the time for him to place it so prominently in his discussion. He first presents Wang's position followed by his own rebuttal.

> Wang Qi-Xuan says, "This is a disease of the two vessels of the *ren* and *chong*. I do not know how this could pertain to the *du* vessel."[9]
> Li Bin-Hu says, although the *du* vessel traverses the spine, a diverging network vessel issues from Long Strong (GV-1) to the *ren* vessel, [so the *du* channel] travels from the lower abdomen directly upward, linking with the center of the umbilicus, linking with the heart and entering the pharynx, ascending to the cheeks, encircling the lips and entering the inner canthus of the eye. Hence, [the cause of] all of the above symptoms is obvious. [Wang] Qi-Xuan has not considered this issue very deeply.

Wang's argument may simply be a vehicle for allowing Li to stress the importance of bearing in mind all of the branches of the *du*. Given that the holes recommended in *Basic Questions* are on the *ren* vessel, Li's argument appears to be little more than theoretical posturing. He makes no further mention of heart pain in this chapter and continues with a synthesis of a number of passages from both *Basic Questions* and *Divine Pivot* detailing more familiar *du* vessel symptomatology.

> [Ch. 60 of] *Basic Questions* states: "The *du* vessel [...] when excessive, [it] presents with arched-back rigidity. When deficient, it presents with heavy-headedness such that one wobbles ones head [in an attempt to hold it up], and if there is pathological change [in the diverging network of the *du* vessel] that hugs the spine, select the diverging [hole]."
> Qin Yue-Ren, in his *Classic of Difficulties*, states: "When the *du* vessel becomes diseased, there is spinal rigidity and reversal.

With the help of *Basic Questions* and the *Classic of Difficulties,* Li has painted a general picture of *du* vessel pathology. He then moves on to a discussion of therapy in which he will further develop these ideas. Although Li attributes the following sentence to Wang Hao-Gu, here referred to as Wang Hai-Cang (王海藏), the original source is unknown. This is the only mention in *Exposition on the Eight Extraordinary Vessels* of the use of individual herbal ingredients in the treatment of the extraordinary vessels.

> Wang Hai-Cang says that for this disease, it is appropriate to use medicinals in the class of Notopterygii Rhizoma seu Radix *(qiang huo)*, Angelicae pubescentis Radix *(du huo)*, Saposhnikovia Radix *(fang feng)*, Schizonepetae Herba *(jing jie)*, Asari Radix et Rhizoma *(xi xin)*, Ligustici Rhizoma *(gao ben)*, Coptidis Rhizoma *(huang lian)*, Rhei Radix et Rhizoma *(da huang)*, Aconiti Radix lateralis preparata *(fu zi)*, Aconti Radix *(wu tou)*, and Xanthi Herba *(cang er zi)*.

The *du* vessel, it seems, is unique in that it may be treated with individual herbs even in the absence of associated herbal formulas. These eleven herbs are all Li has to say on the herbal treatment of the *du* vessel. Although his next quote is from *Essentials from the Golden Cabinet,* a book concerned primarily with herbal medicine, Li makes no mention of herbs, discussing only acupuncture therapies.

> Zhang Zhong-Jing, in his *[Essentials from the] Golden Cabinet,* says that spinal rigidity is the general appellation for the five [types of] rigidity. Its symptoms include trismus, arched-back rigidity, and contractures. When medicinals are ineffective for these [symptoms], one may perform moxa on the Body Pillar (GV-12), Great Hammer (GV-14), and Kiln Path (GV-13) holes.

This passage addresses both symptom presentation and treatment. The reference to rigidity *(zhi* 痓*)* is actually a reference to spasmodic disease *(jing* 痙*)*. The original passage in Ch. 2 of *Essentials from the Golden Cabinet* reads:

> Patients with a hot trunk and cold feet, rigidity of the neck, aversion to cold, intermittent heat in the head, facial redness, red eyes, only the head wobbles, sudden jaw clenching, and arched-back rigidity have spasmodic diseases.[10]

This passage is followed by a discussion of formulas that treat such problems. These include Trichosanthes and Cinnamon Twig Decoction *(gua lou gui zhi tang)*, Kudzu Decoction *(ge gen tang)*, and Major Order the Qi Decoction *(da cheng qi tang)*.[11] Given Li's technique of attributing herbal formulas to the extraordinary vessels based on the symptoms they treat, these three prescriptions are conspicuous by their absence from Li's discussion of *du* vessel therapeutics.

The symptom of rigidity provides a segue into a more extensive discussion of the pulses associated with the *du* vessel. Li attributes "the pulse of those with rigidity" (*zhi jia mai* 痙家脈) to Zhang Zhong-Jing, though he has once again substituted the word "rigid" (*zhi* 室) for "spasmodic" (*jing* 痙): "[Zhang Zhong-Jing] also states: 'The pulse of those with rigidity is disturbed and wiry; its movement beats straight up and down'" (又日痙家脈築築而弦直上下行).[12]

Though Li confuses spasms with rigidity, his central point remains valid. Zhang Zhong-Jing has associated a very specific pulse quality with spinal rigidity and spasmodic illness. The pulse is pounding and wiry, and there is no sense of a pulse wave, therefore it "beats straight up and down." Katsuda Masayasu describes this pounding quality as akin to pounding the ground in order to prepare the earth to build a

	OUTSIDE (RADIAL)	MIDDLE	INSIDE (ULNAR)
DISTAL			
MIDDLE			
PROXIMAL			
	DISTAL	MIDDLE	PROXIMAL
SUPERFICIAL	██		
MIDDLE			
DEEP			

Fig. 30-1 *Du* vessel pulse

house.[13]

By including this line in this chapter, Li extends Zhang's original meaning to include the *du* vessel. This is not entirely capricious. Wang Shu-He describes the pulse of the *du* vessel in a very similar, although not identical, manner, citing spinal rigidity and pain as primary symptoms.

> Wang Shu-He in his *Pulse Classic* states: "When the pulses from the proximal to the distal positions are all floating [beating] straight up and straight down, this is the *du* pulse. [When the pulse is] perturbed in this way, [the patient] suffers from rigidity and pain of the entire back and will be unable to bend forward or backward. Adults will have seizures, and children will have wind seizures."

The unifying factor in the pulses associated with the *du* is that they all beat straight up and down. Li goes on to cite another of Wang's *du* vessel pulses that is linked to a related symptom complex and a treatment strategy employing moxibustion.

又日脈來中央浮直，上下動者，督脈也。動苦腰背膝寒，大人癲，小兒癇，宜灸頂上三壯。

[Wang Shu-He] also states: "A pulse that arrives as floating in the middle positions pulsing directly up and down is the *du* pulse. [When the pulse is] perturbed in this way, [the patient] suffers from cold of the back and knees, adults will have seizures, and children will have wind seizures. In such cases, it is appropriate to administer three cones of moxibustion to the vertex."

The floating quality felt in this pulse occurs only down the center of the longitudinal axis of the pulse. Because it beats directly up and down in such a narrow bandwidth, it is not surprising that Zhang described the pulse as "wiry" *(xian 弦)*.

The final two passages are not directly concerned with treatment at all; they address a species of wind affecting the eyes. This pathogenic wind ascends along the *du* vessel to become "brain wind."

[Ch. 42 of] *Basic Questions,* "The Discourse on Wind," states: "Wind qi proceeds to the Wind House (GV-16) and ascends, which then becomes brain wind. Wind may [also] enter and link to the head, which then becomes eye wind and eye cold."

The characteristic symptoms of brain wind are aversion to cold on the nape and neck and a sense of extreme cold at Brain's Door (GV-17), with unbearable pain.[14] Li finds this passage worthy of further comment; however, his contribution of a line by Wang Qi-Xuan is less than enlightening: "Brain's Door (GV-17) is the meeting [hole] of the *du* vessel and the foot greater yang … ."

Wang Bing's comments on the original passage from Ch. 42 of *Basic Questions* explain the relationship between these two statements much more clearly than Li himself.

[Wind qi proceeds to] the Wind House (GV-16) and ascends to the Brain's Door (GV-17). Brain's Door (GV-17) is the meeting of the *du* vessel and the foot greater yang, hence [when wind] travels from the Wind House (GV-16) and ascends, it results in brain wind. The vessel of the foot greater yang vessel arises in the inner corner of the eye … hence, when wind enters and ties up the head, there will be eye wind and eye cold.[15]

The relevance of Wang Qi-Xuan's remark is now more intelligible. The pathology at work here involves wind qi transmitted through the bladder and *du* vessels, entering the brain through both Wind House (GV-16) and Brain's Door (GV-17) and afflicting the eyes. These passages primarily describe a pathological process; the trajectory of the disease is the trajectory of the afflicted channels, and Wind House (GV-16) and Brain's Door (GV-17) are mentioned as landmarks along the way to afflicting the brain. It is unclear whether Li intends for us to interpret them also as treatment holes or whether they are simply way stations where pathogenic wind accumulates, causing discomfort in transit to the eyes. *The Systematic Classic of Acupuncture and Moxibustion,* Li's primary source on acupuncture holes, prohibits moxibustion at Wind House (GV-16) and Brain's Door (GV-17). *The Systematic Classic* identifies Wind House (GV-16) as the transporting hole of the brain, the place where the *du* vessel submerges into the brain, and it does have some ophthalmological indications. In addition to headache with aversion to cold, Wind House (GV-16) treats upturned eyes and confused and dizzy vision, all of which are consistent with the above-mentioned symptoms of brain wind. An alternate name of Brain's Door (GV-17) is Whirling Wind *(za feng* 雜風). Its only related symptom pertinent to this pattern is cold in the brain due to exposure to wind.

Summary

Pathology of the *du* vessel is characterized by pain, stiffness, and spasms in both the channel and the viscera influenced by its trajectory. These symptoms are often, but not invariably, caused by wind. Li's discussion of the herbal treatment of this vessel is remarkable in that he focuses on individual medicinals.

CHAPTER 31

On the *Dai* Vessel

Trajectory

It is fitting that the only channel with a transverse trajectory should appear at the end of the discussion of the extraordinary vessels. Not because the *dai* vessel is incidental, but because it exerts a direct influence on every other channel in the body. Li Shi-Zhen is content to stick to familiar ground in his introductory chapter, limiting himself to a recitation of the channel's trajectory, its intimate relationship to kidney function, and an explanation of why it is called the *dai* vessel. He will develop these ideas further in his subsequent discussion of its pathology, but for now, he presents a concise and tightly knit overview of the *dai*.

> The *dai* vessel arises at the tip of the free ribs at the foot reversing yin hole Camphorwood Gate (LR-13). Together with the foot lesser yang, it travels to the Girdle Vessel (GB-26) hole. (Camphorwood Gate [LR-13] is the confluence of the foot reversing yin and lesser yang, and is located at the tip of the free rib bone. The hole is where the tip of the elbow [touches the side of the thorax]; the Girdle Vessel [GB-26] hole is on the foot lesser yang channel in the depression one *cun* and eight *fen* below the tip of the free ribs.) [This vessel] encircles the entire body like a girdle. [Traveling] with the foot lesser yang, it meets with Fifth Pivot (GB-27) (located three *cun* below Girdle Vessel [GB-26]) and Linking Path (GB-28) (located five *cun* and three *fen* below Camphorwood Gate [LR-13]). There are eight holes in all.

Innovations

This passage opens with an extrapolation on the 28th Difficult Issue of the *Classic of Difficulties*, which states: "The *dai* vessel arises from the ribs and encircles the entire body."[1] Li's inclusion of Camphorwood Gate (LR-13) in the trajectory of the *Dai* is innovative in that *The Systematic Classic* identifies Camphorwood Gate (LR-13) as a meeting hole of the foot greater yin and lesser yang but does not link it with the *dai* vessel.[2] Wang Bing observes in his commentary on Ch. 59 of *Basic Questions* that the Girdle Vessel (GB-26), Fifth Pivot (GB-27), and Linking Path (GB-28) are all "meeting holes of the two channels of the foot lesser yang and *dai* vessel." However, *The*

Systematic Classic again identifies only Linking Path (GB-28) as a meeting hole of the foot lesser yang and *dai* vessels.[3] Li does not adhere to any one authority in selecting the holes that constitute the *dai* vessel, choosing instead to cobble together his trajectory from a variety of sources.

Exposition on the Eight Extraordinary Vessels is the first source to include Camphorwood Gate (LR-13) on the trajectory of the *dai* vessel.[4] Li includes this hole on the *dai* for a good reason. It is central to his understanding of this vessel as a vector for spleen pathology, a thread he will develop in the subsequent chapter. He continues with a passage from Ch. 11 of *Divine Pivot* that is full of implications for our understanding of the role of the *dai* vessel in the channel system at large.

> *Divine Pivot* classic states: "The primary [channel] of the foot lesser yin reaches the popliteal fossa and, diverging, travels to the greater yang to unite with it. It ascends to reach the kidney, and at the 14th vertebra, emerges to home to the *dai* vessel."[5]

This passage is a declaration of physiological function in the guise of a simple statement of trajectory relationships.

Connections of the *Dai* Vessel

Because virtually all the channels in the body are bound by the *dai* vessel, it exerts an influence on them all. Yet, the channel divergence of the foot lesser yin kidney is unique in that once it reaches its source viscera, it "emerges to home to the *dai* vessel." This is more than a tangential relationship. The channel divergence of the kidney and the *dai* vessel are effectively grounded in one another. The channel divergence of any channel is the deepest and arguably most direct facet of its channel matrix, conveying the most potent aspect of its influence. This suggests a proportionately deeper degree of communication than, for instance, the association of the *yin qiao* with the network vessels. In a very real sense, the *dai* vessel may be conceptualized as an immediate extension of the channel divergence of the kidney.

Another aspect of the relationship between the channel divergences and the *dai* vessel is that they share the same terminology. As Li notes in Ch. 2 of the *Exposition*, "The *dai* vessel horizontally binds all the vessels so it is referred to as the six directions." The six directions or confluences (*liu he* 六合) include the four compass points plus what is above and what is below. They define the conceptual boundaries that organize our perception of space. Similarly, the *dai* vessel defines the outer perimeter of the channels' influence, and it girds the extraordinary channels into a unified whole.

The bladder and kidney channel divergences are the first to be discussed, and their trajectories are the most detailed. The description of the first confluence in Ch. 11 of *Divine Pivot* can be understood as a template onto which the other five confluences may be mapped, allowing the reader to fill in the ambiguities inherent in the less detailed descriptions of the other confluences.[6] Though not explicitly stated, Ch. 11 of *Divine Pivot* leaves the reader with a sense of the first confluence as the archetypal channel divergence. In linking the *dai* vessel to the channel divergence of the foot lesser yin and the notion of the six confluences, this passage establishes the *dai* vessel's influence on the deepest levels of physiological function. It extends this influence to the most external aspects of structural organization and beyond to the relationship of the human body with the world at large. By skillfully placing this passage in his discussion, Li packs a wealth of resonances into just a few sentences.

Meaning and Basic Practical Applications

> Mr. Yang says that the *dai* vessel binds together all of the vessels, preventing them [from] being misaligned, like a man who ties together a belt which he hangs in front; hence the name. A woman's lochia follows the *dai* vessel and is discharged. Therefore, [similar vaginal discharges] are called *dai.*

This passage is a paraphrase of Yang Xuan-Cao's commentary on the 28th Difficult Issue of the *Classic of Difficulties,* which states: "The word for *dai* means to bind or to bunch up. It binds all of the channels and makes them supple. … It encircles the body like a girdle."[7]

The image of belt-like girding has become the standard understanding of *dai* vessel function, just as leukorrhea has become its benchmark symptom. The *dai* vessel functions like a belt or band encircling a sheaf of wheat. If the band is too tight, communication above and below is interrupted. If it is too loose, the entire system lacks the requisite structure for proper functioning.

According to *Elucidations of the Signs and Explications of the Graphs Annotated by Sections (Shuo wen jie zi duan zhu* 說文解字段註), "*dai* is an official's sash *(dai shen ye* 帶紳也), resembling an ornament on an elephant. Such ornaments always have a piece of cloth [designed for special purposes], and [for an elephant, one must use] multiple layers of such cloth." The sash *(shen* 紳) mentioned here means the lower, hanging part of a large girdle. *Dai* (帶) originally referred to a waist belt, and the upper part of the character was derived from its shape on the waist. Various ornaments known as *pei* (佩) hang from these waist belts. The graph 佩 is composed of a pair of 巾, one on top of another, and the lower 巾 was called *shen* (紳).

The *dai* vessel derives its name from its trajectory that encircles the waist. The word 'girdle' *(shu dai* 束帶) was used to describe the *dai* vessel, signifying that all the vertical channels were bunched together, connected, and controlled. Yang Shang-Shan observes: "[When I said that *dai* vessel] already makes a circle, [I meant that] it also encircles [the] waist and the spine. Therefore, at the 14th vertebra, the *dai* vessel bundles up the waist and girdles the belly; that is why it is called the *dai* vessel."[8]

The word *dai xia* (帶下) is indeed commonly translated as leukorrhea, meaning watery vaginal discharges, but it is clear from its association with the term *e lou* (惡

露, 'lochia' here) that we cannot be too narrow in our interpretation. Lochia may be both watery and bloody by virtue of its relationship to both blood and fluids. Hence, Li's rather idiosyncratic use of the term here suggests that vaginal discharges of any sort may be associated with the *dai* vessel and so referred to as *dai xia* (帶下).

Although Li has identified the channel divergence of the kidneys as an important facet of *dai* vessel function and leukorrhea as the benchmark of *dai* pathology, the etiology of this symptom lies with the spleen. He takes up this thread of *dai* vessel pathodynamics again in the next chapter.

CHAPTER 32

On Diseases of the *Dai* Vessel

Although the kidney is the predominant viscera in *dai* physiology, the spleen is the principal viscera in *dai* vessel pathology. The channel divergence of the kidney may be a direct vector for the transmission of essence to the *dai* vessel, but a disordered spleen is much more likely to produce a disease of the *dai* vessel.

Dissolution

Exposition on the Eight Extraordinary Vessels opens its discussion on diseases of the *dai* with another quotation from the now familiar 29th Difficult Issue from the *Classic of Difficulties.* It broadly sketches out two different but related types of symptoms associated with the *dai:* abdominal fullness of an internal nature and complaints of a more structural nature such as an odd sense of discomfort in the low back.

> When the *dai* is diseased, there is abdominal fullness, and there will be [a sense of structural] dissolution in the low back as if sitting in water (dissolution, as in seeming to be lax or sluggish).

Lu Guang explains this passage using syntax that clarifies the causal relationship between these two symptoms:

> The *dai* vessel girds a person's body. When it becomes diseased, there will be abdominal laxness, and hence, there will be a sense of [structural] dissolution in the low back, as if sitting in water.[1]

The failure of the *dai* to properly gird the torso allows the abdomen to become hypotonic, and this produces the low back discomfort. Li Shi-Zhen's own annotation links the sense of dissolution *(rong rong* 溶溶*)* to laxness *(huan* 緩*)* to evoke a sense of expansiveness, lack of structural coherence, and sluggishness.[2] He goes on to describe this sensation in a slightly different way that further stresses its lack of structural coherence.

> *Luminous Court* states: The *dai* vessel has two holes; "it masters low back and abdominal dissolution, [lacking structure] like a bag of water. In women, there will be lower abdominal pain and tenesmus, contractures, menstrual irregularity, and red and white vaginal discharge." [These holes] may

be needled to a depth of six *fen,* and moxibustion can be applied seven times.

Luminous Court (*Ming tang* 明堂) refers to Xi Fang-Zi's (西方子) *Luminous Court Moxibustion Classic* (*Xi fang zi ming tang jiu jing* 西方子明堂灸經) written during the Yuan dynasty (1271–1368). The passage also appears in Gao Wu's *Gathering of the Blossoms of Acupuncture* (*Zhen jiu ju ying* 針灸聚英) and *Comprehensive Recording of Sagely Beneficence* (*Sheng ji zong lu* 聖濟總錄, 1117).

The *Dai* and the Spleen

Li continues by paraphrasing Zhang Jie-Gu: "Zhang Jie-Gu says that for diseases of the *dai* vessel, the greater yin masters them. One should moxa both Camphorwood Gate (LR-13) holes three times." The source of this passage is unclear. It may have originated as his annotation of the *Classic of Difficulties,* which states: "The *dai* vessel runs through the foot greater yin spleen and Camphorwood Gate (LR-13) is the alarm hole of the spleen, hence, one should moxa it."

Zhang Jie-Gu's passage establishes a central tenet of *dai* vessel pathology: The *dai* is intimately related to diseases of the spleen. Li stretches this point with a passage from Ch. 63 of *Basic Questions* that makes no mention of the *dai* vessel, although it describes symptoms that are consistent with its trajectory.

> [Ch. 63 of] *Basic Questions* states: "When pathogens invade the networks of the greater yin, this causes a person to experience lumbar pain radiating to the lower abdomen and up to below the free ribs such that one cannot catch one's breath." ([The word] *chao* refers to the soft hollow spot below the free ribs.)

The original passage from Ch. 63 makes no mention of a specifically seasonal pathogen, nor does it mention the *dai* vessel. Li infers that lumbar pain radiating to the lower abdomen and the subcostal region occurs along the trajectory of the *dai,* which intersects the foot lesser yang in the lateral lumbar region and then the foot greater yin.

Most intriguing is Li's failure to mention the treatment technique associated with network vessel disorders. Ch. 63 of *Basic Questions* is concerned with cross needling (*miu ci* 繆刺), a technique in which one typically pricks a point in the vicinity of the well (*jing* 井) holes on the opposite side of the affected channel. In the case of the greater yin network, however, we are instructed to "Prick the recesses [in the sacral foramen] on the coccyx on the twin mounds of flesh next to the spine" (刺腰尻之解兩胂之上).[3]

In commenting on this passage, Wang Bing identifies the hole referred to here as Lumbar Transport (GV-2). He makes the very legitimate point that the entire question of picking holes on the left hand for problems on the right and vice versa makes little sense in this case since the sacral foramen are on the midline.[4]

Li's interest in the symptoms of "lumbar pain radiating to the lower abdomen and up to below the free ribs such that one cannot catch one's breath" is two-fold. They are not only related to the *dai* vessel, they are also associated with the spleen and some facet of the spleen channel matrix. This combination serves to further bind the *dai* to the spleen.

If, as Li suggests, spleen network pathology is linked to *dai* vessel disorders, then why would he fail to include the treatment for the problem he was discussing? One possibility is that, in omitting a prescription for treatment, he keeps his message focused on the dynamic between the spleen and *dai*. He also maintains his tacit principle of limiting the treatment of *dai* vessel disorders to holes on its trajectory, a standard that will become more apparent as this chapter unfolds.

Wang Bing provides a description of the trajectory of the greater yin network that more closely resembles the channel divergence of the spleen than the *dai* vessel.

> The network of the greater yin travels from the spleen [channel] to meet with the yang brightness. It ascends to link with the coccyx and binds to the terminal yin and lesser yang at the lower bone hole [in the sacrum]. Proceeding from the coccyx, it enters the abdomen and ascends to network with the throat and penetrate the tongue. Hence, the lumbar pain it produces radiates to the lower abdomen and pours into the free ribs. 足太陰之絡從脾合陽明上貫尻骨中與厥陰少陽結于下骨髎而循尻骨內入腹上絡嗌貫舌中故腰痛則引少腹控於中也.[5]

Although the trajectory described here by Wang Bing indeed approximates the spleen's channel divergence, it is inconsistent with the trajectory presented in Ch. 11 of *Divine Pivot*, which traverses neither the coccyx nor the sacral foramen. Still, there is at least one reason to believe that Li may have understood the above-mentioned passage from *Basic Questions* as a reference to the channel divergence of the spleen. After all, Li's passage makes no mention of the sacral foramen, either as a pathway for the channel's trajectory or as a treatment site, and he has already linked the *dai* vessel to the kidney channel divergence in the previous chapter.

Some commentators, Zhang Zhi-Zong among them, consider the network vessels in Ch. 63 of *Basic Questions* to be synonymous with the channel divergences.[6] This is the basis for the opinion of some commentators that cross needling is the treatment of choice for channel divergence disorders.

Interpreting the network vessel of the spleen as its channel divergence sustains a number of symmetries in Li's overall view of the channel divergences. In this scenario, both of the central players in *dai* vessel pathology would have channel divergence resonances. This is consistent with Li's attribution of the *dai* as the six confluences (*liu he* 六合), a term closely associated with the channel divergences. In Li's scheme, the *wei* and *qiao* vessels structure the networks, and the *chong, ren,* and, *du* control the deepest aspects of the physiological function and pathology. The latter vessels are three branches with a single source, and the *dai* vessel is aligned with them. It therefore makes sense that the *dai* would draw from the deeper wells of the channel divergence system rather than from those of the networks.

Admittedly, this analysis is highly speculative. What is not in question, however, is Li's focus on the relationship between the spleen, dampness, and the *dai*.

The *Dai* and the Lower Extremities

Li continues with a passage from the *Discussion of Cold Damage*, in the chapter on "Yin-Yang Exchange and Exhaustion Relapse" *(Bian yin yang yi cha hou lao fu bing mai zheng bing zhi* 變陰陽易差後勞復病脈證病治):

> Zhang Zhong-Jing states: "If after a severe illness there is water qi from the lumbar region down, Oyster Shell and Alisma Powder *(mu li ze xie san)* masters it." If it does not stop, then perform moxibustion at Camphorwood Gate (LR-13).

Once again, the *dai* is not mentioned by name. Here the *Exposition* expands the *Classic of Difficulties'* symptom of "dissolution" to include edema in the lower extremities. This is one of the few mentions of acupuncture in the *Discussion on Cold Damage*, and, as always, it is administered only as a last resort. The acupuncture treatment of the *dai* vessel is limited only to holes along its trajectory. Despite its influence on pathology of the extremities, distal treatment is apparently not an option. Citing passages from Wang Shu-He and Wang Hai-Cang, Li continues with more circumstantial evidence for the involvement of the lower extremities in *dai* vessel pathology.

> Wang Shu-He states: Diseases of the *dai* vessel "extend to the left and right encircling the umbilicus [and the entire torso] with pain in the lumbar spine that surges down the inside of the thighs."
> Wang Hai-Cang says that for pediatric protuberant bulging, one may moxa Camphorwood Gate (LR-13) three times, and this will effect a cure because the *dai* vessel passes through the region of terminal yin, and the greater yin masters it.

In this context, protuberant bulging *(tui shan* 癲疝) probably refers to scrotal swelling without pain or itching, usually due to living in a damp climate.[7] Wang Hai-Cang reiterates the supervisory capacity of the spleen over both the *dai* and the liver, which explains why that hole is so effective in treating this symptom. Scrotal swelling may be understood as a species of abdominal laxness, arising from a failure of the *dai* to gird the middle and allowing things to fall down. The external genitals are also nourished by the liver channel. The spleen-strengthening, dampness-transforming influences of Camphorwood Gate (LR-13) are transmitted along both the liver and *dai* vessels.

Wang also discusses the herbal treatment of profuse uterine bleeding that Li attributes to a *dai* vessel imbalance.

> He [Wang Hai-Cang] also says, "For women's menstrual diseases such as heavy uterine bleeding that becomes chronic and causes withering, one should bind [the blood] and augment [the qi]. For blood obstructions that become chronic and cause exhaustion, one should augment [the qi] and break up [blood stasis]. There are three treatments that break up blood [stasis]. Initially, one may use Four-Substance Decoction *(si wu tang)* with the addition of Carthami Flos *(hong hua)* and suitable amounts of Astragali Radix *(huang qi)* and Cinnamoni Cortex *(rou gui)*. Next, one may use Four-Substance Decoction *(si wu tang)* with the addition of Carthami Flos *(hong hua)*, suitable amounts of Persica Semen *(tao [ren])*, Cinnamoni Cortex *(rou [gui])*, and Urinae Hominis *(tong zi xiao bian)*, which are decocted in wine and administered. Finally, one may use Four-Substance Decoction *(si wu tang)* with the addition of Carthami Flos *(hong hua)* and suitable amounts of Myrrha Powder for Easy Aging *(yi lao mo yao san)*."

Li uses an abbreviated gloss of a passage by Zhang Zi-He to present the pathomechanism involved in leukorrhea, the symptom most commonly associated with the *dai* vessel. It also highlights the particularly close relationship between the *dai* and the *chong, ren,* and *du*. This relationship is the means by which pathologies of the *dai* may spill over into these other channels, which in turn produce abnormal discharges.

> Zhang Zi-He says that the 12 channels and seven of the extraordinary vessels all flow up and down. Only the *dai* vessel arises from the sides of the lateral abdomen below the free ribs and encircles the body, networking with the lumbar region and passing on like a tightly-tied belt. The two vessels of the *chong* and *ren* travel along the abdomen, hugging the umbilicus and flowing from the qi thoroughfare [hole], which belongs to the *dai* vessel, and networking with the *du* vessel. The three vessels of the *chong, ren,* and *du* have the same origins, but their trajectories differ. They are of a single source but have three branches and all network with the *dai* vessel. Since all of the [other] channels move upward and downward, when heat is left in the *dai* vessel, this lodged heat becomes constrained and oppressed, causing white substances to become full to overflowing. They follow the urine and are discharged in a continuous and unbroken manner [known as] white *dai* [disease in women].

The *Exposition* follows this 'thread' of thought back to Ch. 44 of *Basic Questions*, which discusses an analogous pathodynamic in males. The etiological factors cited in *Basic Questions* are consistent with a debilitation of both spleen qi and kidney essence: "When obsessive thoughts persist indefinitely, when one fails to attain what one aspires to, when one engages in wanton thoughts or when one engages in excessive bedroom activity, ... this causes a withering of the [ancestral] sinew [penis] leading to white excess [in men]."

Li reiterates that the above-mentioned emission of white substances may occur in both men and women. He then takes the novel position that these conditions are all due to damp-heat. Pathogenic cold as an etiological factor in leukorrhea or seminal emission is apparently not an option. Moreover, these conditions should be remedied using methods appropriate for the treatment of dysentery.

> This excess emission of white is the excess emission of white substances, which take the form of semen. In men, it is discharged with the urine, and in women there will be a continuous [vaginal] discharge. All of these [conditions] are treated as damp-heat and are addressed using the same methods that one would apply in treating dysentery. Red and white dysentery is [an expression of] pathogenic heat being transmitted to the large intestine, while red and white vaginal discharge is an expression of pathogenic heat being transmitted to the small intestine [channel]. In later times, everyone attributes redness to heat and whiteness to cold. This error has been perpetuated in thousands of writings, and this is a mistake that doctors make.

Of Ghosts and Artemesia

Li continues with a case history involving ghosts and the timely use of the Girdling Vessel (GB-26) hole in the treatment of a species of leukorrhea known as red and white *dai*.

> [Zhang Zi-He] also says that in *Classic of Nourishing Life* there was a woman who suffered from red and white *dai* [disease] and someone applied moxibustion to the Sea of Qi (CV-6) [hole], which proved ineffective, so the next day I [Zhang] did moxa on the Girdling Vessel (GB-26) hole. A ghost attached itself to my ear and said "Yesterday's moxibustion [on the Sea of Qi (CV-6)] was good, but it did not get to me [and] cleave to me, but today's moxibustion [where I am residing] did cleave to me so I will leave now. You may offer wine and food to propitiate me." [The patient's] family performed the propitiation as instructed, and she thereupon recovered.
>
> At first, I [Li Shi-Zhen] was taken aback by this affair as I was reminded of the two ghosts who resided in the Gao Huang (BL-43) [holes] of Duke Jing of Jin [during the Warring States period]. That is to say, [the prince was suffering from] such severe exhaustion that the ghosts were able to take advantage of this deficiency and take up residence there. This woman [with red and white *dai* disease] may also have suffered deficiency and harm from

overexertion by the heart, hence, ghosts could have taken up residence in the Girdling Vessel (GB-26) [hole]. Once moxibustion had cleaved to [the ghost] in the hole, it could not help but depart.

Since this [experience], whenever a patient has a disease such as this, I always palpate these holes and they are invariably sore when pressed. I have them return to apply moxibustion over [this hole], and they are invariably cured.

Taking the High Road

Li Shi-Zhen recommends the addition of Hundred Convergences (GV-20) to the acupuncture treatment and explains his reasoning with a few lines from the *Inner Classic*.

> *Inner Classic's [Divine Pivot]* states: "When the upper [part of the body] is diseased, then select [holes] in the lower [part of the body to treat it]; when the lower [part of the body] is diseased, then select [holes] to treat [it in the upper part of the body]. It also says for that which is above, cause it to descend, and for that which is below, raise it.

This passage reflects a rudimentary premise of acupuncture theory, that of treating problems using holes distal to the location of the disease. From this perspective, the addition of Hundred Convergences (GV-20) to the acupuncture prescription seems straightforward enough, and it may indeed be as simple as that. Yet it is worth noting that the lines used to substantiate this addition, if interpreted in their original context, raise some questions as to the precise nature of the pathodynamics involved in red and white *dai* disease, and tacitly contradict Li's previous statement that they are invariably due to damp-heat.

Though they appear to be saying precisely the same thing, the two sentences in the previous passage derive from two separate sources and reflect two quite different approaches to treatment. The first sentence is a paraphrase of Ch. 9 of *Divine Pivot*: "When the upper [part of the body] is diseased, then select [holes] in the lower [part of the body to treat it]; when the lower [part of the body] is diseased, then select [holes] to treat [it in the upper part of the body]."[8]

The second sentence is a reference to Ch. 70 of *Basic Questions,* which states:

> When the qi moves in a contrary manner, and the disease [is] in the upper [part of the body], then select [acupuncture holes] in the lower [part of the body]. When a disease is in the lower [part of the body], then select [acupuncture holes] in the upper [part of the body]. When a disease is located in the middle and sides, then select [acupuncture holes] there.[9]

This passage has been interpreted in a number of ways, all of which suggest that the pathogen involved is cold in nature. Wang Bing explains this passage in terms of cold accumulations in the lower part of the body.

> To select the lower [part of the body] means that cold has counterflowed to the lower [part of the body], and heat has attacked the upper [part of the body] such that there is inhibition below and a fullness of qi above, hence, one should warm the lower [part of the body] below to regulate it. To select the upper [part of the body] means that cold has accumulated in the lower [part of the body], and that warming [therapies] have not expelled it and the yang in the viscera has become insufficient, hence, one should supplement the yang. To select [acupuncture holes] on the sides means that if the [pathogenic] qi has occurred on the left, then one should apply medicinals with a fire-iron on the right, and if the [pathogenic] qi is on the right, then one should apply medicinals with a fire-iron on the left to harmonize [the condition]. [All of these therapies] must be administered in accordance with various manifestations of cold and heat.[10]

By contrast, Ma Shi's interpretation focuses primarily on the directional influence of therapy, as opposed to the specific location at which the therapy is administered.

> It is like this. In the treatment of contrary qi, if the disease is above, then one should select [treatments causing the qi] to descend so that when qi is obstructed in the upper [part of the body], then one should direct it downwards. If the disease is in the lower [part of the body], then one should select [treatments causing the qi] to ascend so that when qi is obstructed in the lower [part of the body], then one should raise it. If the disease is in the middle and [the afflicted] channels and vessels travel to the left and right [sides], then whether one is administering moxa, needling, fire-iron, or manual [therapies], one should select [acupuncture holes] on the sides.[11]

Zhang Jing-Yue provides a complementary interpretation in *The Classified Classic (Lei jing* 類經*):*

> Selecting above or selecting below means that one must examine whether the disease is located above or below. Selecting the inside or selecting the outside means that one must examine whether the disease is in the interior or the exterior. By means of these four [parameters], the location of the progression of disease can be determined, and then on the basis of its strength or weakness, one can carry out a robust or a delicate treatment [strategy]. ...
>
>   If the disease is in the upper [part of the body], then one should lower it [which] means that for yang diseases, one should treat the yin so that the obstruction above is coursed downward. If the disease is in the lower [part

of the body], then one [should] raise it [which] means that for yin diseases, one should treat the yang so that the stagnation below may be diffused upward. If the disease is in the middle, then the sides should be selected [which] means that the disease is engendered in the inside and connects by way [of] the channels to the outside so that one should prick or moxa, or administer fire-iron, or manual [therapies] on the [channel corresponding to the area affected on the interior].

To select [acupuncture holes] in the lower [part of the body] means that cold has counterflowed to the lower [part of the body], and heat has attacked the upper [part of the body] such that there is inhibition below and a fullness of qi above, hence, one should warm the lower [part of the body] below to regulate it. [12]

In the light of these commentaries, one of which is from Zhang Jing-Yue, a rough contemporary of Li Shi-Zhen's, the use of Hundred Convergences (GV-20) is a reasonable choice for treating red and white *dai* regardless of which channel is affected, as long as a cold pathogen is involved, hence, the emphasis on warming and yang supplementation. The implication is that the woman in the case history noted above suffered from red and white *dai* due to cold. This tempers Li's earlier statement that red and white *dai* disease is invariably due to damp-heat.

Li seems to be saying that damp-heat vaginal discharge can be precipitated by any number of factors. He amplifies his point with a quote from Liu Zong-Hou describing a dual debilitation of yin and yang. This pathology merely establishes the ground for the accumulation of dampness and heat in the lower warmer.

Liu Zong-Hou says that vaginal discharge is most often due to yin deficiency and yang exhaustion. The nutritive qi does not ascend, and the channels and vessels become congealed and bound up; the protective qi collapses; [and] the essence qi accumulates and stagnates in the lower burner in the area of the extraordinary channels with accumulation and fermentation that leads [to this problem]. It gets its name because the *dai* vessel becomes diseased and also because of the form it takes. The white type pertains to the qi while the red type pertains to the blood. These are most often caused by drunkenness, overeating, exhaustion from sexual excess, and the consumption of drying and hot foods. There are also cases due to damp-phlegm pouring into the lower burner, or the kidney and liver yin being overwhelmed by excessive dampness. In other instances, [one may experience] fear and fright such that wood overwhelms the seat of earth, and turbid fluids flow downward; or persistent lamentation may produce a withering of the [ancestral] sinew, and this is what is referred to as diseases of the two yang developing in the heart and spleen; or the other channels have damp-heat that concentrates and stagnates in the inferior aspect of the lower abdomen. In other instances, the primal [qi] of the lower [burner] may be deficient and chilled, causing the womb to become excessively damp. The methods for treating [these conditions] include purgation, or emesis, or simultaneously supplementing while discharging, simultaneously promoting [urination] while supplementing the middle, simultaneously raising and discharging while drying, simultaneously warming and nourishing while moistening, or warming and tonifying, or restraining and binding. All cases require different [treatment techniques] as well as their flexible application based on the [particular expression] of the pathodynamic.

Sitting in Water

The final illness identified by Li as a disease of the *dai* vessel is kidney fixity (*shen zhuo* 腎著). It bears many of the ear marks of a *dai* vessel problem, including a sensation that "one's back is weighed down by a belt containing five-thousand coins," and a feeling "as if one were sitting in water."

> Chao Yuan-Fang, in his *[Discussion of the] Origins of the Symptoms of Disease,* says that [in the case of] fixed kidney disease, the lower back is painful and as cold as ice, [there is] generalized heaviness, a feeling like one's back is weighed down by a belt containing five-thousand coins, absence of thirst, and uninhibited urination, due to profuse sweating after exertion such that one has become cold and damp inside one's clothes. When this has lasted a long time, then it turns into a water [disease].

According to *Discussion of the Origins of the Symptoms of Disease*:

> When the kidney qi becomes fixed inside, it is unable to diffuse and penetrate, hence, there is low back pain. Its symptoms include a heavy [feeling] body, and a cold lower back, the abdomen is heavy as if one were wearing a belt of five-thousand coins, as if one were sitting in water, its appearance is watery, there is an absence of thirst, the urine flows freely, and one's intake of drink and food are normal. When this has lasted a long time, then it turns into a water [disease].

The water disease referred to here is edema. Sun Si-Miao and Li Dong-Yuan provide the therapies of choice for this condition in their prescriptions Kidney Fixity Decoction *(shen zhuo tang)*, Dampness Leaching Decoction *(shen shi tang)*, and Pubescent Angelica Decoction *(du huo tang)*.

Conclusion

Li Shi-Zhen's discussion of *dai* vessel pathology draws from a broad range of sources, the majority of which do not mention *dai* at all. Emphasizing the role of the spleen, dampness, and water metabolism in *dai* vessel pathology, he nevertheless manages to present a reasonably coherent picture of the ways in which this vessel can become imbalanced.

CHAPTER 33

On the Pulses of the Extraordinary Vessels

Introduction

Over the course of its history, the medicine traditions of China have shown a remarkable capacity to embrace a broad range of mutually contradictory ideas. China has also produced a sizeable body of literature devoted specifically to organizing and systematizing these disparate ideas and treatment strategies. These efforts remain an essential part of the process of transmitting the medicine from one generation to another.

The ongoing attempts to integrate nearly two-thousand years of medical writings into something approximating a coherent system of thought must inevitably leave some things by the wayside. This may or may not have any bearing on their clinical utility. Even useful and engaging strains of thought may be relegated to the periphery simply because they do not fit the standard model or because they failed to gather enough historical momentum to penetrate the inner circle of Chinese medical knowledge. Moreover, cultural and political pressures were no less responsible for shaping the terrain of Chinese medicine in the 16th century than they are in defining medicine in the West today.

Li Shi-Zhen's perspectives on the extraordinary vessels' applications in the areas of acupuncture, herbal medicine, and Daoist meditative practices are poignant examples of this phenomenon. Only the facets of Li's book that blend smoothly into the established body of knowledge regarding the extraordinary vessels have been retained. The rest, although not repudiated, is simply ignored. Li's failure to rise through the ranks of the Confucian examination system may also be a factor in why only some, but by no means all, of his ideas have gained popular currency. Despite the veneration he is accorded today, he was not considered a true literati by his peers. His lifelong work on the *Comprehensive Outline of the Materia Medica* may be rightly interpreted as at least partially motivated by a desire to overcome his humiliation at failing his exams and to gain some legitimacy in the upper echelons of Confucian scholarship.

Whatever the dynamics that shaped its development, extraordinary vessel pulse diagnosis falls somewhere between the extremes of mainstream orthodoxy and the outer fringes of medical praxis. Because this system of diagnosis originally appeared in Wang Shu-He's *Pulse Classic*, it probably enjoyed some degree of legitimacy during the Han (206 BCE–220 CE). Yet by Li Shi-Zhen's own account, the extraordinary vessel pulses remained virtually ignored until his time in the Ming dynasty (1368–1644).

Since then, they have received only sporadic attention among those interested in all facets of pulse diagnosis. For reasons that remain unclear, a review of the premodern pulse literature reveals very little interest in the extraordinary vessels. Li Zhong-Zi, Shen Jin-Ao, and Zhou Xue-Hai are among the few who have acknowledged its place in the larger scope of pulse diagnosis. Yet, their contributions on the pulses of the extraordinary vessels have had only nominal influence on the core material presented in modern texts on pulse diagnosis.

Extraordinary vessel pulse diagnosis has certainly garnered a consistent, if modest, following in Japan and the United States over the past twenty years, yet it has by no means reached the popularity accorded the other ideas surrounding the extraordinary vessels, such as the use of the eight confluent holes or the notion that the extraordinary vessels convey original/primal qi. This would probably have come as something of a disappointment to Li Shi-Zhen because he clearly felt a strong affinity for this style of diagnosis, devoting an entire chapter of *Exposition on the Eight Extraordinary Vessels* to pulses.

Here in the final chapter of the *Exposition,* he recapitulates much of a chapter from the *Pulse Classic* that presents the extraordinary vessel pulses in their original milieu within the arcane system of pulse diagnosis known as the "The Hand Diagram of the Thirty-One Locations" *(Shou jian tu san shi yi bu* 手檢圖三十一部). This chapter of the *Pulse Classic* contains a great deal of difficult and contradictory material. Commentators over the centuries have gone to great lengths to reconcile these inconsistencies, yet the general consensus is that by the time of Li's writing in the Ming dynasty, the "Hand Diagram" material had definitely become corrupt. Even the title is problematic and has long been a source of debate in that Wang Shu-He discusses far fewer than 31 positions. The modern *Pulse Classic* commentator Shen Yan-Nan (沈炎南) believes that the number of locations in the title is a typographical error and should actually be 21. He suggests that these 21 locations refer to the 12 primary channels excluding the triple burner, the eight extraordinary vessels, all of the yang networks, and all of the yin networks. According to Shen, the triple burner is omitted from this tally because it has no definite pulse position of its own but is reflected throughout the pulse, with the upper burner in the distal position, the middle burner in the middle position, and the lower burner in the proximal position.[1]

Whatever its difficulties, this chapter of the *Pulse Classic* provides the larger context for Wang's discussions of the extraordinary vessel pulses elsewhere in his book. According to Li himself, he included this material in his own book on the extraordinary vessels because of its clinical value. Whatever Li's reasons for including this "Hand Diagram" material, the arrangement of nearly all the extraordinary vessel pulses in one place provides the reader with an opportunity to consider them as a group. It is an ideal venue for comparing and contrasting similar extraordinary vessel pulses and for understanding their place within the larger context of Li's work on pulse studies. In this chapter, we will discuss some of the broader considerations involving extraordinary vessel pulse diagnosis. We will examine how extraordinary vessel pulses are differentiated from one another, and how they are discerned from the other pulses in the system from which they originate. Finally, we will consider the place of pulse diagnosis in Li's overall approach to the extraordinary vessels.

We have no way of knowing to what extent Li actually used the extraordinary vessel pulses himself. He makes no mention of them in any of the case records presented in his *Comprehensive Outline of the Materia Medica (Ben cao gang mu* 本草綱目), and an anthology of his case records compiled by him has been lost. His *Pulse Studies of the Lakeside [Recluse]*, written around the time he was working on the *Exposition*, contains Cui Jia-Yan's (崔嘉彥, late 12th century) précis on extraordinary vessel pulses. This material is itself based on the *Pulse Classic*, and because it is presented in four-line rhymed verse to facilitate memorization, it is considerably more concise. As an introductory learning tool, its synopsis of extraordinary vessel pulses may actually be a superior model for students interested in implementing the extraordinary vessel pulses. A translation of this material appears in Appendix V.

Had Li contented himself with a recapitulation of Cui's rhymes, we would most likely be far more confident of our understanding of extraordinary vessel pulses today because it is much less ambiguous than the material presented in the *Pulse Classic*. Yet Cui's overview is really just a sketch of a much more complex and nuanced body of information, and Li's introduction to his chapter on pulses strongly endorsed the fully developed system presented in the *Pulse Classic*.

Li's chapter on pulse diagnosis suggests that he believed something essential had been omitted from the previous summaries of the material. The excerpts earlier in the *Exposition* individually referencing each extraordinary vessel pulse tend to blur their relationship to one another. His final chapter may be understood as an attempt to tie things together in a more comprehensive manner.

There is no question that Li was intimately familiar with the material. His father, Li Yue-Chi, was the author of a critical essay on the *Pulse Classic*. Yet, Li himself has little to add to the discussion, contenting himself largely with shaping the organization of the existing material to fit his tacit interpretation and then leaving it to his readers to discern the details of that interpretation.

It must be admitted that Li's advocacy of extraordinary vessel pulses is among his least remarkable contributions to pulse studies. As the man whose basic pulse scheme had been adopted by the majority of modern practitioners and the person responsible for standardizing the pulses to the 27 images we recognize today, his thoughts on the extraordinary vessel pulses are remembered by most as little more than a footnote. Li did not hesitate to stretch the bounds of pulse diagnosis in other ways as well. He developed the method of interpreting the distal position as a general indicator of the condition of the upper burner, the middle position as a general indicator of the middle burner, and the proximal position as a general indicator of the lower burner. He also divided the pulse into three depths, attributing various viscera to each depth, again along the lines of the triple burner. In this system, the most superficial aspect of the pulse corresponds to the heart and lungs, the middle level corresponds to the spleen and stomach, and the deepest level of the pulse corresponds to the liver and kidneys. The first of these two innovations is still used widely, the latter less so.

All of Li's major innovations reflect a willingness to approach the pulse as an indicator of broad trends in the system. For him, the pulse is a means of evoking a three-dimensional image of the qi terrain. This characteristic of his thought is particularly evident in the extraordinary vessel pulse images, which are necessarily defined in three-dimensional terms.

Drawing heavily from Wang Shu-He's "Hand Diagram" chapter throughout his *Exposition*, Li considers this obscure style of pulse diagnosis to be a lost jewel, foolishly ignored by his contemporaries and predecessors alike. By presenting this material as a coherent unit, both Li and Wang lay out the overall system in which the extraordinary vessels are embedded. Despite its unwieldy nature, it is essential to have at least a rough understanding of the entire system if we hope to make sense of its descriptions of extraordinary vessel pulses.

Li Shi-Zhen's Introductory Remarks to His Chapter on the Pulse

Li begins where Wang begins, with an introductory statement outlining pulse diagnosis according to a now-lost text known as Qi Bo's secret teaching of *Yellow Emperor's Rhyme*. He rationalizes the juxtaposition of two apparently contradictory pulse systems, asserting, "Although they pass through the three [standard] positions, the nine pathways are submerged [within it]." That is to say, the extraordinary vessel pulse system is not separate from the three standard positions used to diagnose the 12 primary channels, but rather is embedded within it.

According to Li, he is resurrecting a diagnostic method that has been lost for millennia.

> Because nobody in the world knows the pulses for the eight extraordinary vessels, I have now decided to draw a diagram [of this pulse diagnosis system] and append an explanation after it to transmit the secrets that have remained unknown throughout the ages.

Li did not in fact "draw" a diagram at all, and neither Wang's nor Li's original chapters contain any graphic material. According to Shen Yan-Nan, the first commentator to illustrate the relationships depicted in the "Hand Diagram" was He Meng-Yao (何蒙 瑤) sometime during the Qing dynasty. It is his drawing that appears in most modern editions of the *Pulse Classic* and is reproduced at the end of this chapter.[2]

Li Shi-Zhen goes on to assert that, "When [the pulse is] examined in this manner, one may know where the disease pathogen lies." This statement differs slightly but perhaps meaningfully from Wang's original: "The floating, sinking, bound, and scattered [pulse qualities] [allow one to] know where the pathogen lies."[3]

Li's failure to mention these latter pulse qualities as an essential component of this system of pulse diagnosis may be a consequence of an imperfect memory, but it highlights a unique feature of extraordinary vessel diagnostics. Wang's sentence stresses that proper diagnosis requires one to consider the location of the pulse within the "Hand Diagram" scheme and an additional set of specific pulse qualities. In nearly all of the individual pulse qualities presented in the "Hand Diagram", the above-mentioned pulse qualities are integral to making proper use of the system. As in the more familiar forms of Chinese pulse diagnosis, pulse position tends to define the location of the disease, and pulse quality identifies the pathodynamic. The "Hand Diagram" chapter attributes a channel and a set of symptoms to each of the nine pulse locations in the system. Wang then distinguishes the pathogenic factors contributing to the condition based on whether the pulse is "floating, sinking, bound, or scattered," though this is by no means a comprehensive list.[4]

Li's interests lie specifically with the extraordinary vessels, which are defined by two criteria that differ slightly from the other pulses in this system. The first is that every extraordinary vessel pulse occupies more than one of the nine positions of the "Hand Diagram." The second is that, with the exception of the *du* vessel pulse which is "floating in all three positions," the extraordinary vessels rely on an entirely different set of pulse qualities to define them. The pill-like, tapping, hard, and confined qualities used to describe the extraordinary vessels are unique to them, and these terms are not associated with individual pulse positions within the "Hand Diagram" system.

Unlike individual positions, most extraordinary vessels have one or more core pulse qualities that distinguish them from the surrounding pulse terrain. *Yin wei* pulses may be sinking, *yang wei* pulses may be floating, and *chong* pulses may be sinking and faint, but these are not their defining characteristics. Whatever Li's reasons for framing his remarks in the way he did, in excluding such secondary pulse qualities from his introductory remarks, Li focuses his reader's attention on the essential pulse qualities characterizing the extraordinary vessels.

Evidently anticipating some controversy over the adoption of such an obscure system of pulse diagnosis, Li's introduction establishes its pedigree beyond Wang Shu-He's claim that "Each [position] has its own diagnostic presentation according to Qi Bo's secret teaching of the *Yellow Emperor's Rhyme*."

Characteristics of the "Hand Diagram" Scheme and Li's Interpretation of It

If Li's interest in the "Hand Diagram" system were limited to its capacity to describe the extraordinary vessel pulses, Li could easily have saved himself some effort and simply cited the introductory section at the beginning of that chapter of the *Pulse Classic*. It concisely outlines the location of each of the nine pulse positions on the wrist. Yet Li omits this entirely. He seems to have gone out of his way to catalogue many but not all of the symptoms associated with each pulse position.

Despite Li's attention to the details of the "Hand Diagram," extraordinary vessel pulse symptoms correlate poorly with the symptoms attributed to the pulse positions they traverse. For example, the *yang wei* pulse passes through the bladder, heart master, and kidney positions in the "Hand Diagram" system (see Table 33-1), and yet these channels and their representative symptoms have little bearing on *yang wei* pathology. Just as the nine-position pulse system is conceptually submerged within the standard pulse system, the extraordinary vessel pulses appear to be further embedded within the nine positions. Li's rhetoric notwithstanding, on initial inspection, his only apparent use for the "Hand Diagram" system is as an anatomical reference grid for describing the extraordinary vessels. Indeed, with the exception of the distinctive oblique trajectories of the *wei* vessel pulses, the remaining extraordinary vessel pulses are more easily described using more conventional means.

	OUTSIDE (RADIAL)	MIDDLE	INSIDE (ULNAR)
DISTAL			
MIDDLE			
PROXIMAL			

	DISTAL	MIDDLE	PROXIMAL
SUPERFICIAL			
MIDDLE			
DEEP			

Fig. 33-1 Pill-like *ren* pulse in the distal position

For example, it is unnecessary to resort to a nine-position pulse scheme to adequately describe a *ren* pulse that is "pill-like across all of the distal positions" 前部橫于寸口丸丸者住脈也. Any pulse quality that covers all of the distal positions in the nine-position pulse scheme simply occupies the conventional distal (*cun* 寸) position.

Whatever his reasons, Li Shi-Zhen carefully presents the iconoclastic terminology of the "Hand Diagram" despite the fact that he has already described the extraordinary vessel pulses themselves in much simpler terms in his *Pulse Studies of the Lakeside [Recluse]*, written in 1564, 13 years before the publication of his work on the extraordinary vessels. In his book on the pulse, Li describes the *yang wei* pulse as traveling "from the inside of the proximal position and ascending obliquely, to reach the distal position." Shen Jin-Ao, the writer who adhered most closely to Li's vision of the extraordinary vessels, also dispenses with the nine-position jargon, clearly and succinctly describing the *yang wei* pulse as "traveling obliquely to the outside of the distal position."[5] These descriptions are far more accessible than those presented in the *Pulse Classic*.

The *Pulse Classic* scatters its descriptions of the extraordinary vessel pulses throughout its discussion of each of the nine pulse positions. Li arranges his material differently, describing all of the individual pulses before dealing with the extraordinary vessels. He works proximally from the lateral side of the distal position, then proximally from the medial side of the distal position, and finally down the midline. This arrangement is summarized in the table.

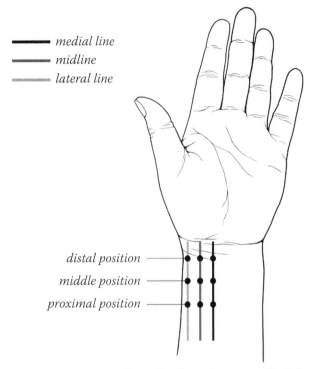

medial line
midline
lateral line

distal position
middle position
proximal position

Fig. 33-2 Pulse positions from the "Hand Diagram" of the *Pulse Classic*

	LATERAL	MIDLINE	MEDIAL
DISTAL	Bladder	Heart	Liver
MIDDLE	Stomach	Heart master	Spleen
PROXIMAL	Gallbladder	Lung/Large intestine	Kidney

Table 33-1 Channel correspondences from the "Hand Diagram" of the *Pulse Classic*

He Meng-Yao (何蒙瑤, Qing dynasty) offers a different interpretation of the terminology in this chapter of the *Pulse Classic*. In the section of his *Medical Writings (Yi bian* 醫編, 1730) titled "Diagnostic Methods of the Eight Extraordinary Vessels" *(qi jing ba mai zhen fa* 奇經八脈診法), he concurs that the anterior, middle, and posterior positions correspond to the three distal, middle, and proximal locations, respectively, but then goes on to claim that lateral *(wai* 外) indicates floating *(fu* 浮), medial *(nei*

內) means sinking *(chen* 沉), and midline or center *(zhong yang* 中央) denotes neither floating nor sinking *(bu fu bu chen* 不浮不沉). By this reckoning, a *yin wei* pulse described as "moving obliquely from the lesser yang to the terminal yin" is floating in the distal position and becomes sinking in the proximal position.[6] This interpretation obviously reads a great deal into Wang's original text, and seems unlikely.

Pulse images for the *ren, du,* and *chong* pulses are conspicuously absent from most editions of Wang's chapter on the "Hand Diagram," though they appear in an earlier chapter of the *Pulse Classic* devoted specifically to diseases of the extraordinary vessels. Li discusses all references to extraordinary vessel pulses under the rubric of the "Hand Diagram" regardless of where they originally appear in the *Pulse Classic.*[7]

	OUTSIDE (RADIAL)	MIDDLE	INSIDE (ULNAR)
DISTAL			
MIDDLE			
PROXIMAL			

Fig. 33-3 "Hand Diagram" bladder pulse

	OUTSIDE (RADIAL)	MIDDLE	INSIDE (ULNAR)
DISTAL			
MIDDLE			
PROXIMAL			
	DISTAL	MIDDLE	PROXIMAL
SUPERFICIAL			
MIDDLE			
DEEP			

Fig. 33-4 *Yang wei* pulse

Each extraordinary vessel cuts across a large swath of the channel system, establishing an organizing principle among the channels it influences. This characteristic is similarly reflected on the wrist. Extraordinary vessel pulses do not occupy a single pulse position; rather, they are topological features consuming significant portions of the radial pulse. As already mentioned, this is one of the two ways that they may be differentiated from ordinary channel pulses, particularly within the "Hand Diagram" system. Compare, for instance, the bladder and *yang wei* pulses. "On the lateral side of the distal position is the foot greater yang urinary bladder." The *yang wei* pulse travels "obliquely from the [foot] lesser yin to the [foot] greater yang."

These two pulses appear to be quite distinct, yet in practice, they may be confused when the examiner focuses exclusively on the lateral deviation in the distal position. A pulse that is identified only on the lateral side of the distal position is not, strictly

	OUTSIDE (RADIAL)	MIDDLE	INSIDE (ULNAR)
DISTAL			
MIDDLE			
PROXIMAL			
	DISTAL	MIDDLE	PROXIMAL
SUPERFICIAL			
MIDDLE			
DEEP			

Fig. 33-5 *Yang wei* pulse along a generalized gradient

speaking, a *yang wei* pulse. A *yang wei* pulse must also be felt on the medial aspect of the proximal position, establishing the oblique trajectory of the pulse. Pulses that are medially or laterally deviated in a single position are fairly common, particularly in the distal position; pulses that genuinely travel obliquely are less so. This same distinction holds true for liver and *yin wei* pulses. The pulse of the foot reversing yin liver channel is located "on the medial side of the distal position," and the *yin wei* pulse is located "from the [foot] lesser yang obliquely to the [foot] terminal yin." This pulse is the inverse of the *yang wei*. Interpreted rigorously, it must be felt in both the medial aspect of the distal position and the lateral aspect of the proximal position.

Though they are the focus of Li's interest, the extraordinary vessel pulses originally described by Wang Shu-He constitute a relatively small part of larger system of pulse diagnosis. In using this system, it is therefore necessary to discriminate between extraordinary vessel pulses and pulses pertaining to the primary channels. It is equally important to discriminate between a number of somewhat uncommon pulse qualities associated with the extraordinary vessels, and it will become apparent that this is easier said than done.

Between a Rock and a Hard Place: Tapping and Pill-like Pulses

Extraordinary vessel pulses that initially seem unambiguous become difficult to parse when their descriptions are transposed from paper to wrist. This is particularly true when distinguishing between pulses that are tapping *(tan* 彈*)* and pulses that are rolling, pill-like *(wan* 丸*)*, both of which are hard, though in different ways. Tapping and pill-like pulse qualities comprise half of the extraordinary vessel pulses and therefore merit some discussion. It is a testament to their place on the periphery of pulse lore that neither quality is among the standard 27 pulses established by Li Shi-Zhen, though it is essential to comprehend these two qualities if one hopes to understand the pulse images of the extraordinary vessels.

The word *tan* (彈) is generally used adverbially in the early Chinese medical literature to denote a percussive sensation of hardness. In Ch. 75 of *Divine Pivot*, when palpating for excess and deficiency in the channels, "one presses and percusses them" (*an er tan zhi* 按而彈之). In pulse diagnosis, *tan* (彈) typically denotes a peculiar sensation of hardness "like a finger tapping on stone." The medical commentary literature establishes that there are multiple layers of meaning associated with this pulse quality. Wang Bang-Fu's (王幫傅) relatively recent discussion of *tan* (彈) pulses provides one of the clearest explanations that this pulse actually has two facets. In his *Nurturing Sea of the Pulse Rhymes (Mai jue ru hai* 脈決乳海, 1891), Wang states:

彈字，當作平聲讀，不當作去聲讀. 彈石者，如指彈於石上，劈劈而
堅硬也. 若誤作去聲讀則為彈丸之彈，失其劈劈之旨矣

The word 彈 (*tan*) should be read with an even tone and not a falling tone. *Dan shi* refers to [the quality of] a finger tapping on a stone. It is shredded and hard. If erroneously read with a falling tone, this refers only to the pill-like pebble quality and loses its meaning of being shredded.

In describing the 'tapping stone' pulse like a finger tapping against a rock, Wang Bang-Fu further specifies that it feels as if it has been chopped up or shredded (*pi pi* 劈劈). This means that the pulse not only strikes with hardness, but with a bouncing quality, creating the impression that the pulse has also been chopped up (*pi pi* 劈劈), as if the radial artery had been divided into smaller threads along its long axis. The modern commentator Katsuda Masayasu, for instance, describes the *yang qiao* pulse as contacting only the bladder and liver positions as a means of emphasizing that the pulse bounces around from side to side, never arriving at the center of the finger.[8] The presence of this chopped or shredded quality is the key indicator that the condition is serious and distinguishes a *tan* (彈) pulse from one that is simply hard (*jian* 堅).

The tapping stone (*tan shi* 彈石) pulse is one of the unusual pulses (*guai mai* 怪脈) originally described in *Basic Questions*. Such pulses generally portend a very poor prognosis. Wang Shu-He cites an earlier pulse text that also describes other unusual pulses as having a tapping-on-stone quality, suggesting that it is one the fundamental characteristics of ominous pulse presentations. For instance, he describes the two original unusual pulses first mentioned in *Basic Questions* in terms of their tapping. 'Roof leaking' (*wu lou* 屋漏) and 'sparrow pecking' (*que zhuo* 雀啄) pulses both indicate a severe and likely fatal impairment of spleen and stomach function.

又經言得病七八日脈如屋漏雀啄者死（脈彈人手如黍米也）脈來如彈
石去如解索者死（彈石者辟辟急也解索者動數而隨散亂無複次緒也）

Bian Que said ... Furthermore, the classic states that "when seven or eight days after contracting a disease, the pulse is like a leaky roof, or sparrows pecking, this is fatal. (This pulse hits the hand like a grain of millet.) When the pulse arrives like a tapping on stone, and leaves like an unraveled rope, this is fatal. (A pebble bouncing on stone [has a quality that is] is hard and urgent. A pulse like an unraveled rope pulses rapidly but is chaotic and without rhythm.)[9]

In this passage, *tan* (彈) is described as *bi bi* (辟辟), an onomatopoeia for fingers tapping on stone in an urgent manner.[10] It is also associated with the quality of an unraveled rope, amplifying its chaotic and fragmented nature. Wang Shu-He, however, also recognizes the tapping pulse as a distinct quality in its own right, one that is typically associated with kidney debilitation. In the following passage, the tapping on stone pulse is identified as the true visceral pulse of the kidney, an indicator of imminent organ failure and death.

腎脈來發如奪索辟辟如彈石曰腎真腎脈至搏而絕如以指彈石辟辟然色
黃黑不澤毛折乃死

When the kidney pulse arrives like a taut rope and is hard as if bouncing on stone, this means kidney death. "When the genuine kidney pulse arrives balled up and exhausted, like the fingers tapping stone, the patient's complexion will be yellow-black and lusterless, the hair will be brittle and, thus, the condition is fatal."[11]

The clinical relevance of distinguishing between the two aspects of a tapping pulse is immediately apparent in Wang's chapter on the "Hand Diagram." Here, although a purely tapping pulse in the kidney position is ominous, it does not necessarily portend death. The condition is only fatal when this tapping quality is followed by a sense of the pulse unraveling or having become shredded. This passage clearly separates the two qualities, placing the tapping pulse at the beginning of the pulse wave and the unraveled quality at the end.

腎脈之來也微細以長曰平來如彈石曰病去如解索者死

When the kidney pulse arrives faint, thin, as well as long, this is normal. It is said that when it arrives like a tapping stone, this is said to be diseased. When it departs like an untied rope, then this is fatal.[12]

In a similar discussion, the *Pulse Rhymes* reverses the order in which each of these pulse qualities appears on the pulse wave, though the clinical outcome is the same.

腎乎則若上大下銳滑如雀啄腎之病脈啄啄連屬連屬之中然而微曲來如
解索去如彈石已死之腎

The kidney [pulse] is like this.
It is large above and sharp below.

It is slippery like a sparrow pecking.
The pulse of a diseased kidney,
Is linked to pecking
And within this [pecking]
It is linked to
A faint and crooked pulse,
Arriving like an unraveled rope
And departing like a tapping on stone
Meaning that the kidney has perished.

Which of these two qualities is perceived first is evidently not a critical factor in identifying a pebble tapping on stone pulse. More often than not, the tapping and unraveled pulse qualities are described as occurring concurrently, making them two aspects of the same perception. A tapping pulse that bounces from left to right across the width of the artery is another way of expressing a bouncing, shredded quality. Wang Shu-He uses this image of transverse bouncing in his "Hand Diagram" and elsewhere for pulses that indicate severe though not fatal conditions, as in the following statement.

脈直前左右彈者病在血脈中瘀血也脈後而左右彈者病在筋骨中也

When the pulse arrives distally, striking like a stone against its left and right sides, the disease is in the blood vessels, and there is stagnant blood. When the pulse arrives proximally and strikes the left and right side like a pebble, the disease is in the sinews and bones.[13]

Li's *Pulse Studies of the Lakeside [Recluse]* reflects a more streamlined and considerably less ominous understanding of tapping pulses. In some passages, Li recognizes the tapping stone pulse as a potential death pulse; however, he also routinely refers to this pulse quality as an indicator of less grave conditions. For instance, a tapping stone pulse that is sinking may simply mean that the disease lies in the external aspect of the body.

太過則如彈石按之益堅病在外也

[A sinking pulse] that is excessive like a tapping on stone, and is strong and hard when pressed, means that the disease is located in the outside of the body.[14]

The word *tan* is also used in the sense of plucking a string. Li utilizes this connotation to both expand and simplify the meaning of this pulse quality. Here the condition is not necessarily grave, and the pulse quality is simply tense.

When the pulse is rapid in comparison to a healthy person's, it may be tense, arriving like the plucking of a string. A few hundred years later, He

Meng-Yao also interprets tapping pulses moving to the left and right as simply meaning that they are "wiry, tense, and tapping" (*xian jin tan* 絃緊 彈).[15]

The modern commentator Shen Yan-Nan, probably noting Li Shi-Zhen's linkage of the two terms in his *Pulse Studies of the Lakeside Master* and He Meng-Yao's opinion, claims that a tapping pulse is simply a tense (*jin* 緊) pulse. This perspective is problematic in that the "Hand Diagram" system uses the descriptors tense and tapping in close proximity, hence, it is unlikely that they mean the same thing in that context.[16] Another modern commentator, Li Min-Shou (黎民壽), provides a more helpful insight in reducing the description of the pebble tapping on stone pulse to its essential parts.

彈石之狀堅而促來遲去速指下尋之至搏而絕喻為指彈石此真腎脈也

The tapping stone pulse is hard and rough. It arrives slowly and departs quickly. One seeks the pulse beat under the finger, and then it is gone, which is comparable to a finger tapping a stone. This is the true pulse of the kidney.[17]

Although the extraordinary vessels' pulses in the "Hand Diagram" chapter and later in Li's *Exposition* are invariably described as tapping *(tan* 彈*)* and not specifically as tapping on stone *(tan shi* 彈石*)*, the *qiao* pulses are still described as moving from left to right across the width of the artery. Or at least, this is how Shin Jin-Ao interprets Li's description of the *qiao* vessel pulses, which appear in the "distal left and right positions." The rebounding quality of the pulse causes it to bounce back and forth and from left to right across the three distal positions on the wrist "regardless of whether it occurs on the left or right hand" *(bu lun zuo you shou* 不論左右手*)*.[18] Each of the three distal pulses associated with individual channels in the "Hand Diagram" may have a wide variety of qualities, but in this system, only the *qiao* and *dai* pulses are described as tapping. Katsuda Masayasu concurs in this assessment. He also defines a tapping *qiao* vessel pulse as bouncing to right and left and uses the classic image of a stone bouncing on a hard surface to describe its rebounding quality.[19]

Li Min-Shou concludes that the biomedical implications of a tapping are "indicative of sclerotic changes in the radial artery consistent with arteriosclerotic cardiac disease and syphilitic cardiopathy." Li also attributes a dire prognosis with these pulses, which "undoubtedly reflects a desiccation of kidney water causing a hyperactive flaring of wind fire. Although it is not necessarily fatal, it is difficult to treat."[20]

The tapping quality associated with extraordinary vessels is clearly more ominous than pulses that are merely hard or tense. The presence of tapping pulses that bounce transversely in extraordinary vessel patterns suggests that the extraordinary vessel pathologies they reflect are commensurately severe, although not necessarily fatal.

The symptoms associated with these pulses are also relatively severe. For instance, a tapping *yang qiao* pulse appears with such unpleasant complaints as "low back and [mid]back pain, seizures with falling down, sheep-like bleating, hemilateral withering, recalcitrant obstruction, and generalized rigidity." We may surmise that the back pain referred to here is more severe than garden-variety lumbago. However one chooses to

	OUTSIDE (RADIAL)	MIDDLE	INSIDE (ULNAR)
DISTAL			
MIDDLE			
PROXIMAL			

	DISTAL	MIDDLE	PROXIMAL
SUPERFICIAL			
MIDDLE			
DEEP			

Fig. 33-6 *Yang qiao* pulse

	OUTSIDE (RADIAL)	MIDDLE	INSIDE (ULNAR)
DISTAL			
MIDDLE			
PROXIMAL			

	DISTAL	MIDDLE	PROXIMAL
SUPERFICIAL			
MIDDLE			
DEEP			

Fig. 33-7 *Yin qiao* pulse

	OUTSIDE (RADIAL)	MIDDLE	INSIDE (ULNAR)
DISTAL			
MIDDLE			
PROXIMAL			

	DISTAL	MIDDLE	PROXIMAL
SUPERFICIAL			
MIDDLE			
DEEP			

Fig. 33-8 *Dai* pulse

interpret the tapping, its association with extraordinary vessel patterns unambiguously suggests that the eight vessels were typically used for a more serious class of illness than the primary channels.

In summary, when interpreted most strictly, tapping pulses are hard, strike the finger like a stone, and bounce back and forth across the width of the radial artery. In some instances, however, Li appears to interpret 'tapping' to merely mean tense. However one elects to interpret the tapping pulse, the *yang qiao* pulse is tapping in the proximal position, the *yin qiao* pulse is tapping in the distal position, and the *dai* is tapping in the middle position.

Pill-like Pulses

Where the tapping pulse is nuanced in its definition and clinical interpretation, the pill-like pulse is relatively straightforward. Li devotes the final section of his *Exposition on the Eight Extraordinary Vessels* to a gloss of key terms appearing in the book, providing information as to how they should be pronounced and his interpretation of their meaning. There he describes the *wan wan* (丸丸) pulse as "round like a pearl" *(wan wan mai ru zhu wan ye 丸丸脈如珠丸也)*. Pill-like *(wan wan 丸丸)* is not a common descriptor in the pulse literature, but where it does appear, its meaning is clear. Aside from its association with the *ren* vessel, its use in the *Pulse Classic* is linked to unmistakably morbid prognoses.

> 腎死臟浮之堅按之亂如轉丸益下入尺中者死

> The [pulse of the] mortal kidney viscera is floating and hard. It is chaotic when pressed, like rolling a pill, and when it spills down into the forearm, it is fatal.[21]

Like the tapping pulse, the pill-like pulse is closely associated with both kidney insufficiency and stomach-spleen debilitation.

	Outside (radial)	middle	Inside (ulnar)
Distal			
Middle			
Proximal			
	Distal	Middle	Proximal
Superficial			
Middle			
Deep			

Fig. 33-9 Rolling pill-like pulse

脈至如泥丸是腎精予不足也榆莢落而死

When the pulse arrives like a ball of mud, this is due to an insufficiency of kidney essence. [It is like] the falling of elm seeds and is fatal.[22]

Both of these descriptions are consistent with one another. The above-mentioned mud ball (*ni wan* 泥丸) quality is not mushiness, but a slippery hardness.

In discriminating the pill-like *ren* pulse and the tapping *yang qiao* pulse, we may say that both pulses are hard and both move under the finger in the distal position. The slippery rolling of the *ren* pulse occurs along the long axis of the pulse, whereas the tapping quality bounces transversely across the pulse.[23]

Hard *Ren* and *Chong* Pulses

The second *ren* pulse described in the pulse chapter of the *Exposition* also closely resembles the second of the *chong* pulses, which is described as arriving hard and excessive on the midline position, reaching the middle. By contrast, the second *ren* pulse is "tight, fine, excessive, and long that reaches from below [the proximal position] to the middle position."[24] Both pulses are defined as excessive in the middle and presumably proximal positions. The *chong* pulse is felt only in the midline position, which might reasonably be interpreted more conventionally as a thin, wiry pulse. This does not leave a great deal of difference between the *chong* and *ren* pulses, but the most easily discernible distinction between them is that the *ren* pulse is longer than that of the *chong*. It extends proximally beyond the proximal position.

	OUTSIDE (RADIAL)	MIDDLE	INSIDE (ULNAR)
DISTAL			
MIDDLE			
PROXIMAL			

	DISTAL	MIDDLE	PROXIMAL
SUPERFICIAL			
MIDDLE			
DEEP			

Fig. 33-10 A tight, excessive, and long *ren* pulse

The above-mentioned *chong* pulse must be differentiated from yet another of the extraordinary vessel pulses. The pulse of the *dai* vessel is described as "tapping in the middle left and right positions." Both pulses are excessive in nature; however, the *dai* pulse is expressed almost solely in the middle position, whereas the *chong* pulse is presumably also palpable to some degree in the proximal and middle positions. Both the *dai* and the *chong* are hard, but the *dai* has that transverse 'tapping' or bouncing quality.

The *chong* vessel holds the distinction of having more pulses attributed to it than any other extraordinary vessel. There are the two permutations in the "Hand Diagram" already discussed above, not to mention a pulse that is simultaneously floating and sinking, denoting a mixed *du* and *chong* vessel disorder.

	OUTSIDE (RADIAL)	MIDDLE	INSIDE (ULNAR)
DISTAL			
MIDDLE			
PROXIMAL			
	DISTAL	MIDDLE	PROXIMAL
SUPERFICIAL	███████████████████████████		
MIDDLE			
DEEP	███████████████████████████		

Fig. 33-11 Combined *du* and *chong* pulse

Li has imported these pulses, along with those of the *ren* and *du,* from an earlier chapter in the *Pulse Classic* into his own version of the "Hand Diagram." Then there is a *chong* pulse that even Li omits from the "Hand Diagram." His reasons for this omission are unclear because it is described in a manner consistent with "Hand Diagram" terminology and it appears in Li's own chapter on diseases of the *chong*. This *chong* pulse is "firm from the proximal to distal positions, beating straight up and down" *(zhi shang zhi xia* 直上直下). The quality of beating straight up and down means that there is no sense of a pulse wave. The pulse hits the fingers all at once. This *chong* pulse must be differentiated from the *du* pulse, which also beats straight up and down, but in addition is floating.

Are the *chong* pulse and the *du* pulse simply components of the combined *du* and *chong* pulse? Perhaps. Stripped of their characteristic pulse qualities, these individual extraordinary vessels pulses roughly resemble the combined pulse. It is simultaneously sinking and floating, but is not defined by any further pulse quality. Yet the *du* pulse is not only floating, it also lacks a waveform. It feels rigid; therefore, it "[beats] perpendicularly up and down." A *chong* pulse that is firm throughout its length, also beating straight up and down, could be at any depth. Finally, Wang stipulates that the combined *du* and *chong* pulse must be felt in both hands, whereas the individual *du* and the *chong* pulses may be felt on either wrist. In the final analysis, there are more differences than similarities among these pulses.

Auxilliary Pulse Qualities

Only three of the extraordinary vessel pulses from the *Pulse Classic* have auxiliary qualities that are associated with specific symptom presentations, and none of these are described in the "Hand Diagram" chapter. These include the *yang wei* and *yin wei* pulse images and the *yang qiao* pulse. Just as in ordinary pulse diagnosis, pulse qualities provide more specific information regarding the nature of the pathodynamic involved. For instance, when a *yang wei* pulse floats, the patient may experience "vertigo [that] will occur with standing. This is due to the yang being overabundant and overfull [so the patient also] suffers from raised-shoulder breathing and shivering as if cold." A sinking, large, and excessive *yin wei* pulse implies the presence of "pain in the chest, propping fullness below the hypochondrium, and heart pain." The clinical implication of a *yin wei* pulse that feels like a string of pearls is gender specific. "In men there will be an excess below both rib-sides and lumbar pain, while in women there will be genital pain as if sores have formed."

Because they have no pulse qualities of their own, the *wei* pulses are less complicated than the *yang qiao* pulse. The *wei* pulses are defined entirely by their oblique trajectory whereas the *yang qiao* is defined primarily by its tapping quality across the breadth of the distal position. According to Wang and Li, this tapping quality may also be "faint and choppy," which is indicative of wind seizures. As we have seen, part of the definition of a tapping pulse is that it is rough or choppy yet it stretches the imagination to conceive of it as simultaneously faint. We can only conjecture that however weak a faint, tapping pulse would be, it would still be perceived as tapping rather than as a pulse wave, and the examiner might experience the pulse as bouncing back and forth across the width of the artery.

There are a few pulses in the *Exposition* that do not appear in the *Pulse Classic* and yet are associated with patterns that Li has identified as extraordinary vessel pathologies. Most prominent among these is a pulse pattern described by Sun Si-Miao.

> In his [*Important*] *Formulas Worth a Thousand Gold Pieces*, the True Man Sun [Si-Miao] says that when there is a cough that causes one to spit up saliva accompanied by frigidly cold extremities, qi from the lower abdomen surges upward into the chest, mouth, and throat, [and] the face will be flushed and boiling hot as if one were intoxicated. [The patient feels] as if she will experience either urinary or fecal incontinence that will flow down the inner thigh, [and] there will be difficult urination [although the patient] remains anxious about the possible return of these symptoms. The distal pulse will be deep, and the proximal pulse will be faint. It is appropriate to use Poria and Schisandra Decoction *(ling wu wei zi tang)* to treat this surging of qi. The formula contains Poria *(fu ling)*, Schizandrae Fructus *(wu wei zi)*, 2 qian [each], Cinnamon Cortex *(rou xin)*, and Glycyrrhizae Radix *(gan cao)*, 1 qian [each]. This is decocted in water and administered. If there is chest fullness, omit the Cinnamon Cortex *(rou gui)*.

Li's discussion of pulses in the *Exposition* seems to go in two directions at once. He first appeals to the authority of the *Pulse Classic* in establishing a well-defined set of extraordinary vessel pulses. Then, in his efforts to expand the scope of extraordinary vessel diagnostics and therapeutics, he muddies the waters by bringing other pulses into his discussion. Are the "Hand Diagram" pulses the only legitimate extraordinary vessel pulses or can the other pulse images in the *Exposition* also be properly classified as extraordinary vessel pulses?

One has to wonder how the pulse qualities described in the previous passage by Sun Si-Miao are fundamentally any different from the extraordinary vessel pulses described in the "Hand Diagram." The more carefully one examines these questions, the less clear such distinctions become. It seems that Li's intention was to actively extend the bounds of pulse diagnosis beyond the standard images of the "Hand Diagram." Elsewhere in the *Exposition,* Li presents criteria for a *yang wei* pulse derived from a passage in the *Discussion On Cold Damage (Shang han lun* 傷寒論*)*.

> This means that if after [administering] Cinnamon Twig [Decoction], the patient presents with spontaneous sweating, feverishness, and chills, his pulse is floating in the distal position and weak in the proximal position and [the patient] is irritable, then this disease is located in the *yang wei.*

This passage raises the question of whether or not we are to interpret this pulse image as pathognomonic for the *yang wei.* It is described as occupying multiple pulse positions, a defining characteristic of an extraordinary vessel pulse, and Li explicitly associates it with an extraordinary vessel pathology. It seems most reasonable to conclude that, taken by themselves, the pulses described in the above-mentioned *chong* and *yang wei* patterns are no more or less extraordinary vessel pulses than those described in the "Hand Diagram." By extension, it would seem that any definable pulse pattern covering multiple pulse positions might, in the right circumstances, reflect an extraordinary vessel pathology, and therefore be considered an 'extraordinary vessel pulse.' Such a proposition challenges the very notion of an independently identifiable extraordinary vessel pulse. That leaves us with the question of what, if anything, defines an extraordinary vessel pulse.

If an examiner were to perceive a tapping pulse in the distal position of the right wrist accompanied by chest pain, persistent cough, exhaustion, and spontaneous sweating, would this be an indicator of a *yang qiao* disorder or of a binding accumulation in the lungs profoundly damaging the qi? In this situation, the latter diagnosis fits the presentation more closely than the former. This example illustrates how inextricably bound extraordinary vessel pulse presentations are to their accompanying symptoms.

Each pulse image discussed in the "Hand Diagram" is accompanied by a list of symptoms that might occur when that pulse is present. This same format is found throughout the *Pulse Classic.* The syntax of these descriptions suggests that an accurate pulse evaluation enables the skilled physician to predict a patient's symptom presentation; however, this is not necessarily the case.

The symptoms described are no less a part of the diagnosis than the pulse image itself, and together they represent a bimodal diagnostic picture. Moreover, the symptoms provide a practical means of cross-referencing their respective pulses. For instance, notwithstanding Katsuda Masayasu's neat differentiation, pill-like and tapping qualities can be challenging to discriminate from one another in real patients. Fortunately, the symptoms associated with each of these pulse images leaves little room for doubt. The pill-like *ren* pulse is accompanied by "lesser abdominal pain and counterflow qi that pierces the heart ... a sense of gripping urgency in the thorax that prevents forward or backward bending." The tapping *yang qiao* presents along with "low back and [mid]back pain, seizures with falling down, and sheep-like bleating, hemilateral withering, recalcitrant obstruction, and generalized rigidity."

Symptoms associated with the first *ren* pulse are more internal than those attributed to the *yang qiao*, although they may be equally severe. The symptoms associated with the *chong* and second *ren* pulses are similar. Both indicate the presence of abdominal pain, accumulations, and bulging disorders. Nevertheless, *chong* disorders are most typically characterized by counterflow, and this is evident in the *chong's* symptom picture of lesser abdominal pain "ascending to the heart."

So, then, is it at all meaningful to discuss extraordinary vessel pulses in the absence of their accompanying symptom presentations? The evidence provided by Wang and Li suggests that it is not. Neither the *Pulse Classic* nor the *Exposition on the Eight Extraordinary Vessels* ever mentions an extraordinary vessel pulse without an accompanying symptom presentation. Their message is not that the "Hand Diagram" is a useful method of pulse diagnosis; rather, that the "Hand Diagram" is a valuable tool for assessing pulse and symptom complexes. This may be a reason why Li elected to include the symptom complex associated with each of the nine pulse positions in his introductory material. It reinforces the point that the system is nearly meaningless without an accompanying symptom picture. A laterally oblique distal pulse is only a bladder pulse when there are also symptoms of bladder channel pathology such as visual dizziness and rigid pain in the head, neck, low back, and back. Of course, the mutually dependent nature of the relationship between signs and symptoms is true throughout Chinese medical history: neither is truly meaningful without the other.

If this assessment is correct, then we must conclude that Li's *yang wei* pulse from the *Discussion on Cold Damage* is no more or less an extraordinary vessel pulse than the descriptions presented in the *Pulse Classic*. Both are irrelevant to the extraordinary vessels if they are not accompanied by their associated symptom presentation from one of the eight vessels.

Once we acknowledge the necessity of the relationship between the extraordinary vessel pulses and their respective symptom presentations, another set of questions presents itself. Must these pulses present exclusively with the symptoms described in the "Hand Diagram" or within the *Exposition* at large? If not, then how severe do these symptoms have to be? We have to wonder whether a patient must present with "lesser abdominal pain and counterflow qi that pierces the heart" when one feels a pill-like pulse in the distal positions, or whether a broader range of symptom presentations is possible. Certainly, anything that might be construed as a species of bulging (疝 *shan*) disorder would reasonably fall within the rubric of a *ren* vessel pattern, particularly if accompanied by a pill-like pulse in the distal position. But how much farther can one realistically take this rationale? Li leaves it to us to decide these matters for ourselves.

Conclusion

Both Wang and Li excerpt pulse-symptom complexes from the "Hand Diagram" and position them elsewhere within the flow of more general discussions of extraordinary vessel pathology. We have demonstrated that Li's *Exposition* is more than a laundry list of pertinent quotations punctuated by the occasional annotation. It is a carefully composed document that presents an integrated vision of extraordinary vessel physiology, pathology, and treatment. It is unlikely that Li means for us to interpret any single component of his treatise outside of the context of the whole. If this is correct, then we must infer that, for Li, a *ren* vessel pulse-symptom complex is determined by a pill-like pulse in the distal position presenting with any of the symptoms he has identified as pertaining to the *ren*, and so on.

In most cases, the nature of the extraordinary vessel pulses themselves reflects the presence of relatively deep-seated conditions so one would expect to see symptoms of a similar gravity. For instance, it is unlikely that an examiner would observe a truly tapping pulse in the absence of a significant confirming symptom presentation. As previously mentioned, although it is not a death pulse, this quality most definitely signals an ominous situation.

The pulses and symptoms in the *Exposition* must be considered together as basic units of information comprising an overall picture of extraordinary vessel function. Li blends them to further define the general landscape of extraordinary vessel pathology. They reflect a number of tacit assumptions concerning extraordinary vessel function, pathology, and treatment, and provide a means for understanding his integration of extraordinary vessel material from a wide range of sources.

Part IV

LEGACY OF
Exposition on the Eight Extraordinary Vessels

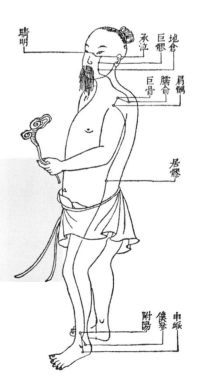

In Part IV, a selection of writings is presented that reflects the direct influence of Li Shi-Zhen's perspectives on the extraordinary vessels, ranging in time from the 17th century to the present. The writings illustrate how Li's ideas have been applied and expanded upon in the realms of acupuncture and herbal medicine, and even how they inform our understanding of the historical development of the extraordinary vessels in the realm of internal cultivation.

Along the Grand Thoroughfare: Luo Dong-Yi's Vision of Extraordinary Vessel Function

The relationship between original or source (*yuan* 原), primal *(yuan* 元), or essence *(jing* 精) qi and the extraordinary vessels has in recent years been the subject of some debate. Early Chinese medical sources describe the extraordinary vessels as functioning to absorb spillover from the primary channels and as broad regulators of yin and yang throughout the channel system as a whole. Neither of these roles requires the involvement of original/primal qi. Indeed, neither the *Inner Classic* nor the *Classic of Difficulties* makes any general statements regarding the relationship between original qi and extraordinary vessels. Still, the *Inner Classic* does discuss the role of the *chong* and *ren* vessels in the process of maturation and decline, another key function of these two vessels. This strongly suggests their involvement with some deeper, prenatal aspect of qi than what is generally at play in the rest of the channel system.

A closer look at the Chinese medical literature reveals that although source and essence qi figures more prominently in later discussions of extraordinary vessel function, these discourses are far from unanimous on the extent of this role. The essential acupuncture texts dealing with extraordinary vessel therapeutics, such as *An Acupuncture Hole Diagram Based on the Bronze Model, A Gathering of the Blossoms of Acupuncture*, and *Grand Compendium of Acupuncture and Moxibustion,* remain silent on the topic. Li Shi-Zhen's *Exposition on the Eight Extraordinary Vessels* is probably the first text to truly address this issue.

Using medical sources and texts drawn from internal alchemy, Li presents a nuanced, if not entirely consistent, vision in which original/primal qi figures more prominently in some extraordinary vessels than in others. Here, the *chong, ren*, and *du* are unambiguously involved in the regulation and transmission of original/primal qi, and the *wei* vessels regulate the protective and nutritive qi, apparently to the exclusion of any other type of qi. The *Exposition* is of two minds with regard to the *qiao* vessels. It presents the opinion expressed in Ch. 80 of *Divine Pivot,* that the *qiao* vessels facilitate the transmission of protective qi, and possibly even nutritive qi, between the interior and the exterior. In addition, it presents a principle drawn from the internal alchemical tradition that the extraordinary vessels are not generally open or available and must be actively cultivated prior to being utilized.

This is a testament to the esteem in which the extraordinary vessels were held in the internal alchemical traditions and to the precious nature of their contents. According to Li Shi-Zhen, the extraordinary vessels are the "root of the great way of former heaven, which is the ancestor of a Unitary Qi."[1] Curiously, this perspective on the cultivation of the extraordinary vessels requires that the *yin qiao* be 'opened' first. The arcane nature of this material leaves a great deal of room for interpretation.

For better or worse, Li Shi-Zhen left it largely to his readers to sort out the precise role of original/primal qi in the extraordinary vessels for themselves. A number of perspectives have been presented, and original/primal qi figures prominently among some of the most influential of these. Writing approximately one-hundred years after the publication of Li's *Exposition on the Eight Extraordinary Vessels*, Luo Dong-Yi presented what may be the most concise and unambiguous statement about the role of original qi in extraordinary vessel function in the medical literature. In his *Critical Interpretation of the Inner Classic (Nei jing bo yi* 內經博義, 1675), Luo describes the extraordinary vessels primarily in terms of their respective roles as mediators of primal qi. He envisions the eight vessels as strands of a single grand thoroughfare *(tai chong* 太衝) dedicated to the communication of original qi throughout the body. Although he is not generally remembered as an authority on extraordinary vessel physiodynamics, his short discussion is a valuable contribution to the evolution of ideas concerning the extraordinary vessels and therefore merits discussion.

The term 'grand thoroughfare' *(tai chong* 太衝) is typically accorded a rather narrow range of meaning in Chinese medicine. Although it has a number of philosophical and esoteric resonances, its modern medical usage is largely limited to the acupuncture hole LR-3 and to the descending trajectory of the *chong* vessel.[2]

In Luo Dong-Yi's interpretation, however, the grand thoroughfare has a much broader scope of meaning that varies with the context in which it is used. Few medical writers have been quite so explicit in stating the importance of the grand thoroughfare in any context, much less in terms of the extraordinary vessels.

One common theme in Luo's use of the term is that the grand thoroughfare is invariably associated with the transmission of prenatal qi. It is the medium by which the primal qi is communicated through the body from some external source. The direction of this transmission is always upward from below. The trajectory of the *chong* along the lower extremity is merely the most obvious expression of this function. However, the source literature describes the trajectory of this branch from the top down, as does Li Shi-Zhen. His discussion of the grand thoroughfare contains a variety of passages emphasizing its downward trajectory, culminating in the well-known passage from Ch. 38 of *Divine Pivot* that specifically addresses this question.

> [Ch. 38 of] *Divine Pivot* classic states: "The Yellow Emperor said: Only the lesser yin vessel travels downward, why is this?"
>
> Qi Bo said: It is not so. [It is not the lesser yin that goes downward, it is the *chong*]. The *chong* vessel is the sea of the five yin viscera and the six yang receptacles. ... Its upward [trajectory] emerges at the juncture of the hard and soft palates,[3] percolating into all the yang [channels] and irrigating the various essences. Its downward [trajectory] pours into the great network of

the lesser yin, arising below the kidneys to emerge at the qi thoroughfare. It continues along the posterior medial aspect of the thigh and obliquely enters the popliteal fossa. It then travels concealed along the medial aspect of the tibia to adhere to the lesser yin channel. From here it descends to penetrate behind the inner ankle and penetrate to the bottom of the foot. A diverging branch [of the network vessel] adheres to the lesser yin and percolates into the three yin, obliquely entering the ankle, and traveling concealed through the instep, it continues downward along the instep to enter into the big toe. From here it percolates into the network vessels and warms the flesh [of the foot], so therefore this vessel normally pulsates.[4]

This passage leaves little doubt that qi is supposed to flow out of the qi thoroughfare and down the leg. It is certainly consistent with the assumption that the wellspring of the *chong* vessel is in the womb, yet the overall flow of qi in the *chong* is unclear. The most definitive statement that can be made regarding this is that it counterflows upward when the vessel becomes diseased. Luo Dong-Yi effectively reverses the flow of qi in his 'grand thoroughfare,' at least as far as the transmission of primal qi is concerned. This is in itself less remarkable than the fact that he is so clear as to which way any type of qi should be traveling in the extraordinary vessels. Nutritive and protective qi may circulate through the extraordinary vessels in a tide-like manner in keeping with their function of regulating the primary channels and networks, but for Luo Dong-Yi, original qi flows uniformly upward through these vessels.

A translation of Luo's discussion of the extraordinary vessels is presented below. In this passage, Luo Dong-Yi explains that the grand thoroughfare may also be used as a collective term for the *chong*, *ren,* and *du* vessels. The *du* organizes the yang, the *ren* organizes the yin, and at the very core, the *chong* organizes the blood and all of the vessels. More importantly, the grand thoroughfare is a general term for the role of all of the extraordinary vessels in transmitting and regulating primordial qi, each of which does so in its own specific manner. So the grand thoroughfare may refer to the *chong,* the vessel that conveys primal qi upward to the root extraordinary vessel; it may refer to the triad of core extraordinary vessels; or it may refer to all of the extraordinary vessels.

According to Luo, the *dai* vessel organizes the vessels around the periphery. It functions like a lock that secures the essence qi and is rooted in the spine. The *wei* vessels maintain and preserve the yang throughout the body, but their proper function is dependent on a healthy abundance of qi. Luo delegates the role of regulating the nutritive qi to the *wei* and the protective qi to the *qiao*, establishing a much cleaner division of influence between them than the model presented by Li Shi-Zhen. With their greater emphasis on the organization and maintenance of nutritive and protective qi, the role of the primordial essence is less apparent in these peripheral extraordinary vessels. Both of these vessel pairs are closely affiliated with the network vessels, a stratum of the channel system not typically associated with original qi. According to Luo, even the name *qiao* suggests a quality of a vigorous upsurge of qi. With the obvious exception of the *dai* vessel, all the extraordinary vessels ascend from the 'lower pillars' (*xia zhu* 下柱), which most likely refers to the lower extremities.[5] The *dai* vessel has its own relationship with the essence qi. It fulfills the role of securing the essence as it is expressed in all of the extraordinary vessels. In Luo's view, the grand thoroughfare is an expression of the transmission of primordial essence through the body as an eight-fold unity.

Translation

奇經八脈原[6]

人身陰陽元氣皆起於下故內經以廣明之後即為太衝太衝之地屬之少陰
少陰之前乃為厥陰其部為血海常與太衝騰精氣而上灌滲陰陽斯則人之
元氣精氣皆起於下也而由下而起則分三道而上其陽者從少陰之後行太
陽夾脊之中道以總統諸陽其名為督其陰者由前陰地道而上行陽明之表
中以總統諸陰其名為任而中央一道則脈起血海騰精氣而上積於胸中為
宗氣以司呼吸其名為衝是氣則與陽明胃氣俱住中州亦與營俱行十二經
者也

On the Origins of the Extraordinary Vessels

The human body's yin, yang, and primal qi all arise from below. Therefore, the *Inner Classic* takes what is behind the vast brilliance as the grand thoroughfare. The ground of the grand thoroughfare pertains to the lesser yin. In front of the lesser yin is reverting yin, which is the location of the sea of blood. The essence qi invariably soars up along the grand thoroughfare and ascends to irrigate the yin and yang. Thus, a person's primal qi and essence qi all arise from below. Moreover, in arising from below, they divide into three pathways and ascend. Its yang [aspect] travels from behind the lesser yin, hugging the middle pathway of the spine with the greater yang to organize all of the yang, so it is called the governor. Its yin [aspect] travels from the location of the genitals, ascending in the middle of and along the exterior of the yang brightness [channels] to organize all of the yin, so it is called the *ren*. There is a pathway in the center, and this vessel arises from the sea of blood, and it conveys essence qi upward to accumulate in the chest, which is the ancestral qi that controls respiration. It is called the *chong*.

蓋嘗考之督脈起胞中上巔歷百會神庭任脈起中極之下胞中循關元歷承
漿上與督脈會衝脈起胞中上行伏臍會於咽喉三脈同起於下極一源而三
歧故聖人不日衝督任而總名日太衝是太衝者以一身之精氣上升言之不
獨為血海言之也。

One must consider that the *du* vessel arises from the gestational membranes and ascends to the vertex, passing through Hundred Convergences (GV-20) and Spirit Court (GV-24). The *ren* vessel arises from the gestational membranes below Central Pole (CV-3), and proceeds from the Origin Pass (CV-4) through to the Sauce Receptacle (CV-24), ascending to meet with the *du* vessel. The *chong* vessel arises from the womb and ascends, traveling hidden beneath the umbilicus to meet [the *ren*] at the throat. The three vessels together arise from the lower pole, having a single origin but three branches. Hence, the sages did not call them *chong*, *du*, and *ren*, but referred to them [collectively] as the grand thoroughfare. The name grand thoroughfare refers to the rising ascent of essence qi within the body and does not only mean the sea of blood.

中外之間橫者為帶脈帶脈橫於季脅統於章門五樞總束諸脈使上下有常
而要約營束之毋令懶散其脈如人束帶而前垂亦精氣關鎖也此處為脊
人之全力出焉脊力不衰殆為此也

Among those [vessels] peripheral to the center, the horizontal one is the *dai* vessel. The *dai* vessel moves horizontally to the lateral ribs to unite with Camphorwood Gate (LV-14) and Fifth Pivot (GB-27). Overall, it binds all of the vessels and promotes their normal ascent and descent. Its vessel is like a person's girding belt that hangs in front and also closes and locks the essence qi. This is located on the spine, and the entirety of a person's strength issues from here! That the spine is strong and not debilitated is nearly due to this [lock].

二維者維持維係之義人身陽脈統於督陰脈統於任矣而諸陽諸陰之散見
而會又有所必維係而持之故有陰維以維於諸陰陽維以維於諸陽

The two *wei* have the significance of preserving and holding together. The human body's yang vessels are organized by the *du*, and the yin vessels are organized by the *ren*, and all of the yin and all of the yang [networks] that are seen scattered throughout [the body] meet [at the *wei* and] must be held together and preserved. Therefore the *yin wei* holds together all the yin, and the *yang wei* holds together all the yang.

然而能為維者必從陰陽之根柢具盛氣之發而後能維陽維從少陰至太陽
發足太陽之金門而與手足少陽陽明五脈會於陽白陰維從少陰斜至厥陰
發足少陰之築賓至頂前而終少陰少陽為陰陽根足少陰之築賓至頂前而
終少陰少陽為陰陽根柢之氣維於陽者必從少陰以起之是陰為陽根也維
於陰者必從少陽而起之是陽為陰致也故二脈又為營氣之綱領焉

While they are able to hold together [the yin and yang], it is because they must be rooted deeply in the yin and yang. They are able to hold [these] together only once an abundance of qi is present. The *yang wei* travels from the lesser yin to reach the greater yang, issuing from the foot lesser yang's Metal Gate (BL-64), and along with the hand and foot lesser yang and yang brightness, these five vessels meet at Yang White (GB-14). The *yin wei* travels from the lesser yin obliquely to the terminal yin, issuing from the Guest House (KI-9) to arrive in front of the vertex and terminate.[7] The lesser yin and lesser yang are deeply rooted in the qi of the yin and yang. That the binding of the yang must arise from the lesser yin means that the yin is the root of the yang. That the binding of the yin must arise from the lesser yang means that the yang is the ultimate result of yin. Therefore, these two vessels also constitute the framework of the nutritive qi.

兩蹻脈者蹻以矯舉為義其脈之剽悍同於衛氣而皆上於目然有孔道與衛
不同其脈則陰出陽而交於足太陽陽入陰而交於足少陰其氣其行每從陰
陽根柢和合以為矯舉而上榮大會於目故目之瞑開皆宜

As for the two *qiao* vessels, *qiao* means vigorously uplifting. Its vessels are nimble and fearless like the protective qi, and they both ascend to the eye. However, their passageways differ from those of the protective qi. Its vessels issue from the yin to the yang and intersect at the foot greater yang, [and conversely enters] the yin from the yang to intersect at the foot lesser yin. Both the qi and trajectory of each [*qiao* vessel] is harmoniously grounded in the yin and yang to vigorously uplift and upwardly nourish in their grand meeting at the eye, and therefore the opening and closing of the eyes is normal.

其曰陰脈榮其臟陽脈榮其腑者入陰則榮臟入陽則榮腑也男女脈當其數
者男子陽用事其蹻在陽故男子數斷其陽女子陰用事其蹻在陰故女子數
斷其陰

In saying that the yin vessels nourish the viscera and the yang vessels nourish the receptacles, [this means that the qi] enters the yin [*qiao*] to nourish the viscera and enters the yang [*qiao*] to nourish the receptacles. Which vessel is counted depends on whether one is a male or a female. Because males have yang activity, their *qiao* vessel is the yang; thus, in males, one counts the yang [*qiao*]. Because females have yin activity, their *qiao* vessel is the yin; thus, in females, one counts the yin [*qiao*].

總之八脈唯帶脈橫束手脊而七脈皆自下柱而上雖有孔道宗眾會然當起
於太陽少陰則皆所謂太衝之義也故聖人止言太衝而不及督任維蹻蓋有
分之而不分者矣

Of all the eight vessels, only the *dai* vessel is horizontally bound to the spine, whereas the other seven vessels ascend from the lower pillars. Although their passageways have many meeting places, they nevertheless arise from the greater yang and lesser yin, and thus the term grand thoroughfare refers to them all. Therefore, the sages only used the word grand thoroughfare and did not bother with the *du, ren, wei,* and *qiao.* They have been divided and yet remain indivisible.

Conclusion

Luo Dong-Yi's use of the term *tai chong* suggests that the primal qi is not transmitted through the extraordinary vessels as part of a closed system. Original qi flows into the human organism as well as within it. As previously noted, the *tai chong* has been associated with primordial forces since at least its first known appearance in *Zhuang zi.* Here, the term was used in reference to Absolute Emptiness or Great Vastness.[8] This is the ground from which all things issue, and it is the state of consciousness that is capable of perceiving it. The *tai chong* evokes an agency that is the source of all things. There is literally nothing more original, more primordial, than this. In calling the extraordinary vessels *tai chong,* Luo Dong-Yi frames them as the embodied expression of fecund emptiness. From this perspective, the extraordinary vessels may be understood as reducing an agency of cosmic proportions down to a more human scale and of giving it a tangible and more immediately meaningful structure.

A central tenet of Luo's description of the grand thoroughfare of the extraordinary vessels is that it transmits its influence upward from below. Where Li Shi-Zhen's portrayal of the extraordinary vessel circulation is much more ambiguous in its overall directionality, suggesting something more akin to tidal forces, Luo Dong-Yi is very clear on the ascending vector of primal qi. Though this influence is cosmic in origin, it is transmitted not downward from heaven above, but upward from the earth. Insofar as original qi pervades all things, why must it be absorbed from any particular direction? An agency as potent as original qi must be further filtered through the earth for humans to properly assimilate it.

By linking all of the extraordinary vessels to primal qi, Luo also tacitly redefines their essential pathological expression as one of deficiency. In his view, the extraordinary vessels are the fundamental conduits of essence qi, which by definition, there can never be too much of. Such reasoning demands that extraordinary vessel pathologies are therefore necessarily defined by deficiencies. There are clear echoes of this perspective in the case histories of Ye Gui, arguably the most influential proponent of the extraordinary vessel theory of his time.[9] Ye Tian-Shi's *Case Records as a Guide to Clinical Practice,* dating 70 years after Luo's commentary, exhibits a lucid appreciation for the importance of essence qi in extraordinary vessel therapeutics. For Ye, a debilitation of essence qi is the defining characteristic of extraordinary vessel pathology. His case records are typified by his identification of multiple extraordinary vessel pathologies in complex symptom presentations. Moreover, Ye's most common extraordinary vessel diagnosis identifies a generalized pathology in all of the extraordinary vessels in which a debilitation of essence qi is a central component.

Ye Gui's herbal prescriptions are a concrete expression of Luo's observation that the extraordinary vessels "have been divided and yet remain indivisible," and that they are the primary conduits of essence qi in the channel system. Luo's vision of extraordinary vessel function may be understood as a transitional step between the positions staked out by Li Shi-Zhen and Ye Gui. It provides a crucial bit of clarity to the theoretical framework of the extraordinary vessels, and in doing so, it reframes extraordinary vessel pathologies as deficiency patterns.

CHAPTER 35

Ye Tian-Shi's Contributions to Extraordinary Vessel Therapeutics

The only other physician to approach Li Shi-Zhen's influence on the development of extraordinary vessel strategies in herbal medicine is the master clinician of the Qing dynasty, Ye Gui (葉桂), who is better known to physicians by his style name, Ye Tian-Shi (葉天士). Where Li Shi-Zhen formalized the theoretical basis for the application of the extraordinary vessels, Ye Gui demonstrated their potential in clinical practice. Drawing on a comprehensive understanding of the medical knowledge of his time, Ye used an impressive range of methods to treat extraordinary vessel disorders, always remaining flexible in his application of ideas and never limiting himself to a single therapeutic doctrine.

Biography

Ye Gui was born in Suzhou province in 1667 into a family of physicians. His style name was Tian-Shi and his nickname was Xiang-Yan (香岩). His grandfather, Ye Shi (葉時), and his father, Ye Chao-Cai (葉朝采), both practiced medicine. In early life, he studied the classics with a teacher while learning medicine from his father. After his father's death, when Ye was 13, he continued his medical studies with one of his father's disciples, quickly surpassing his teacher's knowledge. From the ages of 11 to 17, Ye is reported to have changed masters 17 times. He would discover who was skilled at treating a particular condition and then apprentice himself to that physician, moving on as soon as he had mastered that physician's methods. According to one of his biographers, it was the scope of his training that enabled him to make a name for himself.[1]

Ye became a scholar of Confucian learning who was also well-versed in the *Book of Changes,* and he applied this knowledge to his medical practice. Another of Ye's biographers praised Ye's diagnostic abilities and the fact that he "did not hold fixed opinions for treatment."[2] Ye himself was quite vocal in his criticism of physicians with a predilection for one method of practice, such as Liu Wan-Su's (劉完素) preference for cooling methods or Li Dong-Yuan's (李東垣) preference for nourishing the spleen and stomach rather than simply seeking to master a comprehensive body of knowledge. Although he was intimately familiar with the medical literature of the canons, Ye's genius was has ability to adapt ideas throughout medical history to the conditions of the time. According to Hua Xiu-Yun (華岫雲, 1679–1773), who wrote a preface to Ye's *Case Records as a Guide to Clinical Practice,* "Ye was able to alter the ancient methods, rounding them off with a centered compass, and transforming the newest ones, splitting [i.e., moderating] them with a centered square."[3]

Ye practiced medicine during a time when all physicians were seeking to elevate the status of their profession in the hopes of being considered Confucian scholars, as opposed to mercenary healers. In this, he was apparently quite successful, and his sons and grandsons, many of whom were physicians, also had official careers in the civil service. Ye Gui was a respected scholar as well as an adept physician. Notwithstanding Ye's quest for social legitimacy, he had at least one less than reputable pastime. Another of Ye's biographers, Wang You-Liang (王友亮 1741–1797), describes Ye as someone who was a skilled doctor but sought wealth through gambling, a preoccupation that apparently consumed much of his time. At least once, this passion caused him to arrive late to treat a patient who was in critical condition. Yet because Ye always managed to achieve miraculous cures, his name continued to be highly regarded even after his death.[4]

An Overview of Ye's Case Records

Following his death in the spring of 1746, a wide range of texts were published bearing Ye's name, yet there is no credible evidence that he produced even one medical text during his lifetime. When he wasn't gambling, Ye apparently devoted all his energies to practicing medicine and expressed little interest in writing about it. Physicians who claimed to be his followers compiled his case records, which were published under the title *Case Records as a Guide to Clinical Practice* about 20 years after Ye's death.

Like most case records of the time, *Case Records as a Guide to Clinical Practice* is written in a terse, telegraphic, almost short-hand style that developed out of the legal notation of 16th century China. It assumes that the reader is sufficiently conversant with the medical theories at play that he can follow the flow of ideas with little or no explanation as to what is transpiring. Consequently, the only data included in these case records is the information that most directly pertains to the point the author is trying to make. Almost nothing is spelled out for the reader, and it is up to him or her to make sense of the case. Despite the challenges the book posed for its readers, *Case Records as a Guide to Clinical Practice* was among the most popular medical texts of the Qing dynasty. The book was so popular that one contemporary physician voiced concern that medical students of the time were reading nothing but the *Case Records*, and that, failing to develop their skills with such classics as *Basic Questions*, *Divine Pivot*, and the *Discussion on Cold Damage*, they would "inevitably end up making serious mistakes."[5] Publishers during the Qing printed more editions of the *Case Records as a Guide to Clinical Practice* than any other text of its kind, attesting to its pervasive influence.

Ye's *Case Records* contains numerous accounts of illness treated from the perspective of the extraordinary vessels, and it provides some of the most extensive information available regarding how one master physician actually used the extraordinary vessels in clinical practice. Although clearly influenced by Li Shi-Zhen's perspectives on extraordinary vessel therapeutics, Ye integrated a wide range of ideas to produce a methodology uniquely his own. Zhang Jie-Bin's (張介賓, 1563–1640) emphasis on supporting kidney function is especially evident in Ye's prescriptions, although his approach to the extraordinary vessels is nothing if not versatile. In light of this, Ye Tian-Shi's contributions to extraordinary vessel therapeutics are every bit as significant as Li Shi-Zhen's.

Ye Tian-Shi's Case Records involving the Extraordinary Vessels

Ye extrapolated on the principles of extraordinary vessel prescriptions presented in *Exposition on the Eight Extraordinary Vessels*. In Li's book, the pivotal piece linking an extraordinary vessel to a treatment was its core set of pathodynamics, which were then further differentiated according to the specific pattern being expressed. Ye's case records subtly but significantly turn this equation around, first emphasizing the overall presenting pattern, and only then attending to the pathodynamics characteristic of each vessel. The ramifications of this conceptual shift were significant. It meant that Ye first attended to the extraordinary vessels as an integrated whole, asking himself, "How has the entire extraordinary vessel system become disordered?"

Far and away the most common extraordinary vessel diagnosis in Ye's *Case Records* is a generalized debilitation of the extraordinary vessels presenting as an obstruction in the free flow of qi and blood. For Ye, the eight vessels were an integrated package, often best conceptualized and treated as a functional unit. Such a perspective is reminiscent of Luo Dong-Yi's (羅東逸) model of the extraordinary vessels as the "grand thoroughfare" of primal qi, described in the previous chapter. When Ye describes a patient's situation in this manner, he is invariably referring to an overall weakening of their kidney, source, and essence qi with at least some background stagnation.

To be sure, Ye also identified diseases in a single extraordinary vessel and treated them independently of the others. As already noted, he was particularly fond of diagnosing certain types of insomnia as an insufficiency of the *yang qiao*. More often than not, however, his case records identify pathologies in multiple extraordinary vessels. Consistent with the methodology established by Li Shi-Zhen, it was not uncommon for Ye to identify an extraordinary vessel pathology based on the presentation of a single key symptom representative of its overall pathodynamic. Ye took this principle a step further, mixing and matching these as he saw fit. In a single case history, he identified chills and fever as a *yang wei* pathology, heart pain as a disease of the *yin wei*, and counterflow presenting as nausea accompanied by abdominal masses as a disorder of the *chong* vessel. Nevertheless, his differentiation of extraordinary vessel pathology according to each of the eight vessels still occurred in the larger context of the extraordinary vessels as a unified "grand thoroughfare" of qi.

In determining precisely how the eight-vessel system had become disordered, Ye would typically frame his diagnosis in terms of some sort of imbalance in the viscera or receptacles. He then finely tuned his treatment strategies to the specifics of the presentation. The range of approaches Ye brought to treating extraordinary vessel disorders is evident in the *Case Records'* summary of treatment strategies for wilting *(wei 痿)*.

> 無一定之法。用方無獨執之見。如衝任虛寒而成痿者。通陽攝陰。兼實奇脈為主。

One cannot use a fixed methodology, and in the use of formulas, one cannot latch onto a single opinion. ... For instance, when there is deficiency cold in the *chong* and *ren* producing wilting, the main strategy is to open the yang and absorb the yin, while simultaneously replenishing the extraordinary vessels.

> 腎陽奇脈兼虛者。用通納八脈。收拾散越之陰陽為主。

When the kidney yang and the extraordinary vessels are both deficient, the main strategy is to open and nourish the eight vessels, while repairing and disseminating the yin and yang.

> 胃陽腎督皆虛者。兩固中下為主。

When the stomach yang, kidney, and *du* are all deficient, the main strategy is to jointly secure both the middle and lower [burners].

> 奇脈入絡而成痿者。以解毒宣行為主。精血內奪。奇脈少氣而成痿者。以填補精髓為主。

When [a disease of] the extraordinary vessels enters the networks producing wilting, the main strategy is to resolve toxicity, [and] diffuse and circulate [the qi and blood]. When there is an internal deprivation of essence and blood and a lack of qi in the extraordinary vessels producing wilting, the primary strategy is to replenish and tonify the essence and marrow.[6]

If extraordinary vessel pathologies can be modeled in such a wide variety of patterns, then this once again raises the question of how useful it really is to think in terms of the extraordinary vessels in prescribing herbs. In his attention to the broader pathodynamics involved in extraordinary vessel disorders, Ye identified a few commonalities in extraordinary vessel patterns. He recognized that these problems often occur in the context of a deep debilitation compounded by stasis in the network vessels. Ye's attention to opening *(tong 通)* the eight vessels is a hallmark of his therapeutic approach. In this, Ye added a further criterion to the core pathodynamics used by Li Shi-Zhen to identify extraordinary vessel pathologies.

Ye's approach to treatment therefore strongly emphasized the tonification of the liver and kidneys, and the replenishment of essence, while simultaneously opening the networks. Toward this end, his case records rely heavily on animal products, which he understood as providing the deepest level of nourishment necessary to influence the extraordinary vessels. Although they are not present in all of his case records concerning the eight vessels, Ye's use of animal products is another defining characteristic of his extraordinary vessel therapeutics.

Most of Ye Gui's extraordinary vessel case records contain at least one essence-enriching animal product, though they are integrated into a wide range of treatment strategies, all of which include a component of opening. In this, he shared Li Shi-Zhen's appreciation for the myriad ways in which extraordinary vessel disorders might present themselves. Among the methods he favored for treating the extraordinary vessels were astringing the essence, warming and opening the yang, using shells to restrain the yang, and transforming phlegm, again to open the yang.

Ye sometimes employed a two-phased approach in his extraordinary vessel prescriptions, first clearing away pathogenic factors, and then directly tonifying the underlying deficiencies. This strategy is particularly evident in his treatment of insomnia due to an obstruction of the *yang qiao*. A more thorough description of this mechanism of disease and Ye's approach to treating it appears in Appendix IX below.

Subsequent editors and commentators have collated the drugs Ye used in treating extraordinary vessel pathologies into lists linking individual drugs with each of the eight vessels. Though a convenient reference, lists such as these obscure the fact that Ye's prescriptions are defined by the precision with which he matched his treatment strategies to the presenting pattern, and not by his use of individual herbs. Nevertheless, Ye's methodology has gradually fostered an increased emphasis on individual drugs in extraordinary vessel prescriptions that continues today.

The case records that follow illustrate the salient aspects of Ye's approach to extraordinary vessel treatment. Given the terse style in which they were written, we have edited our translations for clarity and style.

Ye Directly Adopted Li's Methodology

There are a few instances in which Ye simply recapitulated the formulas prescribed by Li Shi-Zhen for extraordinary vessel treatment, testifying to his familiarity with Li's work. The following case record by Ye could have been written by Li himself.

> 陳（二八）寒熱時作。經歲不瘥。且產後病起。陽維為病明矣。（陽維病寒熱）歸桂枝湯。

> Chen (28 years of age) suffered from intermittent chills and fever. The condition had persisted for years and she still had not recovered. Moreover, the present illness had originated after giving birth. The *yang wei* was clearly diseased. (*Yang wei* diseases are characterized by fever and chills.) The patient was given Cinnamon Twig Decoction *(gui zhi tang)*.

Adapting Li's Principles to the Presenting Condition

Even when he cleaved closely to the formulas advocated by Li Shi-Zhen, Ye Tian-Shi adapted his treatment strategy to more effectively accommodate the underlying deficiencies he believed were at the root of all extraordinary vessel pathologies. Where Li's discussions of *wei* vessel disharmonies are concerned only with the regulation of the protective and nutritive qi, in the following case, Ye acknowledges that these imbalances may arise out of a deeper insufficiency of the kidney and lung yin.

> 經云：陽維為病苦寒熱，陰維為病苦心痛。此陰陽營衛之偏虛也。擬黃芪建中法，和中臟之陰陽而調營衛。復合生脈保肺之陰，復脈保腎之陰。通盤合局，頭頭是道矣。

The *Classic* states, "When the *yang wei* is diseased, [the patient] suffers from chills and fever; when the *yin wei* is diseased, [the patient] suffers from heart pain." This reflects a tendency toward deficiency of the yin and yang, nutritive and protective. The goal was to administer methods such as Astragalus Decoction to Construct the Middle *(huang qi jian zhong tang)* to harmonize the yin and yang of the viscera and to regulate the nutritive and protective qi. This [formula] was combined with Generate the Pulse [Powder] *(sheng mai san)* to protect the lung yin and Restore the Pulse Decoction *(fu mai tang)* to protect the kidney yin, thereby establishing a comprehensive treatment plan.[7]

Supplementing the Essence and Marrow with Animal Products

While the previous case acknowledged the role of kidney deficiency in many of Ye's extraordinary vessel cases, it relies entirely on plant-based drugs for tonification. Although plant materials such as Ginseng Radix *(ren shen)*, Cuscutae Semen *(tu si zi)*, and Eucommiae Cortex *(du zhong)* are pervasive in Ye's extraordinary vessel cases, he commonly includes at least one animal product in each of his prescriptions in recognition of the affinity these drugs have for the eight vessels. The following case highlights the strategy of replenishing the essence marrow using animal products. The formula contains Ox Bone Marrow *(niu gu sui)*, Goat Bone Marrow *(yang gu sui)*, and Pig Bone Marrow *(zhu gu sui)*, all of which act to directly open the *du* vessel. These substances are also considered gentle yang drugs, which are more appropriate for tonification than harsh, warming drugs such as Cinnamomi Ramulus *(gui zhi)* and Aconiti Radix *(fu zi)* that directly activate the yang.

> 王（二二）此少壯精氣未旺。致奇脈網維失護。經云。形不足者。溫之以氣。精不足者。補之以味。今納谷如昔。當以血肉充養。（陰虛）牛骨髓羊骨髓豬骨髓茯神枸杞當歸湖蓮芡實．

Wang (22 years of age), the essence qi in this young and vigorous man had yet to flourish. Therefore, the overall binding functions of the extraordinary vessels lost their protective capacity. The *Classic* states, when the body is weakened, then warm it by means of qi [tonics]. When the essence is insufficient, tonify it by means of [the five] flavors. Today we still nourish the grain [qi] as in the past. By means of [medicinals comprised of] blood and flesh, one should replenish and nourish [the qi]. (This was a case of yin deficiency.)

Ox Bone Marrow *(niu gu sui)*, Ovis Capris Marrow *(yang gu sui)*, Pig Bone Marrow *(zhu gu sui)*, Poria Sclerotium paradicis *(fu shen)*, Lycii Fructus *(gou qi zi)*, Angelica sinensis Radix *(dang gui)*, Coptidis Rhizoma *(huang lian)*, and Euralyes Semen *(qian shi).*[8]

Simultaneously Treating All the Extraordinary Vessels

As the previous case demonstrates, Ye Gui's attention to systemic weakness in the extraordinary vessels is evident in many of his case records. This theme continues in the following case records where Ye again makes use of gentler yang tonics to replenish the extraordinary vessels.

郭（二四）產後下元陰分先傷。而奇經八脈。皆麗于下。肝腎怯不固。八脈咸失職司。經旨謂陽維脈痛。苦寒熱。陰維脈病。苦心痛。下損及胃。食物日減。然產傷先傷真陰。忌用桂附之剛。溫煦陰中之陽。能入奇經者宜之。（下損及胃奇脈虛）人參鹿茸紫石英當歸補骨脂茯苓

Guo (24 years of age). After giving birth, the yin aspect of the lower origin first became damaged and the eight extraordinary vessels have all collapsed in the lower [warmer]. Hence, the liver and kidneys were weak and insecure. The eight vessels had lost their controlling duties. When it speaks of *yang wei* vessel disease, the *Classic* means that [the patient] suffers from chills and fever. When the *yin wei* vessel becomes diseased, one suffers from heart pain. The detriment in the lower [warmer] extended to the stomach, and the patient's food intake diminished daily. Although the damage from childbirth initially damaged the true yin, and harsh medicinals such as Cinnamon Ramulus *(gui zhi)* and Aconiti Radix *(fu zi)* were to be avoided, it was nevertheless appropriate to warm the yang within yin [with medicinals] capable of entering the extraordinary vessels. (Lower detriment extending to the stomach means that there is an extraordinary vessel deficiency.)

Ginseng Radix *(ren shen)*, Cervi Cornu pantotrichum *(lu rong)*, Fluoritum *(zi shi ying)*, Angelica sinensis *(dang gui)*, Psoralea Fructus *(bu gu zhi)*, and Poria *(fu ling).*[9]

某（二十）少壯形神憔悴。身體前後牽掣不舒。此奇經脈海乏氣。少
陰腎病何疑。淡蓯蓉甘枸杞當歸牛膝沙苑茯苓

A certain 20-year-old young and robust man was weak in spirit, and his
entire body, front and back, was tense and not at ease. This was a case of the
tiring of the qi in the sea of the extraordinary vessels. Could there be any
doubt that this was a lesser yin kidney disease?

Cistanches Herba (*rou cong rong*), Lycii Fructus (*gou qi zi*), Angelica sinensis Semen (*dang gui*), Achyranthes bidentatae Radix (*niu xi*), Astragali
complanati Semen (*sha yuan zi*), and Poria (*fu ling*).[10]

Treating the Extraordinary Vessels by Astringing the Essence

Seminal emission is an obvious expression of a loss of kidney essence. In the following
case, the patient's persistent seminal emission debilitated the yin, impairing the *yang
qiao*, which in turn produced insomnia. For Ye, this was a case of heart and kidney yin
insufficiency and an empty *yang qiao* vessel. Li's discussion of the *yang qiao* acknowledges the possibility that this vessel may be pathologically empty, despite the fact that
the only formula he recommends treats insomnia due to phlegm congestion, suggesting the *yang qiao* was in this case pathologically full. In this and many other case records, Ye believes that the *yang qiao* is deficient and focuses entirely on supplementing
and astringing.

胡，遺精四年。精關久滑不固。陰久傷。陽氣不入陽蹺。夜晴不寐。
前以鎮攝小效。獨心中徵悸不已，以桑螵蛸散。從心腎治。

Mr. Hu had suffered from seminal emission for four years. His essence was
chronically loose and insecure. When the yin becomes chronically damaged, the yang qi is unable to enter the *yang qiao* vessels. At night, he could
not sleep. Previous prescriptions to promote calming and containment
were of little effect. His only other symptom was incessant palpitations. He
was given Mantis Egg-Case Powder (*sang piao xiao san*) to treat the heart
and kidneys.[11]

Sleep disturbance is the key indicator of a *yang qiao* disease. In the following case, Ye
conceptualizes seminal emission in terms of the *ren* and *du*. Plant-based tonification is
insufficient to influence the extraordinary vessels. Animal products are needed to get
the job done.

任脈、督脈，分行乎身之前後，自覺熱蒸，不夢自遺，皆奇經虛也。
辛濕藥頗效。六味加五味於不應

The *ren* vessel and *du* vessel divide and travel to the anterior and posterior aspects of the body. The spontaneous appearance of a steaming fever and spontaneous [seminal] emissions without dreams indicate that all of these extraordinary channels are deficient. Acrid, moistening herbs are quite effective. Administration of Six-Ingredient Pill with Rehmannia *(liu wei di huang wan)* with the addition of Schizandrae Fructus *(wu wei zi)* was inappropriate.

方藥僅僅達下，未能約束奇經，議用聚精固攝之法。

The medicinals in this prescription would simply run through the patient [presumably causing diarrhea] and so would be unable to control the extraordinary vessels. Hence, the plan was to use methods of accumulating the essence, and securing it.

桑嫖峭，龜板，芡實，刺蒺藜線魚膠，胡連龍骨，金櫻子，覆盆子

Mantidis Oötheca *(sāng piāo xiāo)*, Testudinis Plastrum *(guī bǎn)*, Euryales Semen *(qiàn shí)*, Tribuli Fructus *(cì jí lí)*, Piscis Vesica Aeris Colla *(xiàn yú jiāo)*, Coptidis Rhizoma *(huang lian)*, Fossilia Ossis Mastodi *(long gu)*, Rosae laevigatae Fructus *(jin ying zi)*, Rubi Fructus *(fu pen zi)*.[12]

Treating the Extraordinary Vessels by Opening the Yang

Li Shi-Zhen's discussion of the diseases of the *du* vessel is one of the rare places in the *Exposition* where he discusses treatment in terms of individual drugs. The drugs associated by Li with the *du* resolve obstructions primarily by expelling wind and secondarily by opening the yang. Ye again modifies this strategy by emphasizing the use of harsh drugs that vigorously open the yang. The animal products so prevalent in other case records involving the *du* vessel are absent here. The issue is not fundamentally one of deficiency, but of stagnant cold impairing kidney function and obstructing the yang along the trajectory of the *du* vessel. Consequently, such conditions require mobilization as opposed to tonification.

孫（二四）腎氣攻背項強。溺頻且多。督脈不攝。腰重頭疼。難以轉側。先與通陽。川椒（炒出汗三分）川桂枝（一錢）川附子（一錢）茯苓（一錢半）生白朮（一錢）生遠志（一錢）

Sun (24 years of age). The kidney qi attacks the spine causing rigidity of the neck and frequent urination. The *du* vessel is not absorbing so that the low back is heavy, the head is sore, and it is difficult to turn sideways. First, open the yang.

Zanthoxyli Pericarpium *(hua jiao)* (blast fried until it sweats), 3 *fen*,

Cinnamomi Ramulus *(gui zhi)*, 1 *qian*, Aconiti Radix lateralis preparata *(zhi fu zi)*, 1 *qian*, Poria *(fu ling)* 1.5 *qian*, unprepared Atractylodis macrocephalae Rhizoma *(bai zhu)*, 1 *qian*, and unprepared Polygalae Radix *(yuan zhi)*, 1 *qian*.[13]

In the next case involving a *yang wei* disorder presenting as rib side pain radiating to the low back and hip, the supple, warm, essence-nourishing Cervi Cornu degelatinatum *(lu jiao shuang)* is added to the primary treatment method of opening the yang to harmonize the networks. In general, the drugs in this prescription enter the liver and kidney channels while Cinnamomi Ramulus *(gui zhi)* opens the yang qi in the foot greater yang.

唐（嶇）右後脅痛連腰胯。發必惡寒逆冷。暖護良久乃溫。此脈絡中氣血不行。遂至凝塞為痛。乃脈絡之痹症。從陽維陰維論病

The case of Tang: Right, posterior rib pain radiating to the low back and hip producing aversion to cold and icy-cold extremities. [The patient was so cold that] it took a long time to get the patient warm. This was a lack of movement of qi and blood within the vessels and networks, culminating in congealed cold producing pain that was an obstruction pattern of the vessels and networks and is understood in the context of a *yang wei* and *yin wei* disease.

鹿角霜，小茴香，當歸，川桂枝，沙苑，茯苓

Cervi Cornu degelatinatum *(lu jiao shuang)*, Foeniculi Fructus *(xiao hui xiang)*, Angelica sinensis Radix *(dang gui)*, Cinnamomi Ramulus *(gui zhi)* from Sichuan, Astragali complanati Semen *(sha yuan zi)*, and Poria *(fu ling)*.[14]

Using Shells to Restrain the Yang in Extraordinary Vessel Therapies

In addition to providing the deep fortification necessary to influence the extraordinary vessels, animal products may contribute to an overall treatment strategy in a variety of other ways. Testudinus Plastrum *(gui ban)*, a drug of choice for Ye when yin enrichment and essence nourishment is indicated in extraordinary vessel therapy, also restrains the yang, addressing two interrelated aspects of a common disease presentation. This effect is amplified by the addition of Mytillae crassitesta Herba *(dan cai)*, as illustrated in the following case record.

田臟液內耗。心腹熱灼。陽氣不交于陰。陽蹺穴空。令人寤不成寐。靈樞有半夏秫米法。但此病乃損及肝腎。欲求陽和。須介屬之鹹。佐以酸收甘緩。庶幾近理。（肝腎陰虧陽浮）龜膠淡菜熟地黃柏茯苓萸肉五味遠志

Mr. Tian suffered from an internal consumption of visceral fluids and burning epigastric heat. The yang qi was unable to communicate with the yin. The *yang qiao* holes were empty, causing him to be wakeful and unable to get to sleep. *Divine Pivot* contains the treatment method of Pinellia and Millet Decoction *(ban xia shu mi tang)*, however in this disease, the detriment had reached the liver and kidney so the plan was to rescue and harmonize the yang with the use of salty shells, assisted by sour, restraining and sweet, relaxing [medicinals]. This is the proper way to approach such a condition. (The liver and kidney yin were depleted and the yang was floating [upward].)

Testudinus Plastri Colla *(gui ban jiao)*, Mytillae crassitesta Herba *(dan cai)*, Rehmannia Radix preparatae *(shu di huang)*, Phellodendri Cortex *(huang bai)*, Poria *(fu ling)*, Corni Fructus *(shan zhu yu)*, Schizandrae Fructus *(wu wei zi)*, and Astragali complanati Semen *(yuan zhi)*.

又咸苦酸收已效。下焦液枯。須填實肝腎。龜鹿膠熟地蓯蓉天冬萸肉五味茯苓羊內腎

While the salty, bitter, sour, restraining [medicinals] proved effective, the fluids in the lower warmer were still desiccated. It was necessary to replenish the liver and kidneys.

Testudinus Plastri Colla *(gui ban jiao)*, Rehmannia Radix preparatae *(shu di huang)*, Cistanches Herba *(rou cong rong)*, Asparagi Radix *(tian men dong)*, Corni Fructus *(shan zhu yu)*, Scheizandrae fructus *(wu wei zi)*, Poria *(fu ling)*, Ovis Capris Kidney *(Yang nei shen)* 羊內腎.

[The anthologist's comment explains:] This case makes use of shells to restrain the yang. The *yang qiao* fails to communicate with the yin so the patient is wakeful and cannot sleep. It makes use of Testudinus Plastri Colla *(gui ban jiao)* and Mytillae crassitesta Herba *(dan cai)* to boost the yin, Rehmannia Radix preparatae *(shu di huang)* and Corni Fructus *(shan zhu yu)* to bank and boost the liver and kidney, Phellodendri Cortex *(huang bai)* to drain kidney fire, and all of these primarily treat the kidneys.[15]

Treating the Extraordinary Vessels by Eliminating Qi Constraint and Blood Stasis

As already mentioned, the concept of opening the eight vessels was central to Ye's understanding of them. In some cases they may have an almost purely excessive presentation. In the following case record, the counterflow manifesting as nausea, vomiting, and obstructions in the throat is all a result of amassment in the abdomen. Even so, the largest ingredient in the formula is Trionycis Carapax *(bie jia)*, which, in addition to resolving accumulations, substantially tonifies the yin. Here Ye identifies the patient's chills and fever as an indicator of *yang wei* involvement and epigastric pain as a symptom of *yin wei* involvement.

> 鈕（吉安州，三十五歲）保和丸女科肝病為多，產後必病及八脈，即
> 如少腹瘕聚，衝氣攻心，必嘔吐。逆上則喉間閉塞，經水半年不來，
> 越日常有寒熱。凡下焦多屬血病，症屬氣聚，瘕為血痹。病在衝脈，
> 陰維陽維混混施治，焉得入奇經。

Mrs. Niu (from Ji An province , age 35). Liver diseases are the most common disorders in gynecology, and postpartum diseases invariably involve the eight vessels. If there are concretions and amassments in the lateral lower abdomen, qi may surge to attack the heart, which will inevitably cause nausea and retching. [In this case,] a counterflow ascent of qi resulted in throat obstructions. The patient's menses had not arrived for a year-and-a-half [after giving birth] and she experienced daily chills and fever. [Diseases] of the lower burner are most commonly blood diseases, and this illness was a concretion of qi and an amassment, producing blood obstruction. When a disease is mingled within the *chong* vessel, *yin wei*, and *yang wei* [vessels], how [can a physician guide one's medicine] into the extraordinary vessels?

> 地鱉蟲（一兩）延胡（一兩）山楂（一兩）桃仁（五錢）莪術（五
> 錢）金鈴子（五錢）麝香（三錢）供為末，用青鱉甲（五六兩），祛
> 衣搗碎，用無灰酒煮汁一杯，和前藥末為丸，每服二錢，益母草湯送
> 下．

Eupolyphaga/Steleophaga *(tu bie chong)*, 1 *liang*, Corydalis Rhizoma *(yan hu suo)*, 1 *liang*, Cratagae Fructus *(shan zha)*, 1 *liang*, Persicae Semen *(tao ren)*, 5 *qian*, Curcumae Rhizoma *(e zhu)*, 5 *qian*, Toosendan Fructus *(jin ling zi)*, 5 *qian*, [and] Moschus *(she xiang)*, 3 *qian*. All of the above [medicinals] were ground into powder. The shell was then removed from an immature turtle (Trionycis *bie jia)*, 5-6 *liang*, and pounded into pieces and cooked with wine down to one cup of liquid. This was used as a binder to make pills from the above powder. Two *qian* were administered each time along with a decoction of Leonuri Herba *(yi mu cao)*.[16]

In this final case record, Ye treats a patient with constrained heat impairing the extraordinary vessels and the lower burner exclusively by dredging the qi in the upper burner.

> 吳（氏）氣血鬱痹。久乃化熱。女科八脈失調。漸有經阻瘕帶諸疾。
> 但先治其上。勿滋膩氣機。（鬱熱先清上焦）黑山梔皮炒黃川貝枇杷
> 葉栝蔞皮杏仁鬱金橘紅

Wu suffered from constrained impediment of qi and blood that over time transformed into heat. In gynecology, when the eight vessels become unregulated, this gradually produces all sorts of diseases such as menstrual obstructions, amassments, and leukorrhea. However, one must first treat the [upper burner] and not administer enriching, cloying [drugs that congest] the qi mechanism. (When there is constrained heat, first clear the upper burner.)

Charred Gradenia Fructus Peel (*zhi shan zi pi*), dry-fried until yellow Fritillariae cirrhosae Bulbus (*chuan bei mu*), Eriobotryae Folium *(pi pa ye)*, Trichosanthis Pericarpium *(gua lou pi)*, Armeniacae Semen amarum *(xing ren)*, Curcumae Radix *(yu jin)*, and Citri reticulatae Exocarpium rubrum *(ju hong)*.[17]

Conclusion

Ye Tian-Shi's case records are among the clearest examples of how subsequent physicians actually made use of the extraordinary vessels in clinical practice. His approach to extraordinary vessel herbal prescriptions integrates the ideas of both Li Shi-Zhen and Luo Dong-Yi even as it represents a perspective unique to himself. This, along with his emphasis on the use of animal products, established a major current in modern extraordinary vessel therapeutics.

CHAPTER 36

Shen Jin-Ao's Contributions to Extraordinary Vessel Therapeutics

At around the same time that Ye Tian-Shi was taking Li Shi-Zhen's perspective on the herbal treatment of the extraordinary vessels in entirely new directions, Shen Jin-Ao (沉金鰲) was consolidating Li's approach. Extrapolating on Li's fundamental therapeutic methods yet never straying too far from them, Shen helped to expand the range of established herbal formulas associated with the extraordinary vessels. Although Ye Tian-Shi's case records place him on equal footing with Li Shi-Zhen in terms of their contributions to extraordinary vessel therapeutics, Shen is in many ways the true heir of Li's thought. As a logical extension of Li's ideas, Shen Jin-Ao's writings on the extraordinary vessels hint at how Li might have developed them himself.

Shen Jin-Ao's courtesy name was Qian-Lu (芊綠), and his nickname was Ji-Men (汲門). He was born in 1717 in the city of Wuxi in Jiangsu province, and died in 1776 at the age of 59. He also went by the name Life-Worshiping Old Man (Zun Sheng Lao Ren 尊生老人).

As a young man, Shen devoted himself to Confucian studies. Like many people who became physicians in the latter half of Chinese history, he never passed his civil examinations, although he received an excellent education. Nevertheless, before taking up the practice of medicine at age 40, he produced collections of poems, annotated Confucian classics, and compiled books on history. He practiced medicine for 19 years during which time he published seven books.[1] These include *Systematic Classifications of Pulse Images (Mai xiang tong lei* 脈象統類), *Verses on All Pulses and Their Disease Indications (Zhu mai zhu bing shi* 諸脈主病詩), *Wondrous Lantern for Peering into the Origin and Development of Miscellaneous Diseases (Za bing yuan liu xi zhu* 雜病源流犀燭), *The Comprehensive Outline of Cold Damage (Shang han lun gang mu* 傷寒論網目), *Explanation of the Puzzles of Pediatrics (You ke shi mi* 幼科釋謎), *Jade Ruler* of *Gynecology (Fu ke yu chi* 婦科玉尺), and *On Essential Medicines and Discriminating Prescriptions (Yao yao fen ji* 要藥分劑).

Three of these works made significant contributions to the Chinese medical literature. Shen's *Systematic Classifications of Pulse Images* is a brief, and as the name suggests, systematic text that subdivides the 27 pulses into six categories. His *Verses on All Pulses and Their Disease Indications* is based on Li Shi-Zhen's *Pulse Studies of the Lakeside Recluse (Bin hu mai xue* 瀕湖脈學), and its well-crafted poetic prose facilitates memorization. Finally, Shen's *Wondrous Lantern for Peering into the Origin and Development of Miscellaneous Diseases* is his magnum opus. Quoting from 82 medical classics, it discusses the conceptual development of 92 miscellaneous diseases *(za bing*

雜病). This work showcases the depth of Shen's knowledge of the medical classics and his capacity for making sense of complex pathological concepts. All seven of his writings were published together in 1775, which subsequently obscured the original publication dates of the individual texts.

Shen presents his extraordinary vessel material in a crisp style consistent with his other medical writing. In volume 11 of *Wonderous Lantern for Peering into the Origins of Various Diseases (Za bing yuan liu xi zhu* 雜病源流犀燭, 1773), titled "On The Eight Extraordinary Vessels," he discusses each of the eight vessels, presenting their origins in the classics, trajectories, clinical indications, and the herbal formulas associated with them. Unfortunately, he published no case records, but instead focused entirely on theoretical concerns, leaving later generations with little sense of how he might have actually made use of his ideas in practice.

Like Li Shi-Zhen, Shen Jin-Ao's treatment strategies are based primarily on formulas directly linked to the core mechanisms and symptoms of each vessel. Shen references all of the formulas in Li's *Exposition on the Eight Extraordinary Vessels*, listing ingredients and methods of preparation, and often commenting on their relevance to extraordinary vessel treatment. Yet it must be said that Shen's insights into extraordinary vessel therapeutics seem to focus more strongly on some areas than on others. He adds nothing to Li's original list of formulas for the *wei* and *qiao* vessels, but expounds at length on bulging disorders as expressions of *ren* vessel pathologies.

Additional Formulas for the Various Vessels

Shen's herbal contributions begin with the five new formulas he attributes to the *dai* vessel. These are summarized as follows: Clove and Persimmon Pill for Spleen Accumulation *(ding xiang pi ji wan)*, Root-Invigorating Elixir *(zhuang ben dan)*, Secretly Transmitted Evodia Powder to Dissolve Internal Accumulation *(mi chuan wu zhu nei xiao san)*, Modified Dragon Tiger Decoction *(jia wei long hu tang)*, and Fast-Acting Powder *(su xiao san)*.

Shen Jin-Ao adds four formulas to the 11 herbs that Li associates with *du* vessel disorders: Liquid Styrax Pill *(su he xiang wan)*, Patchouli/Agastache Powder to Rectify the Qi *(huo xiang zheng qi san)*, Chuanxiong Powder to Be Taken with Green Tea *(chuan xiong cha tiao san)*, and Angelica Pill *(bai zhi wan)*.

Shen apparently had either an intense fascination or extensive experience with bulging disorders and their relationship to the *ren* vessel. Where Li Shi-Zhen lists no formulas for the *ren* vessel, Shen posits 41 possible patterns and prescriptions.[2] Three of these are indicated for *ren* vessel disorders in general, and 37 are for bulging disorders of one sort or another.

Shen suggests four formulas for general disorders of the *ren* vessel, all of which also treat bulging syndromes. These include Elixir to Seize Destiny *(duo ming dan)*, One Pinch of Gold Powder *(yi nie jin san)*, Aucklandiae Radix Powder to Smooth the Flow of Qi *(mu xiang shun qi san)*, and Harmonize the Qi Decoction *(he qi tang)*.

In addition to his attention to herbal medicine, Shen Jin-Ao also stressed the importance of acupuncture and 'pulling and drawing' exercises *(dao yin* 導引*)*. This latter interest is reminiscent of Li Shi-Zhen's attention to internal alchemy, although it is unclear how deeply Shen was actually involved in Daoist practices per se. Be that as it may, there are striking similarities in the messages Li and Shen drew from their respective material. In quoting the longevity text *The Secret Essentials of Preserving Life (bao sheng mi yao* 保生秘要*)*, Shen expresses two of the central themes developed by Li in his *Exposition*.

> The origin of all illness is stagnation of qi. Beyond using medicinal herbs, [one must also] include longevity practice *(tiao yang* 調養*)* so that one can eliminate [illness] and prolong one's life. Did not the ancient [sages] say that the path of medicine leads to the path of immortality, which is part of longevity practice, by training [one's] qi and body in order to transform them into spirit? The first volume of *Basic Questions* also states that [being] tranquil, cheerful, and without cares[3] contains the spirit inside and [that being] replete with quiet meditation harmonizes and nourishes the true spirit.

The majority of the extraordinary vessel patterns discussed in the *Exposition* involve a significant component of excess or stagnation. As already noted, this is a perspective that goes back at least as far as the *Classic of Difficulties*. Li recognized that some element of deficiency generally lies beneath such stagnation, and this is evident in his choice of herbal formulas. The passage above reflects an attention to stagnation consistent with Li's understanding of extraordinary vessel pathology. Although this paragraph fails to acknowledge this crucial aspect of deficiency, it is evident in Shen's choice of herbal formulas, just as it is in Li's use of herbal medicines.

This passage is remarkable in that it once again acknowledges that the primary means for remedying disease is grounded in quietude. Activity in the form of exercise or activation in the form of internal cultivation or herbal therapy is an essential ingredient in health and longevity, but it must arise out of a place of stillness. This is the essential message conveyed in the *Exposition's* passages dealing with internal alchemy.

The following section details the herbal strategies Shen Jin-Ao advocated for the treatment of the extraordinary vessels. Shen omits dosages and ingredients from many of the more common herbal formulas, but he often specifies very precise dosages and methods of preparation for less common prescriptions. A comprehensive list of the standard ingredients of the following formulas, along with Shen's preparation instructions, appear in Appendix 2 of the present text.

Shen Jin-Ao's Herbal Strategies for the Extraordinary Vessels[4]

Herbal Strategies for Pathologies of the *Chong* Vessel

Shen posits 12 individual drugs that treat the *chong* vessel by reversing a counterflow of qi and dispersing pathogenic heat. These include Citri reticulatae Pericarpium *(chen pi)*, Angelicae sinensis Radix *(dang gui)*, Moschus *(she xiang)*, Evodiae Fructus *(wu zhu yu)*, Astragali Radix *(huang qi)*, Rehmanniae Radix *(sheng di huang)*, Arecae Semen *(bing lang)*, Atractylodis macrocephalae Rhizoma *(bai zhu)*, Coptidis Rhizoma *(huang lian)*, Scutellariae Radix *(huang qin)*, Phellodendri Cortex *(huang bai)*, and Anemarrhenae Rhizoma *(zhi mu)*.

The following formulas treat diseases of the *chong* vessel:

- Regulate the Middle Pill *(li zhong wan)* treats cold reversal.

- Modified Tonify the Yin Pill *(jia wei bu yin wan)* treats counterflow of fire. This pill tonifies deficiencies of yin and discharges yin fire.

- Five-Ingredient Powder with Poria *(wu ling san)* is used to treat protruding disorders due to seasonal imbalances of the seven emotions.

- Saposhnikovia, White Atractylodes, and Oyster Shell Decoction *(fang feng bai zhu mu li tang)* treats aortic pulsing left of the umbilicus. This formula specifically treats aortic pulsing after erroneously causing the patient to perspire, making the sinews jerk and the flesh twitch.

- Licorice and Ailanthus Decoction *(gan li gen tang)* treats aortic pulsing above the umbilicus.

- Major Tangerine Pip Decoction *(da ju pi tang)* treats aortic pulsing above the umbilicus.

- Harmonize the Middle and Augment the Qi Decoction *(tiao zhong yi qi tang)* treats qi counterflow.

- Tonify the Middle to Augment the Qi Decoction *(bu zhong yi qi tang)* treats internal damage.

- Raise the Yang and Drain Heat Decoction *(sheng yang xie re tang)* treats surging qi.

- Miraculously Effective Pill *(shen gong wan)* treats surging qi.

- Generate the Pulse Powder *(sheng mai san)* treats restlessness with heat.

- Four-Ingredient Powder with Poria *(si ling san)* treats surging qi.

- Poria and Schizandra Decoction *(fu ling wu wei zi tang)* treats surging qi.

Herbal Strategies for Treating Disorders of the *Ren* Vessel

According to Shen Jin-Ao, the primary manifestation of *ren* vessel pathology is bulging *(shan 疝)*, and he has a great deal to say on this topic. (For an overview of bulging disorders, see Ch. 28 of the present text.) In Shen's opinion, although the liver is always involved in the pathogenesis of bulging patterns, it is rarely the source of the problem. He identifies the Central Pole (CV-3), which is located in the middle of the lower abdomen and the meeting hole of all yin channels, as the source of all bulging disorders. This hole may suffer from excessive heat, cold, or wind, producing painful conditions that resemble a mountain protruding from the area, hence the name *shan* (疝), which contains the graph for mountain (山). Upon identifying its central pivotal role in all bulging disorders, Shen narrows the scope of the *ren* vessel's involvement to its influence on the lower abdomen.

Notwithstanding his emphasis on the liver and the central pivot, Shen nevertheless acknowledges that diseases in other channels or viscera may produce bulging. He quotes Ch. 64 of *Basic Questions*: "When the lesser yin pulse is slippery, the lungs are sick with wind bulging (*feng shan* 風疝). When the greater yang pulse is slippery, the kidneys are sick with wind bulging." Shen points out that since these imbalances all eventually affect the *ren* vessel, it is the *ren* that is central to the pathogenesis of the bulging.

For Shen Jin-Ao, all bulging disorders are synonymous with an imbalance in the *ren* vessel. Given the scope of these parameters, the resulting category of diseases associated with the *ren* vessel is at best unwieldy, and at worst, meaningless.

At the very least, Shen's discussion contains a wealth of treatment strategies for a wide range of urogenital and abdominal complaints. By associating them with disorders of the *ren* vessel, he facilitates the conceptual integration of acupuncture and herbal therapies. In his discussion of diseases of the *ren* vessel, Shen suggests 37 herbal formulas for the treatment of approximately 15 different types of bulging disorders. The latter count of 15 is somewhat imprecise, however, because, by his own admission, there is substantial overlap between categories. Shen also includes running piglet syndrome as a species of bulging, a syndrome that is generally regarded as being its own disease entity. Shen's attribution of running piglet syndrome to the *ren* vessel contrasts with Li Shi-Zhen, who considered it to be a disorder of the *chong* vessel.

Shen Jin-Ao organizes the material in this discussion of the *ren* first according to herbal formula, and later according to species of bulging. We have consolidated his presentation considerably, placing his explanations of each species of bulging with the formula in which they are first mentioned.

- Aucklandia Powder (*mu xiang san*) treats surging bulge (*chong shan* 衝疝), which originates in the lateral abdominal region and surges to the heart, causing pain and resulting in urinary and fecal incontinence.

- Spider Powder (*zhi zhu san*) treats fox-like bulging (*hu shan* 狐疝). According to Shen Jin-Ao, fox-like bulging may have multiple causes but is expressed in the liver channel; it therefore affects the lateral abdomen and genitalia. Like the movements of a fox, fox-like bulging comes and goes, often depending on the position of the body.

- Two Fragrance Pill (*er xiang wan*) treats fox-like bulging.

- Pain-Curing Pill (*juan tong wan*) treats protuberant bulging (*tui shan* 癩疝). This formula treats all kinds of bulging due to qi surging from the small intestines and bladder. According to Shen, this condition presents as a painful protrusion in the abdomen that is large, swollen, and flaccid.

- Master Yang's Musk Pill *(Yang shi she xiang wan)* treats protuberant bulging as well as all kinds of pain in many parts of the body. It is particularly effective when qi surges up from the bladder, causing severe rib pain. This formula is extremely effective.

- Evodiae Internal Mass-Dissolving Powder *(zhu yu nei xiao san)* treats symptoms of kidney deficiency and cold bulging, swelling of the testes causing a drawing pain, running piglet disease, and indigestion.

- Melia Toosendan Powder #1 *(jin ling zi san)* treats prominent bulging. According to Shen, this formula is also effective for qi bulging from the bladder and the small intestines. Qi bulging is characterized by abdominal pain of varying intensity and/or painful sagging of the scrotum.

- Peach of Immortality and Scallion Decoction *(pan cong tang)* treats reversal bulging. This formula specifically treats deficiency cold of the spleen and stomach, causing severe pain in the heart and the abdomen, and kidney qi *shan*, causing pain along the costal areas, in the bladder, and in the lateral abdomen. Shen explains that reversal bulging is due to the liver overcontrolling the spleen. This causes the spleen pulse *(huang mai* 黃脈*)* to become so empty that it feels large and deficient. The condition is also characterized by an accumulation of qi *(ji qi* 積氣*)* in the abdomen. Finally, the liver qi also counterflows upward as it does when a person is angry. Therefore, the word 'reversal' refers to the spleen's contraction of pathogenic liver qi, resulting in the accumulation of qi and ascending counterflow, hence the term 'reversal bulging.'

- Aconite and Cinnamon Twig Decoction *(wu tou gui zhi tang)* treats reversal bulging. According to Shen, this formula also specifically treats wind-cold bulging qi *(feng han shan qi* 風寒疝氣*)* entering the abdomen to cause stabbing pains, shrinkage of the genitalia, and counterflow coldness of the four extremities.

- Four Miracle Pill *(si shen wan)* treats reversal bulging.

- Modified Heart-Penetrating Powder *(jia wei tong xin san)* treats conglomeration bulging *(shan jia* 疝瘕*)* as well as obstructive protrusion *(long* 癃*)*. This formula treats both hot pain due to bulging qi of the small intestines and inhibited urination. Shen Jin-Ao explains that, according to the *Inner Classic (Nei jing* 内经*)*, when pathogenic liver qi is transmitted to the spleen and then to the kidneys, it is called 'bulging amassment.' In this condition, the lateral abdomen becomes so hot and painful that the patient's face turns white. Naturally, the spleen's digestive function is impaired. Because this condition often enters the cold, water-related viscus of the kidneys and lodges there, it forms a mobile mass *(jia* 瘕*)* like a cucumber *(huang gua* 黃瓜*)*.

- Master Shen's Mass-Dissolving Decoction *(Shen shi san jia tang)* treats conglomeration bulging. According to Shen, "This is my own formula, and I use it to treat conglomeration amassment and qi pain in the small intestine and the bladder in patients who cannot urinate. It always works." He also cites Zhu Dan-Xi in describing bulging concretions as a contraction of excessive damp-heat in the yang brightness and greater yang channels, causing feverishness, aversion to cold, and stifling pain in the lateral abdomen.

- Lichee and Tangerine Pip Decoction *(xie zhi ju he tang)* treats prominent bulging. According to Shen, "The *Classic* states that the sinews of the foot yang brightness channel is called prominent bulging, causing abdominal muscle spasms." "The *Classic* also says that 'If the liver pulse is extremely slippery, it is a sign of prominent bulging, because the liver wood generally overrides the stomach. This is why it is not only called a yang brightness disease, but also liver disease.'"

- Tangerine Pip Pill *(ju he wan)* treats prominent bulging.

- Tangerine Pip Powder *(ju he san)* treats prominent bulging.

- Clove and Toosendan Fruit Pill *(ding xiang lian shi wan)* treats fox-like bulging. This treats all seven bulgings in men and leukorrhea in women because they are all due to wind. Scorpio *(quan xie)* is a miraculous medicine for wind disorders. Toosendan Fructus *(chuan lian zi)* and Foeniculi Fructus *(xiao hui xiang)* both enter the small intestine. Angelicae sinensis Radix *(dang gui)* and Corydalis Rhizoma *(yan hu suo)* harmonize the blood and stops pain. Since bulging qi and leukorrhea are all caused by accumulation of cold pathogen in the small intestines, Aconiti Radix lateralis preparata *(zhi fu zi)*, Caryophylli Flos *(ding xiang)*, and Aucklandiae Radix *(mu xiang)* all help to guide the medicines.

- Four-Part Sublime Toosendan Fruit Pill *(si miao chuan lian wan)* treats fox-like bulging. This formula will treat all forms of qi bulging and swelling pain. It will shrink the swelling, and if taken for a long time, it will eradicate the problem.

- Two-Aged [Herb] Decoction *(er chen tang)* treats fox-like bulging.

- Aristolochia Pill *(qing mu xiang wan)* treats cold bulging *(han shan* 寒疝). Shen quotes Zhang Zhong-Jing, who explains that in cold bulging, "the scrotum gets cold and the testicles become hard like stones. The penis cannot become erect, and the testicles are painful when held [in one's hands]. This condition may be due to lying on the damp ground or walking though water during the winter months, or from being exposed to snow and rain, or by sitting in cold wind."[5]

- Tangkuei Decoction for Frigid Extremities *(dang gui si ni tang)* treats cold bulging *shan*.

- Kidneys Powder *(yao zi san)* treats water bulging *(shui shan* 水疝). According to Shen, in the case of water bulging, the scrotum is swollen and painful, or swollen and translucent. Alternately, the scrotum may be damp and itchy and exude a yellow fluid. There may be a fluid sound in the abdomen upon palpation, which is probably due to the fluid retention from excessive drinking of alcohol followed by exposure to wind-cold, which later accumulates in the scrotum.

- Secretly Transmitted Evodiae Fructus Powder to Dissolve Internal Accumulation *(mi chuan wu zhu nei xiao san)* treats water bulging.

- Modified Bupleurum and Poria Decoction *(jia jian chai ling tang)* treats sinew bulging *(jin shan* 筋疝*)*. This formula not only treats water bulging, it also treats many bulging disorders due to damp-heat causing swelling and discharge. Shen again quotes Zhu Dan-Xi, who explains that "sinew bulging is characterized by painful swelling of the penis, exudation of pus [from the penis], urge to urinate with muscle spasms, extreme pain and itchiness, inability to maintain an erection, or white discharge from the penis. This condition is probably due to sexual excess causing damage to wood and should be treated with Augmented Bupleuri Radix and Poria Decoction *(jia jian chai ling tang)* and Gentiana Decoction to Drain the Liver *(long dan xie gan tang)*." [6]

- Gentiana Decoction to Drain the Liver *(long dan xie gan tang)* treats water bulging.

- Restore the Origin Unblock the Qi Powder *(fu yuan tong qi san)* treats blood bulging *(xue shan* 血疝*)*. Shen again quotes Zhu Dan-Xi, who explains that "blood bulging looks like a cucumber on both sides of the lower abdomen in the fold of skin on either side of the pubic bone. … This type of bulging is probably caused by engaging in sexual activity during hot summer days, which causes qi and blood to rush into the genitals. If [the qi and blood] fail to completely leave the area, it will result in abscesses and swelling with more blood and less pus. If one experiences excessive sexual desire that cannot be satisfied, then this may also cause blood bulging and should be treated by Restore the Origin Unblock the Qi Powder *(fu yuan tong qi san)* or Powder of the Divine Sage that Replaces the Needle *(Shen sheng dai zhen san)*." [7]

- Powder of the Divine Sage that Replaces the Needle *(shen sheng dai zhen san)* treats blood bulging.

- Qi Bulging Drink *(qi shan yin)* treats qi bulging *(qi shan* 氣疝*)*. According to Shen, "Master Zhang [Zi-He] explains 'qi bulging involves the area from Kidney Transport (BL-23) down to the scrotum, which becomes extremely congested and may or may not be painful.' This condition is probably due to excessive anger and loud crying, resulting in qi stagnation, and should be treated with Qi Bulging Drink *(qi shan yin)* or Collected Fragrant Herbs Drink *(ju xiang yin zi)*." [8]

- Collected Fragrant Herbs Drink *(ju xiang yin zi)* treats qi bulging.

- Top-Quality Lindera Powder *(tian tai wu yao san)* treats protuberant bulging.

- Regulate the Middle Pill *(li zhong wan)* treats running piglet disorder *(ben tun* 奔豚*)*.

- Elixir to Seize Destiny *(duo ming dan)* treats running piglet disorder. This formula is also called Four Processed Evodiae Fructus Pill *(si zhi zhu yu wan)*.

- Fenugreek Pill *(hu lu ba wan)* treats running piglet disorder.

- One Pinch of Gold Powder *(yi nie jin san)* treats running piglet disorder. This formula also treats pain in the small intestine and qi pain around the umbilicus.

- Tangkuei and Mutton Decoction *(dang gui yang rou tang)* treats cold bulging.

- Aconite and Gardenia Decoction *(wu tou zhi zi tang)* treats cold bulging due to deficiency.

- Aucklandia and Melia Toosendan Powder *(mu xiang lian zi san)* treats chronic bulging *(jiu shan* 久疝*)*

Herbal Strategies for Treating Disorders of the *Du* Vessel

Shen Jin-Ao attributes six individual medicinals to the *du* vessel. These are Nototerygii Rhizoma *(qiang huo)*, Schizonepetae Herba et Flos *(jing jie)*, Gentianae Macrophyllae Radix *(qin jiao)*, Asari Radix et Rhizoma *(xi xin)*, Cotidis Rhizoma *(huang lian)*, and Aconiti Tuber Laterale *(fu zi)*. Herbal formulas that treat disorders of the *du* vessel include:

- Styrax Pill *(su he xiang wan)* treats spasm due to wind strike *(qiang jue* 強厥*)*.[9]

- Chuanxiong Powder to Be Taken with Green Tea *(chuan xiong cha tiao san)* treats spasm due to wind strike.

- Angelica Pill *(bai zhi wan)* treats heaviness of the head.

Herbal Strategies for Treating Disorders of the *Dai* Vessel

- Clove Powder for Spleen Accumulation *(ding xiang pi ji san)* treats abdominal distention.

- Root-Invigorating Elixir *(zhuang ben dan)* treats coldness in the waist.

- Secretly Transmitted Formula for Leukorrhea *(mi chuan dai xia fang)* treats leukorrhea. Mild cases require eight or nine doses, and severe cases require 12 doses. This formula is never ineffective. If the leukorrhea is red, add 1 *qian* of Gypsum fibrosum *(shi gao)*. Once the patient recovers, she can take these pills to fortify herself.

- Modified Augmented Dragon Tiger Decoction *(jia wei long hu tang)* treats attack of yin cold *(yin xi* 陰襲*)*. This formula also treats waist pain due to wind-cold evil and spasms of the tendons and muscles.

- Fast-Acting Powder *(su xiao san)* treats external pathogens *(ke xie* 客邪*)*.
- Aucklandia and Melia Toosendan Powder *(mu xiang lian zi san)* treats water qi *(shui qi* 水氣*)*.
- Fixed Kidney Decoction *(shen zhuo tang)* treats fixed kidney *(shen zhuo* 腎著*)*.
- Dampness Leeching Decoction *(shen shi tang)* treats heaviness in the lower back.
- Pubescent Angelica Decoction *(du huo tang)* treats heaviness in the lower back. This formula also treats sprains and strains, and severe back pains.

Herbal Strategies for Treating Disorders of the *Wei* Vessels

- Cinnamon Twig Decoction *(gui zhi tang)* treats the *yang wei* vessel.
- Ephedra Decoction *(ma huang tang)* treats the *yang wei* vessel.
- Eight Substances Decoction *(ba wu tang)* treats the *yang wei* vessel.
- Regulate the Middle Decoction *(li zhong tang)* treats the *yin wei* vessel.
- Frigid Extremities Decoction *(si ni tang)* treats the *yin wei* vessel.
- Tangkuei Decoction for Frigid Extremities *(dang gui si ni tang)* treats the *yin wei* vessel.
- Evodia Decoction *(wu zhu yu tang)* treats the *yin wei* vessel.
- Melia Toosendan Powder #2 *(jin ling zi san)* treats the *yin wei* vessel. Administer 2 qian of this prescription with wine until the pain stops. Then administer Unripe Bitter Orange and Atractylodes Pill *(zhi zhu wan)* to remove the remaining pathogens.
- Corydalis Powder *(yan hu suo san)* treats the *yin wei* vessel. This formula also treats blood binding in the chest in women, abdominal and chest pains, and costal pains radiating up and down the body, causing severe muscle spasms.
- Sudden Smile Powder *(shi xiao san)* treats the *yin wei* vessel.
- Nourish the Nutritive Decoction *(yang ying tang)* treats the *yin wei* vessel.
- Four Substance Decoction *(si wu tang)* treats the *yin wei* vessel.

Herbal Strategies for Disorders of the *Qiao* Vessels

- Cinnamon Twig Decoction *(gui zhi tang)* treats the *yang qiao*.
- Ephedra Decoction *(ma huang tang)* treats the *yang qiao*.
- Major Order the Qi Decoction *(da cheng qi tang)* and Minor Order the Qi Decoction *(xiao cheng qi tang)* treat the *yang qiao*.
- Pinellia Decoction *(ban xia tang)* treats the *yang qiao*.
- Licorice and Ginger Decoction *(gan cao gan jiang tang)* treats the *yin qiao*.

CHAPTER 37

Modern Extraordinary Vessel Case Records

Acupuncture Cases

The following four acupuncture cases are excerpted from Mei Jian-Han (梅建寒) and Yang Yu-Hua's (楊玉華) *Clinical Application of the Eight Extraordinary Vessels in Acupuncture and Moxabustion — Illustrated, Collated and Verified (Qi jing ba mai yu zhen jiu lin chuang-tu kao zu he yan zheng* 奇經八脈與針灸臨床–圖考組合驗證).[1] They exemplify an approach to the extraordinary vessels that is consistent with the perspective presented by Li Shi-Zhen in that they do not rely on the so-called master-couple holes. Other examples of this approach can be found in Yitian Ni's *Navigating the Channels of Traditional Chinese Medicine.*[2]

Case No. 1: Panting and Wheezing (Bronchial Asthma): A *Chong* Vessel Disorder[3]

Qian was a 13-year-old male student. Since infancy, he had suffered from panting and wheezing, chest oppression, and rough breathing which, when extreme, would make his lips purple and cyanotic and prevent him from lying down. His Western medical diagnosis was bronchial asthma.

Initial examination. The patient had been suffering from panting and wheezing for 3 days. He reported sensations of qi surging upward from his epigastric region, chest oppression accompanied by a sense of obstruction, and being able to exhale only in rapid bursts. Qian's pulse was floating, slippery, and rapid. His tongue body was red, with a thin yellow coating. [This pattern] was caused by a counterflow of qi and internal urgency along with an ascending surge of phlegm-fire attacking the lungs. The treatment plan was to level the surging [qi] and descend the counterflow, clear fire, and transform phlegm. The holes selected were Great Shuttle (BL-11), Upper Great Hollow (ST-37), Lower Great Hollow (ST-39), and Cubit Marsh (LU-5). After pricking and bleeding Great Shuttle (BL-11) and Cubit Marsh (LU-5), the panting and wheezing diminished and then the chest oppression began to ease as well. The epigastric and abdominal distention and urgency disappeared after needling Upper Great Hollow (ST-37) and Lower Great Hollow (ST-39).

Second examination. The panting and wheezing had stopped, there was a slight sensation of chest oppression, the bowel movements were rough, and his urination was impaired. The original prescription was administered again, omitting Great Shuttle (BL-11) and adding Branch Ditch (TB-6) to smooth and ease the elimination.

Third examination. Qian's appetite had come back, and his elimination was regulated. His pulse was floating and slippery, and his tongue was red with little moisture. Qian received two courses of treatment with six treatments to a course, and his symptoms completely disappeared.

TRANSLATOR'S COMMENT

This case illustrates the *chong's* central pathodynamic of counterflow arising from congestion in the middle or lower burners. The choice of holes is based on Ch. 33 of *Divine Pivot (Ling shu* 靈樞) where the *chong* is identified as the sea of the 12 channels and is linked to Great Shuttle (BL-11) and Upper and Lower Great Hollow (ST-37 and ST-39, respectively).[4] In addition to their influence on the *chong,* Upper and Lower Great Hollow (ST-37 and ST-39) are the lower uniting holes of the large and small intestines, respectively.[5] The decision to bleed Great Shuttle (BL-11) reflects the pathogenic excess in the *chong.* The treatment is a simple, elegant, and apparently effective expression of Li's view of the extraordinary vessels. Cubit Marsh (LU-5) and Branch Ditch (TB-6) are used here to treat the symptoms of asthma and constipation.

Case No. 2: Restless Viscera Syndrome: A Dual *Yin Wei* and *Yang Wei* Disorder[6]

Initial examination. Li was a 27-year-old textile worker. Relations between the patient and her husband become indifferent as a result of her infertility, and in recent years, she had become emotionally tense, absentminded, and distracted. She was melancholy and perpetually on the verge of tears. She would have hallucinations at dusk when she would imagine that she saw young children all around her, playing in front of and behind her. Mrs. Li would call to them, but there was no response; pull them toward her, but there was nothing there. She had difficulty sleeping and had confusing dreams, ate little, and was constipated. Mrs. Li's tongue was red with little coating, and her pulse was deep, fine, and wiry. She had difficulty concentrating and was unable to answer ordinary questions.

The protective is the qi, and the nutritive is the blood. The [protective] qi and nutritive were constrained and damaged, which consequently prevented the *yin wei* from binding the yin and the *yang wei* from binding the yang. The yin and yang could not bind to one another, causing her to become despondent and lose her resolve.

The treatment plan was to soothe the constraint and calm the spirit, and harmonize and regulate the yin and yang. The [acupuncture] prescription included Guest House (KI-9), Cycle Gate (LV-14), Wind Pond (GB-20), Root Spirit (GB-13), and Metal Gate (BL-63). Even tonifying and draining methods were used. The herbal prescription included Glycyrrhizae Radix *(gan cao),* and Jujube Fructus *(da zao),* 9g each, and Tritici levis Fructus *(huai xiao mai),* 30g. This was decocted in water and taken as a tea.

Mrs. Li returned for treatment five times and was cured. She took another ten packets of the herbal prescription to consolidate the treatment.

TRANSLATOR'S COMMENT

Mrs. Li's situation could have been legitimately approached from any number of Chinese medical perspectives, but the acupuncturist focused on the overarching characteristic of her presentation: She seemed to be falling apart.

The *yang wei* arises from Metal Gate (BL-63) and terminates at Spirit Root (GB-13). Both of these holes are indicated for epilepsy and infantile convulsions, two conditions closely associated with disorders of the spirit. Although not typically associated with psychiatric disorders, Wind Pond (GB-20) is sometimes used in this way.[7] Guest House (KI-9) is paired with Cycle Gate (LV-14) to activate the *yin wei*. Guest House (KI-9) is also used to calm fright and quiet the spirit.[8] Cycle Gate (LV-14) does not have any overtly psychiatric indications, but as the alarm hole of the liver, it treats blood-level disorders, particularly those associated with heat.[9] Given the practitioner's choice of herbal formulas, this may be the reason why that hole was selected.

Licorice, Wheat, and Jujube Decoction *(gan mai da zao tang)* is the fundamental prescription for restless viscera syndrome, although it is not specifically associated with the *wei* vessels in Li Shi-Zhen's thinking.

Case No. 3: Dribbling Urinary Obstruction (*long bi* 癃閉):[10] Urinary Retention as a Sequelae to the Surgical Reduction of a Left Femur Fracture

Mr. Zeng was an 18-year-old male student. He sustained a closed fracture to his upper left femur and underwent surgery to reduce the fracture and stabilize it with a steel plate. Subsequent to the surgery, he began to have difficulty urinating and after four days developed urinary retention. He was catheterized seven times, but the urinary retention persisted.

The *yang qiao* vessel arises from the foot greater yang and lesser yang. (The foot greater yang vessel pertains to the urinary bladder, and the foot lesser yang vessel encircles the pubic region.) The *yin qiao* vessel travels along the inside of the thigh, and the *yang qiao* vessel travels along the outside of the thigh, such that the *yin qiao* and *yang qiao* have a mutual exterior-interior relationship. During the surgery to reduce the fracture, an incision was made on the lateral aspect of the thigh, damaging the *yang qiao* and causing it to become slack, and stretching the *yin qiao*, causing it to become tense. The two *qiao* are related to the genitals, and the damage to their network along with blood stasis and a loss of normal tone and flexibility resulted in urinary obstruction and loss of free flow. The plan was to normalize the tension and slackness, open the networks, and disinhibit the [urinary] orifices. The holes selected for treatment were left Squatting Bone (GB-29), to which a tonifying method was applied; right Shining Sea (KI-6), to which a draining method was applied; and Origin Pass (CV-4), which was needled at an oblique angle in the direction of the pubic symphysis using a slow rotation to produce a needle sensation extending directly to the urethra. The needle was manipulated in 10-minute intervals, and the second time the needle was manipulated, the patient felt the urge to urinate. Upon removal of the needles, the patient urinated. He was treated only once and was cured.

TRANSLATOR'S COMMENT

In retrospect, the *qiao* vessel involvement in this case seems obvious, but one has to wonder if one would have thought of it on one's own. It makes use of the central pathodynamic of the *qiao*; the relationship between the slackness and tension in their associated tissues reflects a keen understanding of the terrain they traverse.

The *Systematic Classic of Acupuncture and Moxibustion (Zhen jiu jia yi jing* 針灸甲乙經) describes Squatting Bone-hole (GB-29) as "The intersection hole of the *yang qiao* and the lesser yang."[11] Here, a hole on the *yang qiao* located close to the affected area was tonified to tone the *yang qiao,* and a distal hole, Shining Sea (KI-6), was drained to release the tension in the *yin qiao.* Having reestablished balance between the *qiao* vessels, it was a simple matter to move the qi in the urinary bladder by stimulating Origin Pass (CV-4). It is unclear on theoretical grounds why the acupuncturist chose Origin Pass (CV-4) over Central Pole (CV-3). Both holes address urinary problems, but Central Pole (CV-3) has the added attribute of being the front alarm hole of the urinary bladder, which would, in principle, have made it a better choice.[12]

Case No. 4: Lumbar Pain[13]

Wang, a 46-year-old worker, had suffered from low back pain for three years. He had originally injured his low back as he twisted while carrying a heavy load. Now, he would experience pain when he began to bend his low back, when he coughed, or when he twisted his torso. The patient had already received acupuncture that had helped a little. In recent months, his low back had become particularly sore. It was worse at night or when he got cold; he was unable to bend his back; and when his condition was extreme, he would experience pain when sitting for any length of time. He experienced the pain on the left side of his lumbar spine, between the greater yang and lesser yin [regions] from where it radiated both upward and downward.

His tongue body was dull and red with a thin, white coating, and his pulse was wiry, long, and had strength. The *yang wei* vessel travels upward from the outer ankle, intersecting with and emerging behind the *yang qiao*. It ascends to intersect with the hand greater yang at Upper Arm Transport (SI-10). Its vessel is situated outside the greater yang and inside the lesser yang.

The patient first sustained a trauma that persisted, predisposing him to a contraction of an external pathogen. The pathogenic factor and the stagnant [blood] became bound to one another and subsequently obstructed the networks. The plan was to move the qi and quicken the blood, expel stasis, and open the networks. The points selected were left Wind Pond (GB-20), left Upper Arm Transport (SI-10), left Yang Intersection (GB-39), and left Metal Gate (BL-63), all administered with draining technique. The needles were retained for 30 minutes and manipulated once every 10 minutes.

Follow-up examination. The low back pain gradually decreased following the acupuncture, and he was able to slowly twist his back. There was pressure pain in his low back region and the sides of his tongue were purple. Bend Yang (BL-39) was added to the original prescription. This point was pricked, bled, and then cupped. The patient was treated twice weekly, and after eight acupuncture treatments, his lumbar pain disappeared and his range of motion returned, becoming smooth and unhindered.

TRANSLATOR'S COMMENT

In addition to being an intersection hole of the *yang wei* vessel, Metal Gate (BL-63) is indicated for the treatment of low back pain. Yang Intersection (GB-35) is an intersection hole of the *yang wei* vessel,[14] and Wind Pond (GB-20) and Upper Arm Transport (SI-10) are both intersection holes of the *yang wei* and *yang qiao*, respectively. They are not explicitly indicated for the treatment of low back pain and are used here solely based on their association with these extraordinary vessels.[15]

Herbal Cases

The following case records illustrate how premodern physicians used the *chong* vessel in a variety of ways in their herbal prescriptions.

The *Chong* Vessel as an Organizing Principle[16]

Wei Feng-Pang (female) suffered from a minor cough. There were concretions and hardness inhibiting her abdomen; she vomited foamy drool; and during her menses, she was irritable. Hence, it was appropriate to clear the lungs, balance the liver, and regulate the menses. Four packets of the following herbs were given to Ms. Wei:

Asteris Radix *(zi wan),* 1.5 *qian*
Ostreae Concha *(mu li),* 4 *qian*
Pinelliae Rhizoma preparatum *(zhi ban xia),* 1.5 *qian*
Leonuri Fructus *(chong wei zi),* 3 *qian*
Fritillariae cirrhosae Bulbus *(chuan bei mu),* 1.5 *qian*
Cyperi Rhizoma *(xiang fu),* 3 *qian*
Citri reticulatae Exocarpium rubrum *(ju hong),* 1 *qian*
Rosae rugosae Flos *(mei gui hua),* 5 pieces
Armeniacae Semen dulce *(tian xing ren),* 3 *qian*
Dendrobii Herba *(shi hu),* 3 *qian*
Farfarae Flos *(kuan dong hua),* 3 *qian*
Eriobotryae Folium *(pi pa ye)* [hairs removed], 5 pieces

PHYSICIAN'S COMMENT

When the *chong* vessel becomes diseased, there is qi counterflow with abdominal urgency. In men, there will be internal bulging, and in women, there will be concretions and amassments. When the qi of the *chong* vessel counterflows upward and attacks the stomach, there will be nausea and vomiting of foamy drool. When [the *chong* vessel] surges into the lungs, there will be an incessant hacking cough. Moreover, the *chong* vessel is the sea of blood and extends to the *yang ming*. A careful appraisal of the pathocondition suggested that treatment was indicated to settle the *chong* and nourish the stomach.

Since there are abdominal concretions and nausea, a treatment focused on clearing the lungs and balancing the liver is an extremely good prescriptive method. If one is able to combine this with the use of medicinals to settle the *chong* and nourish the stomach, the result will be especially favorable.

TRANSLATOR'S COMMENT

This case illustrates the use of the *chong* vessel as an organizing concept for treatment. A diagnosis involving the *chong* vessel does not eliminate the need to account for each facet of the pathodynamic condition, yet it provides a structure around which a treatment strategy can be built. In the absence of such a structure, one is left with a laundry list of visceral patterns with little to give them coherence. Though the concretions and amassments ultimately lie at the root of the problem, the *chong* vessel is the vector through which this pathology extends beyond the pelvis. All of the other symptoms are a consequence of the *chong* vessel counterflow.

Shao Lan-Sun covers all of his bases, treating each component of the *chong* vessel disorder. The Asteris Radix *(zi wan)*, Farfarae Flos *(kuan dong hua)*, Eriobotryae Folium *(pi pa ye)*, and Armeniacae Semen dulce *(tian xing ren)* diffuse the lungs, transform phlegm, and clear heat to stop the cough. Pinelliae Rhizoma preparatum *(zhi ban xia)*, Fritillariae cirrhosae Bulbus *(chuan bei mu)*, and Citri reticulatae Exocarpium rubrum *(ju hong)* transform phlegm and redirect counterflow downward. Cyperi Rhizoma *(xiang fu)* and Rosae rugosae Flos *(mei gui hua)* harmonize the liver and regulate the menses while Ostreae Concha *(mu li)* redirects liver counterflow downward. Leonuri Fructus *(chong wei zi)* invigorates the blood and resolves stasis. Finally, Dendrobii Herba *(shi hu)* nourishes stomach yin.

Treating the Root through the *Chong*[17]

The [patient's] pulse was fine, rapid, and rough. This pointed to internal damage to the essence and blood of the liver and kidney. There was cough with vomiting of clear drool and turbid spittle. This represented a counterflow of the qi of the *chong* vessel. What naturally descends, [surged] upward. The qi was unable to grasp and absorb, hence there was asthma and perspiration. One must first pull up the root.

It is difficult to be effective with medicines. If a physician sees bleeding as due to heat or sees a cough and treats the lungs, this can quickly become disastrous.

Ginseng Radix *(ren shen)*
Rehmanniae Radix preparata *(shu di huang)*
Schisandrae Fructus *(wu wei zi)*
Juglandis Semen *(he tao ren)*

TRANSLATOR'S COMMENT

The *chong* vessel disorder in this case has the characteristic symptoms of counterflow occurring in the middle and upper warmers, which are rooted in a liver and kidney vacuity that is evident only in the pulse presentation. In contrast to the previous case, this case reflects a rather minimalist approach of "first pulling up the root."

Treating the *Chong* and *Yang Wei* Together[18]

The [patient's] bodily qi was depleted, and over the years she had suffered from repeated coughs. During the recent spring, she experienced postpartum depression, and her cough had returned. Her spine was cold, but she experienced internal heat. There was qi counterflow with copious phlegm. The pulse was deficient and rapid, and her stools were pasty. This condition had persisted for 100 days, and the disease was weighing heavily on her.

In light of the fact that the patient was postpartum, the blood residence had become empty and deficient, and the qi of the eight vessels was the first to become damaged below.[19] Added to this was grief damaging the lungs, leading to a severe cough. [Hence, there was a] thunderous quaking of the qi of the *chong* vessel counterflowing upward.

The [Systematic] Classic states: "When the *chong* vessel is diseased, there is a counterflow of qi and abdominal urgency," as well as "When the *yang wei* is diseased, [the patient] suffers from cold and heat [effusion]."[20]

Because she had repeatedly received wind-coursing and heat-clearing substances, her stomach and spleen were also damaged, resulting in abdominal pain and pasty stools, diminished food intake, and lack of taste [for food]. All of this is the harm that comes from seeing a cough and treating a cough.

Yue-Ren says that a depletion of ascent is [indicative of] the spleen, while a depletion of descent is [indicative of] the stomach. Both conditions are difficult to treat. The plan was to open and supplement the extraordinary channels, and calm and absorb the *chong* vessel while also assisting the spleen and regulating the lung. This is a common mistake for ordinary practitioners, and it is difficult to avoid.

Rehmanniae Radix preparata *(shu di huang)*,
    char-fried with Amomi Fructus *(sha ren)*
Angelicae sinensis Radix *(dang gui)*, mix-fried with
    3 *fen* Foeniculi Fructus *(xiao hui xiang)*

Paeoniae Radix alba *(bai shao)*, mix-fried with
   3 *fen* Cinnamomi Ramulus *(gui zhi)*

Fluoritum *(zi shi ying)*

Achyranthis bidentatae Radix *(niu xi)*, fried in salt water

Poria Fu Ling *(fu ling)*

Fritillariae cirrhosae Bulbus *(chuan bei mu)*

PHYSICIAN'S COMMENT

The use of Rehmanniae Radix preparata *(shu di huang)*, Angelicae sinensis Radix *(dang gui)*, Foeniculi Fructus *(xiao hui xiang)*, and Fluoritum *(zi shi ying)* warms and absorbs the *chong* and *ren*. Angelicae sinensis Radix *(dang gui)* and Paeoniae Radix alba *(bai shao)* function to regulate the *yang wei*. Then [the following medicinals were] added to the original prescription:

Juglandis Semen *(tu tao ren)*

Ginseng Radix *(ren shen)*

Dioscoreae Rhizoma *(shan yao)*

Astragali complanati Semen *(sha yuan zi)*

Ostreae Concha *(mu li)*

CHAPTER 38

Vessels Wide Shut: Li Shi-Zhen's *Qiao* Vessel Pathodynamics

by Charles Chace

In his discussion of diseases of the *qiao* vessels, Li Shi-Zhen presents two apparently contradictory visions of how the *yang qiao* may become disordered and fail to transmit its qi to the *yin qiao*. The first of these interpretations is consistent with the understanding familiar to most acupuncturists. The latter interpretation, hinging on a single character, adds another dimension to *yang qiao* pathology that bears directly on how we conceptualize and treat these vessels. This chapter will explore these two interpretations of *yang qiao* pathology and their applications in acupuncture and herbal medicine.

Early Chinese medical texts were typically hand written as part of a master-disciple relationship. Nathan Sivin observes that a cornerstone of this relationship was the formal transmission of a text from the mentor and its 'reception' (受 *shou*) by the student.

Reception, we are clearly told, is a formal process that begins only after one has been 'serving' the master as a disciple for some time. When a text is 'received,' it is not simply handed over, but ritually transmitted and taught. At a certain point, the disciple is allowed to copy it out and read it, not necessarily in that order.[1]

Transcription errors were an inevitable part of this process and persisted even with the advent of printing when professional carvers would inadvertently miscopy handwritten documents onto woodblocks. Since memorization was such an integral part of a physician's training, they most probably quoted from memory when writing, though not always accurately. From a scholarly perspective, many of Li Shi-Zhen's citations of classical sources are more akin to paraphrase than actual quotations. These vectors account for some of the variability that has crept into the textual tradition.

As a remedy for these inherent irregularities, the Chinese medical literature has a long history of textual exegesis in which passages are annotated and errors corrected. Most often, these annotations are of more interest to academics than to clinicians. Sometimes, however, a character that had been deemed a transcription error yields a much more interesting reading of a passage than the corrected version. As physicians, our interest in such seemingly arcane matters most often remains little more than a passing curiosity. It soon occurs to us that a team of scholars much better informed than ourselves has decided how the text should be read, and it is best to get on with more productive areas of inquiry. In light of this, Li Shi-Zhen's discussion of diseases of the *qiao* vessels in *Exposition on the Eight Extraordinary Vessels* is particularly intriguing. His rendering of a key passage from *Divine Pivot*, using a character thought to be a transcription error, suggests a more nuanced understanding of *yang qiao* pathology. The Chinese medical literature is full of inconsistencies, and taken on its own, it is difficult to make much of Li's rendering. The interpretation suggested by this reading, however, is also echoed in the case records of Ye Tian-Shi, suggesting that it may be more than a curious anomaly.

Li Shi-Zhen begins his discussion of the diseases of the *qiao* vessels with familiar quotations from the *Classic of Difficulties* and *Pulse Classic*, addressing the relationship of tension and slackness to *qiao* vessel pathology. He proceeds with a recitation of the *Pulse Classic's* description of the pulses associated with each of the *qiao* vessels, and then continues with a series of quotations on seizures. Li then repeats a number of passages from *Basic Questions* pertaining to pathologies and acupuncture treatments involving the *qiao* vessels. Finally, he ties these disparate passages together with a discussion of the role of the *qiao* vessels in the overall circulation of yin and yang.

> [Ch. 21 of *Divine Pivot Classic*] also states: "The *yin qiao* and *yang qiao* are the intersection of the yin and yang. The yang enters the yin, and the yin emerges from the yang. They intersect at the outer corner of the eye. When the yang qi is overly full, then the eyes will stare, and when the yin qi is overly full, then the eyes will be closed. With heat reversal, select the leg greater yang and lesser yang. ..."[2]

The gist of this passage is that when the yang is excessive, the eyes stay open, and when the yin is excessive, the eyes remain closed. This is familiar ground for most students of acupuncture, but there is a catch. Although most of the textual exegesis on this passage simply equates the yin and yang qi with the *yin* and *yang qiao*, respectively, the passage may also be understood as making a much more general statement regarding accumulations of qi in the yin and yang channels.

Li continues with a similar passage from *The Systematic Classic of Acupuncture and Moxibustion*, a passage that is itself derived from Ch. 80 of *Divine Pivot*.

> *The Systematic Classic* states: "When a patient's eyes are shut and they cannot see ..., this is due to protective qi being lodged in the yin and unable to travel to the yang. When it is lodged in the yin, then the yin qi is overly full, and when the yin qi is overly full, then the *yin qiao* is full. [When the protective qi] cannot enter the yang, then the yang qi is deficient and, hence, the eyes are shut.
>
> When a patient's eyes cannot close ... , the protective qi cannot enter the yin and constantly lodges in the yang. If [the protective qi] lodges in the yang, then the yang qi is full. If the yang qi is full, then the *yang qiao* is overly full. [If the protective qi] cannot enter the yin, then the yin qi is deficient, hence, the eyes cannot close."[3]

The two paragraphs make a crucial distinction not apparent in the previous passage. The protective yang may become trapped in the exterior, causing the *yang qiao* to become full. It is not just that the *yang qiao* is full, it is overly full or congested, and this congestion prevents the qi from penetrating into the *yin qiao*. Moreover, the yang qi is not necessarily synonymous with the *yang qiao;* they are separate entities. Although this may appear to be a minor point, it is central to understanding the passages that follow. According to Li,

> [Ch. 71 of] *Divine Pivot* states: "The five grains enter the stomach and are divided into three pathways of dregs, fluids, and the gathering qi. Thus, gathering qi accumulates in the chest and emerges in the throat to link with the heart and lungs and propel respiration there. The nutritive qi secretes the fluids and pours into the vessels. It transforms and becomes blood to nourish the four extremities. Internally, it pours into the five viscera and six receptacles in accordance with the time of the day.
>
> Protective qi emerges with an impetuous ferocity, first in the four extremities in the partings between the flesh and skin, and it does so in a ceaseless manner. During the daytime, it circulates in the yang, and at night, it circulates in the yin from the level of the leg lesser yin, traveling to the five viscera and six receptacles.
>
> When a reversal qi visits the five viscera and six receptacles, then the protective qi alone protects the outside. It travels in the yang but cannot enter the yin. By traveling [only] in the yang, the yang qi becomes overly full, and when the yang qi is overly full, then the *yang qiao* caves in. When [the yang qi] cannot enter the yin, then the yin qi is deficient and the eyes cannot close."[4]

With the exception of a single character, 陷 (*xian*, literally 'collapses'), this passage is in accord with those preceding it. The crux of the third paragraph is "*yang qi sheng ze yang xiao xian*" (陽氣盛則陽蹺陷), that is, "When the yang qi is exuberant, then the *yang qiao* caves in or collapses." This changes the meaning of the passage completely. When read with this character, the yang qi has become congested in the exterior, preventing it from even entering the *yang qiao*, much less the *yin qiao*. Annotators of *Divine Pivot* typically explain away 陷 (*xian*) as a transcription error, asserting that it should properly be read as 滿 (*man*).[5] Thus, this sentence is amended to read, "When the yang qi is exuberant, then the *yang qiao* is full," neatly reconciling it with the others we have already examined.

Li, however, prefers the original reading of 'collapses.' The implication is that, according to Li, two potentially distinct dynamics may be involved in *yang qiao* pathology. In one case, the *yang qiao* becomes congested as a consequence of an exuberance of protective qi in the yang channels. This congestion prevents its descent into the interior and the *yin qiao*. In the second case, the *yang qiao* is deficient, not excessive. The yang qi has become so congested in the exterior that it is unable to even reach the the latter, causing it to collapse.

The discussion in *Divine Pivot* follows with a remedy that is one of the few herbal prescriptions mentioned in the *Inner Classic*, Pinellia and Sorghum Decoction *(ban xia shu mi tang)*, the assumption being that the pathogen congesting the yang channels is phlegm. If we adopt Li's reading of this passage, then it becomes apparent that this formula need not be understood as entering the extraordinary vessels at all. Its focus is on clearing the pathogen that is obstructing the exterior yang. Nevertheless, Pinellia and Sorghum Decoction *(ban xia shu mi tang)* is the only herbal treatment Li Shi-Zhen offers for pathologies of the *yang qiao*, and he makes no mention of herbal formulas for *yin qiao* pathologies at all. At this juncture, it is tempting to dismiss the entire matter as completely irrelevant to clinical practice were it not for the fact that the case records of Ye Tian-Shi (Ye Gui) also discuss the *yang qiao* in terms of deficiency.

The most thoroughly documented case records in the premodern Chinese medical literature dealing with the extraordinary vessels are those of Ye Tian-Shi. As already noted, although he is commonly viewed as the heir to Li Shi-Zhen's lineage of extraordinary vessel herbal prescribing, Ye Tian-Shi most definitely had his own interpretive agenda. His case records are evidence of a remarkable capacity to flexibly integrate a wide range of Chinese medical influences. Li's voice was but one among many. Nevertheless, in his treatment of the extraordinary vessels, Ye, too, almost invariably refers to the *yang qiao* as being empty *(kong* 空*)*. Curiously, however, although Ye Tian-Shi claims that the *yang qiao* vessels are empty, the elimination of phlegm-thin mucus from the yang is still a central component of his treatment strategy. It appears that Ye has taken his cue from Li Shi-Zhen in his understanding of *yang qiao* pathology. The *yang qiao* is empty because the yang is being blocked from entering it. The three cases by Ye Tian-Shi's that follow illustrate this interpretation.

Ye Tian-Shi's Cases

Case No. 1: Wang, age 47, thin mucus is a transformation of turbid yin hindering the yang qi and preventing it from entering the yin. The *yang qiao* is empty, preventing sound sleep at night. *Divine Pivot* advocates the use of Pinellia and Sorghum Decoction *(ban xia shu mi tang)* that is said to unblock the yang and promote communication with the yin, preventing an amassment of the thin mucus pathogen. The use of cold and cool medicinals such as Emperor of Heaven's Special Pill to Tonify the Heart *(tian wang bu xin dan)* is [the wrong] approach for well-established turbid yin [conditions]. During middle age, it is essential to take care of the yang, especially according to *Essentials from the Golden Cabinet (Jīn guì yào lüè* 金匱要略*)*, which says that one must use warming medicinals to harmonize [such conditions].[6]

The treatment strategy in this first case is quite general. Ye's counsel is to incorporate the warming medicinals recommended in *Essentials from the Golden Cabinet* into the basic Pinellia Rhizoma *(ban xia)* prescription presented in *Divine Pivot*. The warming medicinals mentioned by Ye are most likely a reference to a passage in the *Golden Cabinet* that states: "When there is phlegm-thin mucus below the heart with propping fullness of the chest and rib-sides, and dizziness, Poria, Cinnamon Twig, Atractylodes, and Licorice Decoction *(ling gui zhu gan tang)* masters it."[7] The primary ingredients in this formula are Atractylodis macrocephalae Rhizoma *(bai zhu)*, Poria *(fu ling)*, and Cinnamomi Ramulus *(gui zhi)*, which together warm the yang, transform rheum, dis-inhibit water, and settle the heart.

> **Case No. 2:** Mr. Zhu, age 49, was so troubled that he damaged his yang. Thin mucus accumulated over time, therefore the *yang qiao* became empty and the patient became wakeful and unable to sleep. Because the protective yang had lost its protective capacity, the patient's hair fell out. Then, over time, the patient became ever more feeble. First, promote free flow through the rheum turbidity to revive the yang. Administer the Poria Drink from *Arcane Essentials* (*Wai tai fu ling yin*).[8]

The second case represents a further elaboration of this same idea with Ye's use of Poria Drink *(fu ling yin)*, which reflects a more substantial aspect of spleen deficiency. The traditional indications for this formula include fixed phlegm and thin mucus in the chest and vomiting of water, qi deficiency, abdominal fullness, and inability to digest food. It contains Poria *(fu ling)*, 3 *liang*, Ginseng Radix *(ren shen)*, 2 *liang*, Atractylodis macrocephalae Rhizoma *(bai zhu)*, 3 *liang*, Zingiberis Rhizoma recens *(sheng jiang)*, 4 *liang*, Aurantii Fructus immaturus *(zhi shi)*, 2 *liang*, and Citri reticulatae Pericarpium *(chen pi)*, 1.5 *liang*.

> **Case No. 3:** Mr. Gu (age 44), already had graying hair on his temples although the luster on his face remained good. He suffered from emotional irrita-tion and overwork. Because there was an ascendant stirring of yang qi, the phlegm and thin mucus also spilled upward. *Divine Pivot* states, "The yang should descend and enter the yin. When the *yang qiao* vessel is full it allows a person to go to sleep and causes the qi to drain outward. Because the yang was unable to enter the yin, the patient would drink sweet wine until intoxi-cated in the hopes of becoming muddled-headed and thereby falling asleep. This was a poor approach to treating such a disease. In men, during middle age and afterwards, the lower base is the first to become depleted. [The patient] was given Eight-Ingredient Pill with Rehmannia *(ba wei di huang wan)* in the morning and Pinellia and Sorghum Decoction *(ban xia shu mi tang)* in the evening. (The *yang qiao* vessel was deficient).[9]

The treatment strategy in this final case more clearly distinguishes between patho-genic phlegm-thin mucus preventing the yang from entering the *yang qiao* and the underlying deficiency, which in this instance is an insufficiency of yin.

Ye Tian-Shi's preference for a pathodynamic of emptiness with regard to the ex-traordinary vessels may also be viewed in the larger context of his understanding of all extraordinary vessel pathology as being fundamentally one of deficiency. His trade-mark use of medicinals such as Cervi Cornu degelatinatum *(lu jiao shuang)*, Asini Corii Colla *(e jiao)*, Trionycis Carapax *(bie jia)*, and Hominis Placenta *(zi he che)* to treat the extraordinary vessels is well documented. For Ye, the inclusion of these rich and cloying animal products is often the defining feature of an extraordinary vessel treatment strategy.

Implications

An immediate reaction raised by a critical review of all extraordinary vessel herbal prescribing is "so what?" Could we have reached the same conclusion without recourse to an extraordinary vessel diagnosis? In the case of the distinction presented here, the question is even more pointed since the theoretical emptiness or fullness of the *yang qiao* has little impact on the herbal treatment strategy historically used to treat it. It is definitely necessary to clear phlegm-thin mucus from some aspect of the yang, al-though in herbal medicine it is difficult to say with any confidence that one is clearing the congestion from the protective yang or the *yang qiao* itself. In any case, the result is the same. Is this all not an exercise in academic nitpicking? When left in the realm of herbal prescribing, perhaps it is, but the principles implied here clearly extend to the practice of acupuncture. This is particulary true when one considers the context in which this alternative reading first appears. A central characertistic of Li Shi-Zhen's *Exposition on the Eight Extraordinary Vessels* is the integration of alchemy, acupunc-ture, and herbal practice. As we have already seen in Chapters 1 and 2 of that text, Li clearly states that the concepts of one are germain to the others.

Ye Tian-Shi's application of the idea of *yang qiao* emptiness in herbal prescribing is evidence that Li was not alone in this interpretation. Ye's cases also provide a more concrete sense of how all these ideas have been applied clinically. Despite the fact that the crucial passage from Ch. 71 of *Divine Pivot* focuses on herbal treatment, the princ-ple is relevant to acupuncture practice. After all, the source for this notion of a collapse of the *yang qiao* is the *Divine Pivot*, a text primarily concerned with acupuncture. The implications of a pathodynamic of *yang qiao* emptiness are particularly meaningful for acupuncture treatment because, conceptually, the distinction between the networks of the exterior yang and the *yang qiao* is much clearer in the practice of acupuncture. With acupuncture, it is much easier to address the exterior yang and the *yang qiao* as entirely separate, if interrelated, systems.

The fundamental principle implied here is that it may in some instances be nec-essary to open the yang prior to accessing the *qiao* vessels, particulary when there appears to be a significant amount of congestion on the level of the network vessels. This may present as localized muscular soreness and tension, topical redness, inflammation, or poor capillary refilling subsequent to pressure.

There are many eastablished acupuncture techniques for opening the yang in the network vessels. The cross needling method mentioned in Ch. 73 of *Divine Pivot* is a classic example of a therapy intended to specifically clear stagnation of the networks in advance of other treatments. The modern Japanese techniques of Sessokushin, Naso, and Muno, and some of Sugiyama's 18 needling techniques accomplish the same thing with less pain and trauma, although they are by no means universally applied prior to other therapies.[10]

The following case history exemplifies the potential of this idea for guiding acupuncture practice.

A 40-year-old female had recently begun recieving treatment for liver qi constraint with heart and liver blood deficiency presenting as a return of long-standing complaints of insomnia, depression, restless leg syndrome, body aches, mental fogginess, and deep fatigue. Over the course of the past ten days, the Chinese herbal preparation she was taking had been effective in beginning to resolve her situation to the extent that all her symptoms were greatly diminished and she felt better than she had in some time. Encouraged by her progress, she indulged in a single glass of wine at a New Year's Eve party, after which she immediately felt her symptoms return. That night she did not sleep. She returned to the clinic the following afternoon, New Year's day, complaining that her symptoms had returned. Her tongue coating was slightly slimy although she complained of intense thirst. The body of the tongue was slightly dusky. Her left pulse was unambiguously *yang qiao*: it was strong and tapping[11] in the distal position, and otherwise wiry. Both the pulse and symptom presentation were consistent with a *yang qiao* disorder.

I palpated a number of holes to determine optimal availability and selected Instep Yang (BL-59) right, followed by stimulation of Bright Eyes (BL-1) right, with a gold Teishin, which produced a partial softening of the pill-like quality. Unsatisfied with this result, I then performed an extremely superficial needle technique on a few reactive areas on the patient's neck to open the networks. This incrementally improved the overall quality of the pulse but did not impact the fundamental *yang qiao* presentation. I then needled Instep Yang (BL-59) left, and the pulse balanced out completely. Then, I administered a meridian-style root treatment consistent with the patient's liver pattern. When the patient left, she reported that she felt much better and her acute symptoms had resolved. She slept well that night and then resumed her previous course of herbal therapy.

As we have already discussed in the introductory chapters, Li's synthesis of extraordinary vessel therapeutics does not require the use of conventional master-couple holes. Instep Yang (BL-59) is potentially as good a choice as Extending Vessel (BL-62) for accessing the *yang qiao*. In this instance, BL-59 was determined to be energetically more available and was 'coupled' with Bright Eyes (BL-1), the terminal hole on the channel, rather than Back Ravine (SI-3). The response to this pairing, however, was less than optimal until the yang networks were opened. Because nearly all the yang channels transit very superficially through the neck region, the network vessels are particularly accessible here. This, coupled with the fact that the patient's most immediate complaints were localized in her head, made Bright Eyes (BL-1) an obvious choice for treatment.

Li's multivalent interpretation of *yang qiao* pathodynamics is easily overlooked in the midst of his rehearsal of familiar material. One tends to dismiss his discussion of diseases of the *qiao* vessel as little more than an anthology of established ideas to which Li has added no insight of his own. Yet it is apparent that Li's contribution, though subtle, is substantial. Much of the genius of his *Exposition* lies precisely in its careful organization, juxtapositioning, and reinterpretation of orthodox material that is then blended with often iconclastic sources to produce something new. It is a decidedly understated presentation style that demands an informed and attentive reader. The rewards are worth the effort. The case records of at least one other influential physician echo Li's interpretation of *yang qiao* pathodynamics, and it offers a significant possibility for refining one's acupuncture practice.

Apparently anomalous readings such as those discussed here are all too easily swept under the rug or ignored by academics with little interest in their clinical ramifications. Admittedly, these investigations typically fall short of any practical application. Most are dead ends, but every so often the inconsistencies in a text lead us somewhere that enhances our capacity for real treatment. Just when we think we've mined the premodern literature for all it is worth, if we are attentive, we may stumble upon something that may make a difference, something that should not be ignored.

CHAPTER 39

Master Hu's Process: The Seeds of Internal Cultivation through the Extraordinary Vessels

by Charles Chace

The various banches of the *chong* vessel lie at the core of the extraordinary vessel network. They are the hub around which the other seven vessels revolve, the stalk at the center of the primary channels and the sea of blood.[1] Yet if the *chong* are the heartwood of the eight vessels, then their descending branch, known as the *tai chong* (太衝) or Great Thoroughfare, is its taproot. Luo Dong-Yi's vision of the Great Thoroughfare as both the wellspring of and synonym for the extraordinary vessel network as a whole makes the concept of *tai chong* immediately relevant to our understanding of the extraordinary vessels.[2] Although his is a late contribution to the development of the extraordinary vessels writing, as he lived in the 1800s, Luo's ideas are remarkably resonant with how the term was originally used.

The words *tai chong* first appear in the early Chinese philosophical masterpiece known as *Zhuang zi* (late 4th century BCE) as the penultimate phase of internal cultivation and is generally understood to mean something akin to emptiness (*kong* 空) or the great void *(tai xu* 太虛). In light of the intimate relationship between the extraordinary vessels and practices of internal cultivation, it is unlikely that the use of the *tai chong* in relation to the extraordinary vessels is coincidental. Clearly, it merits further consideration. This essay will outline the concept of *tai chong* as it first appears in *Zhuang zi* and discuss its relevance to the extraordinary vessels as a medium for internal cultivation, particularly as it pertains to Li Shi-Zhen's *Exposition on the Eight Extraordinary Vessels.*

The last of *Zhuang zi's* so-called "Inner Chapters" *(Nei pian* 內篇), the "Responses of Emperors and Kings" (*Ying di wang* 應帝王), is concerned with the traits of a truly effective ruler, which in this context can be taken as a proxy for the realized human. Here, a series of seven parables and anecdotes give voice to a variety of sages. They summarize many of the essential points concerning the optimal traits presented in the book as a whole.

At the heart of this chapter is the parable of Master Hu (壺子) and the magus Ji Xian (季咸).[3] This story lays out a clearly sequenced vision of internal cultivation that provides an organizing framework for understanding the related material throughout the rest of the text. In this story, we see concepts that are entirely consistent with those outlined in the alchemical stratum of Li's writing on the extraordinary vessels and that are very similar to those propounded later by Luo Dong-Yi.

That Master Hu's parable contains a recognizable sequence of internal development is apparent in the commentary literature dating back at least to the Daoist commentator Cheng Xuan-Ying (成玄英, fl. 630–660),[4] a thread that continues to the present. In discussing the use of the "Inner Chapters" as a practical manual of meditation in Daoist temples in modern Taiwan, Michael Saso identifies the Hu parable as a general outline for the stages of internal cultivation.[5] The other tales and anecdotes in the "Responses of Emperors and Kings" chapter frame the central message of Master Hu's parable and outline its implications for effective rulership.

The two tales immediately preceding the parable of Master Hu outline how to rule in a manner that transcends humanity and that bypasses governance by externals. The first counsels that the enlightened ruler should "let the mind float in blandness and mingle the qi with vastness. Follow the self-so [nature] of things, do not let any of oneself into it, and all under heaven will be ordered" (汝游心於淡合氣於漠順物自然而無容私焉而天下治矣). In the next tale, the enlightened ruler is described as "established in unfathomability, and wanders in nonbeing" (立乎不測而游於無有者也).[6] The Hu parable that follows describes the sign posts on the path to this concept of wandering in nonbeing.

The Parable of Master Hu[7]

鄭有神巫[8]曰季咸知人之死生存亡禍福壽夭期以歲月旬日若神[9]

In Zheng, there was a magus by the name of Ji Xian who had knowledge of peoples' life and death, whether they would be preserved or perish, whether they would experience calamity or good fortune, and whether they would live long or die young, predicting these things to the year, month, ten-day period, or even day as if he were a divinity.

鄭人見之皆奔而走[10]

Upon seeing him, the people of Zheng all rushed and ran.

列子見之而心醉歸以告壺子曰始吾以夫子之道為至矣則又有至焉者矣

Liezi saw him, and his mind was enchanted. Returning, he reported to Master Hu, proclaiming: "In the beginning, I regarded the Way of you, sir, to be the ultimate! But there is another who possesses something even more supreme than you!"[11]

壺子曰吾與汝既其文[12]未既其實而固得道與

Master Hu said: "Although I have given you its patterns, I have not yet given you its substance, and yet you are confident that you have attained the Way?"

眾雌而無雄而又奚卵

"If you have lots of hens and no roosters, then how could you have any eggs?"

而以道與世亢¹³必信夫故使¹⁴人得而相汝嘗試與來以予示之

"And yet you take this [lesser] way and proclaim it to the world, certain of its veracity. And for this reason you bid people accept it and assist you. Please try to bring [this magus] here and show him to me."

明日列子與之見壺子出而謂列子曰嘻子之先生死矣弗活矣不以旬數矣吾見怪焉見濕灰焉

The next day, Liezi brought him to see Master Hu. Upon leaving, [Ji Xian] said to Liezi: "Ah, your teacher is dying! He has no life left in him! He will not last even ten days! I saw the strangeness¹⁵ in him; I saw damp ashes in him."

列子入泣涕沾襟以告壺子

Liezi went in, sobbing tears that soaked his sleeves, and told Master Hu [what Ji Xian had said].

壺子曰鄉吾示之以地文萌乎不震不止是殆見吾杜德機也嘗又與來

Master Hu said: "Just now I showed my earthly pattern,¹⁶ the sprout [of life] seemed to neither stir nor be still.¹⁷ He probably saw that I had stopped up the power of my dynamic. Try to bring him back again."

明日又與之見壺子出而謂列子曰幸矣子之先生遇我也有瘳矣全然有生矣吾見其杜權矣

The next day, he again brought [Ji Xian] to see Master Hu. [Ji Xian] emerged and said to Liezi: "How auspicious that your teacher met me. He has healed! He has completely come back to life! I saw that this stoppage was only temporary!"¹⁸

列子入以告壺子壺子曰鄉吾示之以天壤¹⁹名實不入而機²⁰發於踵是殆見吾善者機也嘗又與來

Lieze went in and reported to Master Hu. Master Hu said: "Just now I showed him the vitality of heaven and soil,²¹ where neither name nor substance influences me, and my dynamic issued from my heels.²² So he probably saw me with health as my dynamic. Try to bring him back again."

明日又與之見壺子出而謂列子曰子之先生不齊吾無得而相焉試齊且復相之

The next day, [Liezi] again brought [Ji Xian] to see Master Hu. He emerged and said to Liezi: "Your teacher is unstable. I cannot get [any information], so I cannot read him. Try to stabilize him, then I will read him again."

列子入以告壺子壺子曰吾鄉示之以太衝莫勝²³是殆見吾衡氣機也鯢桓
之審²⁴為淵止水之審為淵流水之審為淵淵有九名此處三焉²⁵

Liezi went in and reported to Master Hu. Master Hu said: "Just now I showed him the Great Thoroughfare where nothing is victorious.²⁶ He probably saw me balancing my qi dynamic. The profound depths stirred by leviathans²⁷ are an abyss, the profound depths where there is a stilling of waters are an abyss, the profound depths from where waters flow are [also] an abyss. There are nine kinds of abyss.²⁸ Here then, are three of them."

明日又與之見壺子立未定自失而走壺子曰追之列子追之不及反以報壺
子曰已滅矣已失矣吾弗及已

The next day, [Liezi] again brought [Ji Xian] to see Liezi. [Ji Xian] stood but did not stay. He lost his composure and fled. Master Hu said: "Chase him!" Liezi chased him, but he was too late. He returned and reported to Master Hu saying: "He has already gone! I have lost him! I could not catch him!"

壺子曰鄉吾示之以未始出吾宗吾與之虛而委蛇不知其誰何因以為弟靡
因以為波流故逃也

Master Hu said: "Just now I showed him that my ancestral [influences] had not yet begun to emerge,²⁹ I was empty and entwined with him, so we could not know who was who. Thus were we blown like the wind; thus did we flow like a wave.³⁰ It was for this reason that he fled."

然後列子自以為未始學而歸三年不出為其妻爨食豕如食於事無與親雕
琢復朴塊然獨以其形立紛而封戎一以是終

Afterward, Liezi himself understood that he had not yet even begun to learn [from Master Hu] and returned [to his studies]. He did not go out for three years; cooking for his wife and feeding the pigs [with such care], it was as if he were feeding people; he had little to do with the affairs of the world. From the carved and polished, he returned to simplicity. Clod-like, his singularity became established in his form, he sealed himself off from confusion,³¹ and he uniformly remained like this to the very end.³²

Damp Ashes and the Patterns of the Earth

Ji Xian's first encounter with Master Hu leads Ji to believe that Hu is a dying man. He reports to Liezi that his master looks like "damp ashes." His grim turn of phrase is actually something of a technical term that is part of an entire complex of imagery. In Ch. 22, "Knowledge Wanders North," Quilt Coat (Bei Yi 被衣) proclaims of his compatriot Gnaw Gap (Nie Que 齧缺): "His form is like a withered carcass, his mind like dead ashes" *(xing ruo gao hai, xin ruo si hui* 形若槁骸, 心若死灰). Far from an insult, this is high praise. In *Lao zi*, the imagery of the Way is most familiarly associated with the dark feminine *(xuan pin* 玄牝) womb of fecundity, the suppleness implicit in bending to become straight *(wang ze zhi* 枉則直), and again becoming a newborn child *(fu gui yu ying 'er* 復歸於嬰兒), but this is only part of the equation. *Zhuang zi* commonly evokes the Way using the imagery of death. Although Ji Xian is disconcerted by his ashen presentation, Master Hu is merely expressing the nature of his mind. Precisely what is it that Ji Xian is looking at? Some visual cue apparently. It soon becomes clear that Ji Xian's concern with seeing *(jian* 見) is but a poor substitute for what is described in Ch. 4, "The Human World" *(Ren jian shi* 人間世), as listening *(ting* 聽)[33] with one's qi. In any case, despite the fact that Ji Xian does not see very deeply, his perceptions at each turn in the story illustrate the relationship of the mind, body, and qi in *Zhuang zi*.

Many essayists have written about the relationship between the cognitive and the corporal in *Zhuang zi,* particularly with respect to the concept of heart–mind *(xin* 心).[34] Although mind, body, and qi are clearly understood as distinct and interrelated concepts in *Zhuang zi,* the mind has undeniable primacy. Its relationship with the body and the qi is such that any stage or trait of consciousness must necessarily manifest in both the form and the qi until the final stage where such distinctions ultimately dissolve. It is not only one's mind that ultimately becomes unified with the Way, it is one's entire being. The Hu parable makes this transition clear.

Master Hu explains to Liezi that he had merely embodied the patterns of the earth *(di wen* 地文) for Ji Xian. He had dammed up the power or virtuosity of his dynamic *(de ji* 德機) so that there was neither activity nor the cessation of activity. All of the states described by Master Hu are expressions of his dynamic disposition *(ji* 機). He is not so interested in demonstrating the nature of his mind as he is in demonstrating the nature of his qi as it expresses his mind. The state referred to in this first encounter is described elsewhere in *Zhuang zi* as "fasting of the mind" *(zhai xin* 齋心). It is not described as a final stage of practice, but instead establishes the preliminary conditions for one's unification with the Way.

When not mercilessly ridiculing him, Zhuang zi often puts remarkably Daoist ideas into the mind of Confucius, who first utters the term "fasting of the mind." This practice is what allows one to truly listen to the piping of heaven.

若一志無聽之以耳而聽之以心無聽之以心而聽之以氣聽止於耳心止於
符氣也者虛而待物者也唯道集虛虛者心齋也[35]

Unify your will! Do not listen to it with your ears, listen to [it] with your mind; do not listen with your mind, listen to it with your qi. [Ordinary] listening ceases with the ears and the mind ceases with tabulation. Qi is what is empty and awaits upon things. Only the Way can amass emptiness, and emptiness is the fasting of the mind.

On the Heels of Vitality

When Ji Xian next interviews Master Hu, he is surprised to discover that the master has made a complete recovery. Ji attributes this to his own talents when in actuality Hu has simply showed him a different state of consciousness. Hu explains to Liezi that he has shown Ji a different dynamic or disposition *(ji* 機), a dynamic of the vitality of heaven and earth that springs from his heels. In the previous chapter, the "Great Ancestral Teacher" *(da zong shi* 大宗師), Zhuang zi explains that "the authentic man breathes from his heels, and the common man breathes by means of his throat" (真人 之息以踵衆人之息以喉).[36] Harold Roth has argued that many passages in *Zhuang zi* are concerned with the same kinds of yogic breathing practices mentioned in *Lao zi* (500–200 BCE), the Mawangdui *Huang-Lao* 黃老 (300 BCE) texts, and the *Guan Zi* (26 BCE), and this is clearly one of them.[37] The precise nature of these breathing practices is never specified. *Zhuang zi's* references to breathing through one's heels and letting one's vitality issue through one's heels provide a clue as to the means by which such practices might have been performed.

These references immediately bring to mind the trajectories of the two *qiao* vessels arising from the heels. Master Hu has quite literally put a spring back in his step.[38] At least some of the eight extraordinary vessels are closely associated with the cultivation of original qi in internal alchemy and in Li's *Exposition*, the *yin qiao* being among them. Moreover, the importance of the heels and their associated channels in creating the optimal conditions for the transmission of qi has persisted. As already mentioned, the *yin qiao* was of particular importance to the great Daoist adept of the Song dynasty, Zhang Boduan, who asserted that when cultivating primal influences through the extraordinary vessels, one must first open the *yin qiao*.[39] From this perspective, *Zhuang zi* in general and the parable of Master Hu in particular establishes a primitive model for subsequent systems of internal cultivation.

The Thoroughfare of Neutrality

By Ji's third interview with Master Hu, things are beginning to get out of hand. Hu later explains that he showed Ji the "Great Thoroughfare where nothing is victorious" *(tai chong mo sheng* 太衝莫勝),[40] a state of such perfect balance that Ji does not know what to make of it. He actually interprets Hu's condition as its opposite, a state of instability.

Commentators typically gloss the term Great Thoroughfare as a synonym for emptiness, interpreting Master Hu as becoming one with vacuity.[41] Yet if that is all there is to it, then how does this tranquil emptiness differ from the damp ashes described in the first encounter? There is a crucial difference between the two stages, one that hinges on the larger implications of our understanding of the Great Thoroughfare.

The term *tai chong* (太衝, written slightly later as 太沖), is clearly linked to a similar term in *Zhuang zi, da tong* (大通), which other translators have rendered as Transformational Thoroughfare[42] or Universal Thoroughfare.[43] In Ch. 6, Yan Hui (顏回) explains to Confucius that "going along with the Great Thoroughfare, this is called sitting and forgetting" (同於大通此謂坐忘),[44] a practice closely allied to fasting the mind. The sense of these terms is not exclusively one of passive openness or emptiness. Both words carry the connotation of openness that allows for activity or a blowing free of obstruction. Harold Roth's translation of *da tong* as the 'Great Pervader' captures this sense nicely.[45] The emptiness of the Way obliterates all obstruction. This is clear in the energetic resonances of the Great Thoroughfare.

In both Chinese medicine and internal cultivation, the concept of the *tai chong* is linked to the *chong* vessel as the central conduit of qi in the body around which all other conduits revolve. As part of the triad that includes the *ren* and *du* vessels, the *chong* is intimately involved in the cultivation of primal influences. As already noted, Luo Dong-Yi goes so far as to identify this Great Thoroughfare with the diffusion of primal qi throughout the body.[46]

The *tai chong* is open and empty, yet dynamic and potent; it is the stillness at the center of things that allows for effortless action. Though it is described as a stage of consciousness, it similarly embodies physically and energetically the extraordinary vessels as a whole and, for that matter, the entirety of Master Hu's being. Because his perspective is so limited, the magus Ji Xian is only able to relate to what he perceives to be the state of Master Hu's physical health, and this makes no sense to him.

The progression of Hu's process has a breadth of its own, beginning with the last gasp of a body-mind on its deathbed, followed by a deep invigorating breath issuing from the heels. In the ultimate balance and neutrality of the Great Thoroughfare, there is again a profound stillness. Yet this is a dynamic stillness quickened by the Way and imbued with an aliveness that transcends the 'damp ashes' of the first stage, and what now becomes clear is the relatively superficial vitality expressed in the second stage. When the Way fully pervades the Great Thoroughfare, its calm emptiness enlivens and activates the body, mind, and qi. Hu's display pervades all levels of his being. The perfusion of the Great Thoroughfare with dynamic emptiness establishes the conditions for the final stage of internal cultivation.

What Precedes the Ancestral

Master Hu's final performance so unnerves Ji Xian that he flees. He had shown Ji "that my ancestral [influences] had not yet begun to emerge" *(wei shi chu wu zong* 未始出 吾宗).[47] This is the ultimate unification or entwinement *(wei yi* 委蛇)[48] with the Way, where one loses all sense of the distinction between self and other. There ceases to be anything present that can be differentiated from the Way at large.

In both *Zhuang zi* and *Lie zi*, one's unification with the Way is expressed in one's entire being in a manner that blurs the distinctions between mind, body, and qi. This process of unification, a dissolution of distinctions, or consolidation (*ning* 凝), is typically presented in a piecemeal fashion in *Zhuang zi*. In the chapter titled "Free and Easy Rambling" *(Xiao yao you* 逍遙游), "one's spirit is consolidated" *(qi shen ning* 其神凝),[49] and in the chapter titled "Sunshine" *(Ze yang* 則陽), it takes a more corporal bent: "The sage penetrates bafflement and complication, rounding all into a unified body" *(zhou jin yi ti* 周盡一體).[50] But in the chapter titled "The Great Ancestral Teacher" *(Da zong shi* 大宗師), this process is framed as a sloughing off of all aspects of selfhood such that distinctions of mind, body, and qi become meaningless: "Shed limbs and trunk, dismiss [conventional] consciousness, leave off form and depart from knowing; to unify with the great opening, this is called sitting and forgetting" (墮肢體黜聰明離形去知同於大通此謂坐忘).[51] A similar passage appears in Ch. 2, the "Yellow Emperor," of *Lie Zi*: "My mind consolidated, my form dispersed, my bones and flesh melded together; with no sense of form on which to rely; like trunk and leaves, stem and fruits. Did the wind ride me, or did I ride the wind?" (心凝形釋骨肉都融不覺形之所倚足之所履隨風東西犹木叶干壳竟不知風乘我邪我乘風乎).[52] Insofar as such distinctions are ultimately obliterated, it is therefore meaningless to speak of the cultivation advocated in *Zhuang zi* as a 'spiritual' practice. The end result is ultimately much more encompassing than the spirit.

The Return to Simplicity

Having seen that he had not even scratched the surface of his understanding of the Way, Liezi turns away from the "carved and polished, he returned to simplicity" *(diao zhuo fu pu* 雕琢復朴).[53] His simplicity is a return to wholeness and the unexpressed emergence of his ancestry. Or perhaps it is the unexpressed emergence of what *Lao zi* describes as an abyss that is like the ancestor of the myriad things *(si wan wu zhi zong* 似萬物之宗).[54] In the end, simplicity is the central means by which each of the above stages is realized.

The carved and the polished (*diao zhuo* 雕琢) is an image of refinement and culture. Liezi turns away from this to polish his mind in a different way in the next chapter, making it mirror-like: "The ultimate person's use of his mind is like a mirror. It neither projects nor welcomes; it responds, but it does not hide them, and for this reason, it can be victorious over things without sustaining injury" (至人之用心若鏡不將不迎應而不藏故能勝物而不傷).[55]

In the space of a few paragraphs, the parable of Master Hu and the brief anecdotes surrounding it summarize the progression to unification with the Way and point to the general means by which it is attained. The imagery the parable employs provides the seeds for how the extraordinary vessels were used in internal cultivation. Here, there is as yet no *yin wei, yang wei, yin qiao, yang qiao, chong, ren, du,* and *dai*. There is only a primitive notion of a pathway issuing from the heels, that once opened, allows a Great Thoroughfare of empty awareness to pervade the body, dissolving all distinctions and rounding all into a unified whole.

Part V

APPENDICES

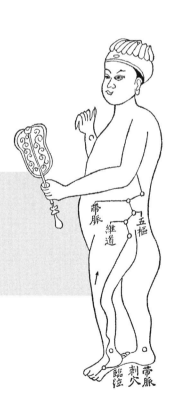

Acupuncture Holes of the Extraordinary Vessels

The following tables list the acupuncture holes occurring on the trajectories of the extraordinary vessels, according to Li Shi-Zhen and the holes he mentions in the treatment of each extraordinary vessel. Those marked with an * denote holes for which an identification is ambiguous or in dispute among commentators.

Acupuncture Holes of the *Yang Wei*	
TRAJECTORY HOLES	TREATMENT HOLES
BL-63	GB-20
GB-35	GV-16
GB-29	GB-3
LI-14	BL-59
TB-13	BL-57*
TB-15	GB-38
GB-21	GB-35*
SI-10	
GB-20 ~ GB-13	

Acupuncture Holes of the *Yin Wei*	
TRAJECTORY HOLES	TREATMENT HOLES
KI-9	Abdomen
SP-13	GB-14
SP-15	BL-61
SP-16	BL-63
LR-14	KI-9
CV-22	
CV-23	

Acupuncture Holes of the *Yang Qiao*

TRAJECTORY HOLES	TREATMENT HOLES
BL-62	BL-59
BL-61	GB-20
BL-59	GV-14
SI-10	BL-62
LI-16	BL-61
LI-15	BL-56
ST-9	BL-64
ST-4	
ST-3	
ST-1	
BL-1	
GB-20	

Acupuncture Holes of the *Yin Qiao*

TRAJECTORY HOLES	TREATMENT HOLES
KI-2	KI-6
KI-6	GB-34
KI-8	KI-8
ST-9	LR-1
BL-1	

Acupuncture Holes of the *Ren*

TRAJECTORY HOLES	TREATMENT HOLES
CV-1 ~ CV-24	CV-22
GV-26	CV-4
ST-1	
ST-9	

Acupuncture Holes of the *Du*

TRAJECTORY HOLES	TREATMENT HOLES
CV-1	CV-2
CV-7	CV-7
BL-35	GV-1
GV-1 ~ GV-28	GV-17
BL-11	GV-16
	GV-14
	GV-13
	GV-8

Acupuncture Holes of the *Chong*

TRAJECTORY HOLES	TREATMENT HOLES
ST-30	Qi thoroughfares
KI-11	BL-11
KI-12	BL-57
KI-13	CV-4
KI-14	CV-17
KI-15	GV-15
KI-16	GV-14
KI-17	GV-20
KI-18	LU-1*
KI-19	ST-36
KI-20	ST-30
KI-21	ST-37
	ST-39
	ST-15*
	ST-16*

Acupuncture Holes of the *Dai*	
TRAJECTORY HOLES	TREATMENT HOLES
LR-13	LR-13
GB-26	GB-26
GB-27	CV-6
GB-28	GV-20

Extraordinary Vessel Herbal Formulas

For a comprehensive list of extraordinary vessel herbal formulas organized by vessel, see Chapter 36 above (starting on page 345).

Aconite and Cinnamon Twig Decoction (*wū tóu guì zhī tāng* 烏頭桂枝湯)

Cook 1 large piece of Aconiti Radix preparata *(zhì wū tóu)* in a small cup of honey down to half of the original amount, and then take the Aconiti Radix preparata *(zhì wū tóu)* out. Stir-fry with Cinnamomi Cortex *(ròu guì)*, 3 *qián* 3 *fēn*; Paeoniae Radix alba *(bái sháo)*, 3 *qián* 3 *fēn*. Divide the cooked herbs into 2 parts, and add to each part 3 pieces of ginger and 2 pieces of Jujube Fructus *(dà zǎo)* or Jujube Fructus *(hóng zǎo)* and boil them in the original honey. If you replace Aconiti Radix preparata *(zhì wū tóu)* with Aconiti Radix lateralis preparata *(zhì fù zǐ)*, it is called Honey and Aconite Decoction *(mì fù tāng)*.

Aconite and Gardenia Decoction (*wū tóu zhī zi tāng* 烏頭梔子湯)

Aconiti Radix *(chuān wū)* (tips); Gardeniae Fructus *(zhī zǐ)*

Angelica Root Decoction (*bái zhǐ tāng* 白芷湯)

Angelicae sinensis Radix *(dāng guī)*, Forsythiae Fructus *(lián qiào)*, 1.5 *qián* each; Notopterygii Rhizoma seu Radix *(qiāng huó)*, Angelicae pubescentis Radix *(dú huó)*, Saposhnikoviae Radix *(fáng fēng)*, Alismatis Rhizoma *(zé xiè)*, Cinnamomi Cortex *(ròu guì)*, 1 *qián* each; Fangji Radix *(fáng jǐ)*, Phellodendri Cortex *(huáng bǎi)*, Rhei Radix et Rhizoma *(dà huáng)*, Glycyrrhizae Radix *(gān cǎo)*, 5 *fēn* each; Persicae Semen *(táo rén)*, 9 pieces (retain tips). Decoct the herbs in a liquid composed of half water and half wine.

Angelica Root Pill (*bái zhǐ wán* 白芷丸)

Angelicae Dahuricae Radix *(bái zhǐ)*, 2 *liǎng*, soaked in Raphani Radix (radish) juice. It is then dried, smashed, and mixed with honey into pills the size of a bullet. Take 1 pill a day.

Aristolochia Pill (*qīng mù xiāng wán* 青木香丸)

Pharbitidis Semen Atrum *(hēi chǒu)*, 3 *liǎng* (tips only); Psoraleae Semen *(bǔ gǔ zhī)*, 2 *liǎng*; Litseae Fructus *(bì chéng qié)*, 2 *liǎng*; Arecae Semen *(bīng láng)*, 2 *liǎng*; Aristolochiae Radix *(qīng mù xiāng)* 1 *liǎng*.

Astragalus Decoction to Construct the Middle
(*huáng qí jiàn zhōng tāng* 黃耆健中湯)

Maltosum (*yí táng*), 6-10 *qián*; Cinnamomi Ramulus (*guì zhī*), 3 *qián*; Paeoniae Radix (*sháo yào*), 2 *qián*; Glycyrrhizae Radix preparata (*zhì gān cǎo*), 2 *qián*; Zingiberis Rhizoma recens (*shēng jiāng*), 3 *qián*; Jujubae Fructus (*dà zǎo*), 12 pieces; Astragali Radix (*huáng qí*) 3 *qián*.

Aucklandia Powder (*mù xiāng sǎn* 木香散)

Aucklandiae Radix (*mù xiāng*), Citri reticulatae Pericarpium (*chén pí*), Zingiberis Rhizoma (*gān jiāng*), Alpiniae officinarum Rhizoma (*gāo liáng jiāng*), Chebulae Fructus (*hē zǐ*), Alpiniae katsumadai Semen (*cǎo dòu kòu*), Gardeniae Fructus (*zhī zǐ*), Chuanxiong Rhizoma (*chuān xiōng*), and Pharbitidis Semen (*qiān niú zǐ*).

Auklandia and Toosendan Fruit Powder (*mù xiāng liàn zǐ sǎn* 木香楝子散)

Acori Rhizoma (*shí chàng pú*), Aristolochiae Radix (*qīng mù xiāng*), Litchi Semen (*lì zhī hé*), Dioscoreae Hypoglaucae Rhizoma (*bì xiè*), Toosendan Fructus (*chuān liàn zǐ*), 2 *qián* each. Add a small amount of Moschus (*shè xiāng*), Foeniculi Fructus (*huí xiāng*), and roasted salt.

Bamboo Leaf Decoction (*zhú yè tāng* 竹葉湯)

Bambusae Folium (*zhú yè*), 3 *liǎng*; Purariae; Radix (*gé gēn*), 3 *liǎng*; Saposhnikoviae Radix (*fáng fēng*), Platycodonis Radix (*jié gěng*), Cinnamomi Ramulus (*gùi zhī*), Ginseng Radix (*rén shēn*), Glycyrrhizae Radix (*gān cǎo*), 1 *liǎng* each.

Chuanxiong Powder to Be Taken with Green Tea
(*chuān xiōng chá tiáo sǎn* 川芎調茶散)

Menthae haplocalycis Herba (*bò hé*), Ligustici Rhizoma (*chuān xiōng*), Schizonepetae Herba (*jīng jiè*), Notopterygii Rhizoma seu Radix (*qiāng huó*), Angelicae dahuricae Radix (*bái zhǐ*), Glycyrrhizae Radix (*gān cǎo*), Saposhnikoviae Radix (*fáng fēng*), Asari Radix et Rhizoma (*xì xīn*). Take 2 *qián* after meals with green tea.

Cinnamon Twig Decoction (*guì zhī tāng* 桂枝湯)

Cinnamomi Ramulus (*guì zhī*), Paeoniae Radix alba (*bái sháo*), Glycyrrhizae Radix (*gān cǎo*), Zingiberis Rhizoma recens (*shēng jiāng*), Jujubae Fructus (*dà zǎo*).

Clove and Toosendan Fruit Pill (*dīng xiāng liàn shí wán* 丁香楝實丸)

Angelicae sinensis Radix (*dāng guī*), Aconiti Radix lateralis preparata (*zhì fù zǐ*), Toosendan Fructus (*chuān liàn zǐ*), Foeniculi Fructus (*xiǎo huí xiāng*), 1 *liǎng* each. Grind all the ingredients and decoct in 3 *shēng* of good wine until the liquid has completely evaporated and only a powder remains. For each *liǎng* of the powder, mix in 2 *qián* of Caryophylli Flos *(dīng xiāng)* and Aucklandiae Radix *(mù xiāng)*; whole Scorpio *(quán xiē)*, 13 pieces; Corydalis Rhizoma *(yán hú suǒ)*, 1 *liǎng*. Grind all the ingredients and mix them with the aforementioned powder. Make this preparation into pills with wine and take 100 pills on an empty stomach with wine.

Clove Powder for Spleen Accumulation (*dīng xiāng pí jī sǎn* 丁香脾積散)

Sparganii Rhizoma *(sān léng)*, Zedoariae Rhizoma *(é zhú)*, Citri reticulatae viride Pericarpium *(qīng pí)*, Caryophylli Flos *(dīng xiāng)*, Aucklandiae Radix *(mù xiāng)*, Alpiniae officinarum Rhizoma *(gāo liáng jiāng)* (cooked in vinegar), Crotinis Semen Pulveratum *(bā dòu shuāng)*, Gleditsiae Fructus *(zào jiá)*, Ustarum fuligo herbarum *(bǎi cǎo shuāng)*. Form into hemp seed-sized pills and take 20–30 pills with hot water.

Collected Fragrant Herbs Drink (*jù xiāng yǐn zǐ* 聚香飲子)

Olibanum *(rǔ xiāng)*, Aquilariae Lignum *(chén xiāng)*, Santali Lignum *(tán xiāng)*, Saussureae (seu Vladminiae) Radix *(mù xiāng)*, Agastaches seu Pogostemi Herba *(huò xiāng)* 8 *fēn* each; Curcumae Longae Rhizoma *(jiāng huáng)*, Linderae Radix *(wū yào)*, Platycodonis Radix *(jíe gěng)*, Cinamomi Cortex *(ròu guì)*, Glycyrrhizae Radix *(gān cǎo)*, Corydalis Tuber *(yán hú* suǒ) 4 *fēn* each; Zingiberis Rhizoma Recens *(shēng* jiang) 3 pieces, Zizyphi Fructus *(dà zǎo)* 2 pieces.

Corydalis Powder (*yán hú suǒ sǎn* 延胡索散)

Corydalis Rhizoma *(yán hú suǒ)*, Angelicae sinensis Radix *(dāng guī)*, Typhae Pollen *(pú huáng)*, Paeoniae Radix rubra *(chì sháo)*, Cinnamomi Cortex Tubiformis *(róu guì)*, 1 *qián* each; Curcumae longae Rhizoma *(jiāng huáng)*, Aucklandiae Radix *(mù xiāng)*, Olibanum *(rǔ xiāng)*, Myrrha *(mò yào)*, 7 *fēn* each; baked Glycyrrhizae Radix *(gān cǎo)*, 5 *fēn*; Zingiberis Rhizoma *(gān jiāng)*, 3 pieces.

Dampness Leeching Decoction (*shèn shī tāng* 滲濕湯)

Poria *(fú líng)*, Polyporus *(zhū líng)*, Atractylodis macrocephalae Rhizoma *(bái zhú)*, Alismatis Rhizoma *(zé xiè)*, Atractylodis Rhizoma *(cāng zhú)*, Citri reticulatae Pericarpium *(chén pí)*, Coptidis Rhizoma *(huáng lián)*, Gardeniae Fructus *(zhī zǐ)*, Gentianae macrophyllae Radix *(qín jiāo)*, Stephaniae Radix *(fáng jǐ)*, Puerariae Radix *(gé gēn)*.

Eight-Substance Decoction (*bā wù tāng* 八物湯)

Ginseng Radix (*rén shēn*), Poria (*fú líng*), Atractylodis macrocephalae Rhizoma (*bái zhú*), Glycyrrhizae Radix (*gān cǎo*), Ligustici Rhizoma (*chuān xiōng*), Angelicae sinensis Radix (*dāng guī*), Paeoniae Radix alba (*bái sháo*), Remmaniae Radix Recens (*shēng dì huáng*).

Elixir to Seize Destiny (*duó mìng dān* 奪命丹)

Evodiae Fructus (*wú zhū yú*), 1 *jīn*. Divide into 4 equal parts. Soak 1 part in wine, 1 part in vinegar, 1 part in hot water, and 1 part in Infantis Urina (*tóng biàn*). Stir-fry everything together and add 2 *liǎng* of Alismatis Rhizoma (*zé xiè*). Form into pills, and take with salt water. This formula is also called Four Processed Evodiae Fructus Pill (*sì zhì zhū yú wán*).

Ephedra Decoction (*má huáng tāng* 麻黃湯)

Ephedrae Herba (*má huáng*), Cinnamomi Ramulus (*guì zhī*), Glycyrrhizae Radix (*gān cǎo*), Armeniacae Semen (*xìng rén*), Zingiberis Rhizoma (*gān jiāng*), Jujubae Fructus (*dà zǎo*).

Evodia Decoction (*wú zhū yú tāng* 吳茱萸湯)

Evodiae Fructus (*wú zhū yú*), Ginseng Radix (*rén shēn*), Zingiberis Rhizoma (*gān jiāng*), Jujubae Fructus (*dà zǎo*).

Evodiae Internal Mass-Dissolving Powder (*zhū yú nèi xiāo sǎn* 茱萸內消散)

Evodiae Fructus (*wú zhū yú*), soak 5 *qián* in half wine and half vinegar overnight and then bake; Corni Fructus (*shān zhū*); Baphicacantis Flos (*mǎ lán huā*), soak in vinegar and then bake; Toosendan Fructus (*chuān liàn ròu*); Cinnamomi Cortex (*ròu guì*); Pharbitidis Semen (*hēi chǒu*), (tips only); salt-stir-fried Foenuculi Fructus (*huí xiāng*); Corydalis Rhizoma (*yán hú suǒ*); Citri reticulatae viride Pericarpium (*qīng pí*), the white part removed; Sargassum (*hǎi zǎo*); Tribuli Fructus (*cì jí lí*); Persicae Semen (*táo rén*); Aucklandiae Radix (*mù xiāng*), 5 *qián* each.

Fast-Acting Powder (*sù xiào sǎn* 速效散)

Toosendan Fructus (*chuān liàn*), (stir-fry with 5 pieces of Crotonis Semen [*bā dòu*] and then remove the beans); salt-fried Foeniculi Fructus (*xiǎo huí xiāng*), honey-fried Psoraleae Fructus (*bǔ gǔ zhī*), 1 *liǎng* each. Take 1 *qián* each time with hot wine.

Fenugreek Pill (*hú lú bā wán* 胡盧巴丸)

Phabitidis Semen alba (*bái chǒu*), tips only, Foeniculi Fructus (*xiǎo huí xiāng*), 2 *liǎng* each; Aconiti Radix preparata (*zhì chuān wū*), Morindae officianalis Radix (*bā jǐ tiān*), Evodiae Fructus (*wú zhū yú*), 0.5 *liǎng* each; Nelumbinis Semen (*lián zǐ*), Foeni-graeci (*hú lú bā*), 1 *liǎng* each.

Five-Ingredient Powder with Poria (*wǔ líng sàn* 五苓散)

Poria (*fú líng*), Polyporus (*zhū líng*), Atractylodis Ovatae Rhizoma (*bái zhú*) 18 *zhū* each; Alismatis Rhizoma (*zé xiè*) 1 *liǎng*, Cinamomi Ramulus (*gùi zhī*) 5 *qián*.

Four-Miracle Pill (*sì shēn wán* 四神丸)

Evodiae Fructus *(wú zhū yú)*, 5 *qián* (soaked in a liquid of half wine and half vinegar and baked over slow fire); Litseae Fructus (*bì chéng qié*), 5 *qián*; Aristolochia Radix (*qīng mù xiāng*), 5 *qián*; Cyperi Rhizoma (*xiāng fù*), 1 *liǎng*. Form into pills with rice paste, and take with salt water.

Four-Ingredient Powder with Poria (*sì líng sǎn* 四苓散)

Poria *(fú líng)*, Polyporus *(zhū líng)*, Atractylodis macrocephalae Rhizoma *(bái zhú)*, Alismatis Rhizoma *(zé xiè)*.

Four-Part Sublime Toosendan Fruit Pill (*sì miào chuān liàn wán* 四妙川楝丸)

Toosendan Fructus *(chuān liàn zǐ)*, 1 *jin*. Divide into 4 equal parts. Wrap the first part in 1 *hé* of bran *(fū pí* 麸皮) with 49 pieces of Mylabris *(bān máo)* and stir-fry until they become brown. Wrap the second part in 1 *hé* of gluten flour skin with 1 *liǎng* of Morindae officinalis Radix *(bā jǐ tiān)* and stir-fry [in the same manner]. Wrap the third part in 1 *hé* of gluten flour skin with 49 Crotonis Semen *(bā dòu)* and stir-fry in the same manner. Wrap the fourth part in 1 *hé* of gluten flour skin with 1 *liǎng* of salt and 1 *hé* of Foeniculi Fructus *(xiǎo huí xiāng)* and stir-fry them until they are brown. Remove only the Toosendan Fructus *(chuān liàn)* and add Saussureae (seu Vladimiriae) Radix *(mù xiāng)* and Psoraleae Fructus *(bǔ gǔ zhī)*, 1 *liǎng* each. Form into pills with rice and wine and take 50 pills each time with salt water 3 times per day.

Four-Substance Decoction (*sì wù tāng* 四物湯)

Chuanxiong Rhizoma *(chuān xiōng)*, Angelicae sinensis Radix *(dāng guī)*, Paeoniae Radix alba *(bái sháo)*, Rehmannia Radix preparata *(shú dì huáng)*, 1 *qián* 2 *fēn* each.

Frigid Extremities Decoction (*sì nì tāng* 四逆湯)

Glycyrrhizae Radix *(gān cǎo)*, 2 *liǎng*; Zingiberis Rhizoma Exsiccatum *(gān jiāng)*, 1.5 *liǎng*; Aconiti Tuber Lateralis *(fù zǐ)*, 1 piece.

Generate the Pulse Powder (*shēng mài sǎn* 生脈散)

Ginseng Radix *(rén shēn)*, Ophiopogonis Radix *(mài mén dōng)*, Schisandrae Fructus *(wǔ wèi zǐ)*.

Gentiana Decoction to Drain the Liver (*lóng dǎn xiè gān tāng* 龍膽瀉肝湯)

Gentianae Radix *(lóng dǎn cǎo)*, Bupleuri Radix *(chái hú)*, Alismatis Rhizoma *(zé xiè)*, 1 *qián* each; Plantaginis Semen *(chē qián zǐ)*, Akebiae Caulis *(mù tōng)*, Poria Rubra *(chì fú líng)*, wine-washed Ramanniae Radix Recens *(shēng dì huáng)*, Angelicae sinensis Radix *(dāng guī)*, Gardeniae Fructus *(zhī zǐ)*, Scutellariae Radix *(huáng qín)*, Glycyrrhizae Radix *(gān cǎo)*, 5 *fēn* each.

Harmonize the Middle and Augment the Qi Decoction (*tiáo zhōng yì qì tāng* 調中益氣湯)

Astragali Radix *(huáng qí)*, 2 *qián*; Ginseng Radix *(rén shēn)*, 1 *qián*; Atractylodis Rhizoma *(cāng zhú)*, 1 *qián*; Honey-fried Glycyrrhizae Radix *(zhì gān cǎo)*, 1 *qián*; Citri reticulatae Pericarpium *(chén pí)*, 4 *fēn*; Cimicifugae Rhizoma *(shēng má)*, 4 *fēn*; Bupleuri Radix *(chái hú)*, 4 *fēn*; Aucklandiae Radix *(mù xiāng)*, 2 *fēn*. Decoct in water and administer.

Kidney Fixity Decoction (*shèn zhuó tāng* 腎著湯)

Atractylodis macrocephalae Rhizoma *(bái zhú)*, 2.5 *qián*; Zingiberis Rhizoma preparata *(páo jiāng)*, Poria Rubra *(chì fú líng)*, 0.5 *qián* each; honey-fried Glycyrrhizae Radix *(zhì gān cǎo)*.

Kidney Powder (*yāo zi sǎn* 腰子散)

Stir-fry equal amounts of Pharbitidis Semen *(hēi chǒu)* (chop off tips). Mince 3 *qián* of pig's kidneys *(zhū yāo zǐ)* and also add Zanthoxyli Pericarpium *(huā jiāo)*, 50 pieces, and Foeniculi Fructus *(xiǎo huí xiāng)*, 100 pieces. Mix all the ingredients, and grind them into a fine mash. Then, wrap this preparation with wet paper, and hold it over fire until an aroma rises. Chew the resulting mixture with wine in the mouth, and swallow the juice on an empty stomach. This will remove toxic waste matter from the intestines.

Lichee and Tangerine Pip Decoction (*lì zhī jú hé tāng* 荔枝橘核湯)

Pyri Succus *(lì zhī)*, Citri reticulatae Semen *(jú hé)*, Persicae Semen *(táo rén)*, Glycyrrhizae Radix *(gān cǎo)*, Poria *(fú líng)*, Crataegi Fructus *(shān zhā)*, Corydalis Rhizoma *(yán hú suǒ)*.

Licorice and Ailanthus Decoction (*gān lǐ gēn tāng* 甘李根湯)

Pruni Salicinae Radicis Cortex *(lǐ gēn pí)*, 5 *qián*; Cinnamomi Ramulus *(guì zhī)*, 1.5 *qián*; Angelicae sinensis Radix *(dāng guī)*, 1 *qián*; Paeoniae Radix alba *(bái sháo)*, 1 *qián*; Poria *(fú líng)*, 1 *qián*; Scutellariae Radix *(huáng qín)*, 1 *qián*; Pinelliae Rhizoma preparatum *(zhì bàn xià)*, 5 *fēn*; GlycyrrhizaeRadix *(gān cǎo)*, 5 *fēn*; Zingiberis Rhizoma Recens *(shēng jiāng)*, 3 pieces.

Licorice and Ginger Decoction (*gān cǎo gān jiāng tāng* 甘草干姜湯)

Glycyrrhizae Radix *(gān cǎo)*, 4 *liǎng;* Zingiberis Rhizoma *(gān jiāng)*, 2 *liǎng.*

Licorice Decoction to Drain the Epigastrium (*gān cǎo xiè xīn tāng* 甘草瀉心湯)

Glycyrrhizae Radix *(gān cǎo)*, 4 *liǎng;* Scutellariae Radix *(huáng qín)*, 3 *liǎng;* Zingiberis Rhizoma Exsiccatum *(gān jiāng)* 3 *liǎng;* Pinelliae Tuber *(bàn xià)*, 0.5 *shēng;* Ziziphi Fructus *(dà zǎo)*, 12 pieces (cracked open); Coptidis Rhixzoma *(huáng lián)*, 1 *liǎng.*

Licorice, Wheat, and Jujube Decoction (*gān mài dà zǎo tāng* 甘麥大棗湯)

Ligustici Rhizoma *(chuān xiōng)*, Angelicae sinensis Radix *(dāng guī)*, Paeoniae Radix alba *(bái sháo)*, Rehmanniae Radix preparata *(shú dì huáng)*, 1 *qián* 2 *fēn* each. In spring, double the amount of Ligustici Rhizoma *(chuān xiōng);* in summer, Paeoniae Radix alba *(bái sháo);* in fall, Rehmanniae Radix preparata *(shú dì huáng);* and in winter, Angelicae sinensis Radix *(dāng guī)*. In spring, add Saposhnikoviae Radix *(fáng fēng);* in summer, Scutellariae Radix *(huáng qín);* in fall, Asparagi Radix *(tiān mén dōng);* and in winter, Cinnamomi Ramulus *(guì zhī)*.

Major Order the Qi Decoction (*dà chéng qì tāng* 大承气湯)

Rhei Rhizoma *(dà huáng)*, 4 *liǎng;* Magnoliae officinalis Cortex *(hòu pò)*, 0.5 *jīn;* Aurantii Fructus Immaturus *(zhǐ shí)*, 5 pieces; Mirabilitum *(máng xiāo)*, 3 pieces.

Major Tangerine Pip Decoction (*dà jú pí tāng* 大橘皮湯)

Citri reticulatae Pericarpium *(chén pí)*, 3 *qián;* Bambusae Caulis in Taeniam *(zhú rú)*, 2 *qián;* Ginseng Radix *(rén shēn)*, 1 *qián;* Glycyrrhizae Radix *(gān cǎo)*, 1 *qián;* Zingiberis Rhizoma recens *(shēng jiāng)*, 5 pieces; Jujubae Fructus *(dà zǎo)*, 3 pieces.

Mantis Egg-Case Powder (*sāng piāo xiāo sǎn* 桑螵蛸散)

Mantis Ootheca *(sāng piāo xiāo)*, 3 *qián;* Os Draconis *(lóng gǔ)*, 4 *qián;* Ginseng Radix *(rén shēn)*, 4 *qián;* Poria *(fú líng)*, 3 *qián;* Acori Rhizoma *(shí chāng pú)*, 2 *qián;* honey-fried Testudinis Plastrum *(guī bǎn)*, 5 *qián;* Angelica Radix *(dāng guī)*, 2 *qián.*

Marvelously Fragrant Powder (*miào xiāng sàn* 妙香散)

Dioscoreae Rhizoma *(shān yào)*, Poria *(fú líng)*, Poria cum Pini Radice *(fú shén)*, Polygalae Radix *(yuǎn zhì)*, Astragali (seu Hedysari) Radix *(huáng qí)* 1 *liǎng* each; Ginseng Radix *(rén shēn)*, Platitycodonis Radix *(jié gěng)*, Glycyrrhizae Radix *(gān cǎo)* 5 *qián* each; Saussureae (seu Vladminiae) Radix *(mù xiāng)* 2.5 *qián*, Cinnabaris *(chén shā)* 3 *qián*, Moschus *(shè xiān)* 1 *qián.*

Master Shen's Mass-Dissolving Decoction (*Shěn shì sǎn jiǎ tāng* 沉氏散瘕湯)

Persicae Semen (*táo rén*), Aurantii Fructus immaturus (*zhǐ shí*), Gardeniae Fructus (*zhī zǐ*), Crataegus Fructus (*shān zhā*), Alisma Tuber (*zé xiè*), Akebiae Caulis (*mù tōng*), Poria Rubra (*chì fú líng*).

Master Yang's Musk Pill (*Yáng shì shè xiāng wán* 楊氏散瘕湯)

Moschus (*shè xiāng*), 1 *qián*; Aucklandiae Radix (*mù xiāng*), 1 *liǎng*; Piperis Fructus (*hú jiāo*), 1 *liǎng*; Scorpio (*quán xiē*), 4 *qián*; Croton tiglium (*bā dòu shuāng*), 4 *qián*. Roll the ingredients with steamed rice into pills the size of a hemp seed and then roll them in Cinnabaris powder (*zhū shā*). Take 5–7 pills per day with hot water. Without the Moschus (*shè xiāng*), this formula is known as Miraculous Preservation Pill (*shén bǎo wán*).

Melia Toosendan Powder #1 (*jīn líng zǐ sǎn* 金鈴子散)

Melia Fructus (*chuān liàn zǐ*), 10 pieces; Crotonis Fructus (*bā dòu ròu*), 30 pieces. Stir-fry together until they become nicely burned, and then remove the Crotonis Fructus (*bā dòu ròu*). Then add Foeniculi Fructus (*xiǎo huí xiāng*) and Aucklandiae Radix (*mù xiāng*), 1.5 *qián* each, and divide into 2 *qián* parts. Each part should be further cooked in a mixture of half wine and half water, and taken with a decoction of Allii fistulosi Bulbus (*cōng bái*).

Melia Toosendan Powder #2 (*jīn líng zǐ sǎn* 金鈴子散)

Melia Fructus (*chuān liàn zǐ*), Corydalys Rhizome (*yán hú sǔo*), 1 *liǎng* each.

Minor Bupleurum Decoction (*xiǎo chái hú tāng* 小柴胡湯)

Bupleuri Radix (*chái hú*), Scutellariae Radix (*huáng qín*), Ginseng Radix (*rén shēn*), Pinelliae Rhizoma preparatum (*zhì bàn xià*), Glycyrrhizae Radix (*gān cǎo*), Zingiberis Rhizoma recens (*shēng jiāng*), Aiziphi Fructus (*dà zǎo*).

Minor Order the Qi Decoction (*xiǎo chéng qì tāng* 小承氣湯)

Rhei Rhizoma (*dà huáng*), 4 *liǎng*; Magnolia Cortex (*hòu pò*), 2 *liǎng*; Aurantii Fructus Immaturus (*zhǐ shí*), 3 pieces.

Miraculously Effective Pill (*shén gōng wán* 神功丸)

Gecko Powder (*gé fěn*), 1 *liǎng*; Eriocaulonis Scapus et Flos (*gǔ jīng cǎo*), 1 *liǎng*; Phaseoli Aurei (*lù dòu pí*), 5 *qián*; Notopterigii Rhizoma (*qiāng húo*), 5 *qián*; Cicadae Peristracum (*chán tùi*), 5 *qián*.

Modified Bupleurum and Poria Decoction (*jiā jiǎn chái líng tāng* 加減柴苓湯)

Bupleuri Radix (*chái hú*), Alismatis Rhizoma (*zé xiè*), 1 *qián* each; Pinelliae Rhizoma preparatum (*zhì bàn xià*), Poria Rubra (*chì líng*), Polyporus (*zhū líng*), Atractylodis macrocephalae Rhizoma (*bái zhú*), CrataegiFructus (*shān zhā*), Gardenia Fructus (*shān zhī*), Litchi Semen (*lì zhī hé*), 7 *fēn* each. If Litchi Semen (*lì zhī hé*) is unavailable, substitute with Citri reticulatae Semen (*jú hé*).

Modified Dragon Tiger Decoction (*jiā wèi lóng hǔ tāng* 加味龍虎湯)

Xanthii Fructus (*cāng zhú*), 1 *liǎng*; whole Scorpio (*quán xiē*), 3 *qián*; Aconiti kusnezoffii Radix preparata (*zhì cǎo wū*), Aconiti Radix lateralis preparata (*zhì fù zǐ*), 2 *qián* each; Gastrodiae Rhizoma (*tiān má*), 3 *qián*. Grind all the ingredients into a fine powder, and take 1 *qián* with a dipper of wine on an empty stomach.

Modified Heart-Penetrating Powder (*jiā wèi tōng xīn sǎn* 加味通心散)

Akebiae Caulis (*mù tōng*), Gardenia Fructus (*shān zhī*), Forsythiae Fructus (*lián qiào*), Scutellariae Radix (*huáng qín*), Glycyrrhizae Radix (*gān cǎo*), Akebia Dianthi Herba (*qú mài*), Aurantii Fructus (*zhǐ ké*), Angelica Sinensis Radicis Extemitas (*dāng guī wěi*), Persicae Semen (*táo rén*), Crataegi Fructus (*shān zhā*), and Toosendan Fructus (*chuān liàn zǐ*), 1 *qián each*; Junci Medulla (*dēng xīn*), 20 long stems; Plantaginis Herba (*chē qián cǎo*), 5 leaves.

Modified Tonify the Yin Pill (*jiā wèi bǔ yīn wán* 加味補陰丸)

Phellodendri Cortex (*huáng bǎi*), 4 *liǎng*; Anemarrhenae Rhizoma (*zhī mǔ*), 4 *liǎng*; Achyranthis bidentatae Radix (*niú xī*), 3 *liǎng*; Eucomiae Cortex (*dù zhòng*), 3 *liǎng*; Morindae officinalis Radix (*bā jǐ tiān*), 3 *liǎng*; Rehmanniae Radix (*shēng dì huáng*), 3 *liǎng*; Evodiae Fructus (*wú zhū yú*), 3 *liǎng*; Cistanches Herba (*ròu cōng róng*), 2 *liǎng*; Poria (*fú líng*), 2 *liǎng*; Lycii Fructus (*gǒu qǐ zǐ*), 2 *liǎng*; Polygalae Radix (*yuǎn zhì*), 2 *liǎng*; Dioscoreae Rhizoma (*shān yào*), 2 *liǎng*; Cornu Cervi (*lù jiǎo*), 2 *liǎng*; Testudinis Plastrum (*guī bǎn*) 2 *liǎng*. [Grind and] roll all the ingredients into pills with honey, and take 80–90 pills a day with water.

Nourish the Nutritive Decoction (*yǎng yíng tāng* 養營湯)

Angelicae sinensis Radix (*dāng guī*), Paeoniae Radix Alba (*bái sháo*), Rehmanniae Radix Exsiccata seu Recens (*shēng dì huáng*), Rehmannia Radix Conquita (*shú dì huáng*), Poria Rubra (*chì fú líng*), Gardenia Fructus (*shān zhī rén*), Ophiopogonis Tuber (*mài mén dōng*), Citri Exocarpium (*chén pí*), 1 *qián* each; Ginseng Radix (*rén shēn*), Glycyrrhizae Radix (*gān cǎo*), 5 *fēn* each; Aiziphi Fructus (*dà zǎo*), 2 pieces; Mume Fructus (*wū méi*), 1 piece.

One Pinch of Gold Powder (*yī niē jīn sǎn* 一捏金散)

Corydalis Rhizoma (*yán hú suǒ*), Toosendan Fructus (*chuān liàn zǐ*), Scorpio (*quán xiē*), Foeniculi Fructus (*xiǎo huí xiāng*). Two *qián* taken with hot wine each time has miraculous effects.

Pain-Curing Pill (*juān tòng wán* 蠲痛丸)

Corydalis Rhizoma (*yán hú suǒ*), 1 *liǎng;* Toosendan Fructus (*chuān liàn zǐ*), 5 *qián;* Foeniculi Fructus (*xiǎo huí xiāng*), 5 *qián;* Phabitidis Semen alba (*qiān niú zǐ*), 2.5 *qián* (tips only); Angelicae sinensis Radix (*dāng guī*), 2.5 *qián;* Alpiniae officinarum Rhizoma (*gāo liáng jiāng*), 2.5 *qián;* Citri reticulatae viride Pericarpium (*qīng pí*), 2.5 *qián;* Aucklandiae Radix (*mù xiāng*), 2.5 *qián;* Linderae Radix (*wū yào*), (2.5 *qián*); Scorpio (*quán xiē*), 7 pieces. Grind all the ingredients, and make [them] into small pills with ginger juice. Take 30–50 pills with warm wine per day.

Patchouli/Agastache Powder to Rectify the Qi (*huò xiāng zhèng qì sǎn* 藿香正氣散)

Arecae Pericarpium (*dà fù pí*), Poria (*fú líng*), Angelicae dahuricae Radix (*bái zhǐ*), Citri reticulatae Pericarpium (*chén pí*), Pogostemonis/Agastaches Herba (*huò xiāng*), Platycodi Radix (*jié gěng*), Glycyrrhizae Radix (*gān cǎo*).

Peach of Immortality and Scallion Decoction (*pán cōng tāng* 蟠蔥湯)

Atractylodis Rhizoma (*cāng zhú*), 1 *qián;* Glycyrrhizae Radix (*gān cǎo*), 1 *qián;* Sparganii Rhizoma (*sān léng*), 7 *fēn;* Curcumae Rhizoma (*é zhú*), 7 *fēn;* Poria (*fú líng*), 7 *fēn;* Citri reticulatae viride Pericarpium (*qīng pí*), 7 *fēn;* Caryophylli Cortex (*dīng xiāng pí*), 5 *fēn;* Amomi Fructus (*shā rén*), 5 *fēn;* Arecae Semen (*bīng láng*), 5 *fēn;* Corydalis Rhizoma (*yán hú suǒ*), 3 *fēn;* Cinnamomi Cortex (*ròu guì*), 3 *fēn;* Zingiberis Rhizoma (*gān jiāng*), 3 *fēn.* Grind all the ingredients, and cook them with a stalk of scallion.

Pinellia Decoction (*bàn xià tāng* 半夏湯)

Boil 8 *shēng* of water drawn from a long stream down to 5 *shēng,* and purify it over a fire of reeds. When the water boils, add 1 *shēng* of sorgham rice and 5 *hé* of Pinelliae Rhizoma preparatum (*zhì bàn xià*). Cook it down to 1.5 *shēng* while scooping off the impurities. Remove the dregs and drink 1 small cupful of the decoction for 3 days, increasing the amount every day, depending on the condition. In acute cases, the patient should lie down after drinking the decoction until perspiration occurs. In chronic cases, drink it only 3 times.

Plum Root Bark Decoction (*lǐ gēn pí tāng* 李根皮湯)

Pruni Saliciae Radicis Cortex *(lǐ gēn pí)*, 5 *qián*; Cinnamomi Ramulus *(guì zhī)*, 1.5 *qián*; Angelicae sinensis Radix *(dāng guī)*, 1 *qián*; Paeoniae Radix alba *(bái sháo)*, 1 *qián*; Poria *(fú líng)*, 1 *qián*; Scutellariae Radix *(huáng qín)*, 1 *qián*; Pinelliae Rhizoma preparatum *(zhì bàn xià)*, 5 *fēn*; Glycyrrhizae Radix *(gān cǎo)*, 5 *fēn*; Zingiberis Rhizoma recens *(shēng jiāng)*, 3 pieces.

Poria and Schizandra Decoction (*fú líng wǔ wèi zǐ tāng* 茯苓五味子湯)

Poria *(fú líng)*, 2 *qián*; Schisandrae Fructus *(wǔ wèi zǐ)*, 2 *qián*; Cinnamomi Cortex *(ròu guì)*, 1 *qián*; Glycyrrhizae Radix *(gān cǎo)*, 1 *qián*.

Poria Drink (*fú líng yǐn* 伏苓飲)

Poria *(fú líng)*, 3 *liǎng*; Ginseng Radix *(rén shēn)*, 2 *liǎng*; Atractylodis Ovatae Rhizoma *(bái zhú)*, 3 *liǎng*; Aurantii Fructus Immaturus *(zhǐ shí)*, 2 *liǎng*; Citri Exocarpium *(jú pí)*, 1 *liǎng*; Zingiberis Rhizoma Recens *(shēng jiāng)*, 4 *liǎng*.

Powder of the Divine Sage that Replaces the Needle (*shēn shèng dài zhēn sǎn* 神聖代針散)

Olibanum *(rǔ xiāng)*, Myrrha *(mò yào)*, Angelicae sinensis Radix *(dāng guī)*, Angelicae dahuricae Radix *(bái zhǐ)*, Ligustici Rhizoma *(chuāng xiōng)*, processed Scutellariae Radix *(huáng qín)*, 1 *qián* each. Grind all the ingredients, and take 1 *fēn*. In severe cases, one may take 5 *fēn*.

Pubescent Angelicae Decoction (*dú huó tāng* 獨活湯)

Angelicae sinensis Radix *(dāng guī)*, Forsythiae Fructus *(lián qiào)*, 1.5 *qián* each; Notopterygii Rhizoma seu Radix *(qiāng huó)*, Angelicae pubescentis Radix *(dú huó)*, Saposhnikoviae Radix *(fáng fēng)*, Alismatis Rhizoma *(zé xiè)*, Cinnamomi Cortex *(ròu guì)*, 1 *qían* each; Stephaniae Radix *(fáng jǐ)*, Phellodendri Cortex *(huáng bǎi)*, Rhei Radix et Rhizoma *(dà huáng)*, Glycyrrhizae Radix *(gān cǎo)*, 5 *fēn* each; Persicae Semen *(táo rén)*, 9 pieces (retain the tips). Decoct the herbs in a liquid composed of half water and half wine.

Qi Bulging Drink (*qì shàn yǐn* 氣疝飲)

Coptidis Rhizoma *(huáng lián)*, soak 2 *qián* in a decoction of Evodiae Fructus *(wú zhū yú)*; Ginseng Radix *(rén shēn)*, Angelicae Dahuricae Radix *(bái zhǐ)*, 1 *qián* each; Paeoniae Radix alba *(bái sháo)*, Citri reticulatae Pericarpium *(chén pí)*, 7 *fēn* each; Glycyrrhizae Radix *(gān cǎo)*, 3 *fēn*; Zingiberis Rhizoma recens *(shēng jiāng)*, 3 pieces.

Raise the Yang Decoction (*shēng yǎng tāng* 升陽湯)

Ephedrae Herba *(má huáng)*, Saposhnikoviae Radix *(fáng fēng)*, Atractylodis Rhizoma *(cāng zhú)*, Glycyrrhizae Radix preparata *(zhì gān cǎo)*.

Raise the Yang and Drain Heat Decoction (*shēng yáng xiè rè tāng* 升陽瀉熱湯)

Bupleuri Radix *(chái hú)*, Citri reticulatae Pericarpium *(chén pí)*, Cimicifugae Rhizoma *(shēng má)*, Poria Rubra *(chì fú líng)*, Aurantii Fructus *(zhǐ ké)*, Cyperi Rhizoma *(xiāng fù)*, Glycyrrhizae Radix *(gān cǎo)*, Paeoniae Radix alba *(bái sháo)*.

Regulate the Middle Decoction (*lǐ zhōng tāng* 理中湯)

Ginseng Radix *(rén shēn)*, Atractylodis macrocephalae Rhizoma *(bái zhú)*, Glycyrrhizae Radix *(gān cǎo)*, Zingiberis Rhizoma *(gān jiāng)*.

Regulate the Middle to Augment the Qi Decoction (*tiáo zhōng yì qì tāng* 調中益氣湯)

Astragali (seu Hedysari) Radix *(huáng qí)* 2 *qián*, Ginseng Radix *(rén shēn)* 1 *qián*, Atractylodis Rhizoma *(cāng zhú)* 1 *qián*, mix-fried Glycyrrhizae Radix *(zhì gān cǎo)* 1 *qián*, Citri Exocarpium *(chén pí)* 4 *fēn*, Cimicifugae Rhizoma *(shēng má)* 4 *fēn*, Bupleuri Radix *(chái hú)* 4 *fēn*, Saussureae (seu Vladminiae) Radix *(mù xiāng)* 2 *fēn*. Decoct in water and administer.

Restore the Origin Free the Qi Powder (*fù yuán tōng qì sǎn* 復元通氣散)

Phabitidis Semen alba *(qiān niú zǐ)*, 2 *liǎng* (tips only); Foeniculi Fructus *(xiǎo huí xiāng)*, Manitis Squama *(chuān shān jiǎ)*, 0.5 *liǎng* each; Citri reticulatae Pericarpium *(chén pí)*, the white part removed, Corydalis Rhizoma *(yán hú suǒ)*, baked Glycyrrhizae Radix *(zhì gān cǎo)*, 5 *fēn* each.

Restore the Pulse Decoction (*fù mài tāng* 復脈湯)/Honey-Fried Licorice Decoction (*zhì gān cǎo tāng* 炙甘草湯)

Honey-fried Glycyrrhiza Radix *(zhì gān cǎo)*, 4 *liǎng*; Ginseng Radix *(rén shēn)*, 2 *liǎng*; Cinnamomi Ramulus Cassiae *(guì zī)*, 3 *liǎng*; Rehmannia Radix Recens *(shēng dì huáng)*, 1 *jīn*; Opiopogonis Tuber *(mài mén dōng)*, 3 *liǎng*; Asini Corii Gelatinum *(ē jiāo)*, 2 *liǎng*; Cannabis Semen *(huó má rén)*, 3 *liǎng*; Zingibeis Rhizoma Recens *(shēng jiāng)*, 3 *liǎng*; Ziziphi Fructus *(dà zǎo)*, 30 pieces.

Root-Invigorating Elixir (*zhuàng běn dān* 壯本丹)

Eucommiae Cortex *(dù zhòng)*, in wine, salted, Psoraleae Semen *(bǔ gǔ zhī)*, Roeniculi Fructus *(huí xiāng)*, 1 *liǎng* each; Cistanches Herba *(ròu cōng róng)*, in wine, Morindae Radix *(bā jǐ tiān)*, in wine, Halitum *(qīng yán)*, 5 *qián* each. Grind all the ingredients and stuff 5 *qián* of herbs into 2 pieces of pork loin. Bind them tightly with thread, and wrap them with paper. Roast them [until they are] well done. Take with wine.

Saposhnikovia, White Atractylodes, and Oyster Shell Decoction (*fáng fēng bái zhú mǔ lì tāng* 防風白术牡蠣湯)

Saposhnikovia (*fáng fēng*), Atractylodis macrocephalae Rhizoma (*bái zhú*), Ostreae Concha (*mǔ lì*). Take 2 *qián* of this powder with wine or rice water, 2–3 times a day.

Secretly Transmitted Evodiae Fructus Powder to Dissolve Internal Accumulation (*mì chuán wú zhū nèi xiāo sǎn* 秘傳吳茱內消散)

Evodiae Fructus (*wú zhū yú*), soak 5 *qián* in half wine and half vinegar overnight and bake it; Corni Fructus (*shān zhū yú*); Kalimeridia Flos (*mǎ lán huā*), soak in vinegar and then bake; Toosendan Fructus (*chuān liàn zǐ*); Cinnamomi Cortex (*ròu guì*); Pharbitidis Semen Atrum (*hēi chǒu*), tips only; salt-stir-fried Foeniculi Fructus (*xiǎo huí xiāng*); Corydalis Rhizoma (*yán hú suǒ*); Citri reticulatae viride Pericarpium (*qīng pí*), with the white part removed; Sargassum (*hǎi zǎo*), Tribuli Fructus (*cì jí lí*), Persicae Semen (*táo rén*), Aucklandiae Radix (*mù xiāng*), 5 *qián* each. Next remove the Toosendan Fructus (*chuān liàn zǐ*) [from each part], and add 1 *liǎng* of Foeniculi Fructus (*xiǎo huí xiāng*) and Psoraleae Fructus (*bǔ gǔ zhī*) into each [part]. [Grind all four parts together and] make them into pills with wine. Take 50 pills with salt water 3 times per day.

Secretly Transmitted Formula for Leukorrhea (*mì chuán dài xià fāng* 秘傳帶下方)

Celosiae Argenteae Semen (*qīng xiāng zǐ*), Cuscutae Semen (*tù sī zǐ*), Gossypii hirsuti Semen (*mián huā zǐ*).[1]

Six Flavor Pill [with Rehmannia] (*liù wèi dì huáng wán* 六味地黃丸)

Rehmanniae Radix (*shú dì huáng*), 16 *liǎng*; Corni Fructus (*shān zhū yú*), 8 *liǎng*; Dioscoreae Radix (*shān yào*), 8 *liǎng*; Poria (*fú líng*), 4 *liǎng*; Moutan Radicis Cortex (*mǔ dān pí*), 8 *liǎng*; Alismatis Tuber (*zé xiè*), 8 *liǎng*.

Spider Powder (*zhī zhū sǎn* 蜘蛛散)

Spider, 14 pieces, lightly stir-fried; Cinnamomi Cortex (*ròu guì*), 5 *fēn*.

Styrax Pill (*sū hé wán* 蘇和丸)

Atractylodes Macrocephalia (*bái zhú*), 2 *liǎng*; Aucklandia Radix (*qīng mù xiāng*), 2 *liǎng*; Rhinocerotis Cornu (*xī jiǎo*), 2 *liǎng*; Cyperi Rhizoma (*xiāng fù zǐ*), 2 *liǎng*; Cinnabaris (*zhū shā*), 2 *liǎng*; Chebuai Fructus (*kē zǐ*), 2 *liǎng*; Santali Lignum (*tán xiāng*), 2 *liǎng*; Benzoinum (*ān xī xiāng*), 2 *liǎng*; Aquilariae Lignum (*chén xiāng*), 2 *liǎng*; Moschus (*shè xiāng*), 2 *liǎng*; Caryophylli Flos (*dīng xiāng*), 2 *liǎng*; Borneolum (*bīng piàn*), 1 *liǎng*; Olibanum (*rǔ xiāng*), 1 *liǎng*; Styrax Liquidus (*sū hé xiāng*), 1 *liǎng*.

---

1. The source text calls this medicinal 棉子肉 (*mián zǐ ròu*). Our best guess is that it is Gossypii hirsuti Semen (*mián huā zǐ* 棉花子*).

Sudden Smile Powder (*shī xiào sǎn* 失笑散)

Trogopterori seu Pteromydis Excrementum *(wǔ líng zhī)*, 2 *qián;* Typhae Pollen *(pú huáng)*, 2 *qián.*

Tangerine Pip Pill (*jú hé wán* 橘核丸)

Stir-fried Citri reticulatae Semen *(jú hé)*, wine-stir-fried Sargassum *(hǎi zǎo)*, wine-stir-fried Eckloniae Thallus *(kūn bù)*, wine-stir-fried Zosterae Marinae Herba *(hǎi dài)*, rice-powder-stir-fried Persicae Semen *(táo rén)*, stir-fried Nelumbinis Semen *(lián zǐ)*, 1 *liǎng* each; wine-stir-fried Corydalis Tuber *(yán hú suǒ)*. Stir-fry equal amounts of Pharbitidis Semen Atrum *(hēi chǒu)*, Phabitidis Semen alba *(bái chǒu)*, and Phabitidis Semen *(qiān niú zǐ)* (chop off tips). Mince 3 *qián* of pig's kidneys *(zhū yāo zǐ)*, and add Zanthoxyli Pericarpium *(huā jiāo)*, 50 pieces, and Foeniculi Fructus *(xiǎo huí xiāng)*, 100 pieces. Mix all the ingredients, and grind them into a fine mash, then wrap this preparation with wet paper and hold it over a fire until its aroma rises. Chew the remaining mixture with wine.

Tangerine Pip Powder (*jú hé sǎn* 橘核散)

Citri Semen reticulatae *(jú hé)*, 1.5 *qián;* Persicae Semen *(táo rén)*, 15 pieces; Gardeniae Fructus *(zhī zǐ)*, 1 *qián;* Aconiti Radix preparata *(zhì chuān wū)*, Evodiae Fructus *(wú zhū yú)*, 5 *fēn* each.

Tangkuei and Mutton Decoction (*dāng guī yáng ròu tāng* 當歸羊肉湯)

Mutton *(yáng ròu)*, 1 *jīn;* Zingiberis Rhizoma recens *(shēng jiāng)*, 5 *liǎng;* Angelicae sinensis Radix *(dāng guī)*, 2 *liǎng.*

Tangkuei Decoction for Frigid Extremities (*dāng guī sì nì tāng* 當歸四逆湯)

Angelicae sinensis Radix *(dāng guī)*, 1.2 *qián;* Aconiti Radix lateralis preparata *(zhì fù zǐ)*, Cinnamomi Cortex *(ròu guì)*, Foeniculi Fructus *(xiǎo huí xiāng)*, 1 *qián* each; Paeoniae Radix alba *(bái sháo)*, Bupleuri Radix *(chái hú)*, 9 *fēn* each; Corydalis Rhizoma *(yán hú suǒ)*, Toosendan Fructus *(chuān liàn zǐ)*, Poria *(fú líng)*, 7 *fēn* each.

Tonify the Middle to Augment the Qi Decoction (*bǔ zhòng yì qì tāng* 補中益氣湯)

Astragali Radix *(huáng qí)*, Ginseng Radix *(rén shēn)*, Angelicae sinensis Radix *(dāng guī)*, Atractylodis macrocephalae Rhizoma *(bái zhú)*, Citri reticulatae Pericarpium *(chén pí)*, Glycyrrhizae Radix *(gān cǎo)*, Cimicifugae Rhizoma *(shēng má)*, Bupleuri Radix *(chái hú)*.

Top-Quality Lindera Powder (*tiān tái wū yào sǎn* 天台烏藥散)

Toosendan Fructus *(chuān liàn zǐ)*, 10 pieces; Crotonis Semen *(bā dòu)*, 14 pieces. Cook them with flour until they get nicely brown. Remove Crotonis Semen *(bā dòu)* and then add Linderae Radix *(wū yào)*, Aucklandiae Radix *(mù xiāng)*, Foeniculi Fructus *(xiǎo huí xiāng)*, Zingiberis Rhizoma *(gān jiāng)*; Citri reticulatae viride Pericarpium *(qīng pí)*, 5 *qián* each, and Arecae Semen *(bīng láng)*, 3 *qián*. Take 1 *qián* of the powdered herbs with wine. For a severe case, take it with stir-fried ginger and hot wine.

Two-Aged [Herb] Decoction (*èr chén tāng* 二陳湯)

Poria *(fú líng)*, 3 *liǎng*; Citri reticulatae Pericarpium *(chén pí)*, 5 *liǎng*; Pinelliae Rhizoma preparatum *(zhì bàn xià)*, 5 *liǎng*; Glycyrrhizae Radix *(gān cǎo)*, 1.5 *liǎng*.

Two-Fragrance Pill (*èr xiāng wán* 二香丸)

Aucklandiae Radix *(mù xiāng)* 3 *liǎng*; Cyperi Rhizoma *(xiāng fù zǐ)*, 3 *liǎng*; Crataegi Fructus *(shān zhā)*, 2 *liǎng*; Cinnamomi Cortex *(ròu guì)*, 2 *liǎng*; Sparganii Rhizoma *(sān léng)*, 1 *liǎng*; vinegar-fried; Curcuma Rhizoma *(é zhú)*, 1 *liǎng*; vinegar-fried Arisaematis Rhizoma preparatum *(zhì tiān nán xīng)*, 1 *liǎng*; Coptidis Rhizoma *(huáng lián)*, 1 *liǎng* [stir-fried with Evodiae Fructus *(wú zhū yú)*]; Raphani Semen *(luó bo zǐ)*, 5 *qián*; Citri reticulatae Semen *(jú hé)*, 5 *qián*; Persicae Semen *(táo rén)*, 5 *qián*; and Gardineae Fructus *(zī zǐ)*, 5 *qián* each. Make them into pills with ginger paste.

Unripe Bitter Orange and Atractylodes Pill (*zhǐ zhú wán* 枳術丸)

Aurantii Fructus immaturus *(zhǐ shí)*, 80 *qián*; Atractylodes Macrocephelae *(bái zhú)*, 160 *qián*.

Various Fragrant Herbs Drink (*jù xiāng yǐn zi* 聚香飲子)

Olibanum *(rǔ xiāng)*, Aquilariae Lignum resinatum *(chén xiāng)*, Santali albi Lignum *(tán xiāng)*, Aucklandiae Radix *(mù xiāng)*, Pogostemonis/Agastaches Herba *(huò xiāng)*, 8 *fēn* each; Curcumae longae Rhizoma *(jiāng huáng)*, Linderae Radix *(wū yào)*, Platycodi Radix *(jié gěng)*, Cinnamomi Cortex *(ròu guì)*, Glycyrrhizae Radix *(gān cǎo)*, Corydalis Rhizoma *(yán hú suǒ)*, 4 *fēn* each; Zingiberis Rhizoma recens *(shēng jiāng)*, 3 pieces; Jujubae Fructus *(dà zǎo)*, 2 pieces.

APPENDIX 3

Single Medicinals Entering the Extraordinary Vessels

From *Materia Medica of Combinations (Dé pèi běn cǎo* 得配本草, 1761)[1]

— Appendix of Medicinals Entering the Extraordinary Vessels
(fù qí jīng yào kǎo 附奇經藥考)

FOENICULI FRUCTUS *(xiǎo huí xiāng)*
Enters the extraordinary vessels

SEMIAQUILEGIAE RADIX *(tiān kuí zi)*
Enters the extraordinary vessels

MORINDAE OFFICINALIS RADIX *(bā jǐ tiān)*
Enters the *chōng* vessel

VERBENAE HERBA *(mǎ biān cǎo)*
Enters the extraordinary vessels

CYPERI RHIZOMA *(xiāng fù)*
Enters the *chōng* vessel

CHUANXIONG RHIZOMA *(chuān xiōng)*
Moves the *chōng* vessel

SCUTELLARIAE RADIX *(huáng qín)*
Moves the *chōng* vessel

TRIONYCIS CARAPAX *(biē jiǎ)*
Moves the *chōng* vessel

AUCKLANDIAE RADIX *(mù xiāng)*
Masters diseases of the *chōng* vessel, counterflow qi, and abdominal urgency

ANGELICAE SINENSIS RADIX *(dāng guī)*
Masters diseases of the *chōng* vessel, counterflow qi, and abdominal urgency;
diseases of the *dài* vessel; abdominal fullness, dripping instability of the lumbar
region, like sitting in water

---

1. Yán Jié (嚴潔), Shī Wén (施雯), and Hóng Wěi (洪煒) 1997.

401

PHELLODENDRI CORTEX *(huáng bǎi)*
Masters diseases of the *chōng* vessel; counterflow qi

ATRACTYLODIS MACROCEPHALAE RHIZOMA *(bái zhú)*
Masters diseases of the *chōng* vessel; counterflow qi and abdominal urgency; umbilical and abdominal pain

ALOE *(lú huì)*
Masters diseases of the *chōng* vessel; counterflow qi and abdominal urgency

ARECAE SEMEN *(bīng láng)*
Masters the *chōng* vessel; counterflow qi and abdominal urgency

EVODIAE FRUCTUS *(wú zhū yú)*
Masters diseases of the *chōng* vessel; counterflow qi and abdominal urgency

XANTHII FRUCTUS *(cāng ěr zǐ)*
Travels to the *dū* vessel

ASARI RADIX ET RHIZOMA *(xì xīn)*
Masters diseases of the *dū* vessel; spinal rigidity and reversal

ACONITI RADIX LATERALIS PREPARATA *(zhì fù zǐ)*
Masters diseases the *dū* vessel; spinal rigidity and reversal

GOAT SPINE *(yáng jǐ gǔ)*
Opens the *dū* vessel

GINGKO SEMEN *(bái guǒ)*
Opens the *dū* vessel

CERVI CORNUS COLLA *(lù jiǎo jiāo)*
Opens the Qi Abode of the *dū* vessel

CERVI CORNU PANTOTRICHUM *(lù róng)*
Opens the Essence Chamber of the *dū* vessel

TESTUDINIS PLASTRUM *(guī bǎn)*
Opens the *rén* vessel

LIGUSTICI RHIZOMA *(gǎo běn)*
Masters the *dū* vessel; spinal rigidity and reversal

PYROLAE HERBA *(lù xián cǎo)*
Supplements and warms the essence blood of the *chōng* and *dū*

LYCII FRUCTUS *(gǒu qǐ zǐ)*
Supplements the essence blood of the *chōng* and *dū*

Astragali Radix *(huáng qí)*
Masters the suffering of feverishness and chills due to disease of the *yáng wéi*, disease of the *dū* vessel, counterflow qi and abdominal urgency

Paeoniae Radix alba *(bái sháo)*
Masters *yáng wéi* feverishness and chills; *dài* vessel abdominal pain

Cinnamomi Ramulus *(guì zhī)*
Travels to the *yáng wéi* vessel

Stephaniae/Cocculi/etc. Radix *(fáng jǐ)*
Enters the *yáng wéi* and *yáng qiāo*

Cinnamomi Cortex *(ròu guì)*
Opens the *yáng wéi*

Manitis Squama *(chuān shān jiǎ)*
Enters the *yīn* and *yáng qiāo*

Tigris Os *(hǔ gǔ)*
Enters the *yīn* and *yáng qiāo*

Dipsaci Radix *(xù duàn)*
Masters diseases of the *dài* vessel

Artemisiae argyi Folium *(ài yè)*
Treats *dài* mai disease causing abdominal fullness; dripping instability of the lumbar region, like sitting in water

Fossilia Ossis Mastodi *(lóng gǔ)*
Treats diseases of the *dài* vessel

Vaccariae Semen *(wáng bù liú xíng)*
Opens the *chōng* and *rén* vessels

Lycopi Herba *(zé lán)*
Regulates diseases and damage to the eight vessels

Cimicifugae Rhizoma *(shēng má)*
Relaxes tension and urgency of the *dài* vessel

Glycyrrhizae Radix *(gān cǎo)*
Harmonizes counterflow of the *chōng* vessel; relaxes urgency of the *dài* vessel

Salviae miltiorrhizae Radix *(dān shēn)*
Boosts the *chōng* and *rén*

Ye Gui's additions to *Principles of Herbal Formulation*[2]

— *Dū* Vessel

PIG SPINAL CORD *(zhū jǐ suǐ)*
Opens the yang, and, according to Ye Gui, "directly enters the extraordinary vessels"

Ye often referred to harsh yang-opening medicinals in terms of the *dū* vessel, including ZINGIBERIS RHIZOMA *(gān jiāng)* and ZANTHOXYLI PERICARPIUM *(huā jiāo)*

— *Rén* Vessel

The *rén* masters the womb.

ASINI CORII COLLA *(ē jiāo)*

FISH PASTE *(yú jiāo)*

DRIED SEA MUSSEL *(dàn cài)*

CLAM *(bàng shuǐ)*

ANEMARRHENAE RHIZOMA *(zhī mǔ)*

SCROPHULARIAE RADIX *(xuán shēn)*

REHMANNIAE RADIX *(shēng dì huáng)*

HOMINIS PLACENTA *(zǐ hé chē)*

FLUORITUM *(zǐ shí yīng)*

ARTEMISIAE ARGYI FOLIUM *(ài yè)*

— *Chōng* Vessel

Ye's case records note that the following medicinals also enter the *chōng* vessel: HOMINIS PLACENTA *(zǐ hé chē)* is blood and flesh and warms and nourishes. Together with FLUORITUM *(zǐ shí yīng)*, it contracts and settles the *chōng* vessel.

— *Dài* Vessel

SCHISANDRAE FRUCTUS *(wǔ wèi zǐ)*

DIOSCOREAE RHIZOMA *(shān yào)*

EURYALES SEMEN *(qiàn shí)*

---

2. Wáng Luó-Zhēn (王羅珍) and Lǐ Dǐng (李鼎), eds., 1985, pp. 129–131.

MELIA FRUCTUS *(chuān liàn zǐ)*

RUBI FRUCTUS *(fù pén zǐ)*

SEPIAE ENDOCONCHA *(hǎi piāo xiāo)*

— *Yáng Qiāo* and *Yīn Qīao* Vessels

For seizures occurring in the morning pertaining to the *yáng qiāo,* use Raise the Yang Decoction *(shēng yǎng tāng).*

EPHEDRAE HERBA *(má huáng)*

SAPOSHNIKOVIAE RADIX *(fáng fēng)*

ATRACTYLODIS RHIZOMA *(cāng zhú)*

GLYCYRRHIZAE RADIX PREPARATA *(zhì gān cǎo)*
   For seizures occurring at night pertaining to the *yīn qiāo,* use Four-Substance Decoction *(sì wù tāng)* with addition of CORYDALIS RHIZOMA *(yán hú suǒ).*

TRICHOSANTHIS FRUCTUS *(guā lóu)*

PINELLIAE RHIZOMA PREPARATUM *(zhì bàn xià)*

ARISAEMATIS RHIZOMA PREPARATUM *(zhì tiān nán xīng)*

ANEMARRHENAE RHIZOMA *(zhī mǔ)*

PHELLODENDRI CORTEX *(huáng bǎi)*

POLYGALAE RADIX *(yuǎn zhì)*

ZIZIPHI SPINOSAE SEMEN *(suān zǎo rén)*

ACORI TATARINOWII RHIZOMA *(shí chāng pǔ)*

— *Yáng Wéi* and *Yīn Wéi* Vessels

Ye used medicinals that harmonized the networks to treat these vessels.

TRIBULI FRUCTUS *(cì jí lí)*

ASTRAGALI COMPLANATI SEMEN *(shā yuàn zǐ)*
   Masters regulation of the liver and kidney by harmonizing the networks

Li Shi-Zhen's Synopsis of Extraordinary Vessel Pulses from *Pulse Studies of the Lakeside Master*

奇經八脈	其診又別	直上直下	浮則為督	牢則為衝	緊則任脈
寸左右彈	陽蹻可決	尺左右彈	陰蹻可別	關左右彈	帶脈當訣
尺外斜上	至寸陰維	尺內斜上	至寸陽維		

The eight vessels are also diagnosed separately [from the other vessels]

[Beating] straight up and down,
Floating is the *du* [vessel].

Confined is the *chong*
And tense is the *ren* vessel.

Tapping in the left and right sides of the distal position,
The yang *qiao* can be discerned.

Tapping in the left and right sides of the proximal position,
The yang *qiao* can be differentiated.

Tapping in the left and right sides of the middle position,
The *dai* should be discerned.

From the lateral aspect of the proximal position ascending obliquely,
To reach the distal position is the *yin wei*.

From the medial of the proximal position ascending obliquely,
To reach the distal position is the *yang wei*.

APPENDIX 5

Editions of
Exposition on the Eight Extraordinary Vessels [1]

▶ Editions of *Exposition on the Eight Extraordinary Vessels (Qi jing ba mai kao* 奇經 八脈考)

1. 清康熙五十六年丁酉 (1717) 刻本(含《本草綱目》內)
2. 清乾隆四十九年甲辰 (1784) 書葉堂刻本(含《本草綱目》內)
3. 清光緒三十三年丁未 (1907) 益元書局刻本(含《本草綱目》內)
4. 清本立堂刻本 (含《本草綱目》內)
5. 1912 年鴻寶齋石印本
6. 書業德刻本
7. 1970 年日本盛文堂影印本
8. 1991 年上海古籍出版社據文淵閣本影印本 (含《本草綱目》內)

▶ Combined Editions of *Pulse Studies of the Lakeside Master (Bin-hu mai xue* 濱湖脈 學), *Exposition on the Eight Extraordinary Vessels,* and *Exposition and Explication of the Pulse Rhymes (Mai jue zheng kao* 脈決証考)

1. 明萬曆三十一年癸卯 (1603) 江西夏良心、張鼎思刻本百瞻樓藏版
2. 明萬曆三十四年丙午 (1606) 晉江楊道會湖北刻本 (含《本草綱目》內)
3. 清順治十二年乙未 (1655) 吳氏太和堂刻本 (含《本草綱目》內)
4. 日本正德四年甲午 (1714) 書林含英豫章堂刻本 (含《本草綱目》內)
5. 清道光六年丙戌 (1826) 務本堂刻本 (含《本草綱目》內)
6. 清道光六年丙戌 (1826) 英德堂刻本 (含《本草綱目》內)
7. 清咸豐九年己未 (1859) 刻本
8. 清同治十一年壬申 (1872) 芥子園刻本 (含《本草綱目》內)
9. 清光緒五年己卯 (1879) 掃葉山房刻本
10. 清光緒五年己卯 (1879) 校經山房刻本
11. 清光緒九年癸未 (1883) 京都文成堂刻本
12. 清光緒十一年乙酉 (1885) 合肥張氏味古齋刻本

---

1. Qian Chao-Chen (錢超塵) and Wen Chang-Lu (溫長路), eds., 2003, pp. 14–15.

13. 清光緒十八年壬辰 (1892) 鴻寶齋書局石印本

14. 清光緒十九年癸巳 (1893) 鴻寶齋書局石印本

15. 清光緒二十二年丙申 (1896) 揚洲文富堂刻本

16. 清光緒二十二年丙申 (1896) 圖書集成印書局鉛印本

17. 清光緒二十九年癸卯 (1903) 刻本

18. 清光緒三十年甲辰 (1904) 上海同文書局石印本 (含《本草綱目》內)

19. 清光緒三十一年乙巳 (1905) 上新書局石印本

20. 清衣德堂刻本 (含《本草綱目》內)

21. 清福文堂刻本 (含《本草綱目》內)

22. 清文會益刻本 (含《本草綱目》內)

23. 清漁古山房刻本 (含《本草綱目》內)

24. 清刻本本衙藏版 (含《本草綱目》內)

25. 清春明堂刻本

26. 清同人堂刻本

27. 清碧梧山房刻本

28. 清芥子園刻本漁古山房藏版

29. 清文聚堂刻本

30. 清聚錦堂刻本

31. 清無錫日升山房刻本

32. 清天德堂刻本

33. 1912 年上海章福記石印本

34. 1912 年鴻寶齋書局石印本

35. 1916 年鴻寶齋書局石印本

36. 1916 年上海錦章書局石印本

37. 1917 年鴻寶齋書局石印本

38. 1928 年江陰寶文堂刻本

39. 民國上海中醫書局鉛印本

40. 日本刻本 (含《本草綱目》內)

41. 1951 年廣益書局鉛印本

42. 1954 年上海錦章書局鉛印本

43. 1955 年上海錦章書局鉛印本

People and Texts Appearing in
Exposition on the Eight Extraordinary Vessels

I. PEOPLE

In this volume we have referred to historical personages by the names that Chinese medical readers in the West are most likely to be familiar with. This is how we have listed them below. In citing other names that are commonly used for that individual, we have omitted their surname unless we are referring to their given (*míng*名) name. Those entries in which there is no alternate name are listed as NA, or not available.

Name used	中文名	Other commonly-used names	常用名	Dates
Chén Nán	陳楠	Nán mù [courtesy] Cuì-Xū [nickname]	南木【字】 翠虛【號】	Died 1213
Chéng Wú-Jǐ	成無己	NA	NA	1066-1156
Cháo Yúan-Fāng	巢元方	NA	NA	550-630
Cuī Xī-Fàn	崔希范	Zhì Yī Zhēn Rén	至一真人 【號】	880-940
Dīng Dé-Yòng	丁德用	NA	NA	1056-1063
Dòu Hàn-Qīng [courtesy]	竇漢卿【字】	Dòu Mò [given]	竇默【名】	1195-1280
Gaō Wǔ	高武	Méi Gū-Zi [courtesy]	梅孤子【字】	
Gaō Shì-Zōng	高士宗	Kè-Xué [courtesy] Zhì-Zhāi [nickname]	克學【字】 志齋【號】	1623-1670
Gaō Yáng-Shēng	高陽生	NA	NA	Five Dynasties
Gāo Yì-Sūn	高儀孫	NA	NA	Song
Gù Jǐng-Xīng	顧景星	Chì-Fāng [courtesy] Huáng-Gōng [nickname]	赤方【字】 黃公【號】	1621-1687
Hé Méng-Yáo	何蒙瑤	Bào-Zi [courtesy] Xī-Chí [nickname]	報子【字】 西池【號】	Fl. 1730
Hé-Shàng Gōng	河上公	NA	NA	2nd century BCE
Huá Shoù	滑壽	Bó-Rén [courtesy] Yīng Níng-Shēng [nickname]	伯仁【字】 櫻寧生【號】	Fl. 1341

Name used	中文名	Other commonly-used names	常用名	Dates
Lǐ Shí-Zhēn	李時珍	Dōng-Bì [courtesy] Bīn-Hú shān rén [nickname]	東壁【字】 瀕湖山人【號】	1518-1593
Lǐ Dōng-Yuán [nickname]	李東垣【號】	Lǐ Gǎo [given] Míng-Zi [courtesy]	李杲【名】 明子【字】	1180-1251
Lǐ Jiàn-Zhōng	李建中	Lǐ Shào-Táng [given]	李邵唐【名】	Qing
Lǐ Lián	李濂	Chuān-Fǔ [courtesy]	川父【字】	1489-1567
Lí Mín-Shoù	黎民壽	Jǐng-Rén [courtesy]	景仁【字】	Northern Song
Lǐ Yùe-Chí	李月池	NA		Ming
Lǐ Zhōng-Zǐ	李中梓	Shì-Cái/Niàn-É [nicknames]	士材/念莪【號】	1588-1655
Lín Zhī-Hàn	林之瀚	Xiàn-Bǎi [courtesy] Shèn-Än, Sháo Dōng-Yì [nicknames]	憲百【字】 慎菴, 苕東逸【號】	Fl. 1723
Liú Wán-Sù	劉完素	Shǒu-Zhēn [courtesy] Hé Jiān Jū Shì, Tōng Xuán Chǔ Shì, Zōng Zhēn Zi, Gāo Shàng Xiān Shēng [nicknames]	守真【字】 河間居士,通玄處士宗真子,高尚先生【號】	1110-1200
Líu Zhōng-Hòu [courtesy]	劉宗厚【字】	Chún, Chún [nicknames]	純,醇【號】	14th century
Luó Dōng-Yì [nickname]	羅東逸【號】	Luō-Měi [given] Dàn-Shēng [courtesy]	羅美【名】 澹生【字】	1662-1722
Lǔ Guǎng	呂廣	NA		Three Kindgom's Period
Mǎ Shì	馬蒔	Zhòng-Huà [courtesy] Xuán-Tái Yuán-Tái [nicknames]	仲華【字】 玄台,元台【號】	15th-16th century
Shào Lán-Sūn	邵蘭蓀	Lán-Shēng [courtesy]	蘭生【字】	1855-1910
Shén Jīn-Aò	沈金奧	Qiān Lù [courtesy] Jí Mén, Zūn Shēng Lǎo Rén [nicknames]	芊綠【字】 汲門,尊生老人【號】	1717-1777
Shì Zhé	蘇軾	Zǐ-Zhān [courtesy] Dōng-Pō Jū-Shì Also known more simply as Dōng-Pō. [nicknames]	子瞻【字】 東坡居士,東坡	1037-1101

Name used	中文名	Other commonly-used names	常用名	Dates
Sūn Sī-Mǐao	孫思邈	Sūn Zhēn Rén [nickname]	孫真人【號】	581-682
Táng Shèn-Wēi	唐慎微	Shěn-Yuán [courtesy]	審元【字】	1056-1136
Wáng Bāng-Fù	王幫傅	Zǐ-Lán [courtesy]	紫瀾【字】	Qing
Wáng Bì	王弼	NA	NA	226 – 249
Wáng Hǎi-Cáng [nickname]	王海藏【號】	Wáng Hào-Gǔ [given]	王好古【名】	1200-1264
Wáng Hóng-Bīn	王宏彬			Modern
Wáng Kěn-Táng	王肯堂	Yǔ-Tài, Sǔn-Zhōng [courtesy] Sǔn-Än, Niàn-Xī Jū Shì [nicknames]	宇泰，損中，【字】損庵，念西居士【號】	1549-1613
Wáng Luó-Zhēn	王羅珍			Modern
Wáng Bīng	王冰	Qǐ-Xuán [nickname]	啟玄【號】	Fl. 762
Wáng Shì-Zhēng	王世禎			Modern
Wáng Tāo	王燾	NA	NA	670-755
Wáng Zhí-Zhōng	王執中	Shū-Quán [courtesy]	叔權【字】	Fl. 1169
Wáng Zǐ-Jiē	王子接	Jìn-Sān [courtesy]	晉三【字】	1658-?
Wéi Wén-Guì	韋文貴	Âi -Táng [courtesy]	靄堂【字】	1902-1980
Wèi Bó-Yáng [courtesy]	魏伯陽【字】	Wèi-Áo [given name] Yún Yá-Zi [nickname]	魏翱【名】雲牙子【號】	1st century
Wèi Huá-Cún	魏華存	Xián-Än [courtesy]	賢安【字】	252-334 BCE
Wú Kūn	吳昆	Shān-Fǔ [courtesy] Hè-gāo, Cān Huáng-zi [nicknames]	山甫【字】鶴皋，參黃子【號】	1552-1620
Wú Qiān	吳謙	Liù-Jí	六吉【字】	1736-1793
Wú Yǒu-Xìng	吳有性	Yòu-Kě [courtesy]	又可【字】	1582-1652
Xú Dà-Chūn [given]	徐大春【名】	Dà-Yè, Huí-Xī Lǎo Rén, Líng-Tāi, [nicknames]	大業，洄溪老人，靈胎【號】	1693-1771
Xú Fèng	徐鳳	Tíng-Ruì [courtesy]	廷瑞【字】	Ming
Xù-Gāo [courtesy]	旭高【字】	Tài-Lín [nickname]	泰林【號】	1798-1862
Yáng Jì-Zhōu	楊繼洲	Yáng Jì-Shí [given]	楊濟時【名】	1522-1619

Name used	中文名	Other commonly-used names	常用名	Dates
Yáng Shàng-Shàn	楊上善	NA		575-670
Yáng Xuān-Cāo	楊玄操	Xuān[nickname]	玄【號】	Late Sui, early Tang
Yè Tiān-Shì [courtesy]	葉天士【字】	Yè Guì [given], Xiāng-Yán [nickname]	葉桂【名】 香嚴【號】	1667-1746
Yú Shù	虞庶	NA	Na	16th century
Yù Yǎn	愈琰	Yù Wú [Courtesy] Quán Yáng Zi [Nickname] Lín Wū Yì Rén [Nickname]	玉吾【字】 全陽子 林屋逸人【號】	1258-1314
Zhāng Jǐng-Yuè [courtesy]	張景岳【字】	Zhāng Jiè-Bīn [given]	張介賓【名】	1563-1640
Zhāng Nán	章楠	Xū-Gǔ [courtesy]	虛谷【字】	C. 1835
Zhāng Shì-Xián	張世賢	Tiān-Chéng [courtesy] Jìng-Zhāi [nickname]	天成【字】 靜齋【號】	1506-1521
Zhāng Yuán-Sù	張元素	Zhāng Jié-Gǔ [courtesy]	張潔古【字】	1151-1234
Zhāng Zhì-Cōng [courtesy]	張志聰	Yǐn-Ān [courtesy]	隱庵【字】	1610-1674
Zhāng Zhòng-Jīng	張仲景	Zhāng Jī [given]	張機【名】	C. 220
Zhāng Zǐ-Hé	張子和	Zhāng Cóng-Zhèng [given] Dài-Rén [nickname]	張從正【名】戴人【號】,	1151-1231
Zhāng Zí-Yáng [nickname]	張紫陽【號】	Zhāng Bó-Dūan [given] Píng-Shū [courtesy]	張伯端【名】 平叔【字】	984-1082
Zhēn Quán	甄權	NA	NA	541-643
Zhōu Xué-Hǎi	周學海	Chéng-Zhī, Ānhuī Jiàn Dé rén [courtesy]	澂之, 安徽建德人【字】	1856-1906
Zhū Dān-Xī [courtesy]	朱丹溪【字】	Zhū Zhèn-Hēng [given] Yàn-Xiū, Dān-Xī Wēng [courtesy]	朱震亨【名】彥修, 丹溪翁【字】	1281-1358
Zhū Xī	朱熹	Yuán-Huì [courtesy] Huì-Ān and Míng Zǐ-Yáng [nicknames]	元晦【字】 晦庵, 明紫陽【號】	1130-1200

II. TEXTS

English Name	中文名	Name in *pīnyīn*	Author	中文名	Date/ Dynasty
Approaching the Refined	爾雅	*Ěr yǎ*	Anonymous		Probably 3rd century BCE
Arcane Essentials from the Imperial Library	外臺秘要	*Wài tái mì yào*	Wáng Tāo	王燾	752
Awakening to the Geniune	悟真篇	*Wú zhēn piān*	Zhāng Bó-Duān Zhāng Zǐ-Yáng	張伯端 張紫陽	1075
Basic Questions	素問	*Sù wèn*	Anonymous		Primarily Eastern Han
Biography of Li Shi-Zhen	李時珍傳	*Lǐ Shí-Zhēn zhuàn*	Gù Jǐng-Xīng Chì-Fāng [courtesy] Huáng-Gōng [nickname]	顧景星 赤方 黃公	18th century
The Blessings of Nature and Destiny	性命圭旨	*Xìng mìng gūi zhǐ*	Traditionally attributed to Yǐn Zhēn-Rén	尹真人	1615
Canon of Poetry	詩經	*Shī jīng*	Anonymous		900 – 700 BCE
Case Records as a Guide to Clinical Practice	臨證指南醫案	*Lín zhèng zhǐ nán yī àn*	Yè Guì/ Yè Tiān-Shì/ Yè Xiāng-Yán	葉桂/ 葉天士/ 葉香岩	1746
Case Records of the Lakeside [Recluse]	濱湖醫案	*Bīn hú yī àn*	Lǐ Shí-Zhēn/ Lǐ Dōng-Bì	李時珍/ 李東壁	16th century

English Name	中文名	Name in *pīnyīn*	Author	中文名	Date/ Dynasty
Classic of Acupuncture and Moxibustion for Nourishing Life	針灸資生經	*Zhēn jiǔ zī shēng jīng*	Wáng Zhí-Zhōng	王執中	Song
Classic of Difficulties	難經	*Nán jīng*	Anonymous; traditionally attributed to Qín Yuè-Rén	秦越人	Probably Eastern Han
Classic of the Changes of Zhou	周易經	*Zhōu yì jīng*	Anonymous		C. 7th century BCE
Classic of the Inner Spirit of the Yellow Court	黃庭內景經	*Húang tíng nèi jīng jīng*	Attributed to Wèi Húa-Cún	魏華存	Possibly 4th century BCE
Classic of Sagely Beneficence	聖濟經	*Shèng jì jīng*	Completed under auspices of Song Emperor Wēi Zóng [given name Zhào Jí]	宋徽宗 【趙佶】	1118
Classified Classic	類經	*Lèi jīng*	Zhāng Jiè-Bīn Zhāng Jǐng-Yuè	張介賓/ 張景岳	1624
Collected and Simplified Prescriptions of the Lakeside Recluse	濱湖集簡方	*Bīn hú jí jiǎn fāng*	Lǐ Shí-Zhēn/ Lǐ Dōng-Bì	李時珍/ 李東璧	1569 [no longer extant]
Collected Annotations on the Yellow Emperor's Inner Classic: Basic Questions and Divine Pivot	黃帝內經素问灵樞集註	*Huáng Dì nèi jīng sù wèn líng shū jí zhù*	Zhāng Zhì-Cōng	張志聰	1672
Collected Treatises of [Zhang] Jing-Yue	景岳全書	*Jīng-Yuè quán shū*	Zhāng Jiè-Bīn/ Zhāng Jǐng-Yuè	張介賓/ 張景岳	1624
Collection of Writings on the Mechanism of Disease, Suitability of Qi, and the Safeguarding of Life as Discussed in Basic Questions	素問病機氣宜保命集	*Sù wèn bìng jī qì yí bǎo mìng jí*	Liú Wán-Sù	劉完素	1186

English Name	中文名	Name in *pīnyīn*	Author	中文名	Date/ Dynasty
Complete Biographies of the Transcendents	列仙全傳	*Liè xiān quán zhuàn*	Wáng Shì-Zhēn	王世貞	Ming
Commentaries on Medical Studies of the Eight Vessels	醫學八脈註	*Yī xué bā mài zhù*	Lǐ Yùe-Chí	李月池	16th century
Compendium of Correct Ancient and Modern Medical Works	古今醫通正脈全書	*Gǔ jīn yī tōng zhèng mài quán shū*	Wáng Kěn-Táng	王肯堂	1601
Comprehensive Compendium of Acupuncture and Moxibustion	針灸大全	*Zhēn jiǔ dà quán*	Xú Fèng	徐鳳	1439
Comprehensive Outline of the Materia Medica	本草綱目	*Běn cǎo gāng mù*	Lǐ Shí-Zhēn/ Lǐ Dōng-Bì	李時珍/ 李東壁	1590
Comprehensive Outline of the General Mirror	通鑒綱目	*Tōng jiàn gāng mù*	Zhū Xǐ/ Yuán-Huì/ Zhòng-Huì/ Lǎo-Tíng/ Huì-Än	朱熹/ 元晦/ 仲晦/ 老亭/ 晦庵	12th century
Comprehensive Recording of Sagely Beneficence from the Zhenghe Era	政和聖濟總錄	*Zhènghé shèng jì zǒng lù*	Song imperial court		1117
Confucians' Duties to Their Parents	儒們事親	*Rú mén shì qīn*	Zhāng Cóng-Zhèng/ Zhāng Zǐ-Hé	張從正/ 張子和	1228
Correcting the Errors of the Pulse Rhymes	脈決刊誤	*Mài jué kān wù*	Dài Qǐ-Zōng	戴起宗	
Diagnosis, Pattern [Discrimination] and Treatment of Pox Diseases	痘診證治	*Dòu zhěn zhèng zhì*	Lǐ Yùe-Chí	李月池	16th century
Difficulties of the Triple Warmer due to Guest [Qi]	三焦客難	*Sān jiāo kè nàn*	Lǐ Shí-Zhēn/ Lǐ Dōng-Bì	李時珍/ 李東壁	16th century
Direct Teaching of the Great Way in Three Chapters	大道三章直指	*Dà dào sān zhàng zhǐ zhǐ*	Anonymous		Ming

English Name	中文名	Name in *pīnyīn*	Author	中文名	Date/ Dynasty
Discourse on the Origins and Presentations of All Diseases	諸病原侯論	*Zhū bìng yuán hòu lùn*	Cháo Yuán-Fāng	巢元方	610
Discussion of Cold Damage	傷寒論	*Shāng hán lùn*	Zhāng Jī/Zhāng Zhòng-Jīng	張機/ 張仲景	C. 220
Discussion of Illnesses, Patterns, and Formulas Related to the Unification of the Three Etiologies	三因極一病證方論	*Sān yīn jí yī bìng zhèng fāng lùn*	Chén Yán	陳言	1174
Discussion of the Origins of the Symptoms of Disease	諸病原侯論	*Zhū bìng yuán hòu lùn*	Cháo Yuán-Fāng	巢元方	610
Discussion of the Spleen and Stomach	脾胃論	*Pí wèi lùn*	Lǐ Gǎo/ Lǐ Dōng-Yuán	李杲/ 李東垣	13th century
Divine Husbandman's Classic of the Materia Medica	神農本草經	*Shén nóng běn cǎo jīng*	anonymous		Probably Eastern Han
Divine Pivot	靈樞	*Líng shū*	anonymous		Probably Eastern Han
Elucidation of the Fourteen Channels	十四經發揮	*Shí sì jīng fā huī*	Huá Shòu/ Bó-Rén	滑壽/ 伯仁	1586
Elucidations of the Signs and Explications of the Graphs	說文解字	*Shuō wén jiě zì*	Xǔ Shèn	許慎	100
Elucidations on the Token for the Agreement of the Three According to the Changes of Zhou	周易參同契發揮	*Zhōu yì cān tóng qì fā huī*	Yù Yǎn	愈琰	1284
The Emerald Emptiness	翠虛篇	*Cuì xū piān*	Chén Nán	陳楠	13th century
Essentials [of Pulse Diagnosis] in Quatrain	四言舉要	*Sì yán jǔ yào*	Cuī Jiā Yàn	崔嘉彦	Song

English Name	中文名	Name in *pīnyīn*	Author	中文名	Date/Dynasty
Essential Knowledge from the Inner Classic	內經知要	*Nèi jīng zhī yào*	Lǐ Zhōng-Zǐ/ Lǐ Shì-Cái/ Lǐ Niàn-É	李中梓/ 李士材/ 李念莪	1642
Essentials of the Channels and holes	經穴纂要	*Keiketu Sanyou*	Kosaka Eishou	小坂營升	1810
Explanation of the Four Diagnoses	四診發明	*Sì zhěn fā míng*	Lǐ Yùe-Chí	李月池	16th century
An Expositsion on the Life Gate	命門考	*Mìng mén kǎo*	Lǐ Shí-Zhēn/ Lǐ Dōng-Bì	李時珍/ 李東璧	16th century
Fine Formulas of Su and Shen	蘇沈良方	*Sū Shěn liáng fāng*	Sū Shì/ Sū Zǐ-Zhān/ Sū Dōng-Pō and Shěn Kuò/ Shěn Cún-Zhōng	蘇軾/ 蘇子瞻/ 蘇東坡and 沈括/ 沈存中	1075
Formulas from Benevolent Sages Compiled during the Taiping Era	太平聖惠方	*Tàiping shèng huì fāng*	Wáng Huái-Yǐn, et. al.	王懷隱	992
Formulas from the Discussion Illuminating the Yellow Emperor's Basic Questions	黃帝素問宣明論方	*Huáng dì sù wèn xuān míng lùn fāng*	Liú Wán-Sù	劉完素	1172
Gathering of the Blossoms of Acupuncture	針灸聚英	*Zhēn jiǔ jù yīng*	Gāo Wǔ	高武	1529
Golden Mirror of the Medical Tradition	醫宗金鑑	*Yī zōng jīn jiàn*	Wú Qiān/ Wú Liù-Jí	吳謙/ 吳六吉	1742
Grand Compendium of Acupuncture and Moxibustion	針灸大成	*Zhēn jiǔ dà chéng*	Yáng Jì-Zhōu	楊繼洲	1601
Grand Essentials [Yellow Emperor's Inner Classic: Grand Essentials]	太素（黃帝內經太素）	*Tài sū [Huáng dì nèi jīng tài sū]*	Yáng Shàng-Shàn	楊上善	7th century

English Name	中文名	Name in *pīnyīn*	Author	中文名	Date/Dynasty
Graphic Addendum to the Categorization of the Classic	類經圖翼	*Lèi jīng tú yì*	Zhāng Jiè-Bīn Zhāng Jǐng-Yuè	張介賓/張景岳	1624
Guan zi	官子	*Gūan zi*	Liú Xiàng	劉向	Compiled in present form in 26 BCE
Guide to Acupuncture	針灸指南	*Zhēn jīng zhǐ nán*	Dòu Hàn-Qīng	竇漢卿	1295
Guide to the Principles [of Meditation]	規中指南	*Gūi zhōng zhǐ nán*	Chén Zhì-Xū/Chén Xū Bái	陳致虛/陳虛白	Yuan
History of Medicine	醫史	*Yī shǐ*	Lǐ Lián/Lǐ Chuān Fù	李濂/李川父	1513
Illustrated and Annotated Classic of Difficulties	圖註難經	*Tú zhù nàn jīng*	Sì Míng-Rén/Zhāng Shì Xīan	四明人/張世賢	1510
Illustrated Classic of Acupuncture and Moxa Holes on the Bronze Man	銅人俞穴針灸圖經	*Tóng rén shū xué zhēn jiǔ tú jīng*	Wáng Wéi-Yī	王惟一	1027
An Illustrated Discourse on the Five [Yin] Organs	五臟圖論	*Wǔ zāng tú lùn*	Lǐ Shí-Zhēn/Lǐ Dōng-Bì	李時珍/李東璧	16th century
Differentiating the Genuine in the Pulse Rhymes, an Illustrated Commentary	圖註脈訣辨真	*Tú zhù mài jué biàn zhēn*	Zhāng shì-Xián/Sì Míng-Rén	張世賢/四明人	1510
Inner Writings of the Master Who Embraces Simplicity	抱樸子內篇	*Bào pǔ zi nèi piān*	Gē Hóng	葛洪	4th century
Inward Training	內業	*Nèi yè*	Liú Xiàng	劉向	Compiled in present form in 26 BCE
Lore of Ginseng	人參傳	*Rén shēn zhuàn*	Li Yùe-Chí	李月池	16th century

English Name	中文名	Name in *pīnyīn*	Author	中文名	Date/ Dynasty
Materia Medica for Decoctions	湯液本草	*Tāng yè běn cǎo*	Wáng Hào-Gǔ/Wáng Jìn-Zhī/Wáng Hǎi-Cáng	王好古/ 王進之/ 王海藏	1306
Materia Medica of Combinations	得配本草	*Dé pèi běn cǎo*	Yán Jié/ Shī Wén/ Hóng Wěi	嚴潔/ 施雯/ 洪煒	1761
Medical Writings	醫編	*Yī Bīan*			1730
Medicinal Notes on the Classic of Difficulties	药注難經	*Yào zhù nàn jīng*	Zhāng Yuán-Sù Jíe-Gǔ [courtesy]	張元素 張潔古	Late 12th, early 13th century
Mind Seal of Profound Subtlety	玄微心印	*Xuán wéi xīn yìn*	Míng Zǐ-Yáng Yù Tài-Zhēn	明紫陽 喻太真	Ming
Nurturing Sea of the Pulse Rhymes	脈訣乳海	*Mài jué rǔ hǎi*	Wáng Bāng-Fù	王帮傅	1891
Penetrating the Mysteries of the Materia Medica	本草通玄	*Běn cǎo tōng xuán*	Lǐ Zhōng-Zǐ/ Lǐ Shì-Cái / Lǐ Niàn-É	李中梓/ 李士材/ 李念莪	Late Ming [17th century]
Precision in the Four Examinations	四診抉微	*Sì zhěn jué wēi*	Lín Zhī-Hàn	林之翰	1723
Prescriptions Worth a Thousand Pieces of Gold for Urgent Care	備急千金要方	*Bèi jí qīan jīn yào fāng*	Sūn Sī-Miǎo	孙思邈	652
Preserving the Genuine in Pulse Theory	脈理存真	*Mài lǐ cún zhēn*	Yú Xiǎn-Yán	余顯延	1876
Pulse Classic	脈經	*Mài jīng*	Wáng Shū-Hé	王叔和	3rd century
Pulse Rhymes	脈訣	*Mài jué*	Cuī Jiā-Yàn	崔嘉彦	Song
Pulse Studies of the Lakeside [Recluse]	濱湖脈學	*Bīn hú mài xué*	Lǐ Shí-Zhēn/ Lǐ Dōng-Bì	李時珍/ 李東璧	1564
Qizhou Gazetteer	蘄州志	*Qí zhōu zhì*	Pān Kè-Pǔ	潘克溥	1852

English Name	中文名	Name in *pīnyīn*	Author	中文名	Date/Dynasty
Records of the Grand Historian	史記	*Shǐ jì*	Sīmǎ Qiān	司馬遷	C. 90 BCE
Records of the Han	漢書	*Hàn shū*	Fàn Yè	范曄	5th century
Records of the Rites of the State of Zhou	周禮	*Zhōu lǐ*	Anonymous		2nd-3rd century BCE
Reverend Cui's Mirror of Medicine	崔公入藥鏡	*Cuī Gōng rù yào jìng*	Attributed to Cuī Xī-Fàn/ Zhì Yī Zhēn Rén	崔希范/ 至一真人	Tang
Seeking Accuracy in the Materia Medica	本草求真	*Běn cǎo qiú zhēn*	Huáng Gōng-Xiù	黃宮秀	1769
Subtle Import of the Jade Key	玉機微義	*Yù jī wēi yì*	Xú Yàn-Chún/ Xú Yòng-Chéng	徐彥純/ 徐用誠	1396
Supplement to Important Formulas Worth a Thousand Gold Pieces	千金翼方	*Qiān jīn yì fāng*	Sūn Sī-Miǎo	孫思邈	7th century
Teachings of [Zhu] Dan-Xi	丹溪心法	*Dān xī xīn fǎ*	Zhū Zhèn-Hēng/Zhū Dān-Xī/Zhū Yàn-Xiū	朱震亨/ 朱丹溪/ 朱彥修	1481
Textual Research on the Pulse Rhymes	脈訣考證	*Mài jué kǎo zhèng*	Lǐ Shí-Zhēn Lǐ Dōng-Bì	李時珍 李東璧	16th century
Token For the Agreement of the Three According to the Changes of Zhou	周易參同契	*Zhōu yì cān tóng qì*	Wèi Bó-Yáng	魏伯陽	142 BCE
Transcendent Mei Zhi's Odes for Collecting Medicinals	梅志仙采藥歌口訣	*Méi Zhì-Xīan cǎi yáo gē kǒu jué*	Attributed to Transcendent Méi Zhì-Xīan	梅志仙	Ming
Wang Shu-He's Pulse Rhymes	王叔和脈訣	*Wáng Shū-Hé mài jué*	Wáng Shū-Hé	王叔和	Attrib. to Wáng Shū-Hé, 3rd century

English Name	中文名	Name in *pīnyīn*	Author	中文名	Date/ Dynasty
The Way and Its Virtue	道德經	*Dào dé jīng*	Anonymous		C. 3rd century BCE
White Thatched Hut Collection	白茅堂集	*Bái máo táng jí*	Gù Jǐng-Xīng Chì-Fāng [courtesy] Huáng-Gōng [nickname]	顧景星 赤方 【字】 黃公 【號】	18th century
Yellow Emperor's Inner Classic	黃帝內經	*Huáng dì nèi jīng*	Anonymous		Probably Eastern Han
Zhong [Li-Quan's] Transmission of the Dao to Lǔ [Dong-Bin]: A Collection	鍾呂傳道集	*Zhōng lǔ chuán dào jí*	Zhōng Lí Yán, Lū Dòng-Bīn, Shī Jiān Wú	鍾離權, 呂洞賓, 施肩吾	Five Dynasties
Zhuang zi	莊子	*Zhuāng zi*	Parts of the text attribtued to an historical figure named Zhuāng zi	莊子	3rd century BCE

Notes

Chapter A: Introduction

1   Paul Unschuld, 1985, p. 163.
2   Huang Huang, 2007, pp. 1-6.
3   Nathan Sivin, 1995.
4   Huang-Fu Mi, 1981, pp. 13–19.
5   Wang Shu-He, 1981, p. 400.
6   Katsuyasu Kido, 1978.
7   Kiiko Matsumoto and Steven Birch, 1986.
8   Neither Wang Luo-Zhen and Li Ding, 1985, nor Katsuda Masayasu, 1995, actually cites the edition they used, but their texts appear to be identical to the *Four Treasuries* edition.
9   For a more detailed discussion of our approach to Chinese medical translation, see Dan Bensky, Jason Blalack, Charles Chace, and Craig Mitchell, 2007.
10   Nigel Wiseman and Feng Ye, 1998.

Chapter B: Biographical Sketch of Li Shi-Zhen

1   *Ling yi* (鈴醫), literally a 'bell doctor,' one who traveled on foot ringing a bell advertising his services.
2   Paul Unschuld, 1986b, p. 148.
3   Ibid., p. 163.
4   Wang Shu-He was the editor of the *Pulse Classic*.
5   Paul Unschuld, 1986b, p. 151.
6   Ibid., p. 162.
7   Ibid., p. 163.
8   A more thorough discussion of Li Shi-Zhen's Daoist influences appears in Part I (Ch. F) of the present text.

Chapter C: Theoretical Considerations

1 See p. 129 of the present text.

2 See, for instance, Ye's case record of the treatment of a bulging disorder wherein he describes the pathogen as first "entering the primary channel," then becoming chronic and "entering the networks and the blood," and over time afflicting the extraordinary vessels, particularly the *wei* and *qiao* vessels. See *juan* 8 on bulging disorders (疝 *shan*) in Ye Tian-Shi, 1997a, pp. 236-240.

3 'Raised shoulder breathing' (*jian xa* 肩息) is characterized by the raising of the shoulders to assist breathing in severe respiratory patterns such as chronic obstructive pulmonary disease.

4 'Propping fullness' (*zha man* 支滿) refers to a subjective sense of fullness in the chest and the lateral costal region. The word *zha*, or propping, refers to a sensation of the chest and diaphragm being propped up from below.

5 The original passage in the *Pulse Classic* reads: "When diagnosis reveals that the *yang wei* pulse … ." Ibid., p. 90.

6 *Divine Pivot*, 1980, vol. 1, p. 278.

7 These holes are generally believed to be Mute's Gate (GV-15) and Great Hammer (GV-14), respectively.

8 Hundred Convergences (GV-20).

9 According to Katsuda Masayasu, the heart envelope master (*xan bao zhu* 心包主) is the heart envelope network vessel (*xan bao luo* 心包絡). Katsuda Masayasu, trans., 1995, p. 116.

10 According to Katsuda Masayasu, ibid., the passage should be punctuated differently, placing a comma after the second 腎 (*shen*, kidney). The passage then reads as follows (with punctuation):

王海藏曰手少陽三焦相火為一府，右腎命門為相火，心包主亦名相火，
其脈同診腎，為生氣之門，出而治臍下，分三歧，上衝夾臍過天樞，上
至膻中兩乳間，元氣所系焉。

Wang Hai-Zang said: The hand lesser yang triple burner is the dwelling place of the ministerial fire, the right kidney life gate is the ministerial fire, and the heart envelope master is also called the ministerial fire. Both vessels are diagnosed in the same [pulse position] as the kidney, [and together] they are the gate of qi generation, emerging from and governing [the area] the below the umbilicus.

11 The original passage appears in the 26th Difficult Issue of the *Classic of Difficulties*. It refers to the constituents of the 15 network vessels. *Divine Pivot* presents a scheme wherein each of the 12 channels has an associated network vessel plus the networks of the *ren*, *chong*, and the great network of the spleen, for a total of fifteen. The *Classic of Difficulties* does not posit networks for the *ren* and *chong* but instead presents a yin network and a yang network. See Wang Jiu-Si et al., eds., 1966, p. 53.

Chapter D: Li Shi-Zhen's Extraordinary Vessel Acupuncture

1 Liu Bing-Quan, 1988, p. 72.

2 Dou Mo, 1997.

3   Another hole, Outer Pass (TB-5), is not mentioned in the *Exposition* at all. Acupuncture texts typically list this hole as treating chills and fever, symptoms associated with the *yang wei* vessel. Nevertheless, Outer Pass (TB-5) was not used in this way until after it was linked to the *yang wei* by Xu Feng. Its theoretical association with the *yang wei* appears to have been responsible for expanding the scope of its application.

4   Kiiko Matsumoto and Stephen Birch, 1988, p. 69.

5   *Basic Questions*, 1980, p. 580.

6   See Ch. 36 in Part IV for extraordinary vessel case records by modern acupuncturists that do not involve the master-couple holes.

7   *Divine Pivot*, 1980, vol. 1, p. 429.

8   Ibid., p. 462.

9   See, for instance, Kiiko Matsumoto and Stephen Birch, 1988, pp. 259–261.

10 For a discussion of this issue as it pertains to the channel divergences, see Charles Chace, 2009, "A Merging of the Ways", in The Lantern, 6 (2): 14-21.

11 See Appendix 4 for Li's synopsis of the extraordinary vessel pulses from his *Pulse Studies of the Lakeside [Recluse]*. Here, the extraordinary vessel pulses are described independently of associated symptoms.

12 See, for instance, Yoshio Manaka, Kazuko Itaya, and Stephen Birch, 1995, and Kazuto Miyawaki, 1997.

Chapter E: Herbal Considerations

1   Although Li Shi-Zhen also uses the symbolic imagery of the deer and tortoise in his discussion of the alchemical uses of the *du* vessel, this is not a literal reference to their use as medicines.

Chapter F: Keeping to the One: Internal Alchemy in *Exposition on the Eight Extraordinary Vessels*

1   See, for instance, Paul Unschuld, 1985 , pp. 191 and 210.

2   For a discussion of the development of the modern concept of *qigong* in the 1930s, see David Palmer, 2007.

3   Isabelle Robinet, 1997, p. 217.

4   See, for instance, Livia Kohn, "Guarding the One: Concentrative Meditation in Taoism," in Livia Kohn, ed., 1989, pp. 125–158; and Isabelle Robinet, "Visualization and Ecstatic Flight in Shangqing Taoism," ibid., 159–192.

5   Isabelle Robinet, 1997, p. 217.

6   Daniel Burton-Rose, 2009, "Integrating Inner Alchemy into Late Ming Cultural History, A Contextualization and Annotated Translation of Principles of the Innate Disposition and the Lifespan" (*xing ming gui zhi* 性命圭旨) (1615). Master's thesis, University of Colorado, Boulder.

7   Livia Kohn, 1992, pp. 84–86.

8   Paul Unschuld, ibid.

9   Paul Unschuld, ibid., p. 191.

10 Li Shi-Zhen, 2004a.

11   This is something of an interpolation of *Lao zi*'s meaning. Ch. 77 of *Lao zi* states: "The way of heaven is to reduce the excessive and increase the insufficient. ... It is thus that sages act on behalf of things but do not make any claim on them." (Robert G. Henricks, trans., 1989, p. 180.) *Lao zi* has long been considered an 'open text' that requires a context for its meaning to emerge. In this instance, Li Shi-Zhen was once again more concerned with what he believed the text meant than what it said.

12   The last sentence of this passage, 肝苦急，以辛補之是矣, may also be read as "The liver is bitter and very tense, so use acridity to tonify it!"

13   Zhen Quan flourished during the late Sui and early Tang dynasties when he wrote annotations to a wide variety of books including *Pulse Classic* and *Arcane Essentials of the Imperial Library.*

14   Li Shi-Zhen (1999b), *Comprehensive Outline of the Materia Medica,* p. 883.

15   Ibid.

16   See the section on woody materials (木部 *mu bu*) in *juan* 36, Acanthopanis cortex (五加 *wu jia),* in Li Shi-Zhen, 1999b, *Comprehensive Outline of the Materia Medica,* pp. 1092–1093.

17   Wang Hong-Bin, 2003.

18   Gu Jing-Xing observed: "I have heard from my great grandfather that [Li] read all day the moment the sun rose and meditated all night long. He was destined to be a divine immortal, and it was not coincidental [that he had become one]!" Ibid., p. 945.

19   Isabelle Robinet, 1997, pp. 25–30.

20   For an argument against an historical personage called Zhuang Zi, see Russell Kirkland, 2004, pp. 33–35.

21   Livia Kohn, 1992, p. 58.

22   Roger T. Ames and David Hall, trans., 2003, p. 99.

23   Ibid.

24   Victor Mair, trans., 1994, p. 32.

25   Guo Qing-Fan, ed., 1961, p. 285.

26   Victor Mair, 1994, p. 64.

27   *Basic Questions,* 1980, vol. 1, p. 5.

28   *Divine Pivot,* 1980, vol. 1, p. 211.

29   Li did acknowledge that lead had some valid medicinal values. However, he remained adamant as to its long-term toxicity and the folly of its use in prolonging life.

30   Wu Lu-Ch'iang and Tenney L. Davis, 1932. Richard Bertschinger, 2002, p. 5, translates the passage as follows:

> In the state of Kuai, a common man,
>
> Alone in a valley barely existing,
>
> Clasps to his bosom rough simplicity,
>
> And pleasures in neither circumstance nor honor.
>
> In rude habit he spends his time,
>
> Careless of either fame or profit,
>
> Grasping onto the quiet and solitude,
>
> Those rare times, so tranquil and still.

> So there, dwelling in idleness and ease,
>
> Then I composed this work
>
> To herald the order of Great Change
>
> The Three Sages' forgotten words…
>
> I looked at their obvious meaning
>
> And saw one thread connecting the whole.

31 Wu Lu-Ch'iang and Tenney L. Davis, 1932, p. 32. Richard Bertschinger, 2002, p. 104, translates the passage as follows:

> Nourish yourself thus within,
>
> Tranquil and still in the void
>
> While at source concealing the brilliance
>
> Which illuminates within your whole body.

32 Richard Bertschinger, 2002, p. 105.

33 The book's title (*Huang ting wai jing jing* 黃庭外景經) itself uses the word *jing* 景 to mean 'spirit,' but it can also be translated as 'light' or even 'landscape.' See Isabelle Robinet, 1993, p. 57.

34 Michael LaFargue, 1992, p. 71.

35 Robert G. Henricks, 1989, p. 198.

36 Ibid.

37 Red Pine, trans., 1996, p. 12.

38 Wang Bi grew up with one of the best private libraries of his time and at a young age became famous for the breadth of his learning. Although he died of a sudden illness at the age of 24, this famous proponent of the Double Mystery *(chong xuan* 重玄*)* school earned enduring fame for his commentaries on *Lao zi* and *Classic of Change*.

39 Ariane Rump and Wing-tsit Chan, trans., 1979, pp. 21–22.

40 Su Zhe was a reclusive man of letters who lived during the Tang and Song dynasties. Although his commentary reflects Neo-Confucian sympathies, it is respected by Buddhists and Daoists alike. His commentary, which is included in Ding Fu-Bao's (丁福保) *Essential Flowers of the Daoist Canon (Dao zang jing hua lu* 道藏精華錄*)* of 1449, professes a commitment to the fundamental unity of the three teachings of Confucianism, Buddhism, and Daoism.

41 He-Shang Gong (d. 159 BCE) was, according to legend, a Daoist master who lived beside the Yellow River, hence his name that means 'riverside master.' His commentary emphasizes internal cultivation and was so popular that it now ranks with that of Wang Bi.

42 Ariane Rump and Wing-tsit Chan, trans., 1979, pp. 12–13.

43 Katsuda Masayasu, trans., 1995, p. 175.

44 Ibid.

45 Ibid.

46 Richard Bertschinger, 2002, p. 96; Wu Lu-Ch'iang and Tenney L. Davis, 1932, p. 245.

47 Richard Bertschinger, 2002, pp. 94–95

48 Ibid.

49　Wang Luo-Zhen and Li Ding, 1985, p. 87. This concept is similar to the later Buddhist idea of the ultimate intermingling of the relative and the absolute.

50　Ibid., p. 78.

51　The author of *Direct Teaching of the Great Way in Three Chapters* is unknown, and its first mention in the literature appears in *Exposition on the Eight Extraordinary Vessels.*

52　Here, "river vehicle" refers to the microcosmic orbit.

53　Wang Luo-Zhen and Li Ding, 1985, p. 88.

54　There is some debate as to whether *Eight Vessel Scripture* can even be legitimately attributed to Zhang Bo-Duan as the text does not appear in any of the standard catalogues of Daoist writings. Nevertheless, the style of writing is consistent with a Song dynasty publication date. *Eight Vessel Scripture* also appears in two later texts of internal cultivation. The first is the Qing dynasty work by Wang Zu-Yuan 王祖源, *An Illustrated Explication of Internal and External (Nei wai gong tu shuo* 內外功圖説*)*, that appears in *Essential Splendors of the Daoist Canon (Dao zang jing hua* 道藏精華*).* Also, in his *Wu-Liu Lineage of Immortality (Wu-Liu xian zong* 伍柳仙宗, 1897), Deng Huiji 鄧徽績 appears to have appended *Eight Vessel Scripture* to Liu Hua-Yang's 柳華陽 famous *Scripture on Wisdom and Potential (Hui ming jing* 慧命經, 1846).

55　尾閭 *(wei lü),* literally the 'caudal funnel,' is here referred to as a focal point for meditation in internal alchemy. The point is located in the perianal region and is most closely associated with Meeting of Yin (CV-1).

56　二節 *(er jie)* literally means the 'two joints.'

57　We are indebted to Professor Li Yuan-Guo 李遠國 for his help in identifying this text.

58　Iwai Yusen, Guo Xiu-Mei, and the Japanese *Inner Classic* Study Group, trans., 2003, p. 1066.

59　Wang Luo-Zhen and Li Ding, 1985, p. 32.

60　Iwai Yusen, Guo Xiu-Mei, and the Japanese *Inner Classic* Study Group, 2003, p. 1066.

61　Here, 'heavenly gate' is another name for the head and is synonymous with the brain.

62　Iwai Yusen, Guo Xiu-Mei, and the Japanese *Inner Classic* Study Group, 2003, p. 1066.

63　Ibid.

64　Roger T. Ames and David Hall, trans., 2003, p. 163.

65　Ibid., p. 154.

66　Isabelle Robinet, 1993, p. 57.

67　In internal cultivation, the dragon is often taken to mean the intellect and the tiger to mean sexual desire, both of which must be tamed and subdued.

68　Richard Bertschinger, 2002, p. 27; Wu Lu-Ch'iang and Tenney L. Davis, 1932, p. 245. Neither of these translations is entirely satisfactory. Bertschinger places the passage at the beginning of the text. Wu and Davis place it in their Ch. XXXVI. It appears in line 41 of the Peng Xiao version.

69　Richard Bertschinger, 2002, p. 29.

70　This theme is developed further in our commentary on the *yin wei* vessel.

71 A more generalized conduction of source qi through the extraordinary vessels in a medical context is also described by Luo Dong-Yi in Ch. 33 of the present text.

Chapter G: An Overview of Extraordinary Vessel Pulse Diagnosis

1 See Katsayasu Kido, 1978.

PART II: *Exposition on the Eight Extraordinary Vessels*

Prefaces

1 Bin Hu is Li Shi-Zhen's pen name.

2 Yi Ya (易牙) is also known as Di Ya (狄牙) or Yong Wu (雍巫). He was the favorite cook of Duke Huan (桓) of Qi (齊) during the Spring and Autumn period (772–481 BCE). In this context, the writer is trying to say that unless one's understanding equals the culinary talent of Yi Ya, it is impossible to understand the true meaning of the eight extraordinary vessels.

3 The mid-autumn solar period is generally in July.

4 The reference to Li Shi-Zhen as "a scholar of our age"(*shi ru* 世儒) may be interpreted in a number of ways. The term originally meant someone of shallow learning, and although Li failed the upper-level imperial exams, he was nevertheless very well-educated, particularly in medicine. By the Tang dynasty, the term simply referred to any well-educated individual.

5 Xuan is another name for the Yellow Emperor (Huang Di 黄帝).

6 Zhu Hui-Weng (朱晦翁) is also known as Zhu Xi (朱熹). He was the person who codified the Neo-Confucian canon.

7 Chun Yu-Yi was a physician during the Western Han Dynasty who stated that he received the pulse writings of Duke Cheng Yang-Qing. This story is recorded in *Records of the Grand Historian (Shi ji* 史記).

8 Note that there are two editions of *Xue Yi's Case Records,* and the first edition does not contain this text.

Chapter 3: The *Yin Wei* Vessel

1 This statement is nearly identical to a passage in the 28th Difficult Issue of the *Classic of Difficulties:* 陰維起於諸陰交也. See Wang Jiu-Si et al., eds., 1966, p. 54.

2 *The Systematic Classic of Acupuncture and Moxibustion* describes the location of Guest House in a similar manner: "The cleft [hole] of the *yin wei* is [located] above the inner ankle in the parting of the flesh of the calf. It is needled to a depth of three *fen* and treated by moxibustion with five cones." Huang-Fu Mi, 1981, vol. 1, p. 465. A note in Ch. 41, "Discourse on Needling Lower Back Pain," locates this point behind the medial malleolus. Li Shi-Zhen has simply added the distance five *cun* to his description.

3 Both *The Systematic Classic* and *Arcane Essentials of the Imperial Library* consider Surging Gate (SP-12) to be a meeting hole of the *yin wei* vessel. *The Systematic Classic* places these holes three-and-a-half *cun* lateral to the midline of the abdomen,

not four-and-a-half *cun*. This location as given by Li is idiosyncratic. Huang-Fu Mi, ibid., p. 417.

4   *The Systematic Classic* describes Great Horizontal as being located "three *cun* below Abdominal Lament directly lateral to the umbilicus; it is the meeting [hole] of the foot greater yin and the *yin wei* channels." The same chapter describes Abdominal Lament as being located "one-and-a-half *cun* below sun and moon; it is the meeting [hole] of the foot greater yin and *yin wei* channels." This location is idiosyncratic. Ibid., p. 416.

5   *The Systematic Classic* describes Cycle Gate as "The liver alarm [hole]. It is located between two ribs one-and-a-half *cun* lateral to Not Contained (ST-13); it is the meeting [hole] of the foot greater yin and *yin wei* [channels]." Ibid., p. 414.

6   *The Systematic Classic* describes Celestial Chimney as "located five *cun* below the pharyngeal prominence on the centerline and in a depression. It is the meeting [hole] of the *yin wei* and *ren* vessels. Lower the head to locate it." Ibid., p. 389. *The Systematic Classic* describes Ridge Spring as "located below the chin, above the throat knot, and below the root of the tongue. It is the meeting of the *yin wei* and *ren* vessels." Ibid., p. 378.

Chapter 4: The *Yang Wei* Vessel

1   *The Systematic Classic of Acupuncture and Moxibustion* describes the location of Metal Gate in a similar manner: "The foot greater cleft is in a hole below the outer ankle and is a branch of the yang wei." Huang-Fu Mi, Shandong zhong yi xue yuan, eds., 1981, vol.1, p. 482.

2   *The Systematic Classic* describes the location of Yang Intersection as: "The cleft of the yang wei is located seven *cun* above the outer ankle in a space located obliquely to the parting of the flesh between the three yang." Ibid., p. 477. Wang Luo-Zhen explains that the "three yang" refers to the foot greater yang. Because this hole is located obliquely to the parting of the flesh between the three yang, this means that Yang Intersection is situated in a posterior position closer to the foot greater yang bladder channel. Li Shi-Zhen's rendering of this passage omits any mention of the "parting of the flesh" *(fen rou* 分肉) and refers to the "two yang," the gallbladder channel upon which Yang Intersection is situated, rather than the bladder channel mentioned in the original passage of *The Systematic Classic*. Wang Luo-Zhen and Li Ding, eds., 1985, p. 15.

3   *The Systematic Classic* describes Squatting Bone-Hole as being the meeting of the *yang qiao* and the foot lesser yang. Huang-Fu Mi, Shangdong zhong yi xue yuan, eds., 1981, pp. 419–420. Wang Luo-Zhen is of the opinion that Li's inclusion of this hole in the *yang wei* is a mistake. Wang Luo-Zhen and Li Ding, eds., ibid., p. 15.

4   *The Systematic Classic* describes the location of Upper Arm as situated "Seven *cun* above the elbow at the end of a muscular mass. It is the meeting of the network of the hand yang brightness." Huang-Fu Mi, ibid., p. 444. This text makes no mention of this hole as a meeting hole of the *yang wei*. Wang Luo-Zhen hypothesizes that the similarity of the graphs 絡 *(luo*, 'network') and 維 *(wei*, 'binding/linking') may have led Li Shi-Zhen to list Upper Arm as a meeting hole of the *yang wei*. Wang Luo-Zhen and Li Ding, ibid., p. 15.

The Illustrated Addendum to the Classified Classic explains that: "The hand meeting [hole] of the network of the hand lesser yin is said to be the meeting hole of the hand and foot *tai yang* and the *yang wei*." Zhang Jie-Bin and Li Zhi-Yong, eds., 1999, p. 747. However, Upper Arm does appear as a meeting hole of the *yang wei* in *The Comprehensive Elucidation of the Fourteen Channels* by Wang Zhi-Zhong and Hua Bo-Ren. Cheng Dan-An, ed., 1973, *The Classic of Acupuncture and Moxibustion for Endowing Life and the Elucidation of the Fourteen Channels in a Combined Edition*, p. 70.

5   *The Systematic Classic* identifies this hole as "located on the front of the arm three *cun* lateral to the acromion. It is the network of the hand *yang ming*." Huang-Fu Mi, ibid., p. 389. This hole is actually located on the posterior aspect of the upper arm.

6   *The Systematic Classic* describes the location of Celestial Bone-Hole as situated "in the supraclavicular fossa in a depression above the clavicle; it is the meeting of the hand lesser yang and the *yang wei* [channels]." Ibid., p. 384.

     The Essentials of the Channels and Holes (Jing xue zuan yao 經穴纂要, 1810) identifies the *bi gu* (蔽骨) as "the prominent bone behind the shoulder well," making it the clavicle. *The Systematic Classic,* ibid., p. 385.

7   *The Systematic Classic* asserts that Shoulder Well is "the meeting of the hand lesser yang and the *yang wei* [channels]." Ibid., pp. 382–383. *Arcane Essentials of the Imperial Library*, Wang Bing's commentary on Ch. 60 of *Basic Questions*, and *An Acupuncture Hole Diagram Based on the Bronze Model* all identify this hole as "the meeting of the hand and foot lesser yang and *yang wei*." Wang Luo-Zhen and Li Ding, eds., ibid., p. 15.

8   *The Systematic Classic* locates this hole "on the shoulder, on the back of the upper arm below the large bone and on the upper border of the scapula." Huang-Fu Mi, ibid., p. 386. The large bone is the scapular crest.

9   *The Systematic Classic* identifies Wind Pond as the meeting hole of the foot lesser yang and *yang wei* channels. Ibid., 342. It also identifies Brain Hollow, Upright Construction, and Eye Window as meeting holes of the foot lesser yang and and *yang wei* channels. Ibid., pp. 337–338.

     The same chapter identifies Overlooking Tears as a meeting hole of the foot greater, lesser yang, and *yang wei* channels. Each hole is located lateral to the hairline and is on the second line of the head in the gallbladder channel. Ibid., pp. 336–337.

10   *The Systematic Classic* identifies Yang White as "the meeting of the foot lesser yang and *yang wei* channels. Ibid., p. 363. Wang Bing's commentary on Ch. 59 of *Basic Questions* erroneously identifies Yang White as the meeting of the two vessels of the foot yang brightness and the *yang wei*. Wang Luo-Zhen and Li Ding, eds., ibid., p. 16. *The Comprehensive Elucidation of the Fourteen Channels* identifies Yang White as the meeting of the five vessels of the hand and foot greater yang and lesser yang and foot yang brightness. Li has followed the pathway laid out in *The Comprehensive Elucidation of the Fourteen Channels.* Hua Bo-Ren, p. 51. The count of five vessels makes no sense.

11   The Spirit Root hole belongs to the foot lesser yang gallbladder channel and is located in front of the hairline, three *cun* beside Spirit Court (GV-24). *The Systematic Classic* says that it is located "one-and-a-half *cun* in front of the hairline. It is the meeting hole of the foot lesser yang and the *yang wei*."

In this book, the *yang wei* ends at this hole, and it is not clear why. The location of the Spirit Root hole is not directly above the eye. Overlooking Tears (GB-15) is more directly above the eye. Huang-Fu Mi, ibid., p. 328.

12   *The Systematic Classic* is in error in deeming Head Binding (ST-8) as "a meeting hole of the foot lesser yang and the *yang wei*." This is a transcriptional error, mistakenly substituting the graph 維 (*wei*) for 明 (*ming*). Ibid., p. 329. Again, in the same chapter of *Basic Questions*, commentator Wang Bing states that "It is the meeting of the two vessels of the foot lesser yang and yang brightness." *Basic Questions*, 1980, vol.2, p. 713.

Wang Luo-Zhen considers this to be correct and asserts that Li based his material on a flawed text. Wang Luo-Zhen and Li Ding, ibid., p. 16.

Chapter 5: Diseases of the Two *Wei*

1   This passage is from line 53 of *Discussion of Cold Damage*, Craig Mitchell, Feng Ye, and Nigel Wiseman, trans., 1999, p. 611.

2   This passage is from line 24 of *Discussion of Cold Damage*. Wind House (GV-16) does not appear as a hole on Li Shi-Zhen's trajectory for the *yang wei* vessel.

3   This is a paraphrase of line 54 of *Discussion of Cold Damage*. Ibid., p. 611.

4   The original sentence in Volume 10 of the *Pulse Classic (Mai jing 脈經)* lacks the word "pulse" or "vessel" (*mai* 脈) at the end of the sentence. Wang Shu-He, Fuzhou shi ren min yi yuan, eds., 1981, p. 650.

5   These symptoms appear in Volume 10 of the *Pulse Classic* in association with the yang network *(yang luo 陽絡)* and not the *yang wei* vessel. It is clear that Li includes pathology associated with the yang networks with *yang wei* vessel pathology. Ibid.

6   In the original passage in the *Pulse Classic,* the word "seizures" (*dian* 癲) precedes the word "fainting" (*jiang pu* 僵僕). Ibid.

7   Guest Host (GB-3) is also known as Upper Barrier (上關 *shang guan*). It is the meeting hole of the hand and foot lesser yang and foot yang brightness channels. It has no direct relationship to the *yang wei* vessel. The original sentence in the *Pulse Classic* reads: "Immediately select Guest Host (GB-3) and treat both *yang wei* vessels located on the outer ankle two *cun* below the fibula." Ibid.

8   The original sentence in the *Pulse Classic* lacks the word "pulse" or "vessel" *(mai* 脈*)* at the end of the sentence. Ibid.

9   When 癲 *(dian)* and 癇 *(xian) a*ppear together as a compound term, they refer to seizure disorders characterized by brief episodes of temporary loss of spirit, turning pale, fixity of the eyes, or sudden clouding collapse, foaming at the mouth, upward-staring eyes, clenched jaw and convulsions of the limbs, and in some cases squealing like an animal. When *xian* appears alone, it refers to seizures, as described in the previous paragraph. When *dian* appears alone it may refer to any pattern characterized by melancholy, indifferent expression, muttering soliloquy, abnormal laughing and weeping, hallucination, and delusions, deranged speech, oblivious to hygiene, and no thought of food and drink.

10   'Raised shoulder breathing' *(jian xi* 肩息*)* is characterized by the raising of the shoulders to assist breathing in severe respiratory patterns such as chronic obstructive pulmonary disease.

11 灑灑 *(sa sa)* is a shivering chill due to exposure to dampness.

12 'Propping fullness' *(zhi man* 支滿*)* refers to a subjective sense of fullness in the chest and the lateral costal region. The word *zhi*, or propping, refers to a sensation of the chest and diaphragm being propped up from below.

13 The original passage in the *Pulse Classic* reads: "When diagnosis reveals that the *yang wei* pulse … ." Ibid., p. 90.

14 This is a reference to the acupuncture hole Yang Intersection (GB-35), which is the cleft hole of the *yang wei* vessel. *The Systematic Classic of Acupuncture and Moxibustion* identifies this hole as Mountain Support (BL-57). Huang-Fu Mi, Shandong zhong yi xue yuan, eds., 1981, vol. 1, p. 482.

15 Mountain Support (BL-57) is not on the *yang wei* trajectory. The hole that should be referred to is Yang Intersection (GB-35).

16 Nigel Wiseman translates 急 *(ji)* as "retracted and tense." Nigel Wiseman and Feng Ye, 1998, p. 606.

17 This passage is referring to Yang Assistance (GB-38).

Chapter 6: The *Yin Qiao* Vessel

1 *The Annotated Systematic Classic of Acupuncture & Moxibustion* substitutes the word 鼽 *(qiu)*, which normally means 'nasal obstruction,' as an alternate character for the word 頄 *(kui)* 'cheekbone.' The two words 内廉 *(nei lian,* inner ridge) appear in Ch. 40 of *Basic Questions*. Wang Bing observes that "This states that both *qiao* head toward the [inner] canthus of the eye." See Katsuda Masayasu, trans., 1995, p. 58.

2 In his *Yellow Emperor's Inner Classic: Grand Essentials*, Yang Shang-Shan comments: "The three vessels of the *yin qiao* along with the greater yang and the *yang qiao* converge and travel upward to Bright Eyes (BL-1) above." *The Systematic Classic* identifies Bright Eyes (BL-1) as the meeting hole of the hand and foot greater yang, the foot yang brightness, and the *yang qiao*. Huang-Fu Mi, Shandong zhong yi xue yuan, eds., 1981, p. 364. In his commentary to Ch. 59 of *Basic Questions*, Wang Bing identifies this hole as "the meeting hole of the five vessels of the hand and foot greater yang, *yin qiao*, and *yang qiao*." See Wang Luo-Zhen and Li Ding, eds., 1985, p. 32.

3 尾閭 *(wei lü)*, literally, the 'end gate,' is here referred to as a focal point for meditation in internal alchemy. The point is located in the perianal region and is most closely associated with Meeting of Yin (CV-1).

4 二節 *(er jie)* is literally the 'two joints.'

Chapter 7: The *Yang Qiao* Vessel

1 The 28th Difficult Issue of the *Classic of Difficulties* states: "The *yang qiao* vessel arises at the heel; it proceeds along the outer ankle, ascends upward, and enters the Wind Pond (GB-20)[hole]." Wang Jiu-Si et al., eds., 1966, p. 55. Neither the *Inner Classic* nor the *Classic of Difficulties* contains the phrase "is a branch vessel of the foot greater yang." The likely rationale for this statement is that Extending Vessel (BL-62) is the meeting hole of the foot greater yang and the *yin qiao* vessels.

2   *The Systematic Classic of Acupuncture and Moxibustion* states: "Extending Vessel engenders the *yang qiao*. It is located below the outer ankle bone in a depression the size of the edge of a fingernail." Huang-Fu Mi, Shandong zhong yi xue yuan, eds., 1981, vol.1, p. 481.

3   In his comments to Ch. 41 of *Basic Questions*, Wang Bing explains that Subservient Visitor (BL-61) is "located in the center of a depression below the heel bone and is the meeting of the two vessels of the foot greater yang and *yang qiao*." Wang Luo-Zhen and Li Ding, eds., 1985, p. 37. *The Systematic Classic* makes no mention of its being an intersection or meeting hole. Given the location of this hole on the outer side of the ankle, it cannot be located by "cupping the foot." Since the *yang qiao* arises from within the center of the heel, this hole is considered the 'root' of the *yang qiao*. Based on this, the trajectory of the *yang qiao* is generally described as traveling from the center of the heel to Subservient Visitor (BL-61) and then arriving at Extending Vessel (BL-62) and traveling upward.

4   *The Systematic Classic* identifies Instep Yang (BL-59) as "the cleft [hole] of the *yang qiao*, located on the foot three *cun* above the outer ankle." Huang-Fu Mi, ibid., p. 482.

5   The trajectory of the *yang qiao* should include Squatting Bone-Hole (GB-29), which *The Systematic Classic* describes as being "the intersection hole of the *yang qiao* and the lesser yang." Ibid., pp. 419–420.

6   *The Systematic Classic* describes Upper Arm Transport (SI-10) as "the meeting [hole] of the hand greater yang, *yang wei*, and [*yang*] *qiao* vessels." Ibid., p. 386.

7   *The Systematic Classic* describes both of these holes as meeting holes of the yang brightness and *yang qiao* vessels. Ibid., p. 384.

8   Man's Prognosis (ST-9) is located level with the tip of the Adam's apple, on the course of the common carotid artery, at the anterior border of the sternocleidomastoid muscle. It is not an intersection meeting hole. Earth Granary (ST-4) is located four *fen* lateral to the corner of the mouth. *The Systematic Classic* describes it as "the meeting of the *qiao* vessels and the hand and foot yang brightness." Ibid., p. 370.

9   Great Bone Hole (ST-3) is located approximately eight *fen* directly below the pupil, at the level of the lower border of the ala nasi, on the lateral side of the nasolabial groove. *The Systematic Classic* describes it as "the meeting of the *qiao* vessels and foot yang brightness." Ibid., p. 368.

10   Tear Container (ST-1) is located between the eyeball and the midpoint of the infraorbital ridge. *The Systematic Classic* describes it as "the meeting of the *yang qiao* and *ren* vessels and the foot yang brightness." Ibid., p. 366.

11   Bright Eyes (BL-1) is located one *fen* superior to the inner canthus. In his commentary to Ch. 59 of *Basic Questions*, Wang Bing explains that this hole is "the meeting of the five vessels of the hand and foot greater yang, foot yang brightness, *yin qiao*, and *yang qiao*." Wang Luo-Zhen and Li Ding, eds., ibid., p. 38.

12   Wind Pool (GB-20) is located on the posterior aspect of the neck, below the occipital bone, in the depression between the sternocleidomastoid muscle and the trapezius muscle. *The Systematic Classic* describes it as "the meeting of the lesser yang and the *yang wei*." Huang-Fu Mi, Shandong zhong yi xue yuan, eds., ibid., p. 342. No mention is made of a meeting with the *yang qiao*. However, the *Classic of Difficulties* states that the *yang qiao* "enters Wind Pool."

13   The 23rd Difficult Issue of the *Classic of Difficulties* states: "[Humans have] in both legs the *chi* vessels that extend from the foot to the eye. They are seven *chi* and five *cun*. Two times seven [*chi*] makes one *zhang* and four *chi*. Two times five [*cun*] makes one *chi*. Altogether, this is one *zhang* and five *chi* long." Paul Unschuld, trans., 1986a, p. 45.

14   The original passage in Ch. 17 of *Divine Pivot* reads: "There is nowhere that the qi does not travel to." *Divine Pivot*, 1980, vol. 1, p. 348.

Chapter 8: Diseases of the Two *Qiao*

1   The original passage appears in the 26th Difficult Issue of the *Classic of Difficulties*. It refers to the constituents of the 15 network vessels. The *Divine Pivot* presents a scheme wherein each of the 12 channels has an associated network vessel plus the networks of the *ren*, *chong*, and the great network of the spleen, for a total of fifteen. The *Classic of Difficulties* does not posit networks for the *ren* and *chong* but instead presents a yin network and a yang network.

2   This is a later interpretation by Lu Guang that did not originate with Wang Shu-He.

3   In the source passage in the *Pulse Classic*, the phrase "generalized body stiffness" (*shen ti qiang* 身體強) is preceded by the word "skin" (*pi fu* 皮膚). Wang Shu-He, Fuzhou shi ren min yi yuan, eds., 1981, p. 646. Depending on how the text is punctuated, the passage may be read as "numbness of the skin and body stiffness," or "stiffness and insensitivity of the skin and body."

4   皮膚淫痺 *(pi fu yin bi),* literally "pernicious obstruction of the skin," refers to obstruction patterns due to the excesses of any of the six qi: wind, cold, fire, summerheat, dampness, or dryness. The source passage in the *Pulse Classic* substitutes the word "stiff" (*qiang* 強) for "pernicious" (*yin* 淫), that is, the skin is stiff and insensitive. Ibid.

5   Bulging diseases *(shan* 疝) are characterized by swelling or pain of the abdomen or scrotum. Yin bulging *(yin shan* 陰疝) is characterized by acute pain in the testicles and genitals attributed to cold pathogen invading the liver channel.

6   Spotting *(lou xia* 漏下) refers to scanty nonmenstrual bleeding from the uterus.

7   As a compound term, 髖窌 *(kuan jiao)* means the pelvis.

8   Li Shi-Zhen's rendering of the phrase "In men, [needle] the yang [*qiao*], and in women, [needle] the yin [*qiao*]" is consistent with both *The Systematic Classic of Acupuncture and Moxibustion* and Ch. 73 of *Divine Pivot*. According to Shou Shan-Ge, the words yin and yang were mistakenly transposed in the carving of the original edition. Given the context in which this reference to the *qiao* vessels occurs, some commentators suggest that the modality being referred to is moxibustion.

9   Our interpretation of this line is based on Katsuda Masayasu, trans., 1995, p. 79.

10   Katsuda Masayasu identifies this location as the medial edge of the cheekbone. Ibid., p. 82.

11   The original passage in *Basic Questions* does not contain the word "person" (*ren* 人).

12   Staring eyes (*chen mu* 瞋目) is contrasted with eyes closed, as if in death *(ming mu* 瞑目). These terms are generally interpreted to mean insomnia and somnolence, respectively.

13   This passage appears in Ch. 21 of *Divine Pivot*, 1980, vol. 1, p. 389.

14 This passage appears in volume 12 of *The Systematic Classic*. The entire passage appears in Ch. 80 of *Divine Pivot*. There, the first sentence reads: "When a patient's eyes are shut and they cannot see, what is the state of the qi that leads to this?" 目閉 而不得視者何氣使然也. *Divine Pivot*, 1980, vol. 2, p. 443. The same passage in *The Systematic Classic* reads: "When a patient's eyes are closed and they cannot see, what [is this condition]?" (目閉不得視者,何也?) Wang Luo-Zhen and Li Ding, eds., 1985, p. 46.

15 This passage appears in Ch. 80 of *Divine Pivot*. The original passage begins with the sentence, "When the patient cannot lie down, what is this condition of the qi?" (病而 不得臥何氣使然.) *Divine Pivot*, 1980, vol. 2, p. 442.

16 According to Katsuda Masayasu, 24 hours were divided into one hundred 刻 *(ke)*, and nutritive qi circulated 50 times throughout the channels every 24 hours of the day, passing each organ at certain times. Katsuda Masayasu, trans., 1995, p. 93.

17 目上綱目下綱 *(mu shang gang, mu xia gang)* refers to the upper and lower eyelids.

18 This sentence appears in Zhang Zi-He's *Confucians' Duties to Their Parents* in the passages dealing with "Afflictions of the Nine Qi" (*Jiu qi gan ji* 九氣感疾). See *A Chinese Encyclopedia of Medicine*, 2004.

19 The third volume of Chao Yuan-Fang's *Discourse on the Origins and Presentations of All Diseases* contains the passage: "If there is heart vexation with inability to sleep, [this is due to] heart heat. If, however, it is only deficiency irritability with inability to sleep, [this is due] only to being chilled." Wang Luo-Zhen and Li Ding, eds., ibid., p. 46.

20 Wang Shu-He, ibid., p. 329.

Chapter 9: The *Chong* Vessel

1 *The Systematic Classic of Acupuncture and Moxibustion* does not list intersection holes for the *chong* vessel per se, although its discussion of the Meeting Yin (CV-1) hole contains the assertion that "[from Meeting of the Yin], a branching network from the *ren* vessel hugs the *du* vessel and it meets with the *chong* vessel." This statement adds the Meeting Yin hole to the trajectory of the *chong* vessel. Huang-Fu Mi, Shandong zhong yi xue yuan, eds., 1981, vol. 1, p. 406.

2 Ch. 60 of *Basic Questions* states: "The *chong* vessel originates from the qi thoroughfare merging with the lesser yin channel, hugging the umbilicus and ascending to reach the chest and disperse in it." *Basic Questions*, 1980, vol. 2, p. 741.

3 Great Manifestation (KI-12), Qi Hole (KI-13), Fourfold Fullness (KI-14), Central Flow (KI-15), and Huang Transport (KI-16) are all holes on the foot lesser yin kidney channel described by *The Systematic Classic* as being meeting holes of the *chong* vessel and the foot lesser yin. They are described there as being located five *fen* lateral to the midline. Huang-Fu Mi, ibid., vol. 1, pp. 407–410.

   An Acupuncture Hole Diagram Based on the Bronze Model (1027) locates these holes one-and-a-half *cun* from the midline. *Comprehensive Compendium of Acupuncture and Moxibustion* locates them one *cun* from the midline. *Arcane Essentials of the Imperial Library* identifies them as "the meeting [holes] of the *ren* vessel, *chong* vessel, and lesser yin." Wang Luo-Zhen and Li Ding, eds., 1985, *An Annotated Exposition on the Eight Extraordinary Vessels*, p. 56.

Also, *The Systematic Classic* states: "Yin intersection is located one *cun* below the umbilicus and is a meeting hole of the *ren* vessel and qi thoroughfare." Huang-Fu Mi, ibid., vol. 1, pp. 403–404. According to Katsuda Masayasu, the characters 氣衝 (*qi chong*, 'qi thoroughfare') are a misprint and should read衝脈 (*chong mai*, 'chong vessel'). Katsuda Masayasu, trans., 1995, p. 106.

4   The original citation appears in Ch. 65 of *Divine Pivot*. Li Shi-Zhen has simplified the original 今婦人之生 (*jin fu ren zhi sheng*, "women who live now") to 婦人 (*fu ren*, "women"). The original also reads: 以其數脫血也任衝之脈不營口唇故須不生焉 "There is repeated desertion of blood. The vessels of the *ren* and *chong* cannot nourish the mouth and lips, hence, hair cannot grow [in these places]." The original also reads: "During their menstrual flow, they repeatedly experience a desertion of blood" (*xia shu tuo xue* 下數脫血). *Divine Pivot*, 1980, vol. 2, p. 230.

5   The Grand Thoroughfare relates to a yin region. Yet according to Zhang Zhi-Cong: "One's back is to the north and is yin. Hence, it is called Grand Thoroughfare." (背北為陰故太衝.) *Basic Questions*, ibid., vol. 1, p. 101.

6   Here we follow Katsuda Masayasu, who interprets 頏顙 (*hang sang*) as "the juncture of the hard and soft palates." Katsuda Masayasu, ibid., p. 110.

7   According to Katsuda Masayasu, the heart envelope master (*xin bao zhu* 心包主) is the heart envelope network vessel (*xin bao luo* 心包絡). Katsuda Masayasu, ibid., p. 116.

8   According to Katsuda Masayasu, ibid., the passage should be punctuated differently, placing a comma after the second 腎 (*shen*, kidney), making the passage read as follows (with punctuation):

王海藏曰手少陽三焦相火為一府，右腎命門為相火，心包主亦名相火，其脈同診腎，為生氣之門，出而治臍下，分三歧，上衝夾臍過天樞，上至膻中兩乳間，元氣所系焉。

Wang Hai-Zang said: The hand lesser yang triple burner is the dwelling place of the ministerial fire, the right kidney life gate is the ministerial fire, and the heart envelope master is also called the ministerial fire. Both vessels are diagnosed in the same [pulse position] as the kidney, [and together] they are the gate of qi generation, emerging from and governing [the area] below the umbilicus.

9   *Pulse Rhymes (Mai jue* 脈訣) was composed during the Five Dynasties period by Gao Yang-Sheng (高陽生) but has been erroneously attributed to Wang Shu-He. It is cited in Dai Qi-Zong's (戴起宗) *Correcting the Errors of the Pulse Rhymes (Mai jue kan wu* 脈決刊誤) in the Yuan dynasty (1271–1368), and in Zhang Shi-Xian's *Illustrated Differentiation of the Pulse Rhymes (Tu zhu mai jue bian zhen* 圖註脈訣辨真) written during the Ming dynasty (1368–1644).

Chapter 10: Diseases of the *Chong* Vessel

1   This passage is from the 29th Difficult Issue of the *Classic of Difficulties*, which lacks the word 'pulse' (*mai* 脈) and substitutes the pronoun *zhi* (之) for it. Wang Jiu-Si et al., eds., 1966, p. 56.

2   This passage is quoted from Ch. 5 of *Basic Questions*. Li Dong-Yuan has altered the passage slightly, substituting the word "counterflow" (*ni* 逆) for the word "reversal" (*jue* 厥).

3   Raise the Yang and Drain Heat Decoction *(sheng yang xie re tang)* does not appear in *Secrets from the Orchid Chamber*. The symptoms described by Li Shi-Zhen are associated with Raise the Yang and Eliminate Dampness Decoction *(sheng yang chu shi tang)*. This formula contains Angelica Sinensis Radix *(dang gui)* 5 *fen*, wine-washed, Angelicae pubescentis Radix *(du huo)* 5 *fen*, Viticus Fructus *(man jing zi)* 7 *fen*, Saposhnikoviae Radix *(fang feng)* 1 *qian*, Glycyrrhizae Radix preparata *(zhi gan cao)* 1 *qian*, Cimicifugae Rhizoma *(sheng ma)* 1 *qian*, Ligustici Rhizoma *(gao ben)* 1 *qian*, Bupleuri Radix *(chai hu)* 1 *qian* 5 *fen*, Notopterygii Rhizoma seu Radix *(qiang huo)* 1 *qian* 5 *fen*, Atractylodis Rhizoma *(cang zhu)* 1 *qian* 5 *fen*, and Astragali Radix *(huang qi)* 1 *qian* 5 *fen*. Li Dong-Yuan, 1981b, p. 204.

4   This is an abbreviated version of the discussion as it appears in Ch. 44 of *Basic Questions*. The original passage reads: "It unites with the yang brightness at the gathering sinew, which is the meeting of the gathering sinews of yin and yang, and meets at the qi thoroughfare, and the yang brightness is the leader [of them all]." *Basic Questions*, vol. 1, p. 578.

5   *Jia yi* 甲乙 are the first and second heavenly stems, *bing ding* 丙丁 are the third and fourth heavenly stems, and *wu ji* 戊己 are the fifth and sixth heavenly stems.

6   Li has transposed the order of the symptoms as they originally appear in the *Pulse Classic*. Wang Shu-He, Fuzhou shi ren min yi yuan, eds., 1981, p. 90.

7   Li has again switched the order of the symptoms, listing enuresis where infertility appears in the original. Ibid., p. 92.

8   *You qi zhu zhu ran er tong* (有氣築築然而痛) refers to pain resulting from severe qi stagnation. This section was one of the sources for abdominal palpation *(fukushin)* and palpation of the aorta around the epigastrium that is still used in Japan, although it is very rare to feel aortic pulsation below the umbilicus.

9   These holes are generally believed to be Mute's Gate (GV-15) and Great Hammer (GV-14), respectively.

10 Hundred Convergences (GV-20).

Chapter 11: The *Ren* Vessel

1   *The Systematic Classic of Acupuncture and Moxibustion* describes a network vessel as issuing from this hole: "[From here] a branching network [vessel] of the *ren* vessel hugs the *du* vessel. It is a meeting hole of the *chong* vessel." Huang-Fu Mi, Shandong zhong yi xue yuan, eds., 1981, vol. 1, p. 406.

2   *The Systematic Classic* describes this hole as "a meeting of the *ren* vessel and the foot reversing yin." Ibid.

3   *The Systematic Classic* describes both holes as "a meeting of the foot three yin and the *ren* vessel." Ibid., p. 405.

4   *The Systematic Classic* describes this hole as "a meeting of the *ren* vessel and the qi thoroughfare." Ibid., p. 403. *Arcane Essentials of the Imperial Library* correctly identifies this hole as: "A meeting of the *ren* vessel, the *chong* vessel, and the lesser yin." Wang Luo-Zhen and Li Ding, eds., 1985, p. 71.

5   *The Systematic Classic* describes this hole as "a meeting of the foot greater yin and the *ren* vessel." Huang-Fu Mi, ibid., p. 403.

6   *The Systematic Classic* describes this hole as "a meeting of the hand greater yang, lesser yang, foot yang brightness, and the *ren* vessel." Ibid., p. 402.

7   *The Systematic Classic* describes this hole as "a meeting of the *ren* vessel, foot yang brightness, and hand greater yang." Ibid., p. 401.

8   *The Systematic Classic* describes this hole as "a branching [network] of the *ren* vessel." Ibid., p. 400.

9   Chest Center (CV-17) was not originally an intersection hole. *A Comprehensive Compendium of Acupuncture and Moxibustion* identifies it as "a meeting of the foot greater yin, lesser yin, foot greater yang and lesser yang, and the *ren* vessel." Wang Luo-Zhen and Li Ding, ibid., p. 71.

10 *The Systematic Classic* describes both holes as "a meeting of the *yin wei* and *ren* vessel." Huang-Fu Mi, ibid., pp. 378–389.

11 *The Systematic Classic* describes this hole as "a meeting of the foot yang brightness and *ren* vessels." It is Li Shi-Zhen's interpretation that this hole is a point of intersection between the *ren* and *du* vessel. Ibid., p. 370.

12 *The Systematic Classic* describes this hole as "a meeting of the *yang qiao, ren* vessel, and foot yang brightness." Ibid., p. 365.

13 This passage appears in Ch. 10 of *Divine Pivot*. The word "branching" *(bie* 別) is a later addition. *Divine Pivot*, 1980, vol. 1., p. 277.

14 This passage appears in Ch. 2 of *Divine Pivot*. In the source text, the last sentence reads: "The pulsing vessel on the sides [of the throat] is the foot yang brightness [hole] that is named Man's Prognosis (ST-9)." Ibid., p. 58.

Chapter 12: Diseases of the *Ren* Vessel

1   This statement originally appears in Ch. 1 of *Basic Questions* where the word "a little" *(shao* 少) follows the word "weakens" *(shuai* 衰). *Basic Questions*, 1980, vol. 1, pp. 7–8.

   Both *The Systematic Classic of Acupuncture and Moxibustion* and the *Yellow Emperor's Inner Classic: Grand Essentials* use the term "hidden thoroughfare" *(fu chong* 伏衝) when alluding to the understood fact that the trajectory of the *chong* vessel is especially deep. Wang Luo-Zhen and Li Ding, eds., 1985, p. 76.

Chapter 13: The *Du* Vessel

1   Ch. 60 of *Basic Questions* states: "It encircles the posterior perianal region, and a diverging branch encircles the buttocks to reach the lesser yin and unite with the middle networks of the great yang." *Basic Questions,* vol. 2, p. 741. The middle networks of the greater yang refer to one branch of the foot greater yang that hugs the lower spine from the waist and links with the buttocks. According to Wang Luo-Zhen, this area refers to the four 'bone holes' on the sacrum and Meeting of the Yang (BL-35) hole. Wang Luo-Zhen and Li Ding, eds., 1985, p. 84.

2   Ch. 60 *Basic Questions* states: "The lesser yin ascends to the posterior aspect inside of the thigh where it links to the spine and homes to the kidney" (少陰上股內後廉,貫脊屬腎). *Basic Questions*, ibid., p. 741. Li Shi-Zhen has followed the trajectory in *The Systematic Classic of Acupuncture and Moxibustion*, which is more specific in its statement that "from the Meeting of the Yang (BL-35), [it] links with the spine" *(*由會陽貫脊). Wang Luo-Zhen and Li Ding, ibid.

3 The 28th Difficult Issue of the *Classic of Difficulties* states: "The *du* vessel arises from the transport [hole] of the lower extremity where it moves upward along the interior to reach Wind House (GV-16) and enter the brain." Wang Jiu-Si et al., eds., 1966, p. 55. Yang Xuan-Cao comments: "The lower extremity is Long Strong (GV-1)." Yang Shang-Shan comments: "The received transmission that the *du* vessel is the only vessel that strikes the spine cannot be correct." Wang Luo-Zhen and Li Ding, ibid., p. 89.

4 The two holes Lumbar Yang Pass (GV-3) and Spirit Tower (GV-10) do not appear in *The Systematic Classic*. Wang Bing mentioned them in a comment to Ch. 59 of *Basic Questions*.

5 *The Systematic Classic* identifies this hole as "meeting of the *du* vessels and the foot greater yang." Huang-Fu Mi, Shandong zhong yi xue yuan, eds., 1981, vol. 1, p. 343.

6 *The Systematic Classic* identifies this hole as "a meeting of the three yang and *du* vessel." Ibid. *Acupuncture Hole Diagram Based on the Bronze Model* and *Comprehensive Elucidation of the Fourteen Channels* expand on this interpretation with the statement that Great Hammer (GV-14) is "a meeting of the three yang of both the hand and foot with the *du* vessel." The latter text also locates this hole above the first thoracic vertebrae. Ibid.

7 *The Systematic Classic* identifies this hole as "the meeting of the *du* vessel and the *yang wei.*" Huang-Fu Mi, ibid., p. 332. The 28th Difficult Issue of the *Classic of Difficulties* states: "The *du* vessel ascends to reach the Wind House (GV-16) and enters, homing to the brain." Wang Jiu-Si et al., ibid., p. 55.

8 *The Systematic Classic* identifies this hole as "a meeting of the *du*, foot greater yang [channels]." The name implies that the trajectory of the *du* vessel diverges and enters the brain. Huang-Fu Mi, ibid., p. 331.

9 *The Systematic Classic* identifies this hole as "a meeting of the *du* [and] foot greater yang." Ibid.

10 *The Systematic Classic* identifies this hole as "a meeting of the *du* and foot greater and yang brightness [channels]." Ibid., p. 327.

11 *The Systematic Classic* identifies this hole as "a meeting of the *du* [and] hand and foot yang brightness [channels]." Ibid., p. 369.

12 In his commentary to Ch. 59 of *Basic Questions*, Wang Bing states that this hole is "a meeting of the two channels of the *du* vessel and *ren* vessel." He also includes this hole as a meeting point of the foot yang brightness channel because this channel "enters at the upper teeth" *(ru shang chi zhong* 入上齒中*)*. Wang Luo-Zhen and Li Ding, ibid., p. 85.

13 See Ch. 6 of the present text.

14 This passage appears in the 23rd Difficult Issue of the *Classic of Difficulties.* The passage originates in Ch. 17 of *Divine Pivot* where it lacks the word *gong* (共, altogether). *Divine Pivot*, vol. 1., p. 342; Wang Jiu-Si et al., ibid., p. 53.

15 The source of this quotation is unknown. It may have originated in his *Medicinal Notes on the Classic of Difficulties* (*Yao zhu nan jing* 藥註難經), which is no longer extant.

16 The source text by Wang Hai-Cang is unknown.

17   This passage is a paraphrase of one that appears in the middle volume of *Comprehensive Elucidation of the Fourteen Channels*. The original passage begins: "The *ren* and *du* are but two branches with a single source. The *du* arises at Meeting of Yin (CV-1) and travels along the back, while the *ren* arises at Meeting of Yin (CV-1) and travels along the abdomen." Wang Zhi-Zhong, Hua Bo-Ren, and Cheng Dan-An, eds., 1973, p. 64.

18   According to Katsuda Masayasu, the yin talisman *(yin fu* 陰符*)* is synonymous with another term, 'original spirit' *(yuan shen* 元神*)*, the activity of conscious thought. Katsuda Masayasu, trans., 1995, p. 175.

19   "When the upper is closed" is a reference to closing the eyes to shut out external stimuli. "When the lower is closed" is a reference to the retention of reproductive essence.

20   This passage appears in *The Inner Landscape Classic of the Yellow Court* in the chapter titled "On the Mind and Spirit" *(Xin shen* 心神*)*. Wang Luo-Zhen and Li Ding, ibid., p. 87.

21   Here, "Water Wheel" refers to the microcosmic orbit.

22   Our interpretation of this line is based on Katsuda Masayasu, ibid., p. 177.

23   The 36th Difficult Issue of the *Classic of Difficulties* refers to the "moving qi between the kidneys below the umbilicus" as "the root of the 12 channels." Daoist meditators also refer to the "root of heaven and earth" as the "gate of the Mysterious Female." This place opens to the foot *jue yin* channel below, to the *du* vessel behind, to the *ren* vessel in front, and to the *chong* in the middle. If the qi is allowed to proceed in these channels in its normal direction, then the body matures and ages normally. However, if the flow of qi is reversed, then this promotes personal cultivation. The statement that the qi "ascends and reunites with *li* and is further enhanced to become *qian*" refers to the guiding of the heart-spirit to the head, the cultivation of the qi of pure yang and its "return to the origin."

Chapter 14: Diseases of the *Du* Vessel

1   The original passage in Ch. 60 of *Basic Questions* contains the word "diseased" *(bing* 病*)* rather than "afflicted" *(ji* 疾*)*. This paragraph is a paraphrase of the original passage as it appears in *Basic Questions*. In the original passage, arch-backed rigidity is mentioned prior to these other symptoms. Li Shi-Zhen has based his own annotation on the original annotation by Wang Bing. *Basic Questions*, 1980, vol. 2, p. 741.

2   For a more thorough discussion of bulging disorders, see Ch. 34, "Ye Tian-Shi's Contributions to Extraordinary Vessel Therapeutics," in the present text.

3   *Nu zi wei* (女子為) is *qi nu zi* (其女子) in *Basic Questions*. Their meaning is the same. *Basic Questions*, ibid., p. 742.

4   Some commentaries identify the barracks *(ying* 營*)* below the umbilicus in a more general way as being any of the transport holes in the lower abdominal region. *The Yellow Emperor's Inner Classic: Grand Essentials* states: "The barracks below the umbilicus is the root of the *du* vessel. The barracks are also an acupuncture hole location." Ibid.

5   The original passage in Ch. 60 of *Basic Questions* reads "directly below both eyes," indicating the intersection hole of the *ren* vessel and the yang brightness channel hole Support Tears (ST-1), and not the inner canthus. Li has confused the two locations. Ibid., p. 741.

6   This is a synthesis of a number of passages from both *Basic Questions* and *Divine Pivot*. The original passage in Ch. 60 of *Basic Questions* reads: "When the *du* vessel becomes diseased, there will be arched-back rigidity." A similar passage in Ch. 10 of *Divine Pivot* reads: "A diverging branch of the *du* vessel is called Long Strong. It ascends the nape and scatters in the head, then descends to pass through both scapulae where branches travel to the greater yang, re-entering the backbone. When excessive, it presents with arched-back rigidity, and when deficient, it presents with heavy-headedness such that one wobbles one's head [in an attempt to hold it up]. For problems with the bone such as this, then select this diverging branch." Li has attributed problems with the 'bone' *(gu* 骨*)* to problems with the spine *(ji* 脊*)*. Ibid.; *Divine Pivot*, 1980, vol. 1, p. 278.

7   The original passage in the 29th Difficult Issue of the *Classic of Difficulties* begins, "Diseases produced by the *du*" *(du zhi wei bing* 督之為病*)*. The meaning is the same. Wang Jiu-Si et al., eds., 1966, p. 58.

8   The original source of this quote is unknown.

9   This passage is from the *Pulse Classic*, Wang Shu-He, Fuzhou shi ren min yi yuan, eds., 1981, p. 92.

10 The original passage in the *Pulse Classic* contains the instruction to moxa the vertex with 三丸 *(san wan)* "three balls" of moxa. Ibid. Another edition adds "right at the top of the head" *(zheng dang ding shang* 正當頂上*)*. Wang Shu-He, 1991b, Shen Yan-Nan et al., eds., p. 62.

11 According to Wang Luo-Zhen, in the original passage in Ch. 42 of *Basic Questions*, above Wind House (GV-16) is the Brain's Door (GV-17): "Brain's Door (GV-17) is the meeting of the *du* vessel and the foot greater yang, hence, [when wind] travels from the Wind House (GV-16) and ascends, it results in brain wind; and the vessel of the foot greater yang vessel arises in the inner corner of the eye, hence, when wind enters and links with the head, there will be eye wind and eye cold." Wang Luo-Zhen and Li Ding, eds., 1985, p. 91.

Chapter 16: Diseases of the *Dai*

1   The 29th Difficult Issue of the *Classic of Difficulties* substitutes the word "if" *(ruo* 若*)* for "like" *(ru* 如*)*. Wang Jiu-Si et al., eds., 1966, p. 55.

2   *Luminous Court (Ming tang* 明堂*)* is mentioned in Gao Wu's (高武) *A Gathering of the Blossoms of Acupuncture*. Although both *An Acupuncture Hole Diagram Based on the Bronze Model* and *Comprehensive Recording of Sagely Beneficence* contain this passage, neither of these two sources contains the words "abdominal urgency" *(hou zhong* 後重*)*. Wang Luo-Zhen and Li Ding, eds., 1985, p. 104.

3   The source of this quote is unclear. It may have originated as Zhang Jie-Gu's annotation of the *Classic of Difficulties* that states: "The *dai* vessel runs through the foot greater yin spleen, and Camphorwood Gate (LR-13) is the alarm hole of the spleen, hence, one should moxa it." The text from which this annotation derives is no longer extant. Ibid.

4   This passage is a quote from Ch. 63 of *Basic Questions.* In the original passage, the word "foot" *(zu* 足) precedes the words "greater yin," and the word "smaller" (xiao 小) is replaced by the word "lesser" *(shao* 少). While the terms *xiao fu* (小腹) and *shao fu* (少腹) are often used interchangeably to mean the smaller, or lower, abdomen, they can denote very distinct regions of the lower quadrant. The part of the abdomen below the umbilicus is referred to as the smaller abdomen while the lateral aspects of the smaller abdomen are referred to as the lesser abdomen. In Ch. 63 of *Basic Questions,* "facing upward" *(yang xi* 仰息) is misprinted as "preserve one's breath" *(yang xi* 養息). *Basic Questions,* vol. 2, p. 810. A similar passage also appears in Ch. 40 of *Basic Questions,* but it does not contain the first sentence or the word breath *(xi* 息). For that matter, the original passage does not mention the *dai* vessel. Li Shi-Zhen has included this citation simply because the etiology of the disease and the location of the pain resemble that of the *dai* vessel. The *dai* intersects the foot lesser yang on the lateral lumbar region and then the foot greater yin, thus moving in an anterior direction. Wang Luo-Zhen and Li Ding, ibid., p. 105.

   The Systematic Classic of Acupuncture and Moxibustion does not say that it intersects *(jiao he* 交合) at all, but notes that Ch. 63 of *Basic Questions* states: "It is a place where the foot greater yang, terminal yin, and lesser yang bind." Huang-Fu Mi, Shandong zhong yi xue yuan, eds., 1981, vol. 1, p. 356. Wang Luo-Zhen observed that greater yang had evidently been made into greater yin and that the eight lower bone holes pertain to the foot greater yin bladder channel. Wang Luo-Zhen and Li Ding, ibid., p. 105.

5   This passage originates in the *Discussion of Cold Damage* in the chapter "Yin-Yang Exchange and Exhaustion Relapse" *(Bian yin yang yi cha hou lao fu bing mai zheng bing zhi* 變陰陽易差後勞復病脈證病治). Craig Mitchell, Feng Ye, and Nigel Wiseman, trans., 1999, p. 601.

6   This originally appears in the *Pulse Classic* in the chapter titled "On Balancing Diseases of the Eight Extraordinary Vessels" *(Ping qi jing ba mai bing* 平奇經八脈病) where the sentence begins, "When diagnosing the *dai* vessel" *(zhen de dai mai* 診得帶脈). In addition, the word "abdomen" *(fu* 腹) appears prior to the word "lumbar" *(yao* 腰). Wang Shu-He, Fuzhou shi ren min yi yuan, eds., 1981, p. 90.

7   For the ingredients of this formula, see Appendix 2.

8   "Of the twenty channels and networks, the number of pathways that circulate up and down is limited to nineteen. Only the *dai* vessel originates in the lesser abdomen and travels to the ends of the ribs at the Camphorwood Gate (LR-13) hole. It encircles the entire body but is not a source of an ascending or descending [trajectory]. Instead, it networks with the gestational membranes and proceeds [around] like a belt binding the body." Wang Luo-Zhen and Li Ding, ibid., p. 104. The latter sentence has been quoted by many sources.

9   In Ch. 44 of *Basic Questions,* the mention of excessive bedroom activity *(ru fang tai shen* 入房太甚) is followed by the phrase "contracture of the ancestral sinew" *(zong jin zhang cong* 宗筋弛縱). *Basic Questions,* vol. 1, p. 74.

10 Wang Bing notes that the original sentence finishes with the words "from within the vagina" *(yin qi zhong* 陰器中), clarifying the source of the discharge. Wang Luo-Zhen and Li Ding, ibid., p. 105.

11   Li has altered Wang Zhi-Zhong's (王执中) original passage from Ch. 7, "On Red and White Dai Disease" *(chi bai dai* 赤白带*)*, of his *Classic of Acupuncture and Moxibustion for Endowing Life (Zhen jiu zi sheng jing* 針灸資生經*)*.

12   Liu Zong-Hou was a Ming dynasty physician. This quotation originates in *Subtle Import of the Jade Key (Yu ji wei yi* 玉機微義*, 1396)* by Xu Yan-Chun (徐彥純) in the chapter discussing red and white *dai* disease. Li has again modified the passage: "This causes the *dai* vessel to become diseased, hence the name *[dai]* as well as the form the disease takes [i.e., leukorrhea]" (以帶脈為病得名亦以病形而名) was originally "This white substance has a consistency of tears, hence the name *dai*, and *dai* also refers to the form the disease takes" (白物如涕之狀故言亦帶者亦病形也). Li has also omitted the sentence "Since the pathodynamic may vary according to depth and severity, there are different [names for this disease]" (盖病机有轻重浅深之异尔). Wang Luo-Zhen and Li Ding, ibid., p. 105.

13   This reading is according to Katsuda Masayasu (勝田正泰), trans., 1995, p. 215.

14   *Discussion of the Origins of the Symptoms of Disease* states: "When the kidney qi becomes fixed inside, it is unable to diffuse and penetrate, hence, there is low back pain. Its symptoms include a heavy [feeling] body, and a cold lower back, the abdomen is heavy as if one were wearing a belt of five-thousand coins, as if one were sitting in water, its appearance is watery, there is an absence of thirst, the urine flows freely, and one's intake of drink and food are normal. If it lasts a long time, it will turn into a water disease because of kidney dampness." Chao Yuan-Fang, 1982, Nanjing zhong yi xue yuan, eds., p. 151. Note that the "water disease" referred to here is edema.

15   Kidney Fixity Decoction *(shen zhuo tang)* appears in the 17th *juan* of *Important Formulas Worth a Thousand Gold Pieces.* Sun Si-Miao, 1982, p. 347. The formula also appears in *Essentials from the Golden Cabinet* where it is known as Licorice, Ginger, Poria, and White Atractrylodes Decoction *(gan cao gan jiang fu ling bai zhu tang).* Liu Yue, 2003, p. 83.

16   Dampness Leaching Decoction *(shen shi tang)* is from Chen Cheng's (陳承) *Formulary of the Pharmacy Service for Benefiting the People in the Taiping Era (Tai ping hui min he ji ju fang* 太平惠民和齊局方*, 1078)*; see Imperial Medical Bureau *(tai yi ju* 太醫局*)*, 2004. Here, Li is citing Chen Yan's *Discussion of Illnesses, Patterns, and Formulas Related to the Unification of the Three Etiologies.*

17   Pubescent Angelica Decoction *(du huo tang)* appears in the "Discussion on Back Pain" *(Yao tong men* 腰痛門*)* in the middle volume of *Secrets from the Orchid Chamber.* Li Dong-Yuan, 1981b, p. 200.

Chapter 17: The Pulses of the Nine Pathways of the Qi Opening

1   "The lungs are the canopy of a person's five yin viscera." Where Li Shi-Zhen uses the words "qi opening" *(qi kou* 氣口*)*, the original passage uses the words "inch opening" *(cun kou* 寸口*)*. Wang Shu-He, Fuzhou shi ren min yi yuan, eds., 1981, p. 641.

2   Translating the words *qian* (前) and *hou* (後) as 'distal' and 'proximal,' respectively, admittedly imparts a modern medical sensibility to the rendering of these passages. Given the multidimensionality of the pulse images described in this chapter, we have chosen these words for the sake of clarity.

3 According to Wang Luo-Zhen, the word "slippery" *(hua* 滑) was originally "blood" *(xue* 血). Wang Luo-Zhen and Li Ding, ibid., p. 112.

4 *Su shi* (宿食), literally 'food left overnight.'

5 The original passage reads: "A pulse that is floating and slightly slippery means that one suffers from disordered bowel movements *(fu wei hua ku da bian bu li* 浮微滑苦 大便不利)." Wang Shu-He, ibid., p. 640. Li has omitted the slippery quality from his pulse description.

6 In the source passage, the word "bound" *(se* 澀) follows the word "qi" *(qi* 氣), thereby clarifying the meaning, that is, the qi is bound up (which is referred to as a choppy pulse). In the source passage, the word "blood" *(xue* 血) follows the word "wind" *(feng* 風), making the phrase read: "A choppy [pulse] means wind and blood [diseases]." Finally, Li appears to have omitted the pulse quality associated with exhaustion. In the source passage, the word "wiry" *(xian* 弦) precedes the words "becomes exhausted" *(wei lao* 為勞), making the phrase read: "A wiry pulse means [exhaustion]." Ibid.

7 In the source passage, the phrase reads: "suffers from lower abdominal pain connecting with the low back." Ibid., p. 644. Abdominal urgency and abdominal pain that connect with the lower back are substantially different symptoms. In the source passage, the symptoms attributed to women are mentioned first, and Li's vaginal obstruction *(zi hu bi* 子戶閉) is extreme internal obstruction of the vagina *(zi men sai jue nei* 子門塞絕內) in the source text.

8 Li has transposed the symptoms. His reads: "frequent [excesses] of joy and anger, and food tasting bitter in the throat" *(duo xi nu shi ku yan* 多喜怒食苦咽). The source passage reads: "food tasting bitter in the throat and frequent [excesses] of joy and anger" *(shi ku yan duo xi nu* 食苦咽多喜怒). Ibid., p. 648.

9 Li has reinterpreted the source passage, attributing *chen* (沉) to a pulse quality rather than reading it as a reference to the overall depth of the heat in this particular condition. The source passage reads: "When tight and choppy, there is accumulated heat in the chest with occasional coughing of blood; [this means] there is sunken heat" (緊澀者胸中有積熱時咳血也有沈熱). Ibid., p. 649.

10 The source passage in the *Pulse Classic* reads: "A stabbing pain radiating downward from the periumbilical area to the pubic bone and into the genitals" *(rao qi xia yin heng gu zhong qie tong* 繞臍下引橫骨陰中切痛). Ibid.

11 We have followed Wang Shu-He in glossing *jun* (帬) with disease radical as "recalcitrant" *(wan* 頑). Katsuda Masayasu translates this as "'paralysis." Katsuda Masayasu, trans., 1995, p. 234.

12 This translation of the text is according to Katsuda Masayasu. Ibid.

13 "Pain that links the low back to the groin" *(yao kua xiang lian* 腰胯相連). In the source text, the passage reads: "low back and groin [pain] linking with pain in the genitals" *(yao ji kua jiao xia xiang lian zhong tong* 腰及胯窌下相連陰中痛). Wang Shu-He, Fuzhou shi ren min yi yuan, eds., ibid., p. 647.

14 Yin bulging *(yin shan* 陰疝) is characterized by acute pain in the testicles and genitals attributed to cold evil invading the liver channel.

15 Spotting *(lou xia* 漏下) refers to scanty nonmenstrual bleeding from the womb.

16 Obstruction and itching *(bi yang* 痺癢). In the source text, the passage reads: "oozing, itching obstruction" *(yin yang bi* 淫癢痺). Ibid., p. 645.

Chapter 18: An Explanation of Pronunciation

1 Wang Luo-Zhen and Li Ding, eds., 1985, p. 114.

2 Ibid., p. 116.

3 Ibid., p. 117 notes that this word may be read either as *chài* or *cuó* specified, their preparation.

4 The modern pronunciation of 瘛瘲 is *chì zòng*.

5 The modern pronunciation of 慄𤷍 is *dié biē*.

Chapter 19: On the Overview of the Eight Extraordinary Vessels

1 The original passage from *Divine Pivot* reads: "The channels and vessels are in the interior while the branches and horizontals are called networks." *Divine Pivot*, 1980, vol.1, p. 342.

2 Wang Luo-Zhen and Li Ding, eds., 1985, p. 2.

3 *Divine Pivot*, vol.2, p. 23. 以上下 *(yi shang xia,* "ascends and descends through them") appears in *The Systematic Classic of Acupuncture and Moxibustion* as 上下行 *(shang xia xing,* "travels up and down").

4 Huang Gong-Xiu (黃宮繡), 2004.

5 *Divine Pivot*, vol. 1, pp. 277–279.

6 Ibid., p. 348.

7 Paul Unschuld, trans., 1986a, p. 327.

8 Wang Jiu-Si et al., eds., 1966, p. 54.

9 Katsuda Masayasu, trans., 1995, p. 13.

10 Wang Luo-Zhen and Li Ding, ibid., p. 3.

11 Ibid., p. 12.

12 Ibid., p. 12.

13 Ibid., pp. 2–3.

14 Paul Unschuld, ibid., p. 322.

15 Ibid., p. 327.

16 Wang Luo-Zhen and Li Ding, ibid., p. 3.

17 Chen Gu-Ying, 1990, pp. 726–727.

Chapter 20: On the Eight Vessels

1 Wang Jiu-Si et al., eds., 1966, p. 54.

2 Ibid.

3 Paul Unschuld, 1986a, p. 327.

4 Charles O. Hucker, 1985, p. 534.

5 Wang Shu-He, Fuzhou shi ren min yi yuan, eds., 1981, p. 85.

6 Ibid., p. 54.

7 *Divine Pivot*, 1980, vol. 1, p. 512.

8   Wang Luo-Zhen and Li Ding, eds., 1985, p. 5.

9   The *ji xie* (季脅, 'costal margin') mentioned above is also an alternate name for Camphorwood Gate (LR-13). See *Grand Encyclopedia of Chinese Medicine*, 1975, p. 927.

10 The symbolism of *qian* and *kun* is discussed at greater length in Part I (Ch. F) of the present text.

11 Robert G. Henricks, trans., 1989, p. 198.

Chapter 21: On the *Wei* vessels

1   Kiiko Matsumoto and Stephen Birch, 1988, p. 219.

2   Paul Unschuld, trans., 1986a, pp. 327–328.

3   Wang Zhi-Zhong, Hua Bo-Ren, and Cheng Dan-An, eds., 1973, p. 70.

4   Wang Luo-Zhen and Li Ding, eds., 1985, p. 9.

5   Huang-Fu Mi, Shandong zhong yi xue yuan, eds., 1981, vol.1, p. 416.

6   Richard Wilhelm and Cary F. Baynes, trans., 1967, pp. 274–275.

7   Wang Luo-Zhen and Li Ding, eds., ibid., p. 9.

8   Ibid., p. 15.

9   Katsuda Masayasu, trans., 1995, p. 51.

10 See Deng Liang-Yue et al., 1993, p. 801.

11 Katsuda Masayasu, trans., ibid., p. 25.

12 Wang Luo-Zhen and Li Ding, eds., ibid., p. 11.

13 Wang Jiu-Si et al., eds., 1966, p. 55.

14 Huang-Fu Mi, Shandong zhong yi xue yuan, eds., ibid., pp. 341–342.

15 Katsuda Masayasu, trans., ibid., p. 30.

16 *Basic Questions*, 1980, vol. 1, p. 713.

Chapter 22: On Diseases of the Two *Wei*

1   Katsuda Masayasu, trans., 1995, p. 20.

2   Ibid.

3   *An Encyclopedia of the Chinese Language (Han yu da ci dian* 漢語大詞典*)*, 2004.

4   Wang Luo-Zhen and Li Ding, eds., 1985, p. 21.

5   Ibid., p. 21.

6   Claude Larre and Elizabeth Rochat de La Vallee, 1997, p. 227.

7   Paul Unschuld, 1986b, p. 333.

8   Wang Luo-Zhen and Li Ding, eds., 1985, p. 21.

9   See Nigel Wiseman and Feng Ye, eds., 1998, p. 268.

10 Wang Luo-Zhen and Li Ding, eds., Ibid., p. 21.

11 Ibid., p. 22; Nie Hui-Min, Wang Qing-Guo, and Gao Fei, eds., 2001, pp. 92–93.

12 Nie Hui-Min, Wang Qing-Guo, and Gao Fei, eds., 2001, 92-93.

13 Ibid.

14 Ibid.

15 Lin Zhi-Han, 2004.

16 Nie Hui-Min, Wang Qing-Guo, and Gao Fei, eds., ibid., p. 93.

17 An excellent discussion of the embodiment of pulse qualities appears in Kuriyama, 1999.

18 See Ch. E, "Herbal Considerations," in the present text.

19 Wang Shu-He, 1981, p. 650.

20 Katsuda Masayasu, trans., 1995, p. 47.

Chapter 23 On the *Qiao* Vessels

1 *Divine Pivot*, 1980, vol. 1, p. 348.

2 Huang-Fu Mi, 1981, vol.1, p. 463.

3 *Divine Pivot*, 1980, vol. 1, p. 348.

4 Huang-Fu Mi, ibid., p. 267.

5 *Divine Pivot*, ibid, p. 348.

6 Ibid, p. 512.

7 Wang Luo-Zhen and Li Ding, eds., 1985, p. 32.

8 Ibid.

9 Ishida Hidemi, 1987, p. 219.

10 Henri Maspero, Yoshio Kawakatsu, trans., 1993, vol. 1, p. 122.

11 The entire poem, by the Song dynasty Daoist, Shao Yong (邵雍), is as follows.

耳目聰明男子身,

To one whose ears and eyes are audiant and clear, and with a male form
[i.e., when one has a sharp mind and a male body],

洪鈞賦予不為貧。

The Vast Hook endows without restraint.
[He is completely endowed by heaven.]

須探月窟方知物,

This one shall explore the Moon Grotto to know things
[He will use his consciousness to understand the truth],

未躡天根不識人。

But if he has not yet paced the Heavenly Root, he cannot comprehend [true]
humanity. [If he has not yet consolidated his *dan tian*, then his perceptions
will fail him.]

乾遇巽時觀月窟,

When *qian* meets *xun*, one can percieve the Moon Grotto
[Only when the head and one's awareness of the movement
of qi unite may one percieve the nature of one's consciousness],

地逢雷處識天根。

And when earth meets the place of thunder, one will know
the heavenly root. [When the abdomen is imbued with yang qi,
one will comprehend the heavenly root.]

天 根 月 窟 閑 來 往，

When there is a languid ebb and flow between the Heavenly Root
and the Moon Grotto,

三 十 六 宮 都 是 春。

Then the the 36 officials are spring-like.
[Then the workings of the entire universe are vital.]

This poem appears in Todo Akiyasu (藤堂明保), 1981, p. 548.

12   Wang Luo-Zhen and Li Ding, ibid., p. 34.

13   Ibid.

14   Huang-Fu Mi, ibid., p. 342.

15   Wang Luo-Zhen and Li Ding, ibid., p. 27.

16   Ibid.

17   *Divine Pivot*, ibid., p. 348.

Chapter 24: On Diseases of the Two *Qiao*

1   Paul Unschuld, 1986b, p. 335.

2   Ibid.

3   Ibid.

4   皮膚淫痹 *(pi fu yin bi)*, literally, "pernicious obstruction of the skin," refers to obstruction patterns due to excess of any of the six qi: wind, cold, fire, summerheat, dampness, or dryness. The source passage in the *Pulse Classic* substitutes the word "stiff" *(qiang* 強) for "pernicious" *(yin* 淫), that is, the skin is stiff and insensitive. Ibid.

5   Bulging disorders *(shan* 疝) are characterized by swelling or pain of the abdomen or scrotum. Yin bulging *(yin shan* 陰疝) is characterized by acute pain in the testicles and genitals attributed to cold pathogen invading the liver channel.

6   Katsuda Masayasu, trans., 1995, p. 234.

7   Li Shi-Zhen's rendering of the phrase "In men, [needle] the yang [*qiao*], and in women, [needle] the yin [*qiao*]" is consistent with *The Systematic Classic of Acupuncture and Moxibustion.* Huang-Fu Mi, Shandong zhong yi xue yuan, eds., 1981, vol. 1, p. 689.

8   Wang Luo-Zhen and Li Ding, eds., 1985, p. 44.

9   In the *Yellow Emperor's Inner Classic: Grand Essentials*, the character for *qiao* lacks the foot radical (足), and yet it retains its meaning of being high or elevated. *Qiao* may be read in the first tone, the second tone, or the fourth tone.

10   Wang Luo-Zhen and Li Ding, ibid., pp. 46–47.

11   *Basic Questions*, 1980, vol. 2, p. 680.

12   Katsuda Masayasu, ibid., p. 20.

13 Ibid, p. 44.

14 Ibid.

15 Paul Unschuld, trans., 1986a, p. 335.

16 Wang Jiu-Si et al., eds., 1966, p. 121.

17 Ibid.

18 Huang-Fu Mi, ibid., p. 946.

19 Katsuda Masayasu, ibid., p. 78.

20 *Basic Questions*, 1980, vol. 1, p. 534.

21 Ibid., p. 533.

22 Ibid.

23 Wang Luo-Zhen and Li Ding, ibid., p. 45.

24 Deng Liang-Yue et al., 1993, p. 814.

25 Ibid.

26 Ibid.

27 Katsuda Masayasu, ibid., p. 82, identifies this location as the medial edge of the cheekbone.

28 Although Li has identified *shu mi* 黍米 as sorghum, most authorities believe that it referred to millet in the *Inner Classic*. Both grains are used at present.

29 This sentence appears in Zhang Zi-He's *Confucians' Duties to Their Parents* in the passages dealing with "Afflictions of the Nine Qi." Wang Luo-Zhen and Li Ding, ibid., p. 46.

30 The third volume of Chao Yuan-Fang's *An Annotated Discussion of the Origins of the Symptoms of Disease* contains this passage: "If there is heart vexation with inability to sleep, [this is due to] heart heat. If, however, [the condition is one of] vacuity vexation, with inability to sleep, [this is due] only to chills" 若心煩不得眠者心熱也．若但虛煩不得眠者但冷也．

31 Wang Shu-He, Fuzhou shi ren min yi yuan, eds., 1981, *The Annotated Pulse Classic*, p. 329.

Chapter 25: On the *Chong* Vessel

1 *Basic Questions*, 1980, vol. 1, p. 578.

2 *Divine Pivot*, 1980, vol. 1, p. 510.

3 *Basic Questions*, ibid., p. 230.

4 Yang Shang-Shan, 2004, *juan* 10: "On the Channels and Vessels" and "On the *Chong* Vessel."

5 Kiiko Matsumoto and Stephen Birch, 1988, p. 36.

6 *Basic Questions*, ibid., vol. 2, p. 741.

7 Wang Jiu-Si et al., eds., 1966, p. 54.

8 Deng Liang-Yue et al., 1993, p. 776.

9 *Basic Questions*, ibid., vol. 2, p. 230.

10 Ibid., p. 757.

11 Ibid., pp. 757–758.

12   Ibid., pp. 758–759.

13   Ibid., p. 759.

14   Shibazaki Yasuzo (柴崎保三著) 1979, p. 4097.

15   Xu Shen, Xu Zhong-Shu, ed., 1981, p. 380.

16   Victor Mair, trans., 1994, p. 70.

17   A. C. Graham, trans., 1981, p. 97.

18   David Hinton, trans., 1997, p. 110.

19   Burton Watson, trans., 1964, p. 93.

20   Claude Larre and Elizabeth Rochat de La Valle, 1997, p. 113.

21   Xu Shen, ibid., p. 380.

22   Wang Luo-Zhen and Li Ding, eds., 1985, p. 56.

23   Wang Jiu-Si, ibid., pp. 55-56.

24   *Basic Questions*, ibid., vol. 1, p. 101.

25   Wang Luo-Zhen and Li Ding, ibid., p. 56.

Chapter 26: On Diseases of the *Chong* Vessel

1   Wang Jiu-Si et al., eds., 1966, p. 27.

2   Nigel Wiseman and Feng Ye, 1998, p. 2.

3   *Annotated Yellow Emperor's Inner Classic: Divine Pivot*, 1980, vol. 1, p. 462.

4   Katsusda Masayasu, trans., 1995, p. 122.

5   Li Dong-Yuan, Yang Shou-Zhong, and Li Jian-Yong, trans., 1993, p. 107.

6   *Annotated Yellow Emperor's Inner Classic: Basic Questions*, 1980, vol. 1, p. 70.

7   Li Dong-Yuan, 2004.

8   Dan Bensky, Stephen Clavey, and Erich Stoger, 2004, p. 268.

9   Cheng Huang-Dun's given name was Min Zheng (敏正). This passage is derived from the *Biography of Master Ju Quan (Ju quan weng zhuan* 橘泉翁傳*)*.

10   Zhu Ju-Quan's given name was Zhong-Ning (仲寧). He was from a family of physicians. This passage was originally cited by Li Lian (李濂) in *juan* 10 of *The History of Medicine*, Wang Luo-Zhen and Li Ding, eds., 1985, p. 64.

11   In volume 17, Chapter 71 of *The Classified Classic*, Zhang Jing-Yue explains the relationship of the gathering sinew to the bones as follows: "The yang brightness is the stomach vessel, and the water and grains that pour into it are transformed to qi and blood to enrich and nourish the interior and the exterior. Hence, it is called the sea of the five viscera and six receptacles, and it also descends to moisten the gathering sinew. The gathering sinew is the sinew that has gathered together at the genitals and is the meeting place for the various sinews. The valleys and streams created by all the sinews of the back and spine home [in] to this place, hence, it masters the binding of the bones and assists the joints." Zhang Jie-Bin, Li Zhi-Yong, eds., 1999, p. 574.

12   Ibid., p. 573.

13   *Annotated Yellow Emperor's Inner Classic: Divine Pivot*, ibid., p. 578.

14   Nigel Wiseman and Feng Ye, 1998, p. 9.

15 Katsusda Masayasu, trans., 1995, p. 127.

16 *Annotated Yellow Emperor's Inner Classic: Basic Questions*, ibid., p. 580.

17 Zhang Zhi-Cong takes this cyclical theme in a different direction, pointing out that seasonal considerations also dictate the depth of needling. One must needle shallowly in the summer and deeply in the winter. Ibid., p. 581.

18 *Annotated Yellow Emperor's Inner Classic: Divine Pivot*, ibid., p. 140.

19 In this regard, Li Dong-Yuan in *On the Spleen and Stomach* also discusses the role of the middle burner *(zhong jiao* 中焦*)* and Astragalus and Ginseng Decoction *(Huang qi ren shen tang* 黃芪人參湯*)*. See Li Dong-Yuan, 2004.

20 In this regard, Zhu Dan-Xi in *Teachings of [Zhu] Dan-Xi* discussed diarrhea *(xie xie* 泄寫*)* and summerheat *(shu* 暑*)*. See Zhu Dan-Xi, 2004.

21 *Annotated Yellow Emperor's Inner Classic: Divine Pivot*, ibid., p. 120.

22 Ibid., vol. 2, p. 118.

23 Katsuda Masayasu, trans., 1995, p. 131.

24 恍 *(huang,* distraction*)* refers to a mental state characterized by ecstatic disengagement.

25 Li has transposed the order of symptoms as they appear in the *Pulse Classic*. Wang Shu-He, Fuzhou shi ren min yi yuan, eds., 1981, p. 90.

26 See, for instance, Donald Edward Kendal, 2001.

27 These final passages are all excerpted and paraphrased from Chapter 33 of *Annotated Yellow Emperor's Inner Classic: Divine Pivot*, ibid., p. 514.

Chapter 27: On the *Ren* Vessel

1 Wang Luo-Zhen and Li Ding, eds., 1985, p. 76.

2 Ibid.

3 Wang Shu-He, Fuzhou shi ren min yi yuan, eds., 1981, p. 87.

4 Wang Luo-Zhen and Li Ding, eds., 1985, p. 71.

5 Basic Questions, 1980, vol. 2, p. 741.

6 Huang-Fu Mi, 1981, vol. 1, p. 406.

7 Li's reference to *hui yin zhi fen* 會陰之分 may also simply refer to the location of Meeting of Yin (CV-1). If this is indeed the correct reading, then Li has deemed it necessary to include the words "between the two yin orifices" *(zai liang yin zhi jian* 在兩陰之間*)* to clarify the ambiguity of his own prose.

8 Ibid., p. 370.

9 *Divine Pivot*, 1980, vol. 1, p. 277.

10 The term 'Windows of the Sky' is a modern invention of the French school of meridian therapy. John Pirog, 1996, pp. 149-150.

11 Some editions of the *Divine Pivot* punctuate the text differently, placing the enumeration at the end of each preceding sentence. This makes the Celestial Chimney (CV-22) the first or primary channel. See, for example, Guo Ai-Chun, ed., 1992, p. 24.

12 Pirog, pp. 149-50.

Chapter 28: On Diseases of the *Ren* Vessel

1   *Basic Questions*, 1980, vol. 2, 741.

2   Wang Jiu-Si et al., eds., 1966, p. 53.

3   Paul Unschuld, trans., 1986a, p. 337.

4   Wang Luo-Zhen and Li Ding, eds., 1985, p. 75.

5   *Basic Questions*, ibid., p. 819.

6   *Basic Questions,* ibid., p. 651. Wiseman and Feng translate *tui shan* as "bulging mounting." This disease may include swelling of the scrotum without pain or itching, abdominal swelling in women, and vaginal prolapse. Nigel Wiseman and Feng Ye, 1998, p. 51.

7   *Basic Questions*, ibid., vol. 1, pp. 7–8.

8   Wang Luo-Zhen and Li Ding, ibid., p. 76.

9   *Basic Questions,* ibid., vol. 2, p. 745.

10 Ibid.

11 In Chapter 17 of the present text, the *ren* pulse is described as "arriving from below [the proximal position] to the middle position" *(xia zhi guan* 下至關).

12 Wang Shu-He, Fuzhou shi ren min yi yuan, eds., 1981, p. 85.

Chapter 29: On the *Du* Vessel

1   *Basic Questions*, 1980, vol. 2, p. 741.

2   Wang Luo-Zhen and Li Ding, eds., 1985, p. 84.

3   Huang-Fu Mi, Shandong zhong yi xue yuan, eds., 1981, vol. 2, p. 1219.

4   Wang Luo-Zhen and Li Ding, ibid., p. 89.

5   *Divine Pivot*, 1980, vol. 1, p. 59.

Chapter 30: On Diseases of the *Du* Vessel

1   Wang Luo-Zhen and Li Ding, eds., 1985, p. 91.

2   Ibid.

3   Ibid.

4   Ibid.

5   Katsuda Masayasu, trans., 1995, p. 189.

6   Charles O. Hucker, 1985, *A Dictionary of Official Titles in Imperial China,* p. 534.

7   Wang Luo-Zhen and Li Ding, ibid., p. 91.

8   Literally, "lumbar [level] horizontal bone."

9   Wang Qi-Xuan comments: "The cause of this illness may be properly sought in the *ren* vessel …." He makes no mention of the *chong* vessel in his discussion.

10 Zhang Ji, 2004.

11 Ibid.

12 The original passage from *Essentials from the Golden Cabinet* reads: "A spasmodic pulse is tense when pressed, like a bowstring moving straight up and down. … It is

disturbed and wiry" (夫瘂脈按之緊如弦直上下行⋯一作築築而弦). Liu Yue, 2003, p. 11.

13　Katsuda Masayasu, ibid., p. 187.

14　Nigel Wiseman and Feng Ye, 1998, p. 50.

15　Wang Luo-Zhen and Li Ding, ibid., p. 91.

Chapter 31:　On the *Dai* Vessel

1　Wang Jiu-Si et al., eds., 1966, p. 54.

2　Huang-Fu Mi, Shandong zhong yi xue yuan, eds., 1981, vol. 1, p. 418.

3　(a) Ibid., and (b) Wang Luo-Zhen and Li Ding, eds., 1985, p. 99.

4　Deng Liang-Yue et al., 1993, *Categorized Collection of Literature on Chinese Channels and Network Vessels*, p. 782.

5　Wang Luo-Zhen and Li Ding, ibid., p. 284. The original passage is from Ch. 11 of *Divine Pivot*, 1980, vol. 1, p. 284.

6　For a further discussion of the channel divergences, see Miki Shima and Charles Chace, 2000, *Channel Divergences: Deeper Pathways of the Web*.

7　Wang Luo-Zhen and Li Ding, ibid., p. 100.

8　Katsuda Masayasu, trans., 1995, p. 106.

Chapter 32:　On Diseases of the *Dai* Vessel

1　Wang Luo-Zhen and Li Ding, eds., 1985, p. 104.

2　*An Encyclopedia of the Chinese Language (Han yu da ci dian* 漢語大詞典), 2004.

3　*Basic Questions*, 1980, vol. 2, p. 810.

4　Ibid.

5　Wang Luo-Zhen and Li Ding, ibid.

6　Wang Zhi-Zhong, Hua Bo-Ren, and Cheng Dan-An, eds., 1973, p. 233. Wang Luo-Zhen is of the opinion that this passage originally had nothing to do with the greater yin. He contends that greater yin *(tai yin* 太陰) is simply a misprint and that the channel referred to is actually the greater yang *(tai yang* 太陽) since the eight sacral foramina are located on this channel. The logic of this argument is somewhat fuzzy. The authors of Ch. 63 of *Basic Questions* discuss each of the network vessels in turn, placing the network of the foot greater yang just after the foot greater yin. If there were a misprint, then the chapter would have two entries for the greater yang networks and none for the greater yin. Wang Luo-Zhen and Li Ding, ibid., p. 105.

7　It can also mean abdominal swelling in women as well as vaginal prolapse. Nigel Wiseman and Feng Ye, 1998, p. 51.

8　This advice is amplified in Volume 22 of *Grand Essentials*: "If the hand greater yin [is afflicted], then turn to the hand yang brightness. If the hand yang brightness [is afflicted], then turn to the foot yang brightness. If the foot yang brightness [is afflicted], then turn to the foot greater yin to connect [the channels] in the upper [part of the body] with those in the lower [part of the body]. Hence, when the hand greater yang and yang brightness are diseased, one should treat the foot greater yin and yang brightness, and this is called selection [of acupuncture holes] in the lower [part of the body]. When the foot greater yang and yang brightness are diseased, one should treat the hand greater yin and yang brightness, and this is called selection [of acupuncture holes] higher in the [the body]." *Divine Pivot*, 1980, vol. 1, p. 206.

9   *Basic Questions*, ibid., p. 1012.

10   Ibid., p. 1013.

11   Ibid., p. 1014.

12   Zhang Jie-Bin, Li Zhi-Yong, eds., 1999, p. 480.

Chapter 33: On the Pulses of the Extraordinary Vessels

1   Wang Shu-He, Fuzhou shi ren min yi yuan, eds., 1981, pp. 395-400.

2   Wang Shu-He, Shen Yan-Nan et al., eds., 1991b, p. 400.

3   Wang Shu-He, Fuzhou shi ren min yi yuan, eds., ibid., p. 640.

4   "The Hand Diagram of the Thirty-One Locations" *(Shou jian tu san shi yi bu* 手檢圖三十一部) also discusses slippery, choppy, tight, urgent, deep, and faint, as well as deficient pulse qualities in association with the individual pulse positions.

5   Shen Jin-Ao, 1999, p. 10.

6   Ibid., pp. 395-400.

7   The *chong, ren,* and *du* pulses are missing from the *Pulse Classic* in the Fuzhou People's Hospital Research Group edition (Wang Shu-He, 1981), but they are included in the Shen Yan-An edition. Wang Shu-He, 1991b, p. 397.

8   Katsuda Masayasu, trans., 1995, p. 234.

9   (1) Yue En-Jian, 2002, p. 295; and (2) Wang Shu-He, Fuzhou shi ren min yi yuan, eds., 1981, p. 246.

10   *An Encyclopedia of the Chinese Language (Han yu da ci dian* 漢語大詞典*)*, 2004.

11   Yue En-Jian, 2002, p. 246.

12   Ibid.

13   Wang Shu-He, 1981, p. 40.

14   From the chapter, "On Deep Yin [Pulses]" *(chen yin* 沉陰), in Li Shi-Zhen *Pulse Studies of the Lakeside [Recluse]*. See *A Chinese Encyclopedia of Medicine*, 2004.

15   Yue En-Jian, p. 400.

16   Wang Shu-He, 1991b, p. 384.

17   Yue En-Jian, ibid., p. 71.

18   Shen Jin-Ao, ibid., p. 11.

19   Katsuda Masayasu, trans., 1995, p. 234.

20   Yue En-Jian, ibid., p. 71.

21   Ibid.

22   Wang Shu-He, Fuzhou shi ren min yi yuan, eds., 1981, p. 255.

23   Ibid., p. 232.

24   The description of the *ren* pulse in Chapter 11 of this book is less specific. In that chapter, the description lacks the words "from below *(xia* 下)" and the pulse simply "arrives at the middle position *(zhi guan* 至關)." The pulse image remains substantially the same.

Chapter 34: Along the Grand Thoroughfare: Luo Dong-Yi's Vision of Extraordinary Vessel Function

1   See Ch. 6 of the present text.

2   Further discussion of the 'grand thoroughfare' appears in Ch. 9 and in Appendix 4 of the present text.

3   Here we follow Katsuda Masayasu, who interprets *hang sang* (頏顙) as "the juncture of the hard and soft palates." Katsuda Masayasu, trans., 1995, p. 110.

4   *Divine Pivot*, 1980, vol. 1, pp. 548-549.

5   The term *xia zhu* (下柱) often refers to any cylindrical support structure, which in the human body would be the lower extremities.

6   The edition used is Luo Dong-Yi, 2004, *Critical Interpretation of the Inner Classic* in *A Chinese Encyclopedia of Medicine*, CD-ROM.

7   See Ch. 3 for a discussion of the termination of the *yin wei* anterior to the vertex.

8   A more thorough discussion of *tai chong* in *Zhuang zi* appears in Appendix 4 of the present text.

9   See Ch. 34 of the present text.

Chapter 35: Ye Tian-Shi's Contributions to Extraordinary Vessel Therapeutics

1   Marta Hansen, 1999, "Inventing a Tradition in Chinese Medicine," p. 244.

2   Ibid.

3   Ibid, p. 245.

4   Ibid.; and Wang You-Liang, Zhou Jun-Fu, eds., 1985, vol. 190, pp. 517–519.

5   Marta Hansen, 1999, p. 247.

6   Ye Tian-Shi, 2004a.

7   Ye Tian-Shi, 2004h, *juan* 1, "Twin Tonification Pills" *(shuang bu wan* 雙補丸).

8   Ye Tian-Shi, 2004a, *juan* 3, "Deficiency Exhaustion" *(xu* lao 虛癆).

9   Ibid., *juan* 9, "Postpartum Diseases" *(chan hou bing* 產後病).

10   Ibid., *juan* 1, "Deficiency Exhaustion" *(xu lao* 虛癆).

11   Ibid., *juan* 3, "Loss of Semen" *(yi jing* 遺精).

12   This case record appears in another anthology containing case records attributed to Ye Tian-Shi, 2004i, *Combined Case Records of Three Physicians*, *juan* 1, Minor Construct the Middle Decoction *(xiao jian zhong tang* 小建中湯).

13   Ye Tian-Shi, 2004a, *juan* 8, "Shoulder, Arm, and Back Pain" *(jian bi ji tong* 肩臂脊痛).

14   Ibid., *juan* 7, "Obstruction" *(bi* 痹).

15   Ibid., *juan* 6, "Insomnia" *(bu mei* 不寐).

16   This case history appears in Ye Tian-Shi, 2004h, *juan* 2, "Quick Fried and Dessicated Kidney Qi Decoction" *(chao ku shen qi tang* 炒枯腎氣湯). A slightly different version of the same case appears in Ye Tian-Shi, 2004h, *juan* 1, "Preserve Harmony Pill" *(bao he wan* 保和丸).

17   Ye Tian-Shi, 2004a, *juan* 6, "On Constraint" *(yu* 鬱*)*.

Chapter 36: Shen Jin-Ao's Contributions to Extraordinary Vessel Therapeutics

1   There are four more books attributed to Shen, but the general consensus is that they are not authentic. For further discussion of this topic, see Tian Si-Sheng, ed., 1999, pp. 119–201.

2   Ibid., pp. 202–204.

3   Literally, 'effortless action' *(wu wei* 無為*)*.

4   The material in this section is derived from Tian Si-Sheng, ed., 1999, pp. 197.

5   Ibid., p. 199.

6   Ibid., p. 200.

7   Ibid.

8   Ibid.

9   Literally, 'rigid reversal' *(qiang jue* 強厥*)*.

Chapter 37: Modern Extraordinary Vessel Case Records

1   Mei Jian-Han and Yang Yu-Hua, 2006.

2   Yitian Ni, 1996.

3   Mei Jian-Han and Yang Yu-Hua, ibid., pp. 37–38.

4   See Ch. 10 of this work.

5   Andrew Ellis, Nigel Wiseman, Ken Boss, 1988, pp. 134–135.

6   Mei Jian-Han and Yang Yu-Hua, ibid., p. 83.

7   Andrew Ellis, Nigel Wiseman, Ken Boss, 1988, p. 311.

8   Ibid., p. 253.

9   Ibid., p. 342.

10   Mei Jian-Han and Yang Yu-Hua, ibid., pp. 56–57.

11   Huang-Fu Mi, 1981, vol. 1., pp. 419–420.

12   Andrew Ellis, Nigel Wiseman, Ken Boss, ibid., pp. 348–349.

13   Mei Jian-Han and Yang Yu-Hua, ibid., pp. 61–62.

14   Andrew Ellis, Nigel Wiseman, Ken Boss, ibid., p. 320.

15   Ibid.

16   Translated from Shao Lan-Sun, 2004, *juan* 2, "On Coughing" *(ke sou* 咳嗽*)*.

17   Translated from Liu Bao-Yi, 2004a, and Liu Bao-Yi, 2004b, *juan* 1, "On Coughing and Wheezing" *(ke chuan men* 咳喘門*)*.

18   Translated from Liu Bao-Yi, 2004a, and Liu Bao-Yi, 2004b, *juan* 3, "On Gynecological Problems" *(fu ren men* 婦人門*)*.

19   The extraordinary vessels influencing the womb are the first to become "damaged below" as a consequence of postpartum debilitation.

20   Although it does indeed in *The Systematic Classic,* the *locus classicus* for these passages is the 29th Difficult Issue of the *Classic of Difficulties.* Paul Unschuld, 1986b, p. 333.

Chapter 38: Vessels Wide Shut: Li Shi-Zhen's *Qiao* Vessel Pathodynamics

1 Nathan Sivin, 1995, pp. 177–204.

2 *Annotated Yellow Emperor's Inner Classic: Divine Pivot*, 1980, Beijing: Ren min wei sheng chu ban she, vol. 1, p. 389.

3 Ibid., pp. 442–443.

4 Ibid., vol. 2, pp. 266–267.

5 Ibid., p. 267.

6 Ye Tian-Shi, 1997a.

7 Ibid.

8 Ibid., p. 161.

9 Ibid., p. 175.

10 See, for instance, Stephen Birch and Junko Ida, 1998, *Japanese Acupuncture— A Clinical Guide.*

11 See Chapter 17 for a discussion of the tapping pulse quality.

Chapter 39: Master Hu's Process: The Seeds of Internal Cultivation through the Extraordinary Vessels

1 See Part I, Ch. A and F, Part II, Ch. 9, and Part III, Ch. 25 for a discussion of *chong* dynamics.

2 See Ch. 33 for a discussion of Luo Dong-Yi's interpretation of the extraordinary vessels and the Great Thoroughfare.

3 This is a well-known story, and a nearly identical version appears in the second chapter of *Liezi* (列子), "The Yellow Emperor" (*Huang di* 黃帝), in Xiao Deng-Fu, p. 187.

4 All references to the *Zhuang zi* are keyed to two sources: (1) Guo Qing-Fan (郭慶藩, 19th century), Wang Xiao-Yu (王孝魚), ed., 1961, *Zhuang zi ji shi* (莊子集釋), Ch. 1, Beijing: Zhong hua shu ju (unless otherwise noted, translations and annotations are based on this edition); and (2) D. C. Lau and Chen Fong Ching, eds., 2000.

5 Michael Saso, 1983, p. 152.

6 (1) Guo Qing-Fan, ibid., p. 296; and (2) D. C. Lau and Chen Fong Ching, ibid., Ch. 7, section 20, line 23.

7 (1) Guo Qing-Fan, ibid., pp. 297–306; and (2) D. C. Lau and Chen Fong Ching, ibid., Ch. 7, section 20, line 25 to section 21, line 19.

8 Guo Qing-Fan's *yi wen* commentary explains that female magicians are known as *wu* (巫, witches) and male magicians are called *xi* (覡, wizards). Most translators, however, assume that Ji Xian is a male. Guo Qing-Fan, ibid., p. 297.

9 Chen Gu-Ying explains that, in *Lie Zi*, the line reads: "There was a magus who was originally from Qi who came [to] Zheng; his name was Ji Xian" (有神巫自齐来处 于郑： 命日季咸). Chen Gu-Ying, 1997, *Zhuang zi, A New Commentary and New Translation*, p. 222.

10 Most commentators have the people flocking to the remarkable magus. Chen Gu-Ying interprets this line differently, noting that the people of Zheng were afraid of

hearing their fortunes, and so they all ran to avoid him. Chen Gu-Ying, ibid.

11 Chen Gu-Ying explains that Master Hu's surname was Lin (林) and his honorific was Hu (壺). He was Liezi's teacher. Ibid.

12 Cheng Xuan-Ying is the author of the standard *shu* (疏, subcommentary) in the Guo Qing-Fan edition. He observes that 與 means 授 (*shou*, to give) and 既 means 盡 (*jin*, complete). Guo Qing-Fan, ibid, p. 298. Bi Xu-Zi reads the line as it is in the *Lie zi*, placing the word 無 (*wu*, lacks) before the word 既 (*ji*), making the line read "What I have given you lacks its pattern" *(wu yu ru wu qi wen* 吾與汝無其文). Liu Wen-Dian, *Supplemental Corrections to the Zhuang zi*, p. 239.

13 Liu Wen-Dian comments that 亢 means 抗 (*kang*, resist). Ibid.

14 In his edition of *Lie zi*, Liu Wen-Dian comments that 必信夫 (*bi xin fu*) should be read as 必信矣 (*bi xin yi*, "assuredly take it as true"). Ibid.

15 In early Chinese medicine, the word 怪 (*guai*) was associated with signs of impending death. For instance, there were strange pulses *(guai mai* 怪脈) that portended death. It is not just that Master Hu looks ill or vaguely strange to Ji Xian; as far as Ji Xuan can tell, Hu is expressing the signs of his imminent demise. For a discussion of strange pulses in early Chinese medicine, see Yue En-Jian, 2002, p. 295, and Chapters 17 and 31 of the present text.

16 Cheng Xuan-Ming explains that 文 means 'appearance' *(xiang* 象). Cui Zhuan explains that 文 means 'principles' *(li* 理). Guo Qing-Fan, ibid., p. 300.

17 Bi Xu-Zi explains that 震 (*zhen*) was originally upright *(zheng* 正). The meaning is essentially the same. In his *Treasury of Antiquities (Gu cang* 古藏), Jiang Nan (江南) argues that 震 (*zhen*) was the original character. According to Cui Zhuan (崔譔, 3rd–4th century), 不誫不止 (*bu shui bu zhi*) means "as if active but not active" *(ru dong bu dong* 如動不動). Liu Wen-Dian, ibid., p. 239.

18 Guo Xiang, the author of the primary commentary in the Guo Qing-Fan edition, explains that 權 means 'dynamic' *(ji* 機), making the line read, "This stoppage had become dynamic." Ibid.

19 Cheng Xuan-Ming explains that 示之以天壤之 means "He expressed an appearance of resonant activity" *(shi yi ying dong zhi rong ye* 示以應動之容也). Ibid., p. 302.

20 According to Cheng Xuan-Ming, 機 is activity' *(dong* 動). "The dynamic of ultimate virtue is blocked and cannot be expressed. So he manifests his congealed blandness *(ning dan* 凝淡), which looks like damp ashes. The lesser shaman is mediocre and trivial *(yong suo* 庸瑣) who sees this narrowly!" Liu Wen-Dian (劉文典), 1980, p. 241.

21 Or perhaps, "heavenly soil," maintaining the parallelism with the "earthly pattern" *(di wen* 地文).

22 According to Chen Xuan-Ming, "Although his capacity to sense things has returned, he has not lost his sense of timeliness, and his spiritual dynamic is like this, issuing from the subtle root, active and yet enduringly quiescent" (雖復物感而動, 不失時宜, 而此之神機, 發乎妙本, 動而常寂). Liu Wen-Dian (劉文典), 1980, p. 241.

23 According to Chen Gu-Ying, in *Liezi*, 勝 is 朕. Chen Gu-Ying (陳鼓應), 1997, p. 223.

24 According to Cui Zhuan, 審 should be read as the "profound depths" *(shen* 瀋). According to Si-Ma Piao (司馬彪, 240–306), it means "amassed" *(ju* 聚). Guo Qing-Fan, ibid., p. 302.

25 According to Chen Xuan-Ming, "He manifests his fundamental traces (*ben ji* 本迹) together, activity and stillness occurring at the same time. Now the ultimate man's virtue is fulfilled (*de man* 德滿), and his wisdom is comprehensive (*zhi yuan* 智圓); his mind is empty, and he has consolidated his illumination (*ning zhao* 凝照); fundamental traces are indistinct (*wu bie* 無別); activity and stillness are undifferentiated. His Way is deep and profound. How could such a lesser magus fathom (*ce* 測) him? Because of the so-called fasting of his mind's traces, when Ji Xian examined him, he did not dare predict his fortune." Guo Qing-Fan, ibid., p. 302.

26 Guo Xiang explains: "Residing in the Ultimate Great Thoroughfare, one definitively harnesses the mind and is profoundly united with the ten thousand directions. For this reason, there is no place for victory and defeat" (居太衝之極, 浩然泊心而玄同萬方, 故勝負莫得厝其間也). Cheng Xuan-Ming explains that 衝 is 'vacuity' (*xu* 虛) and 莫 is 'nothing' (*wu* 無). "Now the sage's illumination is profound and consolidated (*xuan ning* 玄凝), and with the great void (*tai xu* 太虛) in equal measure (*deng liang* 等量), the fundamental traces are manifest in one another (*xiang ji* 相即); activity and quiescence occur at once. Initially, they lack superiority (*you* 優) and lack inferiority (*lie* 劣). How can there be victory or defeat?" Ibid.

27 According to Sima Biao, 鯢 (*ni*) and 桓 (*huan)* are the names of two fish. According to Cheng Xuan-Ming, *ni* is simply a big fish (*da yu* 大魚). Jian Wen states that *ni* is a whale (*jing yu* 鯨魚) and *huan* means "languid or winding around" (*pan huan* 盤桓). According to Cui Zhuan, it was originally *huan ju* (鯢拒). Ibid.

28 According to Cheng Xuan-Ming, the nine kinds of abyss include Lingering Leviathan (*ni huan* 鯢桓), Still Waters (*zhi shui* 止水), Flowing Waters (*liu shui* 流水), Flooding Waters (*xun shui* 汛水), Spilling Waters (*ni shui* 濫水), Fertile Waters (*wo shui* 沃水), Harmonious Waters (*yong shui* 雍水), Patterned Waters (*wen shui* 文水), and Rich Waters (*fei shui* 肥水). Ibid., p. 303.

29 Guo Xiang explains, "Although the transmutations and transformations are inconstant, they are constantly profound and fundamental, abstruse and ultimate" (雖變化無常, 而常深根冥極). Ibid., p. 304.

30 Cui Zhuan explains that "on the flowing waves" (*liu shui* 波流) was originally "along with the waves" (*bo sui* 波隨), meaning that one constantly follows them (*chang sui cong zhi* 常隨從之). Ibid., p. 305.

31 Guo Xiang explains, "Although he was active, his genuine [nature] could not be divided" (*sui dong er zhen bu san* 雖動而真不散). Ibid., p. 306.

32 Guo Xiang explains that Liezi "caused things to each be complete in itself" (*shi wu ge zi dong* 使物各自終). Cheng Xuan-Ming explains that Liezi "held to unity to the end" (*bao yi zhong shi* 抱一終始). Ibid.

33 (1) Guo Qing-Fan, ibid., p. 147; and (2) D. C. Lau and Chen Fong Ching, ibid., Ch. 4, section 10, line 1.

34 (1) Paul Rakita Goldin, 2003, "Nothing Can Overcome Heaven: The Notion of Spirit in *Zhuang zi*," in Scott Cook, ed., *Hiding the World in the World, Uneven Discourses on the Zhuang zi*, New York: SUNY Press, pp. 64–87; and (2) Rur-Bin Yang (楊儒賓), "'Merging the Body with the Mind' and 'Wandering in Unitary Qi': A Discussion of *Zhuang zi*'s Realm of the True Man and Its Corporal Basis," in the same anthology, pp. 88–127.

35   (1) Guo Qing-Fan, ibid., p. 147; and (2) D. C. Lau (劉殿) and Chen Fong Ching, ibid., Ch. 4, section 10, line 1.

36   (1) Guo Qing-Fan, ibid., p. 328; and (2) D. C. Lau and Chen Fong Ching, ibid., Ch. 6, section 16, line 2.

37   Harold D. Roth, 2003, "Bimodal Mystical Experience in the Qiwulun chapter of the *Zhuang zi*," in Scott Cook, ed., *Hiding the World in the World, Uneven Discourses on the Zhuang zi*, ibid., p. 16.

38   One of the most common *qi gong* exercises seen in parks every morning throughout China is the practice of 'swing arms,' where one rocks from heels to toes while swinging one's arms up in the air. It is believed that the maintenance of strength and flexibility in the heels is essential for longevity. The *qiao* vessels are commonly recognized as the mechanism for this.

39   See Ch. 6 of the present text.

40   (1) Guo Qing-Fan, ibid., p. 302; and (2) D. C. Lau and Chen Fong Ching, ibid., Ch. 7, section 21, line 10.

41   See notes 24 and 25 above. Indeed, the word 衝 (*chong*) originally meant 'to be empty.' Axel Schuessler, 2007, *ABC Etymological Dictionary of Old Chinese*, Honolulu: University of Hawaii Press, p. 189.

42   Victor Mair, trans., *Wandering on the Way, Early Taoist Tales and Parables of Chuang Tzu*, p. 64.

43   A. C. Graham, trans., *Chuang Tzu: The Inner Chapters*, p. 92.

44   (1) Guo Qing-Fan, ibid., p. 284; and (2) D. C. Lau and Chen Fong Ching, ibid., Ch. 6, section 19, line 21.

45   Harold D. Roth, ibid., pp. 15–32.

46   See Ch. 33 of the present text.

47   (1) Guo Qing-Fan, ibid., p. 304; and (2) D. C. Lau and Chen Fong Ching, ibid., Ch. 7, section 21, line 15.

48   (1) Guo Qing-Fan, ibid., p. 304; and (2) D. C. Lau and Chen Fong Ching, ibid., Ch. 7, section 21, line 16.

49   (1) Guo Qing-Fan, ibid., p. 28; and (2) D. C. Lau and Chen Fong Ching, ibid., Ch. 1, section 2, line 16.

50   (1) Guo Qing-Fan, ibid., p. 880; and (2) D. C. Lau and Chen Fong Ching, ibid., Ch. 25, section 73, line 17.

51   (1) Guo Qing-Fan, ibid., p. 284; and (2) D. C. Lau and Chen Fong Ching, ibid., Ch. 6, section 19, line 21.

52   Xiao Deng-Fu, ibid., p. 187.

53   (1) Guo Qing-Fan, ibid., p. 306, and (2) D. C. Lau and Chen Fong Ching, ibid., Ch. 7, section 19, line 21.

54   Xiao Deng-Fu, ibid., p. 45.

55   (1) Guo Qing-Fan, ibid., p. 307; and (2) D. C. Lau and Chen Fong Ching, ibid., Ch. 7, section 21, line 21.

BIBLIOGRAPHY

Ames, Roger T. and David Hall, trans., 2003, *Dao De Jing: Making This Life Significant: A Philosophical Translation*. New York: Ballantine Books.

Annotated Yellow Emperor's Inner Classic: Basic Questions (Huáng Dì nèi jīng sù wén jiào shì 黃帝內經素問校釋), 1980. Beijing: Rén mín wèi shēng chū bǎn shè (人民衛生出版社). Cited in this text as *Basic Questions (Su wen* 素問), 1980.

Annotated Yellow Emperor's Inner Classic: Divine Pivot (Huáng Dì nèi jīng líng shū jiào shì 黃帝內經靈樞校釋), 1980. Beijing: Rén mín wèi shēng chū bǎn shè (人民衛生出版社). Cited in this text as *Divine Pivot (Ling shu* 靈樞), 1980.

Bensky, Dan, Jason Blalack, Charles Chace, and Craig Mitchell, 2007, "Toward a Working Methodology for Translating Chinese Medicine," in *The Lantern*, 3(3):10–14.

Bensky, Dan, Stephen Clavey, and Erich Stoger, 2004, *Chinese Herbal Medicine, Materia Medica*, 3rd edition. Seattle: Eastland Press.

Bertschinger, Richard, 2002, *The Secret of Everlasting Life: The First Translation of the Ancient Chinese Text on Immortality*. London: Vega.

Birch, Stephen and Junko Ida, 1998, *Japanese Acupuncture — A Clinical Guide*. Brookline, Massachusetts: Paradigm Publications.

Burton-Rose, Daniel, 2009, *Integrating Inner Alchemy into Late Ming Cultural History: A Contextualization and Annotated Translation of Principles of the Innate Disposition and the Lifespan (Xingming guizhi* 性命圭旨) (1615), Master's Thesis, University of Colorado, Boulder.

Cháo Yuán-Fāng (巢元方), Nánjīng zhōng yī xué yuàn (南京中醫學院), eds., 1982, *An Annotated Discussion of the Origins of the Symptoms of Disease (Zhū bìng yuán hòu lùn jiào shì* 諸病源候論校釋). Beijing: Rén mín yī xué chū bǎn shè (人民醫學出版社).

Chace, Charles, 2009, "A Merging of the Ways," in *The Lantern,* 6 (2): 14-21.

Chén Gǔ-Yīng (陳鼓應), 1990, *Zhuang zi: Modern Annotations with Modern Commentary and Critical Explanations (Zhuāng zi jīn zhù jīn shì* 莊子今註今釋). Beijing: Zhōng huá shū jú (中華書局).

Chén Huì-Chóu (陳惠疇), 2002, *An Illustrated Exposition on the Channels (Jīng mài tú kǎo* 經脈圖考). Shanghai: Shàng hǎi gǔ jí chū bǎn shè (上海古籍出版社).

Chén-Yán (陳言), 1983, *A Unified Discourse on Diseases, Patterns, and Remedies According to the Three Causes (Sān yīn jí yī bìng zhèng fāng lùn* 三因極一病證方論). Beijing: Rén mín wèi shēng chū bǎn shè (人民衛生出版社).

Chinese Encyclopedia of Medicine (Zhōng huá yī diǎn 中華醫典), 2004, CD-ROM. Changsha: Húnán diàn zǐ yīn xiàng chū bǎn shè (湖南電子音像出版社).

Dài Qǐ-Zōng (戴起宗), 2004, *Correcting the Errors of the Pulse Rhymes (Mài jué kān wù* 脈決刊誤) in *A Chinese Encyclopedia of Medicine (Zhōng huá yī diǎn* 中華醫典), CD-ROM. Changsha: Húnán diàn zǐ yīn xiàng chū bǎn shè (湖南電子音像出版社).

Dēng Liáng-Yuè (鄧良月) et al., 1993, *Categorized Collection of Literature on Chinese Channels and Network Vessels (Zhōng guó jīng luò wén xiàn tōng jiàn* 中國經絡文獻通鑒). Qingdao: Qīngdǎo chū bǎn shè (青島出版社).

Dòu Mò (竇默), 1997, *A Guide to Acupuncture (Zhēn jiǔ zhǐ nán* 針灸指南), in Huáng Xiáng-Lóng (黃祥龍), ed., *A Collection of Famous Acupuncture Works (Zhēn jiǔ míng zhù jí chéng* 針灸名著集成). Beijing: Huá xià chū bǎn shè (華夏出版社), pp. 365–387.

———, 2004, *A Guide to Acupuncture (Zhēn jiǔ zhǐ nán* 針灸指南), in *A Chinese Encyclopedia of Medicine (Zhōng huá yī diǎn* 中華醫典), CD-ROM. Changsha: Húnán diàn zǐ yīn xiàng chū bǎn shè (湖南電子音像出版社).

Ellis, Andrew, Nigel Wiseman, and Ken Boss, 1988, *Fundamentals of Chinese Acupuncture.* Brookline, Massachusetts: Paradigm Publications.

Encyclopedia of the Chinese Language (Hàn yǔ dà cí diǎn 漢語大詞典), 2004, CD-ROM. Shanghai: Hàn yǔ dà cí diǎn chū bǎn shè (漢語大詞典出版社).

Gāo Wǔ (高武), 1987, *A Gathering of the Blossoms of Acupuncture (Zhēn jiǔ jù yīng* 針灸聚英). Shanghai: Shànghǎi gǔ jí chū bǎn shè (上海古籍出版社).

Goldin, Paul Rakita, 2003, "The Mind Body Problem in the *Zhuangzi,*" in Scott Cook, ed., *Hiding the World in the World, Uneven Discourses on the Zhuangzi.* New York: SUNY Press, pp. 226–247.

Graham, A. C., trans., 2001, *Chuang Tzu: The Inner Chapters.* Cambridge: Hackett Publishing Company.

Grand Encyclopedia of Chinese Medicine (Zhōng yī dà cí diǎn 中醫大詞典), 1975. Beijing: Rén mín wèi shēng chū bǎn shè (人民衛生出版社).

Guō Âi-Chūn (郭靄春), ed., 1992, *An Annotated and Translated Yellow Emperor's Inner Classic Divine Pivot (Huáng di nèi jīng shū jiào zhù yǔ yì* 黃帝內經靈樞校註語譯). Tianjin: Tiānjīn kē xué jì shù chū bǎn shè (天津科學技術出版社).

Guō Qìng-Fān (郭慶藩), ed., 1961, *The Collated and Annotated Zhuang zi (Zhuāng zi jí shì* 莊子集釋). Beijing: Zhōng huá shū jú (中華書局).

Hansen, Marta, 1999, "Inventing a Tradition in Chinese Medicine," Ph.D. dissertation, University of Michigan Dissertation Services.

Henricks, Robert G., trans., 1989, *Lao-Tzu: Te-Tao Ching, A New Translation Based on the Recently Discovered Ma-wang-tui Texts.* New York: Ballantine Books.

Hinton, David, trans., 1997, *Chuangtzu: The Inner Chapters.* Washington D.C.: Counterpoint.

Huáng-Fǔ Mì (皇甫謐), 1981, Shāndōng zhōng yī xué yuàn (山東中醫學院), eds., *The Annotated Systematic Classic of Acupuncture and Moxibustion (Zhēn jiǔ jiǎ yǐ jīng jiào shì* 針灸甲乙經校釋). Beijing: Rén mín wèi shēng chū bǎn shè (人民衛生出版社).

——, 1997, *The Systematic Classic of Acupuncture and Moxibustion (Zhēn jiǔ jiǎ yǐ jīng* 針灸甲乙經), in Huáng Xiáng-Lóng (黃祥龍), ed., *A Collection of Famous Acupuncture Works (Zhēn jiǔ míng zhù jí chéng* 針灸名著集成). Beijing: Huá xià chū bǎn shè (華夏出版社), pp. 1–164.

Huáng Gōng-Xiù (黃宮繡), 2004, *Discerning the Truth Regarding Pulse Theory (Mài lǐ qiú zhēn* 脈理求真), in *A Chinese Encyclopedia of Medicine (Zhōng huá yī diǎn* 中華醫典), CD-ROM. Changsha: Húnán diàn zǐ yīn xiàng chū bǎn shè (湖南電子音像出版社).

Huáng Huáng (黃煌), 2007, *The Allure of Classic Formulas (Jīng fāng de mèi lì* 經方的魅力). Beijing: Rén mín wèi shēng chū bǎn shè (人民衛生出版社).

Huáng Shòu-Qí (黃壽祺) and Zhāng Shàn-Wén (張善文), eds., 1990, *The Changes of Zhou Explained (Zhōu yì yì zhù* 周易譯註). Shanghai: Shànghǎi gǔ jí chū bǎn shè (上海古籍出版社).

Huáng Yīng-Zhì (黃英志), ed., 1999. *The Complete Medical Writings of Ye Tian-Shi (Yè Tiān-Shi yī xué quán shū* 葉天士醫學全書). Beijing: Zhōng guó zhōng yào chū bǎn shè (中國中藥出版社).

Hucker, Charles O., 1985, *A Dictionary of Official Titles in Imperial China.* Palo Alto, California: Stanford University Press.

Imperial Medical Bureau (Tài yī jú 太醫局), 2004, *Formulary of the Pharmacy Service for Benefiting the People in the Taiping Era (Tàipíng huì mín hé jì jú fāng* 太平惠民和劑局方) in *A Chinese Encyclopedia of Medicine (Zhōng huá yī diǎn* 中華醫典), CD-ROM. Changsha: Húnán diàn zǐ yīn xiàng chū bǎn shè (湖南電子音像出版社).

Ishida Hidemi (石田秀美), 1987, *Qi: The Flowing Body (Ki: Nagareru shintai* 氣-流身體). Tokyo: Hirakawa shuppansha.

Iwai Yusen (巖井祐泉), Guō Xiù-Méi (郭秀梅), and Japanese *Inner Classic* Study Group (日本內經學院), trans., 2003, *Li Shi-Zhen: Research on Qigong Documents Related to His Exposition on the Eight Extraordinary Vessels (Lǐ Shí-Zhēn: Qí jīng bā mài kǎo suǒ yǐn qì gōng wén xiàn kǎo* 李時珍奇經八脈考所引氣功文獻考) in Qián Chāo-Chén (錢超塵) and Wēn Zhǎng-Lù (溫長路), eds., *A Compendium of Research on Li Shi-Zhen (Lǐ Shí-Zhēn yán jiū jí chéng* 李時珍研究集成). Beijing: Zhōng guó gǔ jí chū bǎn shè (中國古籍出版社).

Jì Yún (紀昀) et al., eds., 1983, *Catalog of the Complete Collection of the Four Treasuries (Sì kù quán shū mù lù* 四庫全書目錄), two volumes. Beijing: Zhōng huá shū jú (中華書局).

Katsuda Masayasu (勝田正泰), trans., 1995, *A Modern Language Translation of an Exposition on the Eight Extraordinary Vessels (Gendaigo Yaku Kikei Hachimyaku kou* 現代語訳奇經八脈考校註). Touyou: Gakujutsu Shuppansha (東洋學術出版社).

Katsuyasu Kido (城戶勝康), 1978, *Extraordinary Vessel Treatment (Kikei Chiryo* 奇經療法*)*. Osaka: *Kikei Chiryo Kenkyukai* (奇經治療研究會).

Kendal, Donald Edward, 2001, *Dao of Chinese Medicine: Understanding an Ancient Healing Art.* Oxford: Oxford University Press.

Kirkland, Russell, 2004, *Taoism: The Enduring Tradition.* New York: Routledge.

Kohn, Livia, 1992, *Early Chinese Mysticism, Philosophy and Soteriology in the Taoist Tradition.* Princeton, New Jersey: Princeton University Press.

——, 1989, *Taoist Meditation and Longevity Techniques.* Ann Arbor: University of Michigan Center of Chinese Studies.

Kuriyama, Shigehisa, 1999, *The Expressiveness of the Body and the Divergence of Greek and Chinese Medicine.* New York: Zone Books.

LaFargue, Michael, 1992, *The Tao of the Tao Te Ching.* Albany, New York: State University of New York Press.

Larre, Claude and Elizabeth Rochat de La Vallée, 1997, *The Eight Extraordinary Meridians.* Cambridge: Monkey Press.

Lau D. C. (劉殿) and Chen Fong Ching (陳方正), eds., 2000, *The ICS Ancient Chinese Texts Concordance Series Philosophical Works No. 43, A Concordance to the Zhuang zi.* Hong Kong: Commercial Press.

Lǐ Dōng-Yuán (李東垣), 1981a, *On the Spleen and Stomach (Pí wèi lùn* 脾胃論*)* in Dīng Guāng-Dí (丁光迪) et al., eds., *The Collected Medical Works of Dong-Yuan (Dōng-yuán yī jí* 東垣醫集*).* Beijing: Rén mín wèi shēng chū bǎn shè (人民衛生出版社), pp. 51–132.

——, 1981b, *Secrets from the Orchid Chamber (Lán shì mì cáng* 蘭室秘藏*)* in Dīng Guāng-Dí (丁光迪) et al., eds., *The Collected Medical Works of Dong-Yuan (Dōng-yuán yī jí* 東垣醫集*).* Beijing: Rén mín wèi shēng chū bǎn shè (人民衛生出版社), pp. 133–261.

——, 1993, Yang Shou-Zhong and Li Jian-Yong, trans., *On the Spleen and Stomach (Pí wèi lùn* 脾胃論*).* Boulder, Colorado: Blue Poppy Press.

——, 2004, *On the Spleen and Stomach (Pí wèi lùn* 脾胃論*)* in *A Chinese Encyclopedia of Medicine (Zhōng huá yī diǎn* 中華醫典*),* CD-ROM. Changsha: Húnán diàn zǐ yīn xiàng chū bǎn shè (湖南電子音像出版社).

Lǐ Shí-Zhēn (李時珍), 1999a, *An Exposition on the Eight Extraordinary Vessels (Qí jīng bā mài kǎo jiào zhù* 奇經八脈考*),* in Liǔ Zhǎng-Huà (柳長華), ed., *The Complete Medical Writings of Li Shi-Zhen (Lǐ Shí-Zhēn yī xué quán shū* 李時珍醫學全書*).* Beijing: Zhōng guó zhōng yào chū bǎn, pp. 1623–1644.

——, 1999b, *Comprehensive Outline of the Materia Medica (Běn cǎo gāng mù* 本草綱目*),* in Liǔ Zhǎng-Huà (柳長華), ed., *The Complete Medical Writings of Li Shi-Zhen (Lǐ Shí-Zhēn yī xué quán shū* 李時珍醫學全書*).* Beijing: Zhōng guó zhōng yào chū bǎn shè (中國中藥出版社), pp. 1-1622.

——, 1999c, *Pulse Studies of the Lakeside [Recluse] (Bīn hú mài xué* 濱湖脈學*),* in Liǔ Zhǎng-Huà (柳長華), ed., *The Complete Medical Writings of Li Shi-Zhen (Lǐ Shí-Zhēn yī* *xué quán shū* 李時珍醫學全書). Beijing: Zhōng guó zhōng yào chū bǎn shè (中國中藥出版社), pp. 1645–1662.

———, 2004a, *Comprehensive Outline of the Materia Medica (Běn cǎo gāng mù* 本草綱目), in *A Chinese Encyclopedia of Medicine (Zhōng huá yī diǎn* 中華醫典), CD-ROM. Changsha: Húnán diàn zǐ yīn xiàng chū bǎn shè (湖南電子音像出版社).

———, 2004b, *Bin Hu's Pulse Studies (Bīn hú mài xué* 濱湖脈學), in *A Chinese Encyclopedia of Medicine (Zhōng huá yī diǎn* 中華醫典), CD-ROM. Changsha: Húnán diàn zǐ yīn xiàng chū bǎn shè (湖南電子音像出版社).

Lín Zhī-Hǎn (林之瀚), 2004, *Precision in the Four Examinations (Sì zhěn jué wēi* 四診抉微), in *A Chinese Encyclopedia of Medicine (Zhōng huá yī diǎn* 中華醫典), CD-ROM. Changsha: Húnán diàn zǐ yīn xiàng chū bǎn shè (湖南電子音像出版社).

Liǔ Bǎo-Yí (柳寶詒), 2004a, *Liu Chuang's Case Records from the Four Schools (Liǔ Chuáng sì jiā yī àn* 柳床四家醫案) in *A Chinese Encyclopedia of Medicine (Zhōng huá yī diǎn* 中華醫典), CD-ROM. Changsha: Húnán diàn zǐ yīn xiàng chū bǎn shè (湖南電子音像出版社).

———, 2004b, *The Selected Case Records of Jing Xiang-Lou in Two Juan (Píng xuǎn Jìng Xiāng-Lóu yī àn liǎng juǎn* 評選靜香樓醫案兩卷) in *A Chinese Encyclopedia of Medicine (Zhōng huá yī diǎn* 中華醫典), CD-ROM. Changsha: Húnán diàn zǐ yīn xiàng chū bǎn shè (湖南電子音像出版社).

Liu Bing-Quan, 1988, Wang Qi-Liang, trans., *Optimum Time for Acupuncture, A Collection of Traditional Chinese Chronotherapies*. Shandong: Shandong Science and Technology Press.

Liǔ Huà-Yáng (柳華陽), 1988, *Discussions of the Golden Transcendents (Jīn xiān zhèng lùn* 金仙證論). Taiyuan: Shānxī rén mín chū bǎn shè (山西人民出版社).

Liú Wén-Diǎn (劉文典), 1980, *Supplemental Corrections to the Zhuangzi (Zhuāng zi bǔ zhèng* 莊子補正). Kunming: Yúnnán rén mín chū bǎn shè (雲南人民出版社).

Liú Yuè (劉越), 2003, *An Illustrated Explanation of the Essentials from the Golden Cabinet (Tú jiě jīn guì yào lüè* 圖解金匱要略). Beijing: Rén mín wèi shēng chū bǎn shè (人民衛生出版社).

Liǔ Zhǎng-Huà (柳長華), ed., 1999, *The Complete Medical Writings of Li Shi-Zhen (Lǐ Shí-Zhēn yī xué quán shū* 李時珍醫學全書). Beijing: Zhōng guó zhōng yào chū bǎn shè (中國中藥出版社).

Liu Zheng-Cai et al., 1999, *A Study of Daoist Acupuncture and Moxibustion*. Boulder, Colorado: Blue Poppy Press.

Luó Dōng-Yì (羅東逸), 2004, *Critical Interpretation of the Inner Classic (Nèi jīng bó yì* 內經博義), in *A Chinese Encyclopedia of Medicine (Zhōng huá yī diǎn* 中華醫典), CD-ROM. Changsha: Húnán diàn zǐ yīn xiàng chū bǎn shè (湖南電子音像出版社).

Mǎ Jì-Rén (馬濟人), ed., 1989, *A Practical Dictionary of Medical Qi Gong (Shí yòng yī xué qì gōng cí diǎn* 實用醫學氣功詞典). Shanghai: Shànghǎi kē xué jì shù chū bǎn shè (上海科學技術出版社).

Mair, Victor, trans., 1994, *Wandering on the Way, Early Taoist Tales and Parables of Chuang Tzu.* New York: Bantam Books.

Manaka, Yoshio, Kazuko Itaya, and Steven Birch, 1995, *Chasing the Dragon's Tail.* Brookline, Massachusetts: Paradigm Publications.

Maspero Henri, Yoshio Kawakatsu (川勝義雄), trans., 1993, *The Book of Daoism: The World of Immortal Path and Magical Spells in Search of Anti-Aging and Inmortality; Books Esoterica (Doukyou no Hon—Furou Fushi wo mezasu Sento Jujutsu no Sekai* 道教の本—不老不死をめざす仙道呪術の世界*),* four volumes. Tokyo: Gakushuu Kenkyuu Sha (學習研究社).

Matsumoto, Kiiko and Stephen Birch, 1986, *Extraordinary Vessels.* Brookline, Massachusetts: Paradigm Publications.

———, 1988, *Hara Diagnosis: Reflections on the Sea.* Brookline, Massachusetts: Paradigm Publications.

Méi Jiàn-Hán (梅建寒) and Yáng Yù-Huá (楊玉華), 2006, *Clinical Application of the Eight Extraordinary Vessels in Acupuncture and Moxibustion — Illustrated, Collated and Verified (Qí jīng bā mài yù zhēn jiǔ lín chuáng-tú kǎo zǔ hé yàn zhèng* 奇經八脈與針灸臨床-圖考組合驗證*).* Beijing: Rén mín wèi shēng chū bǎn shè (人民衛生出版社).

Mitchell, Craig, Feng Ye, and Nigel Wiseman, trans., 1999, *Shang Han Lun: On Cold Damage.* Brookline, Massachusetts: Paradigm Publications.

Miyawaki, Kazuto, Masayuki Hamazaki, trans., 1997, *Extraordinary Vessel Treatment Manual*, Ontario, Canada: self-published.

Ni, Yitian, 1996, *Navigating the Channels of Traditional Chinese Medicine.* San Diego: Oriental Medicine Center Press.

Niè Huì-Mín (聶惠民), Wáng Qing-Guó (王慶國), and Gāo Fēi (高飛), eds., 2001, *Collected Commentaries on the Discussion of Cold Damage (Shāng hán lùn jié jiě* 傷寒論集解*).* Beijing: Xué yuàn chū bǎn shè (學苑出版社).

Palmer, David, 2007, *Body, Science and Qigong Fever in Contemporary China.* New York: Columbia University Press.

Pirog, John E., 1996, *The Practical Application of Meridian Style Acupuncture.* Berkeley, California: Pacific View Press.

Qián Chāo-Chén (錢超塵) and Wēn Zhǎng-Lù (溫長路), eds., 2003, *A Compendium of Research on Li Shi-Zhen (Lǐ Shí-Zhēn yán jiū jí chéng* 李時珍研究集成*).* Beijing: Zhōng guó gǔ jí chū bǎn shè (中國古籍出版社).

Red Pine, trans., 1996. *Lao-Tzu's Taoteching.* San Francisco, California: Mercury House.

Robinet, Isabelle, Julian F. Pas and Norman J. Giradot, trans., 1993, *Taoism: The Mao-Shan Tradition of Great Purity.* Albany, New York: State University of New York Press.

———, 1997, Phyllis Brooks, trans., *Taoism: Growth of a Religion.* Palo Alto, California: Stanford University Press.

Roth, Harold D., 2003, "Bimodal Mystical Experience in the Qiwulun Chapter of the *Zhuangzi*," in Scott Cook, ed., *Hiding the World in the World, Uneven Discourses on the Zhuang Zi*. New York: SUNY Press, pp. 15–32.

Rump, Ariane and Wing-tsit Chan, trans., 1979. *Commentary on the Lao Tzu by Wang Pi*. Honolulu: University Press of Hawaii.

Rur-Bin Yang (楊儒賓), 2003, "From 'Merging the Body with the Mind' and 'Wandering in Unitary Qi': A Discussion of Zhuang Zi's Realm of the True Man and Its Corporal Basis," in Scott Cook, ed., *Hiding the World in the World, Uneven Discourses on the Zhuanzi*. New York: SUNY Press, pp. 88–127.

Saso, Michael, 1983, "The Chuang-tzu nei-p'ien: A Taoist Meditation," in Victor Mair, ed., *Experimental Essays on Chuang-tzu*. Honolulu: University of Hawaii Press, pp. 140–157.

Schipper, Kristofer, Karen C. Duval, trans., 1993, *The Taoist Body*. London: University of California Press.

Shào Lán-Sūn (邵蘭蓀), 2004, *The Case Histories of Shao Lan-Sun (Shào Lán-Sūn yī àn 邵蘭蓀醫案)*, in *A Chinese Encyclopedia of Medicine (Zhōng huá yī diǎn 中華醫典)*, CD-ROM. Changsha: Húnán diàn zǐ yīn xiàng chū bǎn shè (湖南電子音像出版社).

Shen Jin-Ao (沈金鰲), 1999, *The Categorized Anthology of Pulse Images (Mai xiang tong lei 脈象統類), Appendix to the Extraordinary Vessels (Fu zai qi jing ba mai 附載奇經八脈)*, in Tian Si-Sheng (田思勝), ed., *The Complete Medical Writings of Shen Jin-Ao (Shen Jin-Ao yi xue quan shu 沈金鰲醫學全書)*. Beijing: Zhong guo zhong yi yao chu ban she (中國中醫藥出版社).

Shima, Miki and Charles Chace, 2000, *Channel Divergences: Deeper Pathways of the Web*. Boulder, Colorado: Blue Poppy Press.

Shǒu Yī-Zǐ (守一子), ed., 1989, *An Anthology of the Essential Writings of the Daoist Canon (Dào zàng jīng huá lù 道藏精華錄)*. Zhejiang: Zhèjiāng gǔ jí chū bǎn shè (浙江古籍出版社).

Sivin, Nathan, 1995, "Text and Experience in Classical Chinese Medicine," in Don G. Bates, ed., *Knowledge and the Scholarly Medical Traditions*. New York: Cambridge University Press, pp. 177–204.

Sūn Sī-Miǎo (孫思邈), 1982, *Important Formulas Worth a Thousand Gold Pieces [for any Emergency] (Bèi jí qiān jīn yào fāng 備急千金要方)*. Beijing: Rén mín wèi shēng chū bǎn shè (人民衛生出版社).

———, 1999, Zhū Bāng-Xián (朱邦賢) et al., eds., *Supplement to The Prescriptions Worth a Thousand Pieces of Gold (qiān jīn yì fang 千金翼方)*. Shanghai: Shànghǎi gǔ jí chū bǎn shè (上海古籍出版社).

Todo Akiyasu (藤堂明保つ), 1981, *A Collection of Poems from More Peaceful Times (Ji rǎng jí 擊壤集)*, in *Chinese-Japanese Dictionary for Study and Research (Gakken Kanwa Jiten學研漢和辭典)*. Tokyo: Gakushuu Kenkyu-sha (學習研究社), p. 548.

Unschuld, Paul, 1985, *Medicine in China: A History of Ideas*. Berkeley, California: University of California Press.

———, trans., 1986a, *Nan-Ching, Classic of Difficult Issues*. Berkeley, California: University of California Press.

———, 1986b, *Medicine in China: A History of Pharmaceutics*. Berkeley, California: University of California Press.

Wáng Hóng-Bīn (王宏彬), 2003, "The Influence of Chinese Daoist Literature on Li Shi-Zhen (*Zhōngguó dào jiā wén huà dui Lǐ Shí-Zhēn de yǐng xiǎng* 中國道家文化對李時珍的影響)," in Qián Chāo-Chén (錢超塵) and Wēn Chǎng-Lù (溫長路), eds., *Compendium of Research on Li Shi-Zhen (Lǐ Shí-Zhēn yán jiū jí chéng* 李時珍研究集成). Beijing: Zhōng guó gǔ jí chū bǎn shè (中國古籍出版社), pp. 187–190.

Wáng Jiǔ-Sī (王九思) et al., eds., 1966, *Collected Annotations on the Classics of Difficulties (Nán jīng jí zhù* 難經集註). Taipei: Táiwān zhōng huá shū jú (臺灣中華書局).

Wáng Jūn (王軍) et al., 1992, *The Four Major [Medical] Currents of the Jin-Yuan [Dynasty]: Their Complete Medical Writings (Jīn yuán sì dà jiā yī xué quán shū* 金元四大家醫學全書). Tianjin: Tiānjīn kē xué jì shù chū bǎn shè (天津科學技術出版社).

Wáng Luó-Zhēn (王羅珍) and Lǐ Dǐng (李鼎), eds., 1985, *An Annotated Exposition on the Eight Extraordinary Vessels (Qí jīng bā mài kǎo jiào zhù* 奇經八脈考校註). Shanghai: Shànghǎi kē xué jì shù chū bǎn shè (上海科學技術出版社).

Wáng Shū-Hé (王叔和), Fúzhōu shì rén mín yī yuàn (福州市人民醫院), eds., 1981, *The Annotated Pulse Classic (Mài jīng jiào shì* 脈經校釋). Beijing: Rén mín wèi shēng chū bǎn shè (人民衛生出版社).

———, 1991a, Fúzhōu shì rén mín yī yuàn (福州市人民醫院), eds., *The Annotated Pulse Classic (Mài jīng jiào zhù* 脈經校註). Beijing: Rén mín wèi shēng chū bǎn shè (人民衛生出版社).

———, 1991b, Shěn Yán-Nán (沈炎南) et al., eds., *The Annotated Pulse Classic (Mài jīng jiào zhù* 脈經校註). Beijing: Rén mín wèi shēng chū bǎn shè (人民衛生出版社).

Wáng Tāo (王燾), 2004, *Arcane Essentials of the Imperial Library (Wài tái mì yào* 外台秘要), in *A Chinese Encyclopedia of Medicine (Zhōng huá yī diǎn* 中華醫典), CD-ROM. Changsha: Húnán diàn zǐ yīn xiàng chū bǎn shè (湖南電子音像出版社).

Wáng Wéi-Yī (王惟一), 2002, *An Acupuncture Hole Diagram Based on the Bronze Model (Tóng rén shū xué zhēn jiǔ tú jīng* 銅人輸穴針灸圖經). Shanghai: Shànghǎi gǔ jí chū bǎn shè (上海古籍出版社).

Wàng Yǒu-Liàng (王友亮), 1985, *A Brief Biography of Ye Tian-Shi (Yè Tiān-Shi xiǎo zhuàn* 葉天士小傳), in *Selected Writings [from the Garden] of the Listening to the Pines Hut (Tīng sōng lú wén chāo* 聽松廬文鈔), repr. Zhōu Jùn-Fù (周駿富), ed., *A Collection of Qing Dynasty Biographies (Qīng dài zhuàn jì cóng kān* 清代傳記叢刊). Taipei: Míng wén shū jú (明文書局), vol. 190, pp. 517–519.

Wáng Zhí-Zhōng (王执中), 2004, *The Classic of Acupuncture and Moxibustion for Endowing Life (Zhēn jiǔ zī shēng jīng* 針灸資生經), in *A Chinese Encyclopedia of Medicine (Zhōng huá yī diǎn* 中華醫典), CD-ROM. Changsha: Húnán diàn zǐ yīn xiàng chū bǎn shè (湖南電子音像出版社).

Wáng Zhí-Zhōng (王执中) and Huá Bó-Rén (滑伯仁), Chéng Dàn-Än (承澹盦), ed., 1973, *The Classic of Acupuncture and Moxibustion for Endowing Life and The Elucidation of the Fourteen Channels in a Combined Edition (Zhēn jiǔ zī shēng jīng. Shí sì jīng fā huī hé kān* 針灸資生經．十四經發揮合刊). Taipei: Xuàn fēng chū bǎn shè (旋風出版社).

Watson, Burton, trans., 1964, *Chuang Tzu: Basic Writings.* New York: Columbia University Press.

Wèi Bó-Yáng (魏伯陽), Péng Xiǎo (彭曉), ed., 2007. *The Token for the Agreement of the Three According to the Changes of Zhou (Zhōu yí cān tóng qì* 周易參同契). Input by Fabrizio Pregadio 1994 and revised 1997. http://venus.unive.it/dsao/pregadio/textbase/ctq_chn. html (accessed May 23, 2008).

Wilhelm, Richard, and Cary F. Baynes, trans., 1967, *The I Ching; or, Book of Changes.* Princeton, New Jersey: Princeton University Press.

Wiseman, Nigel and Feng Ye, 1998, *A Practical Dictionary of Chinese Medicine.* Brookline, Massachusetts: Paradigm Publications.

Wu Lu-Ch'iang and Tenney L. Davis, 1932, "An Ancient Chinese Treatise on Alchemy Entitled Ts'an T'ung Ch'i," in *Isis* 18:210–289.

Xiāo Dēng-Fú (蕭登福), 1990, *Liezi, Ancient Commentaries and a Modern Translation (Liè zi gǔ zhù jīn yì* 列子古注今譯). Taibei: Wèn jìn chū bǎn shè (問津出版社).

Xiāo Tíng-Zhī (蕭廷芝), Dǒng Dé-Nìng (董德寧), ed., 1989, *A Great Compendium of Golden Elixir; composed by Xiao Ting-Zhi; edited by Dong De-Ning. (Jīn dān dà chéng jí; Xiāo Tíng-Zhī zhuàn; Dǒng Dé-Nìng jí lù* 金丹大成集；蕭廷芝撰；董德寧輯錄). Shanghai: Shàng hǎi gǔ jí chū bǎn shè (上海古籍出版社).

Xú Fèng (徐鳳), 2004, *A Comprehensive Compendium of Acupuncture and Moxibustion (Zhēn jiǔ dà quán* 針灸大全), in *A Chinese Encyclopedia of Medicine (Zhōng huá yī diǎn* 中華醫典), CD-ROM. Changsha: Húnán diàn zǐ yīn xiàng chū bǎn shè (湖南電子音像出版社).

Xǔ Shèn (許慎), Xú Zhōng-Shū (徐中舒), ed., 1981, *The Elucidations of the Signs and Explications of the Graphs Annotated by Sections (Shuō wén jiě zì duàn zhù* 說文解字段註), two volumes. Chengdu: Chéngdu gǔ jí shū diàn (成都古籍書店).

Yán Jié (嚴潔), Shī Wén (施雯), and Hóng Wěi (洪煒), 1997, *Materia Medica of Combinations (Dé pèi běn cǎo* 得配本草). Beijing: Zhōng guó zhōng yī yào chū bǎn shè (中國中醫藥出版社).

Yáng Jì-Zhōu (楊繼洲), 1981, *Great Compendium of Acupuncture and Moxibustion (Zhēn jiǔ dà chéng* 針灸大成), in *The Annotated Great Compendium of Acupuncture and Moxibustion (Zhēn jiǔ dà chéng jiào shì* 針灸大成校釋). Beijing: Rén mín wèi shēng chū bǎn shè (人民衛生出版社).

———, 2004, *Great Compendium of Acupuncture and Moxibustion (Zhēn jiǔ dà chéng* 針灸大成), in *A Chinese Encyclopedia of Medicine (Zhōng huá yī diǎn* 中華醫典), CD-ROM. Changsha: Húnán diàn zǐ yīn xiàng chū bǎn shè (湖南電子音像出版社).

Yáng Shàng-Shàn (楊上善), 2004, *Yellow Emperor's Inner Classic: Grand Essentials (Huáng Dì nèi jīng tài sù* 黄帝内經太素*)*, in *A Chinese Encyclopedia of Medicine (Zhōng huá yī diǎn* 中華醫典*)*, CD-ROM. Changsha: Húnán diàn zǐ yīn xiàng chū bǎn shè (湖南電子音像出版社).

Yasuzo Shibazaki (崎保三著), 1979, *The Acupuncture Research Group — The Yellow Emperor's Classic, Basic Questions, Divine Pivot (Shinkyuu Igaku Taikei—Kouteidaikei Somon Reisuu* 鍼灸醫學體系一黄帝内経素問靈樞*)*. Kyoto: Zen Nijuugo Kan (雄渾社).

Yè Tiān-Shì (葉天士), 1997a, Huáng Yīng-Zhì (黄英志), ed., *Case Records as a Guide to Clinical Practice (Lín chuáng zhǐ nán yī àn* 臨床指南醫案*)*, in *The Complete Medical Writings of Ye Tian-Shi (Yè Tiān-Shì yī xué quán shū* 葉天士醫學全書*)*. Beijing; Zhōng guó zhōng yī yào chū bǎn shè (中國中醫藥出版社), pp. 1–336.

——, 1997b, Huáng Yīng-Zhì (黄英志), ed., *On Feverish Disorders (Wēn rè lùn* 温熱論*)*, in *The Complete Medical Writings of Ye Tian- Shì (Yè Tiān-Shi yī xué quán shū* 葉天士醫學全書*)*. Beijing: Zhōng guó zhōng yī yào chū bǎn shè (中國中醫藥出版社), pp. 339–346.

——, 1997c, Huáng Yīng-Zhì (黄英志), ed., *An Official Collection of Zhong Fu-Tang's Cases (Zhòng Fù-Táng gōng xuǎn yī 'àn* 種福堂公選醫案*)*, in *The Complete Medical Writings of Ye Tian-Shi (Yè Tiān-Shì yī xué quán shū* 葉天士醫學全書*)*. Beijing: Zhōng guó zhōng yī yào chū bǎn shè (中國中醫藥出版社), pp. 347–374.

——, 1997d, Huáng Yīng-Zhì (黄英志), ed., *An Official Collection of Zhong Fu-Tang's Superior Formulas (Zhòng Fù-Táng gōng xuǎn liáng fāng* 種福堂公選良方*)*, in *The Complete Medical Writings of Ye Tian-shi (Yè Tiān-Shì yī xué quán shū* 葉天士醫學全書*)*. Beijing: Zhōng guó zhōng yī yào chū bǎn shè (中國中醫藥出版社), pp. 375–444.

——, 1997e, Huáng Yīng-Zhì (黄英志), ed., *Interpretation of Commonly-Used Classical Formulas by Categories (Lèi zhèng pǔ jì běn shì fāng shì yì* 類證普濟本事方釋義*)*, in *The Complete Medical Writings of Ye Tian-Shi (Yè Tiān-Shì yī xué quán shū* 葉天士醫學全書*)*. Beijing: Zhōng guó zhōng yī yào chū bǎn shè (中國中醫藥出版社), pp. 445-575.

——, 2004a, *Case Records as a Guide to Clinical Practice (Lín chuáng zhǐ nán yī àn* 臨床指南醫案*)*, in *A Chinese Encyclopedia of Medicine (Zhōng huá yī diǎn* 中華醫典*)*, CD-ROM. Changsha: Húnán diàn zǐ yīn xiàng chū bǎn shè (湖南電子音像出版社).

——, 2004b, *An Official Collection of Zhong Fu-Tang's Cases (Zhòng Fù-Táng gōng xuǎn yī àn* 種福堂公選醫案*)*, in *A Chinese Encyclopedia of Medicine (Zhōng huá yī diǎn* 中華醫典*)*. Changsha: Húnán diàn zǐ yīn xiàng chū bǎn shè (湖南電子音像出版社).

——, 2004c, *An Official Collection of Zhong Fu-Tang's Superior Formulas (Zhòng Fù-Táng gōng xuǎn liáng fāng* 種福堂公選良方*)*, in *A Chinese Encyclopedia of Medicine (Zhōng huá yī diǎn* 中華醫典*)*, CD-ROM. Changsha: Húnán diàn zǐ yīn xiàng chū bǎn shè (湖南電子音像出版社).

——, 2004d, *Authentic Medical Instructions by Ye Tian-Shi (Yè Tiān-Shì yī àn cún zhēn* 葉天士醫案存真*)*, in *A Chinese Encyclopedia of Medicine (Zhōng huá yī diǎn* 中華醫典*)*, CD-ROM. Changsha: Húnán diàn zǐ yīn xiàng chū bǎn shè (湖南電子音像出版社).

——, 2004e, *On Feverish Disorders (Wēn rè lùn* 溫熱論), in *A Chinese Encyclopedia of Medicine (Zhōng huá yī diǎn* 中華醫典), CD-ROM. Changsha: Húnán diàn zǐ yīn xiàng chū bǎn shè (湖南電子音像出版社).

——, 2004f, *Interpretation of Commonly-Used Classical Formulas by Categories (Lèi zhèng pǔ jì běn shì fāng shì yì* 類證普濟本事方釋義), in *A Chinese Encyclopedia of Medicine (Zhōng huá yī diǎn*中華醫典), CD-ROM. Changsha: Húnán diàn zǐ yīn xiàng chū bǎn shè (湖南電子音像出版社).

——, 2004g, *Principles of Pediatrics (Yòu kē yāo lüè* 幼科要略), in *A Chinese Encyclopedia of Medicine (Zhōng huá yī diǎn* 中華醫典), CD-ROM. Changsha: Húnán diàn zǐ yīn xiàng chū bǎn shè (湖南電子音像出版社).

——, 2004h, *Xu Pi's Authentic Collection of Ye Tian Shi's Case Records from His Later Years (Xú Pī Yè Tiān-Shì wǎn nián fāng yī àn zhēn běn* 徐批葉天士晚年方醫案真本), in *A Chinese Encyclopedia of Medicine (Zhōng huá yī diǎn*中華醫典), CD-ROM. Changsha: Húnán diàn zǐ yīn xiàng chū bǎn shè (湖南電子音像出版社).

——, 2004i, *Combined Case Records of Three Physicians (San jia yi an' he ke* 三家醫案合刻), *juan* 1, Minor Construct the Middle Decoction *(xiao jian zhong tang* 小建中湯), in *A Chinese Encyclopedia of Medicine (Zhong hua yi dian* 中華醫典), CD-ROM. Changsha: Hunan dian zi yin xiang chu ban she (湖南電子音像出版社).

Yuè Ën-Jiǎn (越恩儉), 2002, *A Study of Chinese Medical Pulse Diagnosis (Zhōng yī mài zhěn xué* 中醫脈診學). Tianjin: Zhōng yī mài zhěn xué (中醫脈診學).

Zhāng Jī (張機), 2004, *Essentials from the Golden Cabinet (Jīn guì yào lüè* 金匱要略), in *A Chinese Encyclopedia of Medicine (Zhōng huá yī diǎn* 中華醫典), CD-ROM. Changsha: Húnán diàn zǐ yīn xiàng chū bǎn shè (湖南電子音像出版社).

Zhāng Jiè-Bīn (張介賓), Lǐ Zhi-Yōng 李志庸, ed., 1999, *The Classified Classic (Lèi jīng* 類經), in *The Complete Medical Writings of Zhang Jing-Yue (Zhāng Jǐng-Yuè yī xué quán shū* 張景岳醫學全書). Beijing: Zhōng guó zhōng yī chū bǎn shè (中國中醫出版社), pp. 1–612.

——, 1999, Lǐ Zhì-Yōng 李志庸, ed., *The Illustrated Addendum to the Classified Classic (Lèi jīng tú yì* 類經圖翼), in *The Complete Medical Writings of Zhang Jing-Yue (Zhāng Jǐng Yuè yī xué quán shū* 張景岳醫學全書). Beijing: Zhōng guó zhōng yī chū bǎn shè (中國中醫出版社), pp. 613–769.

Zhāng Zi-Hé (張子和), 2004, *Confucians' Duties to Their Parents (Rú mén shì qīn* 儒門事親), in *A Chinese Encyclopedia of Medicine (Zhōng huá yī diǎn* 中華醫典), CD-ROM. Changsha: Húnán diàn zǐ yīn xiàng chū bǎn shè (湖南電子音像出版社).

Zhū Dān-Xī (朱丹溪), 2004, *Essential Teachings of [Zhu] Dan-Xi (Dān-Xī xīn fǎ* 丹溪心法), in *A Chinese Encyclopedia of Medicine (Zhōng huá yī diǎn* 中華醫典), CD-ROM. Changsha: Húnán diàn zǐ yīn xiàng chū bǎn shè (湖南電子音像出版社).

HERB AND FORMULA INDEX

Hole/Point Index

General Index

487

E